LOSE WEIGHT, EAT GREAT

Affordable
And Time Saving
Macro Friendly
Recipes Designed
To Maximize
Weight Loss Efforts

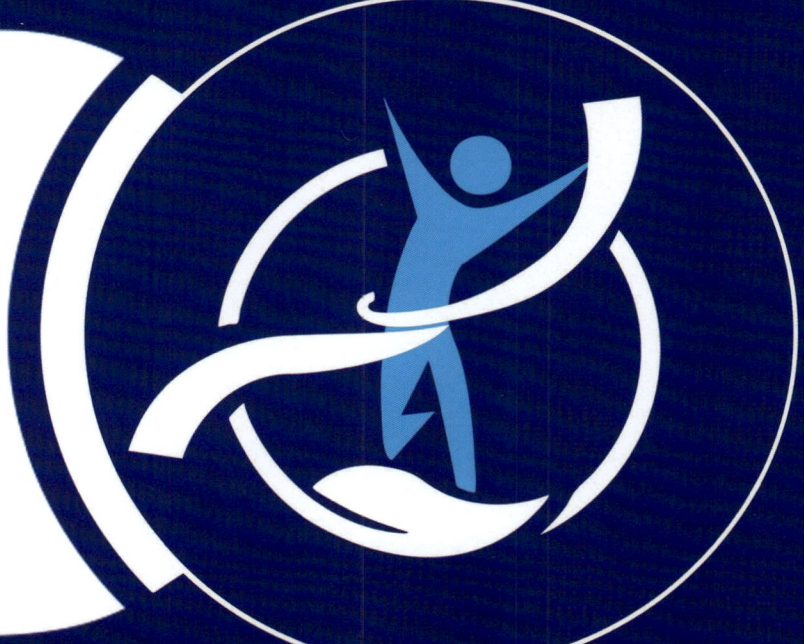

TOTAL WEIGHT LOSS COOKBOOK

2.0 REVISED EDITION

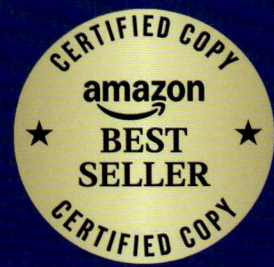

shoptotalweightloss.com

Johnny Hadac, DO

WELCOME SHEET

NUTRITION TIP SHEET

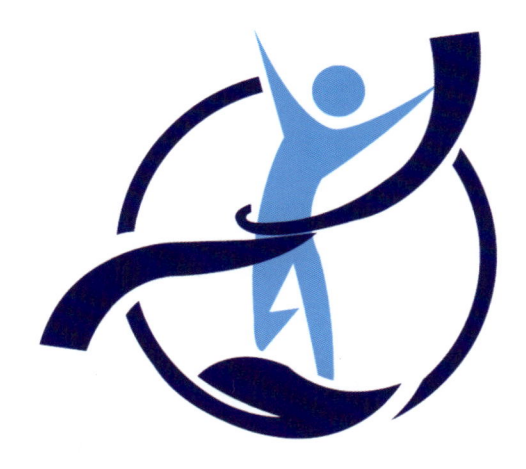

NUTRITION TIP SHEET
LIFE CHANGING NUTRITION 101

Sustainable health and weight loss aren't built on crash diets or quick fixes—they're the result of small, consistent changes that create massive results over time. Life without consistency lacks results!

TOTAL WEIGHT LOSS COOKBOOK 2.4

AFFORDABLE AND TIME SAVING MACRO FRIENDLY RECIPES DESIGNED TO MAXIMIZE WEIGHT LOSS EFFORTS

JOHNNY HADAC

©2025 ALL RIGHTS RESERVED. PRINTED IN CANADA. NO PORTION OF THIS BOOK MAY BE REPRODUCED, STORED IN A RETRIEVAL SYSTEM, OR TRANSMITTED IN ANY FORM OR BY ANY MEANS-ELECTRONIC, MECHANICAL, PHOTOCOPY, RECORDING, SCANNING, OR OTHER-EXCEPT FOR BRIEF QUOTATIONS IN CRITICAL REVIEWS OR ARTICLES WITHOUT THE PRIOR PERMISSION OF THE AUTHOR.

PUBLISHED BY GAME CHANGER PUBLISHING–0625V2.4

PAPERBACK ISBN: 978-1-964811-65-9
HARDCOVER ISBN: 978-1-964811-66-6
DIGITAL: ISBN: 978-1-964811-67-3

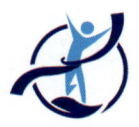

DEDICATION

To my wonderful mother, Tara.
Thank you for all you do and teaching me how to season food with love.

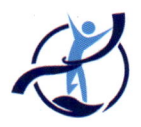

COMING SOON...

TOTAL WEIGHT LOSS APP

Weekly Updated Recipes
All Levels of Workout Programs
Personalized Macronutrient Tracking

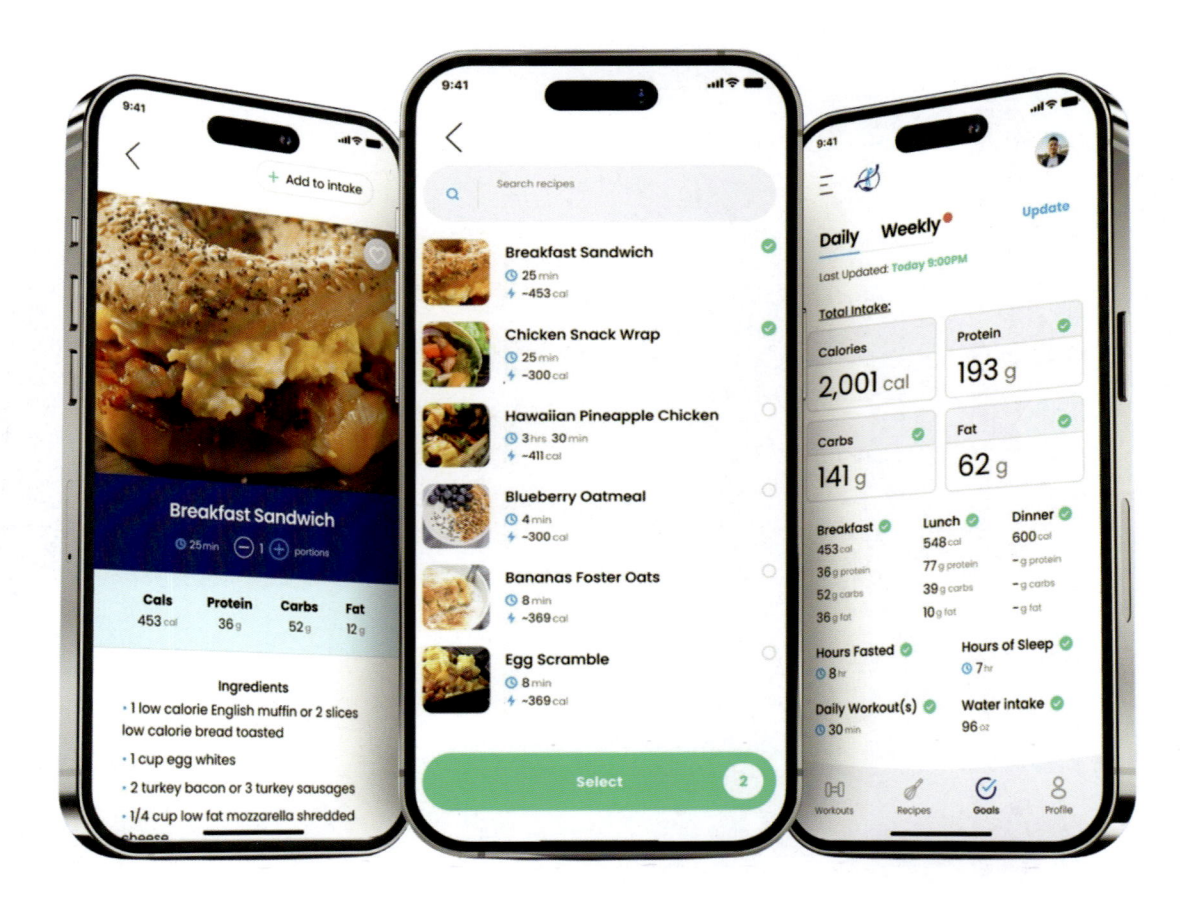

YOUR ALL IN ONE HEALTH APP
COMING SOON!

TABLE OF CONTENTS

- **6** WELCOME
- **7** DISCLAIMER
- **8** NUTRITION TIP SHEET
- **63** BREAKFAST
- **153** MEAL PREPS
- **317** DESSERTS
- **373** SHAKES/SMOOTHIES

WELCOME SHEET

MESSAGE FROM THE AUTHOR: JOHNNY HADAC

The Total Weight Loss Cookbook was created to empower you to take control of your life, health, and happiness. I am proud to have helped thousands of people improve their physical health, weight management, and emotional well-being through these recipes. This cookbook was designed to assist individuals in making healthier food choices and positively contribute to combatting the ongoing health crisis.

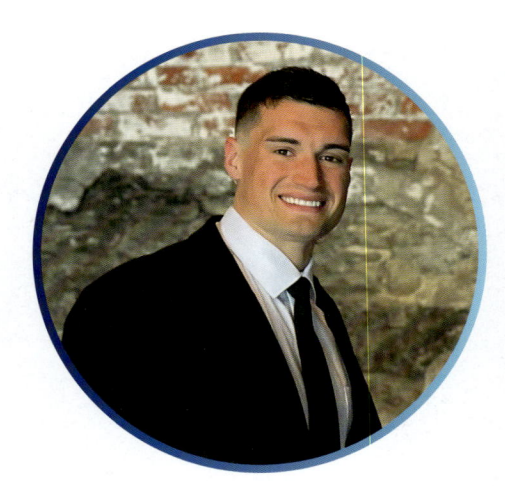

That's why I made sure to create recipes that are easy to prepare utilizing ingredients that are affordable and accessible. With this cookbook, my goal is to empower you to make healthier choices and take control of your health through cost effective nutrition.

Through this cookbook, I hope to provide you with the tools and knowledge to make these positive changes by providing you with nourishing and delicious recipes, along with practical tips and advice. I want to inspire and motivate you to make healthier choices and achieve your goals.

This cookbook was made with love, care, and the desire to help people like you achieve a healthy and fulfilling life.

I would like to express my sincere gratitude to everyone who has supported me in creating this book.

It is my hope that this cookbook will bring joy, health, and happiness to all who use it. Thank you for your trust and for choosing to embark on this journey towards a healthier and happier life.

God bless,
Johnny

WELCOME SHEET

DISCLAIMER

This cookbook is intended for informational and educational purposes only and is not a substitute for professional medical advice, diagnosis, or treatment. The information presented herein is not intended to replace the guidance of a licensed healthcare provider, physician, or registered dietitian. The author, while a medical professional, does not provide personalized medical, nutritional, or dietary advice through this cookbook.

While the author will be a resident physician as of July 1, 2025, this cookbook does not establish a doctor-patient relationship. Any application of the nutritional, dietary, or health information provided in this cookbook is done at the reader's discretion and risk. Readers should consult with their physician or a qualified healthcare provider before making significant dietary, exercise, or lifestyle changes, particularly if they have pre-existing health conditions, take medications, or have specific dietary needs.

The author makes no guarantees regarding the effectiveness, suitability, or accuracy of any recipes, nutritional advice, or health-related content in this cookbook. Individual results will vary based on personal health, medical history, genetics, and lifestyle factors.
The reader assumes full responsibility for any actions taken based on the information in this cookbook. The author, publisher, and any affiliated individuals or entities shall not be liable for any direct, indirect, incidental, or consequential damages, injuries, or losses that may result from the use or misuse of the information presented.

All content in this cookbook—including recipes, nutritional information, and dietary guidance—is protected by copyright law. No part of this cookbook may be reproduced, distributed, or transmitted in any form without prior written permission from the author. Unauthorized use or distribution will result in legal consequences.

The author is affiliated with Muscle Dummies supplement company but does not endorse or guarantee the effectiveness or safety of any specific products, services, or companies mentioned. Readers are encouraged to research and consult with professionals before using any products.
The author reserves the right to modify, update, or remove content in this cookbook at any time without notice. By using this cookbook, the reader acknowledges and agrees to the terms of this disclaimer. If the reader does not agree, they should not use this cookbook.

By purchasing or using this cookbook, the reader agrees to indemnify, defend, and hold harmless the author, its agents, representatives, employees, and affiliates from any claims, liabilities, damages, legal costs, and expenses, including attorneys' fees, that arise from the reader's use of this cookbook or breach of this disclaimer.

IF YOU HAVE ANY MEDICAL CONCERNS OR QUESTIONS REGARDING YOUR HEALTH, ALWAYS CONSULT A LICENSED PHYSICIAN OR HEALTHCARE PROFESSIONAL.

WELCOME SHEET

NUTRITION TIP SHEET

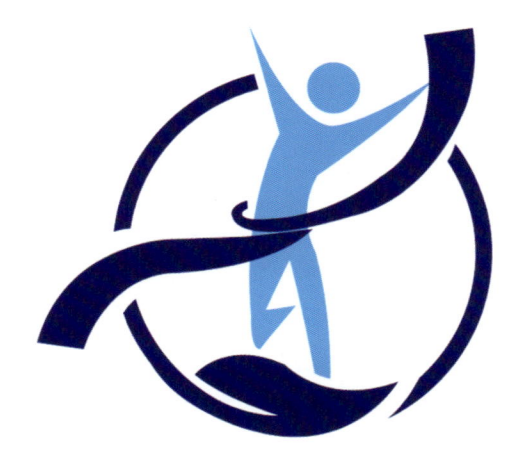

MACRONUTRIENTS, NUTRITION FACTS, & MACRONUTRIENT CALCULATOR

LIFE CHANGING NUTRITION 101

Sustainable health and weight loss aren't built on crash diets or quick fixes—they're the result of small, consistent changes that create massive results over time. Life without consistency lacks results!

NUTRITION TIP SHEET

UNDERSTANDING NUTRITION LABELS

Nutrition Facts		
Serving Size		
Serving Pen Container		
Amount per serving		
Calories	Calories from Fat	
		% Daily Value*
Total Fat		
Saturated Fat	0 g	0 %
Trans Fat	0 g	0 %
Cholesterol	0 g	0 %
Sodium	0 g	0 %
Total Carbohydrate	0 g	0 %
Dietary Fiber	0 g	0 %
Sugar	0 g	0 %
Protein	0 g	0 %
Vitamin A 0 %	Vitamin C 0 %	
Calcium 0 %	Iron 0 %	

*Percent Daily values are based on 2,000 calories diet. Your daily values may be higher or lower depending on your calories needs.

NUTRITION FACTS

- **SERVING SIZE:** Tells you how much is considered one serving.
- **CALORIES:** A unit of energy that measures how much energy food provides to the body when consumed. Weight loss occurs when you consume fewer calories than your body burns, creating a caloric deficit, which forces your body to use stored fat for energy.
- **TOTAL FAT:** Includes both healthy fats (monounsaturated & polyunsaturated) and unhealthy fats (saturated & trans fats).
- **SATURATED FAT & TRANS FATS:** These increase LDL (bad cholesterol) and risk of heart disease. Aim for low saturated fat and zero trans fat (watch for "partially hydrogenated oils" in ingredients)
- **CHOLESTEROL:** Fat-like substance found in animal products that serves as a building block for hormones, cell membranes, and vitamin D production in the body.
- **SODIUM:** Especially important to monitor if you have high blood pressure. American Heart Association recommends aiming for no more than 1,500 milligrams of sodium per day as an ideal limit (~1/2 tsp).
- **SUGARS:** Include both natural sugars (from fruit and dairy) and added sugars (from processed ingredients like corn syrup and sucrose).

<u>FATS</u> are a critical macronutrient that support hormone production, brain function, cell health, and energy balance. Unlike protein and carbohydrates, fat is more calorie-dense (9 cal per gram vs. 4 cal per gram). The right types of fats help reduce inflammation, regulate appetite, and promote heart health, while unhealthy fats can lead to weight gain and increased disease risk.

✅ **Support Hormone Production** – Essential for testosterone, estrogen, and metabolism regulation.
✅ **Provide Long-Lasting Energy** – Fats digest slowly, keeping energy levels stable.
✅ **Support Brain & Heart Health** – Healthy fats improve cognitive function and reduce inflammation.

- **Healthy Unsaturated Fats:** Avocados, olive oil, almonds, walnuts, fatty fish (salmon, tuna)
- **Saturated Fats (Use in Moderation):** egg yolks, grass fed butter, coconut oil, full fat cheese and yogurt
- **Trans Fats** – Found in processed foods, margarine, and hydrogenated oils (increases heart disease risk)
- **Highly Processed Oils** – Soybean/corn oil/vegetable (inflammatory and linked to weight gain)

NUTRITION TIP SHEET

UNDERSTANDING NUTRITION LABELS

CARBOHYDRATES are the body's main energy source, supporting brain function and daily activities. Refined and processed carbs (white bread, sugary snacks, sodas) digest quickly, spike blood sugar, and lead to cravings, energy crashes, and fat storage. On the other hand, complex carbs (whole grains, vegetables, legumes) digest slowly, providing steady energy, fiber, and essential nutrients that support weight management.

✅ **Provide Energy** – Fuel workouts and daily activities but should come from nutrient-dense sources. Best sources: oats, sweet potatoes, bananas, apples, oranges, berries, greek yogurt.
✅ **Impact Blood Sugar & Cravings** – Processed carbs cause insulin spikes, leading to hunger and fat storage. Sources: White bread, sugary cereals, pastries, candy, sodas, syrup.
✅ **Support Digestive Health** – Fiber-rich carbs promote gut health, digestion, and longer-lasting fullness.

- **High-Fiber Whole Grains** – Brown rice, quinoa, whole wheat bread, oats, sprouted grain tortillas
- **Vegetables** – Leafy greens, bell peppers, broccoli, zucchini, carrots, cauliflower, onions
- **Legumes & Beans** – Lentils, black beans, chickpeas, edamame
- **Fruits** – Berries, apples, oranges, bananas

- One serving of carbohydrates is 15 grams.
- NET CARBS = TOTAL CARBOHYDRATES - FIBER (no impact on blood sugar)
- **If you are diabetic or prediabetic, you should be tracking your carbohydrate intake daily.**

FIBER is a type of carbohydrate that the body cannot fully digest, making it essential for gut health, blood sugar control, and weight management. Unlike other carbs, fiber slows digestion, keeps you full longer, and prevents blood sugar spikes that lead to cravings and fat storage. High-fiber diets are linked to better digestion, improved heart health, and sustainable weight loss.

✅ **Increases Fullness & Reduces Hunger** – Slows digestion, helping you eat less and stay satisfied longer.
✅ **Supports Healthy Digestion** – Prevents constipation and promotes gut health by feeding beneficial bacteria.
✅ **Regulates Blood Sugar** – Slows carb absorption, preventing insulin spikes and energy crashes.
✅ **Lowers Cholesterol & Reduces Inflammation** – Helps remove excess cholesterol and supports heart health.

- Fiber is essential for gut health, blood sugar regulation, and appetite control, making it a key nutrient for sustainable fat loss and overall well-being.
- **Daily intake should be 25-30 grams.**

NUTRITION TIP SHEET

UNDERSTANDING NUTRITION LABELS

PROTEIN is the most essential macronutrient for weight loss, as it helps build and preserve lean muscle mass while promoting fat loss. Without enough protein, the body breaks down muscle tissue instead of fat, leading to muscle loss, a slower metabolism, and difficulty maintaining weight loss.

✅ **Prevents Muscle Loss** – During a calorie deficit, protein ensures the body burns fat instead of muscle.

✅ **Boosts Metabolism** – Protein has a high thermic effect, meaning your body burns more calories digesting it compared to carbs or fats.

✅ **Keeps You Full & Reduces Cravings** – Protein slows digestion, stabilizes blood sugar, and keeps hunger in check, reducing the urge to overeat.

✅ **Supports Recovery & Strength** – Essential for muscle repair and growth, especially if you're exercising.

✅ **Preserves Lean Muscle for a Toned Look** – More muscle means a higher resting metabolic rate, helping you burn more calories throughout the day.

Protein is the most important weight loss macronutrient and should be tracked daily. If you aim for 40-50g protein each meal, you will easily hit your daily intake necessary to lose weight and stay full and satisfied.

Nutrition Facts

Serving Size
Serving Pen Container

Amount per serving		
Calories	Calories from Fat	
		% Daily Value*
Total Fat		
Saturated Fat	0 g	0 %
Trans Fat	0 g	0 %
Cholesterol	0 g	0 %
Sodium	0 g	0 %
Total Carbohydrate	0 g	0 %
Dietary Fiber	0 g	0 %
Sugar	0 g	0 %
Protein	0 g	0 %
Vitamin A 0 %	Vitamin C 0 %	
Calcium 0 %	Iron 0 %	

*Percent Daily values are based on 2,000 calories diet. Your daily values may be higher or lower depending on your calories needs.

- Protein sources include chicken, turkey, lean ground beef, steak, turkey sausage/bacon, fish, Greek yogurt, whey, eggs, dairy products, and cheese.
- **Aim for 1 gram per pound of lean body mass.**
- Track daily!

VITAMINS & MINERALS: Listed as a % Daily Value (DV) based on a 2,000-calorie diet. Key nutrients like calcium, iron, potassium, and vitamin D are important for bone health, muscle function, and overall well-being. Aim for at least 20% DV per serving for good sources of these nutrients. Deficiencies in these vitamins and minerals can lead to fatigue, weak bones, and poor immune function, so focus on whole, nutrient-dense foods to meet daily needs.

NUTRITION TIP SHEET

MACRONUTRIENT CALCULATOR: GENERATE YOUR MACROS

WEIGHT LOSS CALCULATOR

Understanding what your daily macronutrient goals are is vital to ensuring effective weight loss. This macronutrient calculator is **based on your current metrics.**

1. Scan QR code with phone camera.
2. Plug in your current height, weight, age, sex, and other information.
3. Write down your macros on a sticky note and place inside book to remind you of daily intake goals.
4. Find any recipe that looks tasty to you and prep.
5. For each recipe you prep, journal the calories, protein, carbs, fats.
6. Add them up at the end of the day.

✅ To prevent plateaus, scan the QR code every 10 pounds lost to receive an updated set of weight loss macronutrients tailored to your progress.

✅ Hitting your daily protein goal should always be the top priority—even if you fall short on total calories. Protein is essential for muscle preservation, recovery, and satiety, making it the most important macronutrient for fat loss and body recomposition.

Example of custom macronutrients

DAILY WEIGHT MACROS	
CALORIES	1800-2000 CALS
PROTEIN	150-180 G
CARBOHYDRATES	120-145 G
FATS	55-65 G
BMI	27

Generate your personalized weight loss macronutrients here.

SCAN ME

If you're in a calorie deficit but meeting your protein needs, you'll maintain muscle mass while losing fat. But if you hit your calories without enough protein, you risk muscle loss and a slower metabolism over time. Your goal is to hit your protein intake and track it daily. It is the **most important macronutrient for weight loss.** In order for results, hit the intake daily.

WELCOME SHEET

NUTRITION TIP SHEET

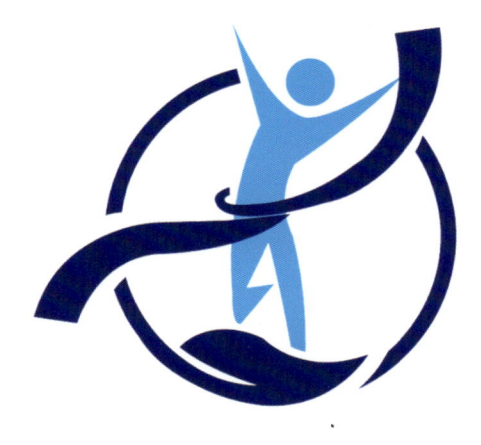

WEIGHT LOSS HACKS
LIFE CHANGING NUTRITION 101

Sustainable health and weight loss aren't built on crash diets or quick fixes—they're the result of small, consistent changes that create massive results over time. Life without consistency lacks results!

NUTRITION TIP SHEET

SIMPLE & EFFECTIVE WEIGHT LOSS HACKS

🚶 WALKING:

Sitting is the new smoking. Aiming for 10k steps a day is an attainable goal for every one of you. Taking walks after lunch, work, or taking a nightly stroll is one of the simplest lifestyle changes that you can start to have a huge impact on your weight loss efforts. Here's why:

✅ **Improves Digestion:** Stimulates digestion, reducing bloating and discomfort.
✅ **Balances Blood Sugar:** Walking after meals helps regulate blood sugar levels, preventing energy crashes and cravings later.
✅ **Enhances Fat Burning:** Regular post-meal walks encourage your body to use stored fat for energy, promoting fat loss over time.
✅ **Elevates Mood:** Walking releases endorphins, reducing stress and emotional eating.

✅ **Goals for you:**

- Walk 5-10 minutes after meals to aid digestion.
- Hit 5,000 steps per day as a starting point
- Walk 3-4 times a week for at least 30 minutes.
- Increase to 7,500-10,000 steps daily
- Add inclines or hills to engage more muscles.
- Make walking a daily habit, even on rest days.

🍽 PORTION CONTROL:

Portion control is just as important as choosing the right foods. By managing portions properly, you can avoid overeating, regulate blood sugar, and maximize fat loss without feeling deprived. If you're following the recipes in the cookbook, you're already set with perfectly portioned meals. But if you're making your own meals, use this simple plate method to stay on track:

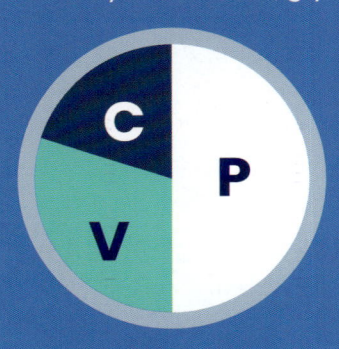

- **50% Protein** – The foundation of every meal (chicken, turkey breast, beef, steak, fish, eggs, egg whites, greek yogurt, cottage cheese, etc)
- **30% Vegetables/Fruit** – Loaded with fiber, vitamins, and minerals, these help digestion and keep cravings in check (onions, peppers, broccoli, spinach, berries, banana, grapes, apples, oranges)
- **20% Carbohydrates** – Fuel your body with healthy, whole-food carbs for sustained energy. (rice, potatoes, oats, beans)

NUTRITION TIP SHEET

SIMPLE & EFFECTIVE WEIGHT LOSS HACKS

💧 HYDRATATION:

Staying hydrated is one of the simplest yet most powerful weight loss hacks. Research shows that even if you are *mildly* dehydrated, your metabolism will slow. If you feel like you are hungry, you may just be dehydrated. Here are some hacks around water:

✅ **REDUCES APPETITE & CRAVINGS** – THIRST IS OFTEN MISTAKEN FOR HUNGER! DRINKING A GLASS OF WATER BEFORE MEALS CAN HELP YOU FEEL FULLER AND EAT FEWER CALORIES.

✅ **ENHANCES FAT BURNING** – YOUR BODY BURNS MORE FAT WHEN WELL-HYDRATED, ESPECIALLY DURING WORKOUTS.

✅ **FLUSHES OUT TOXINS** – PROPER HYDRATION SUPPORTS KIDNEY FUNCTION AND REMOVES EXCESS WASTE, REDUCING BLOATING AND WATER RETENTION

✅ **BOOSTS ENERGY & FOCUS** – DEHYDRATION LEADS TO FATIGUE AND BRAIN FOG, MAKING IT HARDER TO STAY ACTIVE AND MAKE HEALTHY FOOD CHOICES.

✅ **IMPROVES DIGESTION** – WATER HELPS BREAK DOWN FOOD AND PREVENTS CONSTIPATION, KEEPING YOUR GUT HAPPY AND METABOLISM RUNNING SMOOTHLY.

✅ **Goals for you:**

- Start your day before breaking fast with 32 ounces of water.
- Drink at least 1/2 your body weight in ounces of water daily (ex 150 lb = 75 ounces water)
- Carry a 32 ounce water bottle everywhere to stay on track.
- Sip water before meals to reduce overeating.

⚡ ELECTROLYTES:

Electrolytes are essential minerals—like sodium, potassium, magnesium, calcium, and chloride—that help regulate hydration, muscle function, and nerve signaling in your body.

✅ **Regulate Fluid Balance** – Electrolytes help your body absorb and retain water, preventing dehydration.

✅ **Prevent Fatigue & Brain Fog** – Dehydration without electrolytes can lead to dizziness, headaches, and poor concentration.

✅ **Support Muscle Function** – They prevent muscle cramps, weakness, and fatigue by ensuring proper muscle contraction and relaxation.

Scan for electrolytes!

**CODE: JOHNNY
10 % OFF**

NUTRITION TIP SHEET

SIMPLE & EFFECTIVE WEIGHT LOSS HACKS

LIQUID CALORIES:

One of the biggest culprits of weight gain is liquid calories—soda, juice, sweetened teas, energy drinks, and even fancy coffee drinks. These beverages are loaded with sugar and empty calories, leading to blood sugar spikes, increased hunger, and fat storage.

2 SODAS A DAY = 500 CALORIES X 7 DAYS A WEEK = 3,500 CALORIES (1 LB OF FAT GAINED PER WEEK)

OVER 1 YEAR = ~50 LB OF WEIGHT GAINED PER YEAR

Are Diet Soda's Okay? Sort of. Diet sodas don't have calories or sugar, but artificial sweeteners like aspartame and sucralose can trick your brain into craving more sweets or carbs. This can make it harder to control hunger and may lead to eating more later in the day.

While the occasional diet soda isn't likely to ruin your progress, drinking them often can work against your goals. If you're craving something bubbly, try flavored seltzer or sparkling water with lemon instead—hydration and real food always come first.

✅ **Goals for you:**
- Cut out all liquid calories
- Cut out all diet soda
- No more coffee creamer
- Drink 1/2 your body weight in ounces of water each day and utilize zero sugar added electrolytes for taste.

SNACKING:

Snacking can sabotage your weight loss goals without you even realizing it. Most people snack out of habit, boredom, or stress, not true hunger—leading to excess calorie intake and fat storage. Having a snack each day is okay as long as it is a high protein food item.

✅ **BEST SNACKING OPTIONS:**
- ✅ **Greek Yogurt (Plain, Non Fat) + Berries** – High protein, gut friendly.
- ✅ **Hard-Boiled Eggs** – Quick, filling, and packed with nutrients.
- ✅ **Raw Veggies + Hummus** – Fiber-rich and satisfying.
- ✅ **String Cheese or Organic Cheese Stick** – Good protein and fat balance.
- ✅ **Handful of Mixed Nuts** - Provides healthy fats, protein, and fiber.
- ✅ **Protein Shake** - Best bang for your buck. Low in calorie, high in protein.

Protein powder scan here

SCAN ME

NUTRITION TIP SHEET

SIMPLE & EFFECTIVE WEIGHT LOSS HACKS

ALCOHOL:

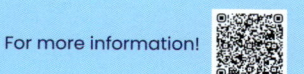

For more information!

While occasional moderate drinking may not have severe effects, frequent or excessive alcohol consumption can harm metabolism, weight loss, cardiovascular health, liver function, mental health, and immune response. Cutting back or eliminating alcohol can significantly improve overall health, energy levels, and fat loss progress.

✅ **REASONS ALCOHOL IS HARMFUL TO HEALTH AND WEIGHT LOSS:**

1. NEGATIVE EFFECTS ON WEIGHT LOSS
- Empty Calories: Alcohol provides 7 calories per gram with little to no nutritional value, leading to excess calorie consumption.
- Slows Metabolism: The liver prioritizes breaking down alcohol over burning fat, slowing fat loss.
- Promotes Fat Storage: Excess alcohol consumption encourages fat accumulation, especially around the abdomen.

2. IMPACT ON METABOLIC AND HEART HEALTH
- Raises Blood Pressure: Regular alcohol intake can increase hypertension risk.
- Increases Risk of Insulin Resistance: Alcohol can impair insulin sensitivity, increasing the risk of type 2 diabetes.
- Liver Damage: Chronic drinking leads to fatty liver disease, impairing the body's ability to detox and metabolize nutrients.

3. EFFECTS ON HORMONES & SLEEP
- Disrupts Sleep Quality: Alcohol reduces REM sleep, leading to poor recovery, fatigue, and increased hunger the next day.
- Affects Testosterone and Estrogen: Alcohol lowers testosterone, which is essential for muscle growth and fat metabolism, and disrupts estrogen balance, increasing fat storage.

4. IMPACT ON MENTAL AND COGNITIVE HEALTH
- Increases Anxiety and Depression: Alcohol disrupts neurotransmitters, contributing to mood swings and depression.
- Memory and Cognitive Decline: Long-term use shrinks brain volume and impairs memory and cognitive function.

5. ALCOHOL AND CHRONIC DISEASE RISK
- Increases Cancer Risk: Even moderate drinking raises the risk of breast, liver, esophageal, and colorectal cancers.
- Weakens Immune Function: Alcohol suppresses immune response, increasing susceptibility to infections.
- Gut Health Disruptions: Alcohol kills beneficial gut bacteria, increasing gut permeability and inflammation.

NUTRITION TIP SHEET

SIMPLE & EFFECTIVE WEIGHT LOSS HACKS

🕐 INTERMITTENT FASTING

For more information!

Fasting is a powerful tool for fat loss, metabolic health, and appetite control. It helps regulate hormones, improve insulin sensitivity, and promote fat burning—all while keeping your body in an optimal state for weight loss.

✅ **Increases Fat Burning** – After about 12-14 hours of fasting, your body shifts from burning glucose to burning stored fat for energy.

✅ **Lowers Insulin Levels** – Lower insulin levels allow your body to tap into fat stores more efficiently (1).

✅ **Reduces Hunger & Cravings** – Fasting naturally helps regulate ghrelin (the hunger hormone), making it easier to eat less.

✅ **Lowers Inflammation** – Fasting triggers cell repair and autophagy, reducing chronic inflammation that contributes to obesity and metabolic diseases (5).

✅ **Improves Sleep** – By finishing meals earlier in the evening, fasting allows the body to focus on recovery instead of digestion, leading to better-quality sleep.

✓ **RULES OF FASTING: RECOMMENDED 14 HOUR FASTS FROM 7PM-9AM**

- 14 hour fasts from 7PM-9AM is recommended.
- The earlier you can push back dinner, the better.
- No calories during fasting periods (liquid/food) including zero calorie foods
- In the morning, drink 32 ounces of water and a cup of black coffee to help boost metabolism.
- 3 meals per day

✓ **MEAL TIMING AND FREQUENCY:** 3 MEALS DAILY PLUS SNACK OR DESSERT IF NEEDED.

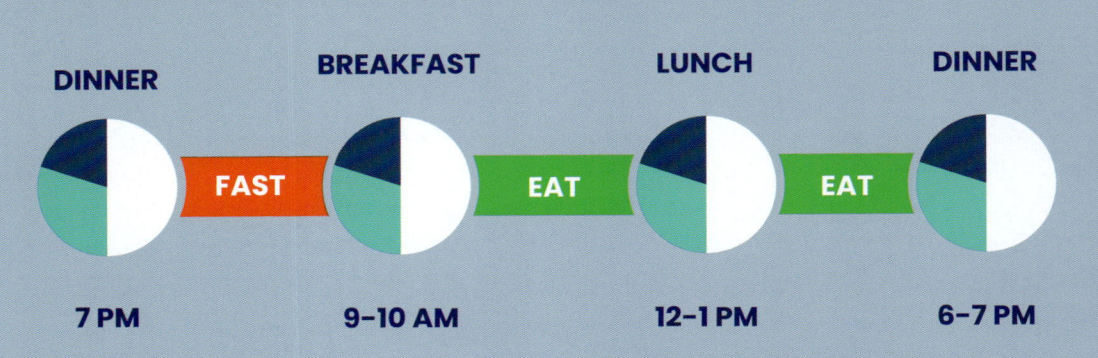

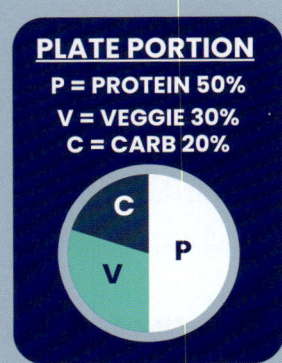

DINNER		BREAKFAST		LUNCH		DINNER
7 PM	FAST	9-10 AM	EAT	12-1 PM	EAT	6-7 PM

PLATE PORTION
P = PROTEIN 50%
V = VEGGIE 30%
C = CARB 20%

NUTRITION TIP SHEET

SLEEP HACKS: UNLOCK UNREAL SLEEP

🌙 SLEEP HACKS:

Sleep is essential for weight loss, muscle recovery, and brain health. Poor sleep disrupts hormones, metabolism, and appetite control, making fat loss harder and increasing cravings. While you sleep, your body repairs muscles, balances hormones, and strengthens brain function, improving focus, mood, and energy. Lack of sleep leads to higher cortisol (stress hormone), increased hunger, slower recovery, and brain fog, all of which can stall progress. Prioritizing 7-9 hours of quality sleep is just as important as nutrition and exercise—without it, your body struggles to burn fat, recover from workouts, and function at its best.

HEALTHY SLEEP HABITS:

✅ **Stick to a Sleep Schedule** – Go to bed and wake up at the same time every day to regulate your body's natural clock.

✅ **Limit Blue Light Exposure** – Avoid screens 1 hour before bed, or use blue light-blocking glasses to boost melatonin.

✅ **Keep Your Room Cool & Dark** – Set your bedroom temperature to 60-67°F and use blackout curtains for better sleep quality.

✅ **Avoid Late-Night Eating** – Stop eating at least 3 hours before bed to support digestion and prevent blood sugar spikes

✅ **No Caffeine After 2 PM** – Avoid coffee, energy drinks, and pre-workout late in the day to prevent restlessness

✅ **Prioritize 7-9 Hours of Sleep** – Proper sleep improves fat loss, muscle recovery, and hormone balance, making it just as important as diet and exercise!

SLEEP SUPPLEMENTS:

💊 **Magnesium Glycinate - 250 mg, 1 hour before bed**
- Natural muscle relaxant that helps lower stress, improve sleep quality, and reduce nighttime cramps. It supports melatonin production and calms the nervous system.

💊 **Ashwagandha - 1300 mg, 1 hour before bed**
- Adaptogen that helps reduce cortisol (stress hormone), improve relaxation, and promote deep sleep. While you can take it during the day to manage stress, it works best at night to enhance sleep and recovery.

Find sleep supplements here
SCAN ME

**CODE: JOHNNY
10 % OFF**

WELCOME SHEET

NUTRITION TIP SHEET

GUT HEALTH
LIFE CHANGING NUTRITION 101

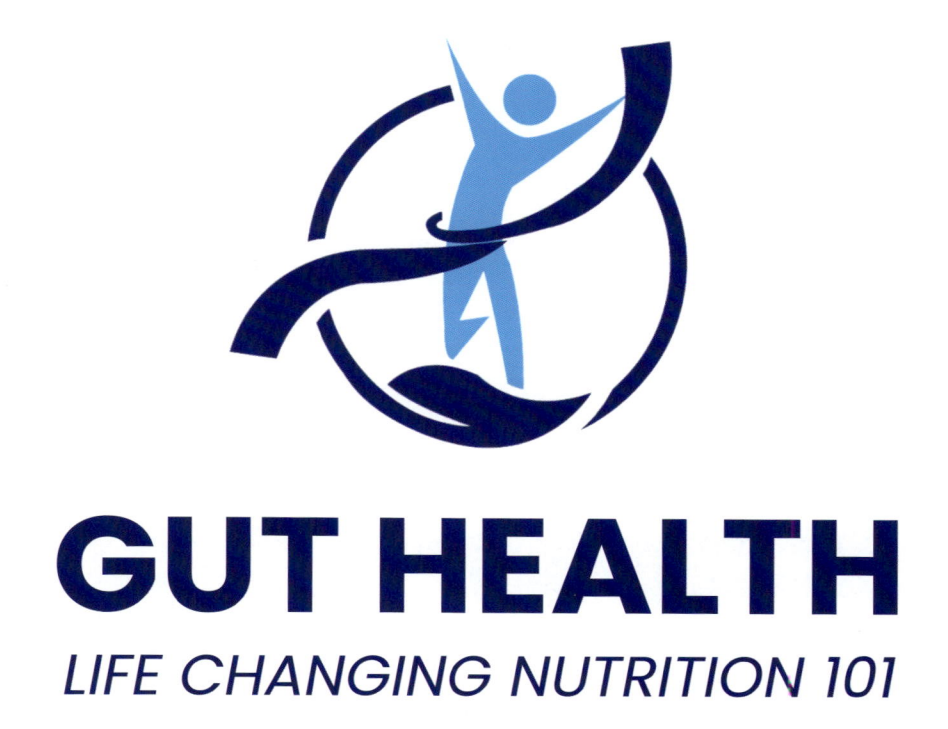

Sustainable health and weight loss aren't built on crash diets or quick fixes—they're the result of small, consistent changes that create massive results over time. Life without consistency lacks results!

GUT HEALTH TIP SHEET

GUT BASICS

GUT HEALTH:

Your gut health plays **a huge role in weight loss, metabolism, and overall well-being.** The gut is home to trillions of bacteria that impact digestion, fat storage, hunger hormones, and inflammation—all of which can make or break your ability to lose weight.

- The "gut" or gastrointestinal tract (GI) includes the stomach, small intestine, large intestine (colon), and gut microbiome—all of which play a direct role in metabolism, fat loss, and overall health.
- It acts as a barrier between your body and potential harmful pathogens from the outside world.
- Your GI tract is the foundation of weight loss. If digestion is slow, gut bacteria are unbalanced, or your body isn't absorbing nutrients properly, fat loss will be much harder.

IMPORTANCE OF GUT HEALTH

✅ **Proper Nutrient Absorption = More Energy, Less Fat Storage** – If your gut isn't absorbing nutrients properly, you'll feel hungrier and crave more food.

✅ **Healthy Digestion = Reduced Bloating & Inflammation** – Poor digestion leads to water retention, bloating, and gut inflammation, making it harder to burn fat.

✅ **Gut Bacteria Control Hunger & Fat Storage** – A balanced gut helps regulate ghrelin (hunger hormone) and leptin (fullness hormone), preventing overeating.

✅ **Regular Bowel Movements = Detox & Fat Elimination** – The body eliminates toxins and excess hormones through digestion, which prevents fat accumulation.

✅ **Better Blood Sugar Control = Less Fat Storage** – A healthy gut prevents insulin spikes and fat storage, making it easier to lose weight.

✅ **70% of Your Immune System is in Your Gut** – Your gut is the first line of defense against illness, helping to fight infections, reduce inflammation, and regulate immune responses. An unhealthy gut weakens immunity, increases inflammation, and can lead to fat retention and low energy levels.

✅ **90% of Your Serotonin is Produced in the Gut** – Serotonin is the "feel-good" neurotransmitter that regulates mood, sleep, and cravings. Poor gut health can lead to low serotonin levels, causing anxiety, poor sleep, emotional eating, and sugar cravings, all of which can make weight loss harder.

GUT HEALTH TIP SHEET

LEAKY GUT

WHAT IS A LEAKY GUT?

Leaky gut, also known as intestinal permeability, occurs when the lining of your intestines becomes damaged, allowing toxins, undigested food particles, and bacteria to leak into your bloodstream. This triggers chronic inflammation, immune system reactions, and metabolic imbalances, making weight loss harder and leading to various health issues. Here are some causes of the damage that can lead to the permeability. Here are some causes:

✅ **Poor Diet** – Processed foods, sugar, refined carbs, artificial additives, and unhealthy fats damage the gut lining.
✅ **Chronic Stress** – Stress weakens the gut barrier and disrupts healthy digestion.
✅ **Excessive Alcohol Consumption** – Alcohol irritates the gut lining, increasing permeability.
✅ **Frequent Antibiotic Use** – Kills beneficial gut bacteria, allowing harmful bacteria to take over.
✅ **Food Sensitivities & Gluten** – Gluten, dairy, and inflammatory foods can weaken the gut barrier over time.
✅ **Toxins & Pesticides** – Chemicals in processed foods, water, and environmental toxins disrupt gut health.
✅ **Low Fiber Intake** – Fiber supports gut bacteria and strengthens the intestinal lining.

SIGNS AND SYMPTOMS:

- Bloating, Gas, or Constipation
- Acid Reflux or Heartburn
- Uncontrollable Cravings for Sugar & Junk
- Unexplained Weight Gain & Fatigue
- Eczema, Acne, or Rosacea
- Anxiety & Depression
- Slow Digestion & Irregular Bowel Movements
- Chronic Inflammation & Stomach Discomfort
- Brain Fog & Low Energy
- Chronic Joint Pain & Inflammation
- Frequent Illnesses

FOODS TO AVOID:

❌ **Gluten (White Bread, Pasta, Cereal, Pastries)** – Can cause gut inflammation and contribute to leaky gut.
❌ **Dairy (Milk, Ice Cream, Processed Cheese)** – May cause bloating, inflammation, and gut irritation.
❌ **Refined Sugar & High-Fructose Corn Syrup** – Feeds bad gut bacteria, causes insulin spikes, and triggers cravings.
❌ **Artificial Sweeteners (Aspartame, Sucralose, Saccharin)** – Disrupts gut bacteria and increases sugar cravings.
❌ **Processed & Fried Foods** – Loaded with inflammatory oils and chemicals that damage the gut lining.
❌ **Alcohol (Especially Beer & Sugary Cocktails)** – Disrupts gut bacteria and slows metabolism.

GUT HEALTH TIP SHEET

HEALING LEAKY GUT

✅ **HOW TO HEAL YOUR GUT:**
By changing your diet with increasing fiber intake, consuming fermented foods, and reducing processed foods, the gut environment can improve. Here are some habits to fix your gut health.

✅ **FOODS TO EAT:**
- **Whole, Unprocessed Foods –** Fresh fruits, vegetables, whole grains, organic meat, fish, yogurt.
- **Lean Protein -** Organic chicken, turkey, grass fed beef, pasture raised eggs, steak, yogurt.
- **Utilize Anti-Inflammatory Fats –** Olive oil, avocado, nuts, and wild-caught fish.
- **Organic Fruits -** Blueberries, apples, strawberries, raspberries, citrus fruits.
- **Fermented Foods -** Sauerkraut, kimchi, kefir, greek yogurt, kombucha
- **Herbs/Spices -** Turmeric, ginger, garlic, cinnamon.
- **High-Fiber Foods –** Raspberries, apples, hummus, onions, celery, black beans, oats, almonds, avocado.
- **Antioxidant-Rich Fruits –** Berries, apples, bananas (prebiotics)
- **Healthy Fats –** Avocados, olive oil, wild-caught salmon, nuts
- **Bone Broth & Collagen –** Heals gut lining and reduces inflammation
- **Fermented Foods –** Kimchi, sauerkraut, kefir, Greek yogurt, miso

✅ **SUPPLEMENTS TO TAKE:**
- 💊 **Probiotic –** A high-quality, multi-strain probiotic for microbiome balance.
- 💊 **Prebiotic Fiber –** Helps feed healthy gut bacteria.
- 💊 **L-Glutamine –** Supports gut lining repair and reduces inflammation.

Find probiotics here
[QR CODE: SCAN ME]
CODE: JOHNNY
10 % OFF

DAILY GUT GOALS:

✅ **Take a Probiotic –** Helps replenish good gut bacteria and improve digestion.

✅ **Eat 25-30g of Fiber Daily -** Fiber feeds good gut bacteria, helps regulate blood sugar, and keeps you full, reducing cravings.

✅ **Eat a Spoonful of Sauerkraut or Fermented Veggies –** Supports gut flora and digestion.

✅ **Drink Water (1/2 body weight in oz.) –** Hydrates your gut and kickstarts digestion.

✅ **Get Sunlight (or Take Vitamin D + K2) –** Essential for immune health and gut function.

✅ **Black Coffee or Green Tea (No Sugar) –** Helps digestion and supports metabolism.

✅ **Magnesium Glycinate Supplement–** Supports digestion and prevents constipation.

✅ **Limit Late-Night Eating –** Finish meals at least 3 hours before bed to improve digestion.

GUT HEALTH TIP SHEET

WHAT IS FIBER?

🌾 FIBER:

Your gut is home to trillions of bacteria that affect digestion, metabolism, and even immunity. Fiber is their main food source! Fiber acts as a prebiotic, providing nourishment to the "good" bacteria. As these bacteria digest fiber, they grow and multiply, which helps create a healthy balance of microbes. When broken down, they promote production of short chain fatty acids which strengthen the gut lining, support immune function, and reduce inflammation.

For more information!

IMPORTANCE OF FIBER:
- **Reduces Hunger:** Fiber slows digestion, keeping you full for longer, which reduces cravings and helps prevent overeating.
- **Lowers Calories Naturally:** High-fiber foods are low in calories but high in volume, meaning you can eat more and stay in a calorie deficit.
- **Controls Blood Sugar:** Fiber slows carbohydrate digestion, preventing blood sugar spikes and crashes that trigger cravings.
- **Boosts Fat Loss:** A high-fiber diet helps regulate insulin, which plays a key role in fat storage and metabolism.

ROLE OF FIBER:

✅ **Feeds Healthy Gut Bacteria –** Fiber acts as a prebiotic, helping good bacteria grow, which improves digestion and nutrient absorption.

✅ **Prevents Bloating & Constipation –** It adds bulk to stool and keeps things moving smoothly, preventing digestive issues.

✅ **Reduces Inflammation –** A healthy gut lowers chronic inflammation, which is linked to obesity and metabolic diseases.

✅ **Fiber and Depression Risk –** A meta-analysis found that higher fiber intake is linked to a lower risk of depression, highlighting its role in mental health. (1)

✅ **Fiber and Immunity –** Dietary fiber nourishes gut bacteria, promoting the production of short-chain fatty acids (SCFAs) that regulate immune responses and reduce chronic inflammation.

✅ **Stronger Gut Barrier –** Fiber strengthens the gut lining, preventing harmful pathogens from entering the bloodstream and lowering the risk of infections and autoimmune conditions.

FOODS TO AVOID

❌ **Gluten** (White Bread, Pasta, Cereal, Pastries) ❌ **Artificial Sweeteners** (Aspartame, Saccharin)
❌ **Dairy** (Milk, Ice Cream, Processed Cheese) ❌ **Processed & Fried Foods**
❌ **Refined Sugar & High-Fructose Corn Syrup** ❌ **Alcohol** (Especially Beer & Sugary Cocktails)

GUT HEALTH TIP SHEET

FIBER SOURCE TIP SHEET

FOOD	SERVING SIZE	CALORIES	FIBER (G)
RASPBERRIES	1 CUP	40	8
APPLE	1 WHOLE	100	4.5
HUMMUS	1/2 CUP	100	7.5
ORANGE	1 WHOLE	80	3
STRAWBERRIES	1 CUP	50	3
BROCCOLI	1 CUP	50	5
CARROTS	1 CUP	40	4
SWEET POTATO	1 MEDIUM	120	4
BRUSSEL SPROUTS	1 CUP	40	4
SPINACH	1 CUP	10	4
BELL PEPPERS	1 CUP	40	3
ONION	1 CUP	40	3
CELERY	1 STALK	10	1
BLACK BEANS	1/2 CUP	90	7
OATS	1/2 CUP	150	4
ALMONDS	1/4 CUP	170	4
WALNUTS	1/4 CUP	180	2
AVOCADO	1/2 MEDIUM	160	5
POPCORN	3 CUPS	100	3.5
CHIA SEEDS	1 TBSP	70	5
WHOLE WHEAT BREAD	1 SLICE	90	2

WELCOME SHEET

NUTRITION TIP SHEET

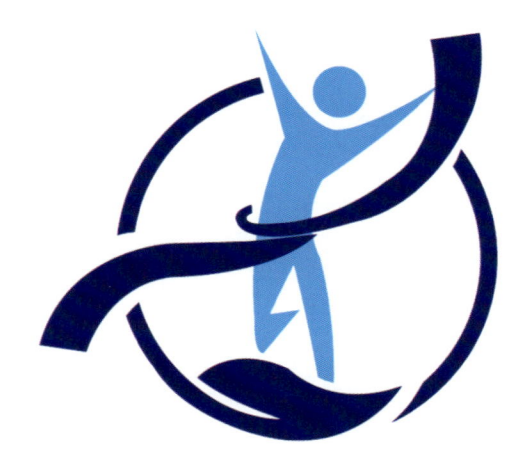

TYPE 2 DIABETES
LIFE CHANGING NUTRITION 101

Sustainable health and weight loss aren't built on crash diets or quick fixes—they're the result of small, consistent changes that create massive results over time. Life without consistency lacks results!

DIABETES TIP SHEET

WHAT CAUSES DIABETES?

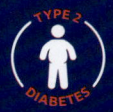

TYPE 2 DIABETES:

For more information!

Type 2 diabetes is a chronic condition where the body either resists the effects of insulin at the cellular level or doesn't produce enough insulin from the pancreas, leading to elevated blood sugar levels. This results in glucose accumulating in the bloodstream instead of being used by the body's cells for energy. AKA insulin resistance. Unlike type 1 diabetes, where the immune system attacks insulin-producing cells, type 2 diabetes develops gradually due to lifestyle factors and genetics. Moving forward, the term diabetes is referring to Type 2 diabetes.

CAUSES OF TYPE 2 DIABETES:

- **Insulin Resistance –** The body's cells become less responsive to insulin, leading to higher blood sugar levels.
- **Pancreatic Dysfunction –** Over time, the pancreas struggles to produce enough insulin to compensate for insulin resistance.
- **Excess Body Fat –** Particularly visceral fat (fat around organs) increases inflammation and worsens insulin resistance.
- **Poor Diet –** Diets high in refined carbohydrates, sugars, and unhealthy fats contribute to blood sugar spikes and metabolic dysfunction.
- **Lack of Physical Activity –** Sedentary lifestyles reduce insulin sensitivity, making it harder for cells to absorb glucose.
- **Chronic Inflammation –** Elevated levels of inflammation interfere with insulin signaling.
- **Genetics & Family History –** Some individuals have a genetic predisposition to insulin resistance.

✅ **MANAGEMENT OVERVIEW:**

- Monitor and balance carbohydrate intake.
- Be consistent with meal timing and consider fasting strategies.
- Exercise regularly to improve insulin sensitivity.
- Incorporate natural blood sugar-lowering supplements like berberine and ACV.
- Support gut health with fiber, probiotics, and prebiotics.
- Stay hydrated and avoid sugary beverages.
- Prioritize quality sleep and manage stress levels..

DIABETES TIP SHEET

TYPE 2 DIABETES: KEY STRATEGIES

PRACTICAL STRATEGIES

Type 2 diabetes is a chronic condition that affects how the body processes blood sugar (glucose). While it can lead to serious health complications if unmanaged, the good news is that lifestyle changes can significantly improve blood sugar control, insulin sensitivity, and overall well-being. By making informed choices about diet, exercise, meal timing, and supplementation, individuals can take control of their health and reduce the impact of diabetes on their daily lives. Below are key strategies to help manage and even improve type 2 diabetes naturally.

While using this cookbook it is important that you are monitoring the servings of carbohydrates you are eating daily. **One serving of carbohydrates is 15 grams.** If you eat 120 grams of carbs in a day, you have eaten 8 servings of carbohydrates. Carbohydrate management is the most important aspect of managing your diabetes and lowering your A1c.

CARBOHYDRATE MONITORING & BLOOD SUGAR CONTROL

- ✅ **Choose Complex Carbs:** Prioritize whole grains, legumes, vegetables, and fiber-rich foods over refined carbs and sugary foods.
- ✅ **Monitor Blood Sugar Responses:** Some diabetics tolerate certain carbs better than others—using a continuous glucose monitor (CGM) can help track individual responses.
- ✅ **Limit Processed Foods:** Avoid white bread, soda, pastries, and ultra-processed snacks that cause blood sugar spikes. Follow the recipes in the book.
- ✅ **Pair Carbs with Protein & Fat:** Adding protein and healthy fats slows down digestion, reducing blood sugar spikes.

MEAL TIMING & CONSISTENCY

- ✅ **Eat at Regular Intervals:** Having meals at the same time daily helps regulate blood sugar and prevents extreme highs/lows. Eat breakfast, lunch, dinner, and a snack/dessert at the same time daily. Get into consistent habits with meal timing.
- ✅ **Avoid Late-Night Eating & Snacking:** Eating late, especially high-carb or sugary snacks, can worsen insulin resistance, disrupt metabolism, and lead to higher fasting blood sugar levels. Opt for a structured meal schedule to maintain stable blood sugar.
- ✅ **Balanced Meal Timing:** Eating four structured meals daily—breakfast, lunch, dinner, and a snack/dessert—helps maintain stable blood sugar levels, prevents extreme highs and lows, and supports better insulin sensitivity.

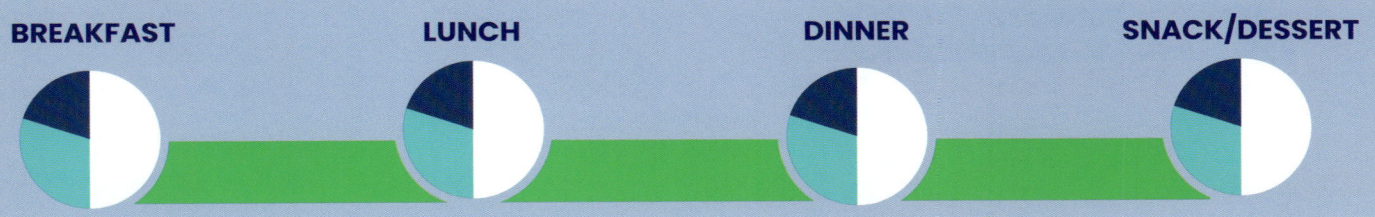

BREAKFAST   LUNCH   DINNER   SNACK/DESSERT

DIABETES TIP SHEET

TYPE 2 DIABETES: KEY STRATEGIES

PURPOSE OF FASTING

Fasting is a powerful tool for improving blood sugar control and insulin sensitivity. During a fasting period, the body reduces its reliance on external sources of glucose (from food) and instead shifts to using stored energy, which can lower blood sugar levels and reduce insulin resistance over time.

- ✅ **Reduces Insulin Resistance:** When we eat frequently, especially carbohydrate-heavy meals, the body is constantly producing insulin. Over time, this can lead to insulin resistance, where cells no longer respond well to insulin, causing high blood sugar levels. Fasting gives the body a break from insulin spikes, allowing cells to become more responsive to insulin.
- ✅ **Lowers Blood Sugar Levels:** By extending the time between meals, fasting naturally helps lower blood glucose, reducing A1c levels and stabilizing overall metabolic health.
- ✅ **Encourages Fat Utilization:** When fasting, the body burns stored fat for energy instead of relying on glucose, which can help with weight loss—a key factor in improving insulin sensitivity.
- ✅ **Reduces Inflammation:** Chronic inflammation contributes to insulin resistance. Fasting has been shown to reduce inflammatory markers, promoting better metabolic function.
- ✅ **Supports Cellular Repair (Autophagy):** Fasting activates autophagy, a process where the body removes damaged cells and regenerates new, healthy ones—helping improve overall metabolic health.

FASTING 101: WHERE TO START

For more information!

- ✅ **Start with a 12-hour fast (e.g., 8 PM - 8 AM)** and monitor blood sugar levels.
- ✅ **Gradually build to 14-hour fasts,** ensuring blood sugar remains stable.
- ✅ Stay hydrated with water, herbal tea, or black coffee (without sugar).
- ✅ **Avoid fasting if on medications that lower blood sugar without consulting a doctor, as prolonged fasting can cause hypoglycemia (low blood sugar), which can be dangerous.**
- ✅ Break the fast with a balanced meal containing protein, healthy fats, and fiber to prevent blood sugar spikes.

By incorporating controlled fasting, individuals with type 2 diabetes can improve insulin function, lower A1c levels, and reduce the risk of diabetes-related complications while promoting long-term metabolic health.

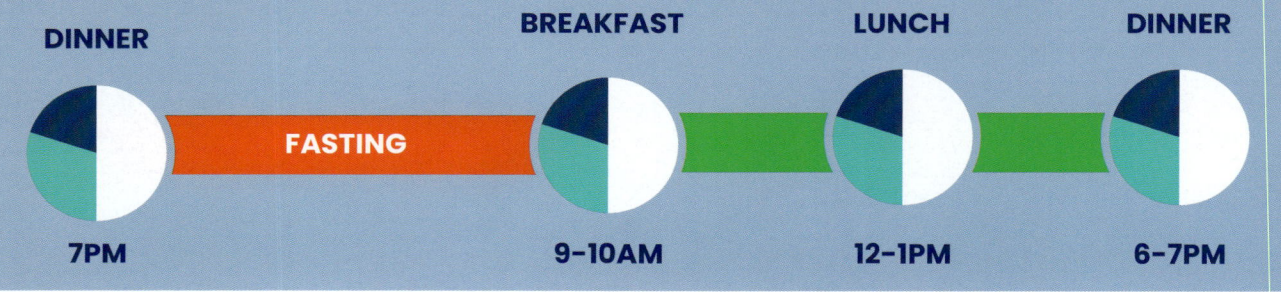

DINNER		BREAKFAST		LUNCH		DINNER
7PM	FASTING	9–10AM		12–1PM		6–7PM

DIABETES TIP SHEET

TYPE 2 DIABETES: KEY STRATEGIES

Regular physical activity is one of the most effective, drug-free ways to improve insulin sensitivity, lower blood sugar levels, and support overall metabolic health. Even small changes, like incorporating post-meal movement, can have a significant impact on blood sugar control.

- ✅ **Post-Meal Walking: 10-Minute Walks After Lunch & Dinner –** A simple 10-minute walk after meals (especially lunch and dinner) can lower post-meal blood sugar spikes by helping muscles absorb glucose more efficiently.
- ✅ **Strength Training for Insulin Sensitivity –** Lifting weights increase muscle mass, which enhances glucose uptake and lowers insulin resistance.
- ✅ **Aerobic Exercise & Cardio for Blood Sugar Control –** Aim for 30 minutes of moderate aerobic exercise, 5 days per week for improving insulin sensitivity (try to move your body 7 days a week).

DIABETIC DAILY GOALS:

✅ **Morning Goals**
- Eat a high-protein, fiber-rich breakfast to stabilize blood sugar (egg scramble and salad)
- Drink 32 ounces of water before eating
- Stretch for 5 minutes

✅ **Meal and Nutrition Goals**
- Eat balanced meals at regular intervals (breakfast, lunch, dinner)
- Include protein, healthy fats, and fiber at every meal (salad or celery/carrots & hummus)
- Avoid processed foods, refined carbs, and added sugars.
- Take apple cider vinegar (ACV) before meals to help regulate blood sugar.

✅ **Fasting and Meal Timing Goals**
- Eat meals at consistent times each day.
- Start with a 12-hour fasting window and build up to 14 hours if tolerated.
- Avoid late-night snacking, especially high-carb or sugary foods.

✅ **Physical Activity Goals**
- Take a 10-minute walk after lunch and dinner to lower blood sugar.
- Strength train 3 times per week for better insulin sensitivity.
- Get at least 30 minutes of movement daily (walking, cycling, swimming, or household chores).

✅ **Monitoring and Tracking Goals**
- Check blood sugar levels regularly and track blood sugar responses to different foods.
- Keep a food and activity journal to track patterns.
- Monitor portion sizes to prevent blood sugar spikes.

PLATE PORTION
P = PROTEIN 50%
V = VEGGIE 30%
C = CARB 20%

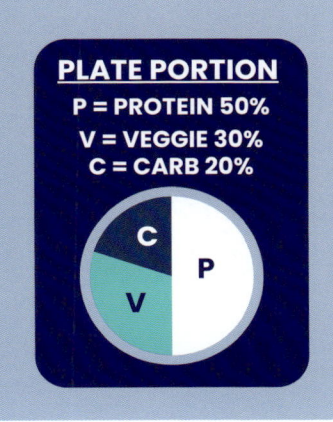

DIABETES TIP SHEET

TYPE 2 DIABETES: KEY STRATEGIES

FOOD (COOKED)	SERVING SIZE	CALORIES	CARBS (GRAMS)
LOW CARB BREAD	1 SLICE	40	13
ENGLISH MUFFIN	1 WHOLE	90	26
LOW CARB TORTILLA	1 WHOLE	81	13
OATS	1/2 CUP	150	27
FAIRLIFE 2%	1 CUP	140	13
RICE	1 CUP	200	44
BLACK BEANS	1/2 CUP	110	19
MIXED NUTS	1/4 CUP	215	7
POTATO	1 (6 OZ)	110	26
SWEET POTATO	1 (6 OZ)	110	26
ONIONS	1/2 CUP	32	7
BELL PEPPER	1/2 CUP	15	3
APPLE	1 WHOLE	100	28
BANANA	1 WHOLE	115	27
GRAPES	1 CUP	100	27
ORANGE	1 WHOLE	70	15
STRAWBERRIES	1 CUP	50	11
BLUEBERRIES	1 CUP	85	22
POPCORN	1 CUP	40	6
HONEY	1 TBSP	60	17
SF MAPLE SYRUP	2 TSBP	10	3

HYPERTENSION TIP SHEET

NUTRITION TIP SHEET

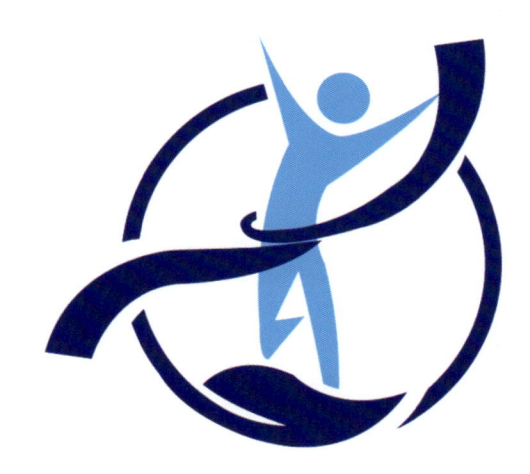

HIGH BLOOD PRESSURE
LIFE CHANGING NUTRITION 101

Sustainable health and weight loss aren't built on crash diets or quick fixes—they're the result of small, consistent changes that create massive results over time. Life without consistency lacks results!

HYPERTENSION TIP SHEET

HIGH BLOOD PRESSURE: KEY STRATEGIES

HIGH BLOOD PRESSURE:

For more information!

High blood pressure (hypertension) occurs when the force of blood against artery walls is too high, increasing the risk of heart disease, stroke, and kidney problems. It often develops without symptoms, making regular monitoring essential.

CATEGORY	SYSTOLIC (UPPER #)	AND/OR	DIASTOLIC (BOTTOM #)
NORMAL	LESS THAN 120	AND	LESS THAN 80
ELEVATED	120-129	AND	LESS THAN 80
STAGE 1	130-139	OR	80-89
STAGE 2	140+	OR	90 OR HIGHER

HYPERTENSION DAILY GOALS

✅ **NUTRITION & DIET**
- Limit saturated and trans fats from processed and fatty meats (follow the book).
    - Fried foods (French fries, fried chicken, deep-fried snacks)
    - Full-fat dairy (butter, cream, whole milk, full-fat cheese)
    - Baked goods and pastries (cookies, cakes, doughnuts, pies)
    - Margarine and shortening (especially hydrogenated oils)
    - Certain coffee creamers (non-dairy creamers often contain trans fats)
- Reduce added sugar intake, including sugary beverages.
- Lower sodium intake to 1,500–2,300 mg daily to help reduce blood pressure (1/2 teaspoon).
- Increase potassium-rich foods like leafy greens, bananas, and beans to balance sodium levels.

✅ **WEIGHT LOSS**
- Blood pressure can drop by about 1 millimeter of mercury (mm Hg) for every 2.2 pounds of weight lost (follow the cookbook).

✅ **PHYSICAL ACTIVITY**
- Engage in at least 30 minutes of aerobic exercise daily to lower blood pressure by 5-8 mm Hg.
- Regular activity is key to keeping blood pressure under control long-term.

HYPERTENSION TIP SHEET

HIGH BLOOD PRESSURE: KEY STRATEGIES

HYPERTENSION DAILY GOALS

For more information!

✅ **ALCOHOL & SMOKING**
- Limit alcohol intake.
- Quit smoking to lower blood pressure and reduce the risk of heart disease.

✅ **SLEEP & STRESS MANAGEMENT**
- Get at least 7 hours of quality sleep each night to support blood pressure regulation.
- Address sleep issues like sleep apnea and insomnia for better heart health.
- Manage chronic stress through relaxation techniques, exercise, or therapy.

✅ **BLOOD PRESSURE MONITORING**
- Check blood pressure at home regularly to track progress and ensure lifestyle changes are working.

EVIDENCE-BACKED SUPPLEMENTS

✅ **MAGNESIUM (1)**
- Helps relax blood vessels and regulate blood pressure.
- Studies show that supplementing with 300-500 mg of magnesium daily can lead to a modest reduction in blood pressure.
- Food sources: Leafy greens, nuts, seeds, whole grains.

✅ **COENZYME Q10 (COQ10) (2)**
- An antioxidant that supports blood vessel function and reduces oxidative stress.
- Studies suggest 100-200 mg daily can help lower blood pressure.
- Food sources: Fatty fish, nuts, seeds.

✅ **OMEGA-3 FATTY ACIDS (FISH OIL) (3)**
- Reduces inflammation, improves blood vessel function, and lowers blood pressure.
- EPA and DHA (1,000-2,000 mg daily) have been shown to reduce systolic and diastolic blood pressure.
- Food sources: Fatty fish (salmon, mackerel, sardines), flaxseeds, walnuts.

✅ **L-ARGININE (4)**
- An amino acid that boosts nitric oxide production, helping dilate blood vessels.
- Studies suggest taking 3-6 grams daily may help lower blood pressure.
- Food sources: Meat, poultry, dairy, nuts.

✅ **VITAMIN D (5)**
- Low vitamin D levels have been associated with higher blood pressure.
- If deficient, taking 1,000-4,000 IU per day may help regulate blood pressure.

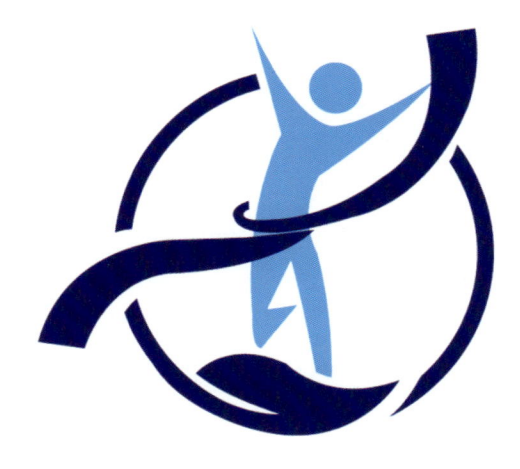

HIGH CHOLESTEROL TIP SHEET

NUTRITION TIP SHEET

HIGH CHOLESTEROL
LIFE CHANGING NUTRITION 101

Sustainable health and weight loss aren't built on crash diets or quick fixes—they're the result of small, consistent changes that create massive results over time. Life without consistency lacks results!

HIGH CHOLESTEROL TIP SHEET

HIGH CHOLESTEROL: KEY STRATEGIES

HIGH CHOLESTEROL:

For more information!

Cholesterol is a fat-like substance essential for cell membranes, hormone production (testosterone, estrogen, cortisol), vitamin D synthesis, and bile salt formation for digestion. It is transported in the blood by lipoproteins:

- LDL (Low-Density Lipoprotein): Known as "bad" cholesterol, high levels contribute to atherosclerosis (plaque buildup in arteries).
- HDL (High-Density Lipoprotein): Known as "good" cholesterol, it helps remove excess cholesterol from the bloodstream.

WHAT CAUSES HIGH CHOLESTEROL?

- Excess saturated and trans fats in the diet.
- High intake of refined carbohydrates (white bread, sugary foods).
- Sedentary lifestyle leading to poor lipid metabolism.
- Genetics and metabolic disorders (hypothyroidism, nephrotic syndrome).
- Chronic inflammation and stress contributing to arterial plaque formation.

IMPORTANCE OF WEIGHT LOSS

Losing weight and exercising regularly can significantly lower LDL (bad) cholesterol and improve overall metabolic health.

✅ **WEIGHT LOSS LOWERS LDL CHOLESTEROL (1)**

- Losing just 2.2 lbs can:
  - Lower LDL (bad cholesterol) by 1.28 mg/dL
  - Reduce triglycerides by 4.0 mg/dL
  - Increases HDL (good cholesterol) by 0.46 mg/dL
- Losing 5-10% of body weight leads to significant reductions in LDL cholesterol and triglycerides.
- Lifestyle changes, medications, and bariatric surgery all contribute to cholesterol reduction, but diet and exercise are the most effective long-term strategies.

✅ **EXERCISE IMPROVES CHOLESTEROL LEVELS (2)**

- Aerobic exercise (walking, jogging, cycling, swimming) can lower LDL by 5-8 mg/dL and improve heart health.
- Resistance training (weight lifting, bodyweight exercises) helps reduce LDL and increases HDL (good cholesterol).
- A combination of aerobic and resistance training is best for long-term cholesterol control.

HIGH CHOLESTEROL TIP SHEET

HIGH CHOLESTEROL: KEY STRATEGIES

CHOLESTEROL FRIENDLY FOODS

For more information!

✅ **INCREASE HEALTHY FATS (MUFAS & PUFAS) (3)**
- Replacing saturated fats with monounsaturated (MUFAs) and polyunsaturated fats (PUFAs) is one of the most effective ways to lower LDL cholesterol.
- MUFAs (Heart-Healthy Fats):
  - Olive oil, avocado oil, almonds, cashews, pecans, pistachios, avocados, olives, dark chocolate.
- PUFAs (Omega-3 & Omega-6 Fats):
  - Walnuts, chia seeds, flaxseeds, fatty fish (salmon, tuna, mackerel).
- MUFAs and PUFAs help reduce LDL cholesterol, improve LDL particle size, and enhance LDL receptor activity, allowing the liver to clear cholesterol from the bloodstream efficiently.

✅ **EAT MORE FIBER**
Soluble fiber binds to cholesterol in the gut, reducing absorption.
- Best Sources: Oats, beans, vegetables, hummus, fruits with skin.
- Goal: Aim for 25-30 grams of fiber daily.

✅ **INCLUDE FOODS RICH IN PHYTOSTEROLS**
Phytosterols compete with cholesterol for absorption in the intestines, lowering LDL by 8-10% when consumed in doses of 2 grams per day.
- Best Sources: Nuts, seeds, whole grains, fortified foods (certain margarines and dairy products).

✅ **CHOOSE LOW-GLYCEMIC, WHOLE CARBOHYDRATES**
- Low-GI Foods: Whole grains (oats, quinoa, brown rice), legumes, vegetables.
- Why? High-glycemic foods increase triglycerides, small LDL particles, and insulin resistance, raising CVD risk.

✅ **LIMIT SATURATED & TRANS FATS**
- High in Saturated Fat: Butter, full-fat dairy, red meat, coconut oil.
- High in Trans Fat: Processed snacks, fried foods, margarine, baked goods.

✓ **HIGH CHOLESTEROL DAILY GOALS**
- ✅ **Meal Prep & Lose weight** – Even small weight loss lowers LDL cholesterol.
- ✅ **Eat nuts** – A handful of almonds, walnuts, or pistachios daily.
- ✅ **Eat healthy fats** – Use olive oil, avocado, nuts, and fatty fish.
- ✅ **Increase fiber** – Eat oats, vegetables, oats, and whole grains, 25-30g daily.
- ✅ **Exercise daily** – 30 min of walking, jogging, or cycling.
- ✅ **Strength train** – Lift weights or do bodyweight exercises minimally 3x per week.
- ✅ **Limit processed foods** – Avoid fried foods, processed meats, and snacks (follow book).
- ✅ **Reduce sugar** – Cut sugary drinks, white bread, and pastries.

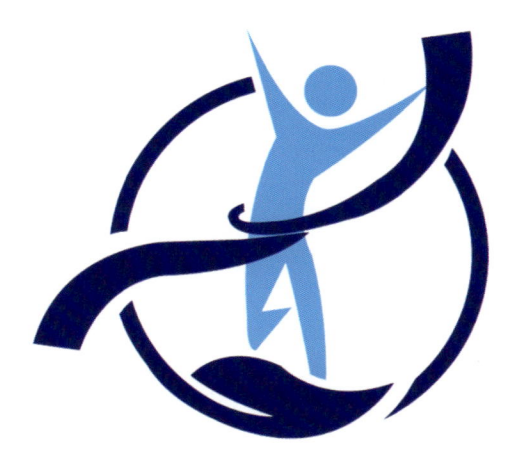

FATTY LIVER DISEASE

NUTRITION TIP SHEET

FATTY LIVER DISEASE
LIFE CHANGING NUTRITION 101

Sustainable health and weight loss aren't built on crash diets or quick fixes—they're the result of small, consistent changes that create massive results over time. Life without consistency lacks results!

FATTY LIVER DISEASE TIP SHEET

FATTY LIVER: KEY STRATEGIES

FATTY LIVER DISEASE

For more information!

Nonalcoholic Fatty Liver Disease (NAFLD) is a condition where fat builds up in the liver not because of alcohol, but because of poor nutrition, obesity, and insulin resistance. It affects 1 in 3 people globally, including kids, and is often silent until advanced stages.

There are two main types:
- Simple steatosis – early stage with just fat accumulation
- Nonalcoholic Steatohepatitis (NASH) – fat + inflammation + liver damage, which can lead to scarring (fibrosis), cirrhosis, or even liver failure

WHAT CAUSES FATTY LIVER?

- NAFLD happens when fat enters or forms in the liver faster than it can leave. The balance gets thrown off by:
- Too much fat being released from belly fat (especially in obesity)
- High sugar and refined carb intake, which turns into fat in the liver (called de novo lipogenesis)
- Poor fat-burning and export from the liver due to metabolic dysfunction and insulin resistance

WHY INSULIN RESISTANCE MATTERS:

- Muscles stop absorbing sugar → extra sugar gets rerouted to the liver → stored as fat
- Fat cells break down more fat than they should → floods the liver with fatty acids
- Liver struggles to send fat out via VLDL particles, so it stores it instead
- Inflammation + stress hormones impair the liver's ability to process fat
- **This creates a metabolic traffic jam inside your liver, increasing your risk for Type 2 diabetes, heart disease, and more.**

✅ THE GUT-LIVER AXIS: A HIDDEN DRIVER OF LIVER DAMAGE

Your gut and liver are closely connected by what's called the gut-liver axis—a two-way communication system through the portal vein, which delivers blood, nutrients, and microbial products from the gut straight to the liver.

When your gut is inflamed or "leaky" from poor diet, stress, or antibiotics:
- Toxins like lipopolysaccharides (LPS) from gut bacteria enter the bloodstream
- These LPS toxins reach the liver and trigger inflammation and oxidative stress
- This cascade promotes fat accumulation and worsens NAFLD, pushing it toward NASH, fibrosis, or cirrhosis

This is why fixing the gut is essential when treating fatty liver—because a leaky gut poisons the liver from the inside out.

FATTY LIVER DISEASE TIP SHEET

FATTY LIVER: KEY STRATEGIES

SIGNS AND SYMPTOMS OF FATTY LIVER DISEASE

- Fatigue and low energy
- Discomfort or pressure in the upper right side of your belly
- Elevated liver enzymes on blood tests (AST, ALT)
- Belly weight gain and difficulty losing fat
- Insulin resistance, pre-diabetes, or full-blown Type 2 diabetes
- High triglycerides and low HDL ("good cholesterol")

Important: Even people who are not overweight can have fatty liver due to poor diet or genetics. This is why liver fat is a better predictor of health risks than BMI alone.

HOW TO FIX OR REVERSE FATTY LIVER—NATURALLY

✅ **LOSE JUST 5–10% OF YOUR BODY WEIGHT**
- Short-term caloric restriction or healthy eating plans can dramatically reduce liver fat
- Studies show this also improves inflammation, liver enzymes, and insulin sensitivity

✅ **TIME-RESTRICTED EATING (TRE)**
Eat all meals within an 10-hour window (e.g., 9am–7pm)
Clinical trials show TRE can:
- Reduce intrahepatic triglyceride (IHTG) levels
- Improve liver stiffness and lower ALT/AST
- Enhance insulin sensitivity, reduce inflammation, and improve cholesterol
- Activate fat-burning pathways like AMPK and ketogenesis
- Improve circadian rhythm for better metabolic efficiency

✅ **CUT SUGAR AND PROCESSED CARBS**
Sugar and refined carbs drive fat production in the liver and worsen insulin resistance
Avoid:
- Soda, pastries,sugary coffee drinks, cereals, white breads
- Replace with protein-rich, whole-food meals from the cookbook

✅ **HEAL THE GUT**
Eat fermented foods (like kefir, sauerkraut), high-fiber veggies, and take quality probiotics
This helps restore the gut barrier and:
- Reduces toxin (LPS) leakage into the liver
- Calms liver inflammation and oxidative damage

✅ **GET MOVING DAILY**
- Walk 15–30 minutes after meals to lower blood sugar and liver fat
- Do resistance training to build muscle and improve insulin sensitivity

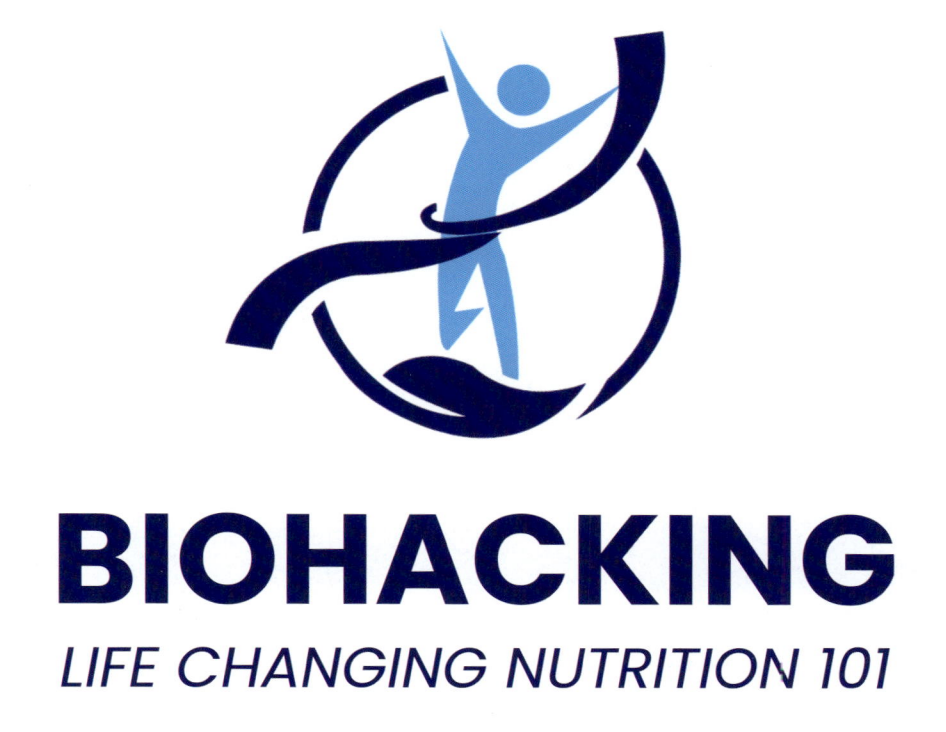

BIOHACKING

NUTRITION TIP SHEET

BIOHACKING
LIFE CHANGING NUTRITION 101

Sustainable health and weight loss aren't built on crash diets or quick fixes—they're the result of small, consistent changes that create massive results over time. Life without consistency lacks results!

BIOHACKING TIP SHEET

BIOHACKING FOR OPTIMAL HEALTH

BIOHACKING:

Biohacking is the practice of making small, science-backed lifestyle adjustments to optimize physical and mental health, boost longevity, and enhance overall performance. By strategically incorporating simple daily habits like sauna therapy, cold exposure, light management, fasting, and breathwork, you can improve energy, sleep, metabolism, and resilience against stress.

BIOHACKING STRATEGIES

- ✅ **Sauna Therapy** – A Finnish study of 2,315 middle-aged men over 20 years found that those who used a sauna 4–7 times per week had a 40% lower risk of all-cause mortality compared to those who used it once weekly (1).
  - Frequent sauna users had a 50% lower risk of fatal cardiovascular diseases and a 63% lower risk of sudden cardiac death due to improved heart health.
  - Sauna therapy helps regulate blood pressure, enhance endothelial function, and support overall cardiovascular health.
  - Incorporating sauna sessions into your routine may increase lifespan, improve stress resilience, and promote overall well-being.

- ✅ **Cold Water Immersion** – Take cold showers or plunges for 1-2 minutes daily to boost insulin sensitivity, metabolic rate, and stress resilience.
  - May reduce muscle inflammation and soreness post-exercise, aiding in quicker recovery.
  - Regular cold exposure can decrease stress and enhance mood.
  - Exposure to cold can elevate metabolic rate as the body works to maintain core temperature, potentially aiding in weight management.

- ✅ **Grounding (Earthing)** – Spend 10-20 minutes barefoot outdoors to reduce inflammation, improve sleep, and enhance recovery.
  - Reduced Inflammation: Some research indicates that grounding can decrease inflammation by neutralizing free radicals in the body (3).

- ✅ **Sunlight Exposure** – Get 10-30 minutes of morning sunlight daily to regulate circadian rhythm, boost vitamin D, and enhance mood.

- ✅ **Breathwork & Deep Breathing** – Practice 5-10 minutes of diaphragmatic breathing to lower cortisol, improve oxygenation, and reduce stress.

- ✅ **Red Light Therapy** – Use red or near-infrared light therapy to support mitochondrial function, skin health, and recovery.
  - Shown to improve skin appearance by reducing wrinkles, scars, redness, and acne.
  - Stimulates mitochondria, increasing adenosine triphosphate (ATP) production, which enhances cellular energy and function.

WELCOME SHEET

NUTRITION TIP SHEET

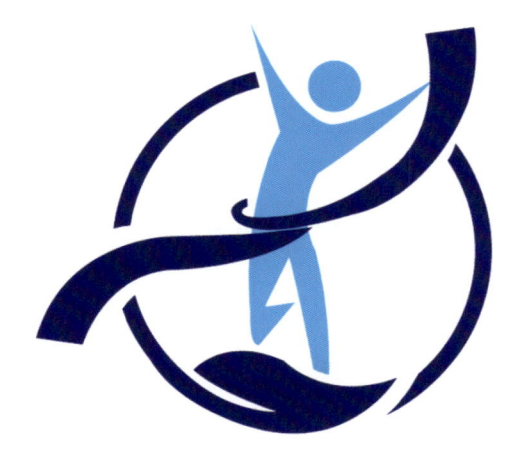

GROCERY LIST & MORE

LIFE CHANGING NUTRITION 101

Sustainable health and weight loss aren't built on crash diets or quick fixes—they're the result of small, consistent changes that create massive results over time. Life without consistency lacks results!

NUTRITION TIP SHEET

COST SAVING GROCERY LIST

PROTEIN	DAIRY	FRUIT	VEGGIES	CARBS	OTHERS
Lean meat: Ground turkey, Ground chicken, Ground beef, Sirloin, Tenderloin, Filet	**Eggs:** Whole eggs, Egg whites	Bananas, Grapes, Apples, Peaches, Pineapple, Avocado	Bell peppers, Onions, Tomatoes, Cucumbers, Garlic	**Low cal/carb:** 647 bread, English muffins, Tortillas	**Powders:** Dummy Supps, Whey, PB2, Cocoa powder
Sausages/Bacon: Chicken sausage, Turkey sausage, Jones Dairy, Turkey bacon	**Yogurt:** Non-fat Greek, Oikos, Fage Lactose free, Kefir	**Berries:** Blueberries, Strawberries, Raspberries, Blackberries	**Cruciferous:** Broccoli, Cauliflower, Brussel sprouts, Cabbage	**Pasta:** Barilla pasta, Chickpea pasta	**Sauces:** G Hughes sugar free sauce, Yellow mustard, Sugar free ketchup
Uncured Deli Meats: Turkey breast, Chicken breast, Roast beef, Ham	**Milk:** Unsweetened Almond, Fairlife, Grass Fed	**Citrus:** Oranges, Grapefruits, Lemons, Limes	**Potatoes:** Sweet potato fries, Shredded hash browns	**Oats:** Quick, Steel cut	**Canned goods:** Black beans, Diced tomatoes, Green chilis
Seafood: Shrimp, Scallops, Lobster, Crab	**Dairy:** Cottage, Ricotta, Sour cream, Whipped cream cheese	**Melons:** Watermelon, Cantaloupe, Honeydew	Carrots, Celery, Green beans, Asparagus, Mushrooms, Sweet potato	**Rice:** White, Brown, Ready rice	**Frozen goods:** Cauliflower rice, Broccoli rice, Mixed vegetable, Fruit, Vegetables
Fish: Cod, Haddock, Tilapia, Salmon, Tuna, Trout	**Low Fat Cheese:** Mozzarella, Cheddar, Pepper jack, Feta, Cheese sticks	**Unsweetened Canned:** Pineapple, Peaches, Mandarin oranges, Applesauce	**Leafy Greens:** Spinach, Arugula, Lettuce, Kale	**Bread:** 647 Low Carb, Sourdough, Multi-grain	**Seasonings:** Fajita seasoning, Ranch seasoning, Taco seasoning

NUTRITION TIP SHEET

PROTEIN SOURCE TIP SHEET

FOOD (COOKED)	SERVING SIZE	CALORIES	PROTEIN (GRAMS)
CHICKEN BREAST	1/2 CUP (4 OZ)	136	25
STEAK	1/2 CUP (4 OZ)	190	24
LEAN GROUND BEEF	1/2 CUP (4 OZ)	170	23
SALMON	1/2 CUP (4 OZ)	200	25
GROUND TURKEY	1/2 CUP (4 OZ)	160	23
TURKEY	4 SLICES	120	20
TURKEY BACON	2 SLICES	70	12
TURKEY SAUSAGE	3 LINKS	100	8
EGG	1 WHOLE	72	6
EGG WHITES	1/2 CUP	63	13
TUNA	1/2 CUP (4 OZ)	120	25
SHRIMP	10 PIECES	140	26
COTTAGE CHEESE	1/2 CUP	90	11
GREEK YOGURT	1/2 CUP	60	11
FAIRLIFE (1%)	1 CUP	100	13
FAIRLIFE CHOCOLATE	1 CUP	140	13
PROTEIN PASTA	1 CUP	190	10
MOZZARELLA CHEESE	1/4 CUP	80	6
STRING CHEESE	1 STICK	80	5
PEANUT BUTTER	2 TBSP	200	7
MIXED NUTS	1/4 CUP	205	8

WELCOME SHEET

NUTRITION TIP SHEET

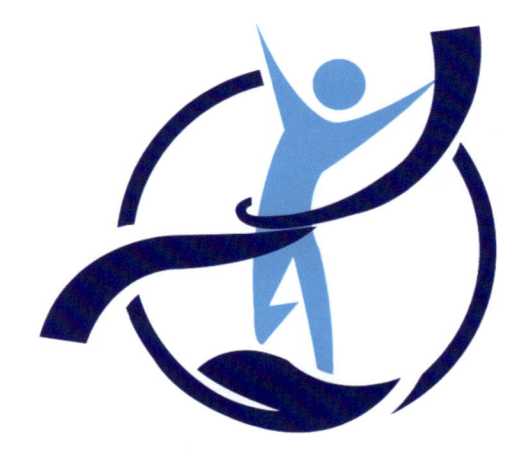

GLUTEN/LACTOSE FREE COOKBOOK + WORKOUT PROGRAMS

LIFE CHANGING NUTRITION 101

Sustainable health and weight loss aren't built on crash diets or quick fixes—they're the result of small, consistent changes that create massive results over time. Life without consistency lacks results!

WELCOME SHEET

NUTRITION TIP SHEET

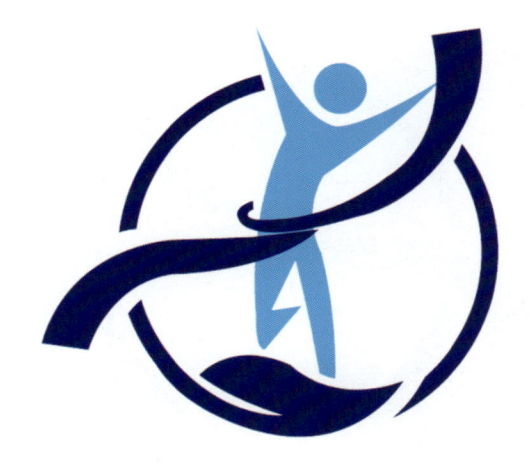

NUTRITION TIP SHEET

LIFE CHANGING NUTRITION 101

Workout programs, gluten/dairy free cookbook & more

Join the Total Weight Loss Community

Sustainable health and weight loss aren't built on crash diets or quick fixes—they're the result of small, consistent changes that create massive results over time. Life without consistency lacks results!

WELCOME SHEET

NUTRITION TIP SHEET

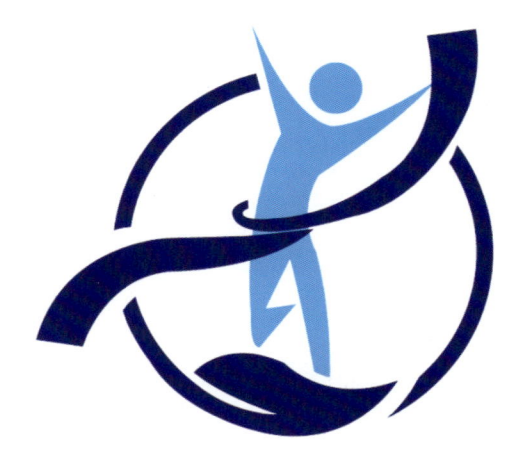

TOTAL 30 WEIGHT LOSS CHALLENGE

LIFE CHANGING NUTRITION 101

Sustainable health and weight loss aren't built on crash diets or quick fixes—they're the result of small, consistent changes that create massive results over time. Life without consistency lacks results!

WELCOME SHEET

30 DAY CHALLENGE

✓ TOTAL 30 RULES:

The Total 30 Challenge is designed to create structure, consistency, and accountability in your weight loss journey. By focusing on high-protein meals, hydration, fasting, clean eating, exercise, and sleep, you'll optimize fat loss, metabolism, and energy levels while eliminating bad habits Following this daily checklist ensures you stay on track, avoid setbacks, and build long-term success—making weight loss simple, effective, and sustainable.

1. **Eat 3 Meals Daily -** Prioritize high-protein, nutrient-dense meals to fuel your body and keep hunger in check. Add a snack or dessert within feeding hours if needed. Meal prep all food.
2. **Hit Your Daily Protein Goals –** Calculate your protein needs using 1g per lb of lean body mass and track intake daily. Hit this goal 7 days a week.
3. **Fast 14 Hours (7 PM - 9 AM)** – Implement a daily fasting window to support digestion and metabolism.
4. **Track Your Daily Macros –** Log all meals/snacks to ensure consistency with calories and macros.
5. **Hydrate–** Stay hydrated by drinking at least 1/2 your body weight in ounces of water daily. Get a 32 ounce water bottle and carry it with you daily.
6. **Incorporate One Salad Daily –** Eat at least one small salads a day with 2 cups of mixed greens, 1 tablespoon olive oil, balsamic vinegar, and some sauerkraut for extra health benefits.
7. **No Alcohol –** Eliminate alcohol to reduce empty calories and improve metabolic health.
8. **No Cheat Meals –** Avoid junk food, processed snacks, and fast food entirely.
9. **Exercise for 30 Minutes Minimum –** Commit to structured workouts or active movement daily.
10. **Read for 10 Minutes –** Choose an educational, motivational, or inspiring book or article.
11. **No Eating Out –** Cook all meals at home for better portion control and ingredient quality.
12. **Prioritize Sleep –** Aim for 7-9 hours of quality rest to support recovery, stress, and hormones
13. **Stretch for 5 Minutes Daily -** Improve flexibility, reduce muscle soreness, and enhance recovery to keep your body feeling strong and mobile.
14. **Be Consistent for 30 Days:** Follow these rules and the checklist to the best of your ability for 30 days. Sign up below and make sure to complete the form when finished.

WELCOME SHEET

30 DAY CHALLENGE

✓ DAILY CHECKLIST:

I challenge YOU to commit to the next 30 days and follow this plan with full dedication—no shortcuts, no excuses. This challenge is designed to reset your metabolism, optimize fat loss, and build lifelong healthy habits that will transform the way you eat, move, and feel.

Morning Routine:
- ✓ Fast until 9-10 AM
- ✓ Drink 32 oz of water upon waking
- ✓ 1 cup black coffee or green tea (no sweeteners/cream)
- ✓ 1 spoonful (2 tbsp) sauerkraut for gut health
- ✓ Eat a high-protein breakfast
- ✓ Take Probiotics, Vitamin D3 + K2
- ✓ Read for 5-15 minutes
- ✓ Stretch for 5-15 minutes
- ✓ Start the day with a positive mindset

Mid-Day Meals:
- ✓ Drink 32 oz of water
- ✓ Eat a high-protein lunch
- ✓ Walk for 10-15 minutes after lunch
- ✓ Eat an optional snack (2-4 PM)

Evening Routine:
- ✓ Workout for 30 minutes
- ✓ Drink 32 oz of water
- ✓ Eat a high-protein dinner
- ✓ Start fasting at 7 PM (or at least 3 hours before bed)
- ✓ Journal to reflect on your day
- ✓ Turn off screens 1 hour before bed
- ✓ Take magnesium & ashwagandha for better sleep

Weekend Focus:
- ✓ Meal prep for the upcoming week
- ✓ 1 cheat day (still hit protein intake!)
- ✓ Hydrate
- ✓ Move your body for 30 minutes

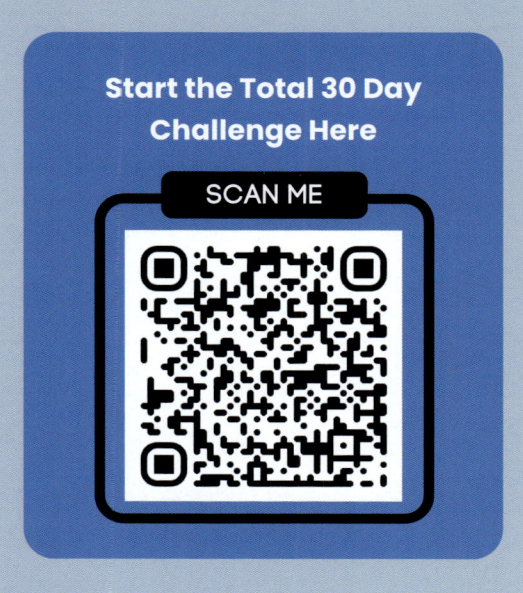

Find probiotics, magnesium and Vitamin D + K2 here

SCAN ME

CODE: JOHNNY 10 % OFF

Start the Total 30 Day Challenge Here

SCAN ME

WELCOME SHEET

30 DAY CHALLENGE

✓ HOW TO START:

Interested in starting the Total 30 Challenge? This is your opportunity to reset your habits, fuel your body with the right foods, and take control of your health in just 30 days! Whether your goal is weight loss, increased energy, or better overall wellness, this challenge is designed to keep things simple, sustainable, and effective—no crash diets, just real results.

Commit to clean eating, smart nutrition choices, and daily movement to build habits that last a lifetime. Are you ready to take on the challenge and see what 30 days of consistency can do for you? Let's get started!

Step 1: To begin the Total 30 Weight Loss Challenge, scan this QR code, plug in your information and download all links for checklists to stay on track.

Step 2: Stay consistent for 30 days.

Step 3: Once you have completed all 30 days of the challenge, scan this QR code and fill out your results. Feel free to join for another month to continue to keep you on track for your most optimal weight loss results.

WELCOME SHEET

REFERENCES

OBESITY:
Ogden CL, Carroll MD, Kit BK, Flegal KM. Prevalence of obesity and trends in body mass index among US children and adolescents, 1999-2010. JAMA. 2012;307(5):483-490. doi:10.1001/jama.2012.40. Available at: https://pubmed.ncbi.nlm.nih.gov/22253364/ (1)

National Heart, Lung, and Blood Institute. Metabolic Syndrome. National Institutes of Health. https://www.nhlbi.nih.gov/health/metabolic-syndrome. Accessed October 29, 2024. (2)

FASTING:
Jamshed H, Beyl RA, Della Manna DL, Yang ES, Ravussin E, Peterson CM. Early time-restricted feeding improves 24-hour glucose levels and affects markers of the circadian clock, aging, and autophagy in humans. Nutrients. 2019;11(6):1234. doi:10.3390/nu11061234. Available at: https://pubmed.ncbi.nlm.nih.gov/31151228/ (1)

Jamshed H, Beyl RA, Della Manna DL, Yang ES, Ravussin E, Peterson CM. Early Time-Restricted Feeding Improves 24-Hour Glucose Levels and Affects Markers of the Circadian Clock, Aging, and Autophagy in Humans. Nutrients. 2019 May 30;11(6):1234. doi: 10.3390/nu11061234. PMID: 31151228; PMCID: PMC6627766. (2)

Paoli A, Tinsley G, Bianco A, Moro T. The influence of meal frequency and timing on health in humans: the role of fasting. Nutrients. 2019;11(4):719. doi:10.3390/nu11040719. Available at: https://pubmed.ncbi.nlm.nih.gov/30925707/

https://www.mountsinai.org/about/newsroom/2019/mount-sinai-researchers-discover-that-fasting-reduces-inflammation-and-improves-chronic-inflammatory-diseases 5)

HYDRATION:
Popkin BM, D'Anci KE, Rosenberg IH. Water, hydration, and health. Nutr Rev. 2010;68(8):439-458. doi:10.1111/j.1753-4887.2010.00304.x. Available at: https://pmc.ncbi.nlm.nih.gov/articles/PMC2908954/ (1)

Bracamontes-Castelo G, Bacardí-Gascón M, Jiménez Cruz A. Effect of water consumption on weight loss: a systematic review. Nutr Hosp. 2020;37(1):46-62. doi:10.20960/nh.02656. Available at: https://pubmed.ncbi.nlm.nih.gov/31657610/ (2)

DIABETES:
1) American Diabetes Association Professional Practice Committee. Standards of medical care in diabetes—2022. Diabetes Care. 2022;45(suppl 1):S17–S38. doi:10.2337/dc22-S002 (1)

https://www.cdc.gov/diabetes/basics/symptoms.html

Javanbakht A, Sadeghi O, Mashinchi S, et al. The effect of apple cider vinegar on lipid profiles and glycemic parameters: a systematic review and meta-analysis of randomized clinical trials. J Diabetes Metab Disord. 2021;20(1):1391-1406. doi:10.1007/s40200-021-00898-y. Available at: https://pmc.ncbi.nlm.nih.gov/articles/PMC8243436/ (3)

BIOHACKING
1) SAUNA: Laukkanen T, Kunutsor S, Kauhanen J, Laukkanen JA. Association between sauna bathing and fatal cardiovascular and all-cause mortality events. JAMA Intern Med. 2015;175(4):542-548. doi:10.1001/jamainternmed.2014.8187.
2) COLD WATER IMMERSION: Tipton MJ, Bradford C. Health effects of voluntary exposure to cold water – a continuing subject of debate. Exp Physiol. 2020;105(1):44-59. doi: 10.1113/EP088251.
(2) Sinatra, S. T., Sinatra, D. S., Sinatra, S. W., & Chevalier, G. (2023). Grounding – The universal anti-inflammatory remedy. Biomedical Journal, 46(1), 11–16. https://doi.org/10.1016/j.bj.2022.12.002

HYPERTENSION:
(1) Zhang, X., Li, Y., Del Gobbo, L. C., Rosanoff, A., Wang, J., Zhang, W., & Song, Y. (2016). Effects of magnesium supplementation on blood pressure: A meta-analysis of randomized double-blind placebo-controlled trials. Hypertension, 68(2), 324–333. https://doi.org/10.1161/HYPERTENSIONAHA.116.07664

(2) Tabrizi, R., Akbari, M., Sharifi, N., Lankarani, K. B., Moosazadeh, M., Kolahdooz, F., Taghizadeh, M., & Asemi, Z. (2018). The effects of Coenzyme Q10 supplementation on blood pressures among patients with metabolic diseases: A systematic review and meta-analysis of randomized controlled trials. High Blood Pressure & Cardiovascular Prevention, 25(1), 41–50. https://doi.org/10.1007/s40292-018-0247-2

(3) Miller, P. E., Van Elswyk, M., & Alexander, D. D. (2014). Long-chain omega-3 fatty acids eicosapentaenoic acid and docosahexaenoic acid and blood pressure: A meta-analysis of randomized controlled trials. American Journal of Hypertension, 27(7), 885–896. https://doi.org/10.1093/ajh/hpu024

(4) Dong, J. Y., Qin, L. Q., Zhang, Z., Zhao, Y., Wang, J., Arigoni, F., & Zhang, W. (2011). Effect of oral L-arginine supplementation on blood pressure: A meta-analysis of randomized, double-blind, placebo-controlled trials. American Heart Journal, 162(6), 959–965. https://doi.org/10.1016/j.ahj.2011.09.012

(5) Beveridge, L. A., Struthers, A. D., Khan, F., Jorde, R., Scragg, R., Macdonald, H. M., & Witham, M. D. (2015). Effect of vitamin D supplementation on blood pressure: A systematic review and meta-analysis incorporating individual patient data. JAMA Internal Medicine, 175(5), 745–754. https://doi.org/10.1001/jamainternmed.2015.0237

CHOLESTEROL
(1) Hasan, B., Nayfeh, T., Alzuabi, M., Wang, Z., Kuchkuntla, A. R., Prokop, L. J., Newman, C. B., Murad, M. H., & Rajjo, T. I. (2020). Weight loss and serum lipids in overweight and obese adults: A systematic review and meta-analysis. The Journal of Clinical Endocrinology & Metabolism, 105(11), dgaa673. https://doi.org/10.1210/clinem/dgaa673

(2) Mann, S., Beedie, C., & Jimenez, A. (2014). Differential effects of aerobic exercise, resistance training and combined exercise modalities on cholesterol and the lipid profile: Review, synthesis and recommendations. Sports Medicine, 44(2), 211–221. https://doi.org/10.1007/s40279-013-0110-5

(3) Mensink, R. P., Zock, P. L., Kester, A. D. M., & Katan, M. B. (2003). Effects of dietary fatty acids and carbohydrates on the ratio of serum total to HDL cholesterol and on serum lipids and apolipoproteins: A meta-analysis of 60 controlled trials. The American Journal of Clinical Nutrition, 77(5), 1146–1155. https://doi.org/10.1093/ajcn/77.5.1146

FATTY LIVER:
Fabbrini, E., Sullivan, S., & Klein, S. (2010).
Obesity and nonalcoholic fatty liver disease: Biochemical, metabolic, and clinical implications. Hepatology, 51(2), 679–689. https://doi.org/10.1002/hep.23280

Lin, X., Wang, S., & Huang, J. (2024).
The effects of time-restricted eating for patients with nonalcoholic fatty liver disease: A systematic review. Nutrients, 16(1), Article 123. https://doi.org/10.3390/nu16010123
(PMCID: PMC10794638)

BREAKFAST RECIPES

EGG SCRAMBLES

DAILY MEAL PREP IDEAS

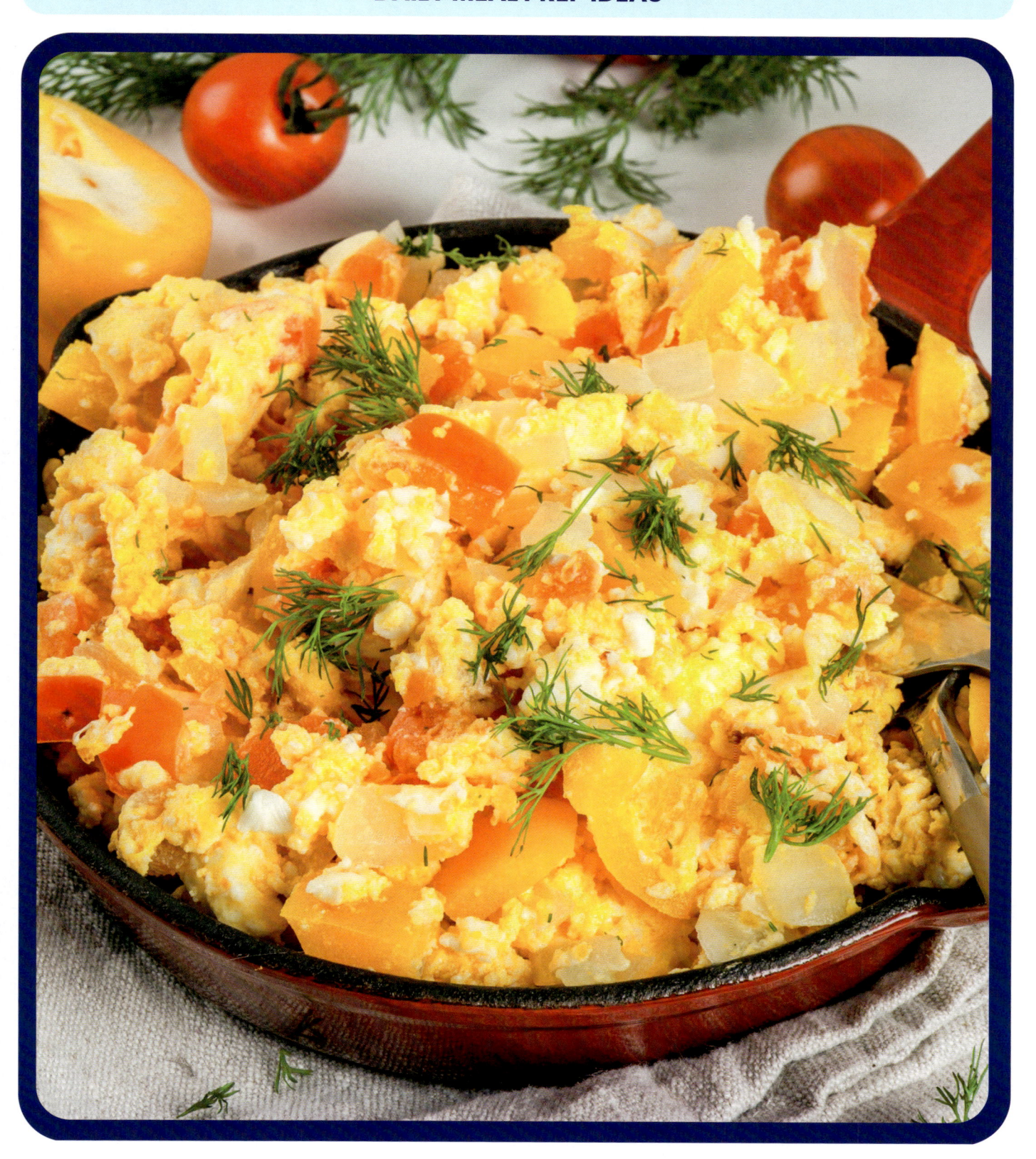

BREAKFAST RECIPES

BACON EGG & CHEESE SCRAMBLE

Calories: 390 **Protein: 52** **Carbs: 8** **Fats: 14**

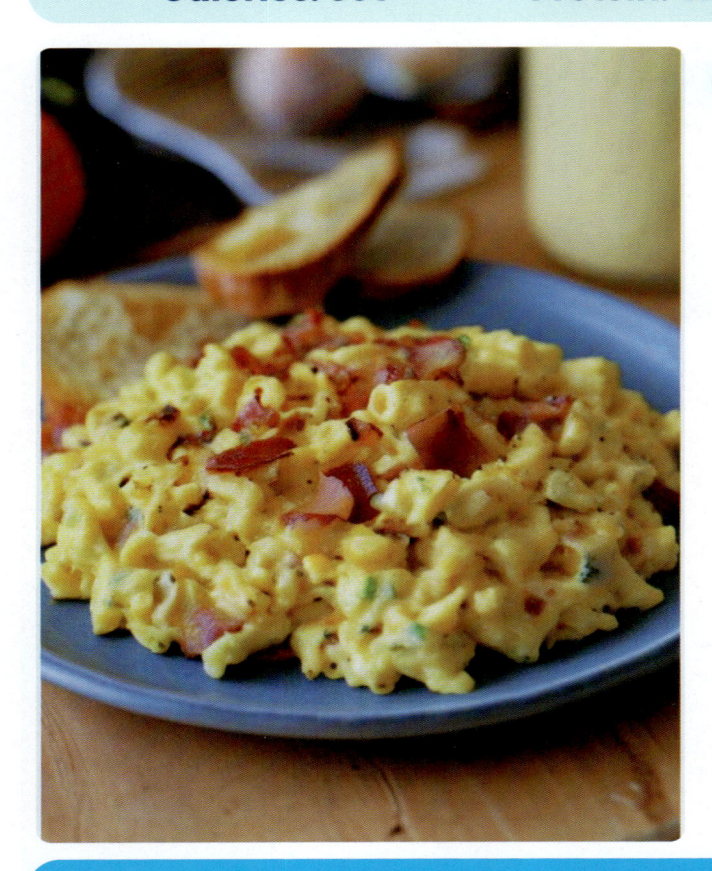

Ingredients Servings: 1

Egg Scramble:

- 1 cup egg whites
- 1 egg
- 1/4 cup shredded cheese
- 2 slices turkey bacon
- 1 tsp garlic powder
- 1 tsp onion powder
- 1/2 tsp black pepper
- 1/4 tsp salt

Optional Sides

- Salad (2 cups greens, 1 tbsp olive oil, 2 tbsp balsamic - 307c, 4P, 11C, 27F)
- Protein shake (2 cups almond milk, 1 scoop Dummy Supps - 200c, 28P, 5C, 7F)
- Toast (1 slice 647 bread- 40c, 2P, 13C, 1F)
- Sugar-free jam (1 tbsp - 10c, 0P, 17C, 2F)
- Salsa (2 tbsp - 10c, 0P, 2C, 0F)
- Hot sauce (1 tsp - 1c, 0P, 0C, 0F)
- Avocado (1/2 whole -120c, 2P, 6C, 11F)

Instructions

1. Heat a non-stick skillet over medium heat with cooking spray, cook turkey bacon for 3-4 minutes per side, then chop.
2. Lower heat to low, add eggs, and scramble for 4-5 minutes, stirring occasionally.
3. Add seasonings and shredded cheese, cook for 1 minute until melted.
4. Mix in chopped bacon, then serve hot.

BREAKFAST RECIPES

SAUSAGE EGG & CHEESE SCRAMBLE

Calories: 410   **Protein: 48**   **Carbs: 21**   **Fats: 5**

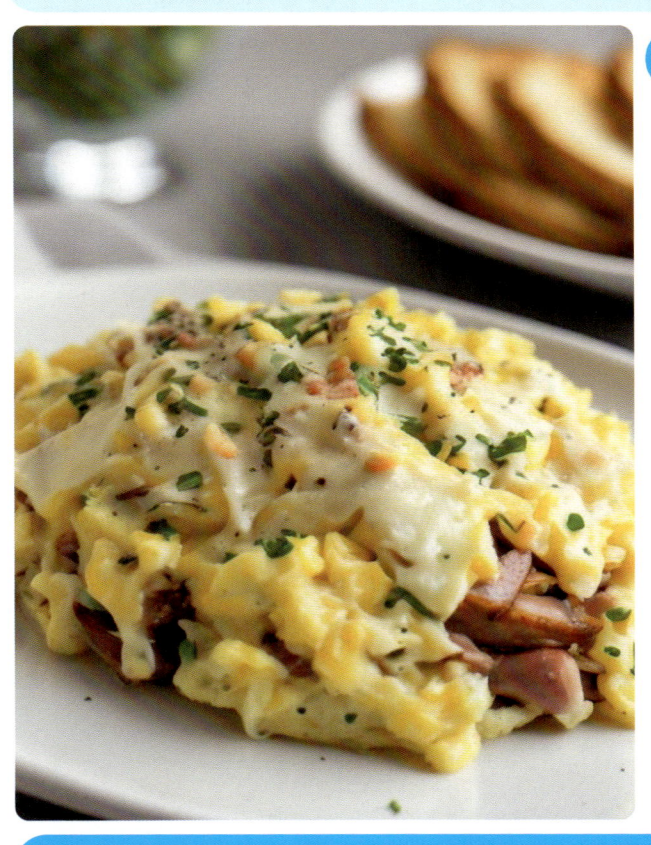

Ingredients   Servings: 1

Egg Scramble:

- 1 cup egg whites
- 1 egg
- 1/4 cup shredded cheese
- 3 frozen turkey sausage links
- 1 tsp garlic powder
- 1 tsp onion powder
- 1/2 tsp black pepper
- 1/4 tsp salt

Optional Sides

- Salad (2 cups greens, 1 tbsp olive oil, 2 tbsp balsamic - 307c, 4P, 11C, 27F)
- Protein shake (2 cups almond milk, 1 scoop Dummy Supps - 200c, 28P, 5C, 7F)
- Toast & Jam (1 slice 647 bread, 1 tbsp SF jam- 50c, 2P, 30C, 1F)
- Salsa (2 tbsp - 10c, 0P, 2C, 0F)
- Hot sauce (1 tsp - 1c, 0P, 0C, 0F)
- Avocado (1/2 whole -120c, 2P, 6C, 11F)

Instructions

1. Microwave turkey sausage for 45-60 seconds, then chop.
2. Heat a non-stick skillet over medium heat with cooking spray, add sausage, and cook for 1-2 minutes.
3. Lower heat to low, add eggs, and scramble for 4-5 minutes, stirring occasionally.
4. Add seasonings and shredded cheese, cook for 1 minute until melted.

65

BREAKFAST RECIPES

SOUTHWEST SCRAMBLE

Calories: 510 **Protein: 58** **Carbs: 6** **Fats: 24**

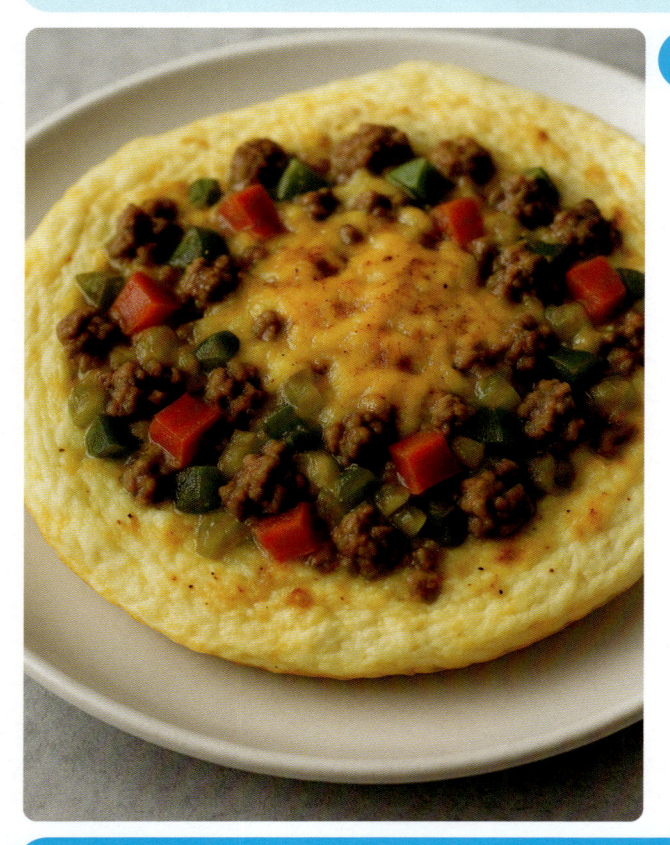

Ingredients **Servings: 1**

Egg Scramble:
- 1 cup egg whites
- 1 egg
- 1/4 cup shredded pepper jack cheese
- 1/2 cup lean ground beef
- 1/4 cup bell pepper (fresh/frozen)
- 1/4 cup sweet onion (fresh/frozen)
- 2 tbsp diced green chilis
- 2 tbsp jalapeno peppers
- 2 tsp taco seasoning

Optional Sides
- Salad (2 cups greens, 1 tbsp olive oil, 2 tbsp balsamic - 307c, 4P, 11C, 27F)
- Protein shake (2 cups almond milk, 1 scoop Dummy Supps - 200c, 28P, 5C, 7F)
- Toast & Jam (1 slice 647 bread, 1 tbsp SF jam - 50c, 2P, 30C, 1F)
- Salsa (2 tbsp - 10c, 0P, 2C, 0F)
- Hot sauce (1 tsp - 1c, 0P, 0C, 0F)
- Avocado (1/2 whole - 120c, 2P, 6C, 11F)

Instructions
1. Chop bell pepper, sweet onion, and jalapeño peppers.
2. Heat a non-stick skillet over medium heat with cooking spray, cook ground beef for 4-5 minutes, breaking it up as it browns.
3. Add chopped bell pepper, onion, green chilies, jalapeños, and taco seasoning, cook for 2-3 minutes, then set aside.
4. Lower heat to low, add eggs and egg whites, and scramble for 4-5 minutes, stirring occasionally.
5. Add shredded pepper jack cheese, cook for 1 minute until melted.

BREAKFAST RECIPES

GREEK SCRAMBLE

Calories: 410 **Protein: 48** **Carbs: 6** **Fats: 15**

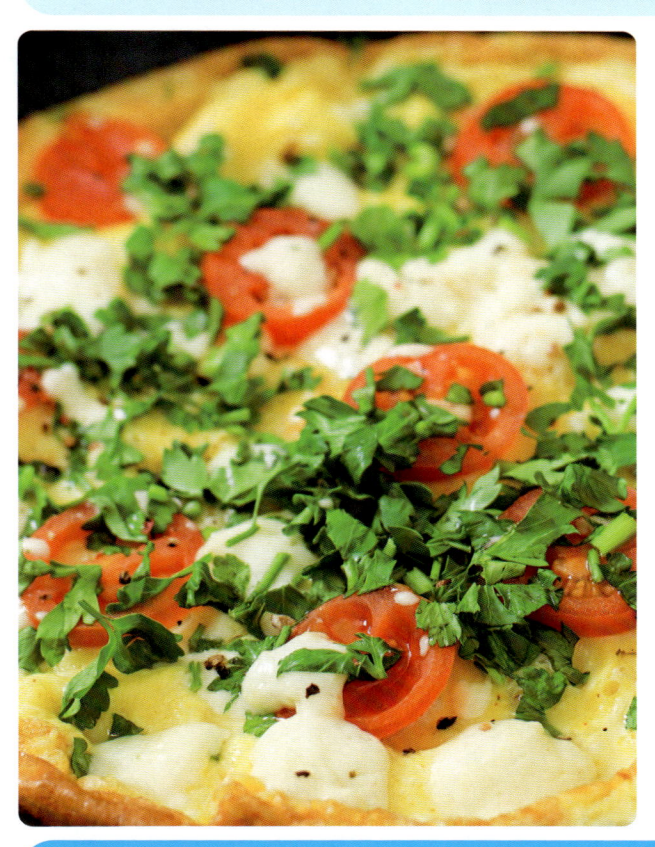

Ingredients **Servings: 1**

Egg Scramble:
- 1 cup egg whites
- 1 egg
- 1/4 cup low-fat feta cheese
- 3 frozen turkey sausage links
- 1/4 cup diced cherry tomatoes
- 1 cup spinach
- 1 tsp garlic powder
- 1 tsp onion powder
- 1/2 tsp black pepper
- 1/4 tsp salt

Optional Sides

- Salad (2 cups greens, 1 tbsp olive oil, 2 tbsp balsamic - 307c, 4P, 11C, 27F)
- Protein shake (2 cups almond milk, 1 scoop Dummy Supps - 200c, 28P, 5C, 7F)
- Toast & Jam (1 slice 647 bread, 1 tbsp SF jam- 50c, 2P, 30C, 1F)
- Salsa (2 tbsp - 10c, 0P, 2C, 0F)
- Hot sauce (1 tsp - 1c, 0P, 0C, 0F)
- Avocado (1/2 whole -120c, 2P, 6C, 11F)

Instructions

1. Microwave turkey sausage for 45-60 seconds, then chop.
2. Heat a non-stick skillet over medium heat with cooking spray, add sausage, and cook for 1-2 minutes.
3. Add diced cherry tomatoes and spinach, sauté for 2-3 minutes until softened.
4. Lower heat to low, add eggs, and scramble for 4-5 minutes, stirring occasionally.
5. Add seasonings and feta cheese, cook for 1 minute until melted.

BREAKFAST RECIPES

MEAT LOVERS SCRAMBLE

Calories: 510 **Protein: 60** **Carbs: 5** **Fats: 26**

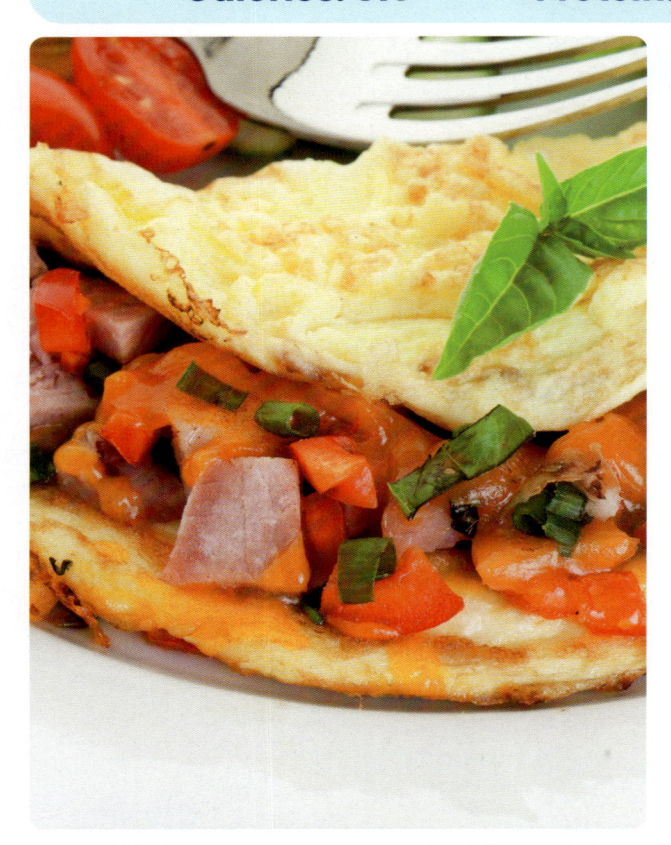

Ingredients **Servings: 1**

Egg Scramble:
- 1 cup egg whites
- 1 egg
- 3 frozen turkey sausage links
- 2 slices turkey bacon
- 2 slices low-fat ham
- 1/4 cup shredded cheese
- 1 tsp garlic powder
- 1 tsp onion powder
- 1/2 tsp black pepper
- 1/4 tsp salt

Optional Sides
- Salad (2 cups greens, 1 tbsp olive oil, 2 tbsp balsamic - 307c, 4P, 11C, 27F)
- Protein shake (2 cups almond milk, 1 scoop Dummy Supps - 200c, 28P, 5C, 7F)
- Toast & Jam (1 slice 647 bread, 1 tbsp SF jam- 50c, 2P, 30C, 1F)
- Salsa (2 tbsp - 10c, 0P, 2C, 0F)
- Hot sauce (1 tsp - 1c, 0P, 0C, 0F)
- Avocado (1/2 whole -120c, 2P, 6C, 11F)

Instructions
1. Microwave turkey sausage for 45-60 seconds, then chop.
2. Heat a non-stick skillet over medium heat with cooking spray, cook turkey bacon for 3-4 minutes per side, then chop.
3. Chop ham, add to skillet with sausage and bacon, and cook for 1-2 minutes.
4. Lower heat to low, add eggs, and scramble for 4-5 minutes, stirring occasionally.
5. Add seasonings and shredded cheese, cook for 1 minute until melted.

BREAKFAST RECIPES

WESTERN SCRAMBLE

Calories: 320   **Protein: 46**   **Carbs: 7**   **Fats: 11**

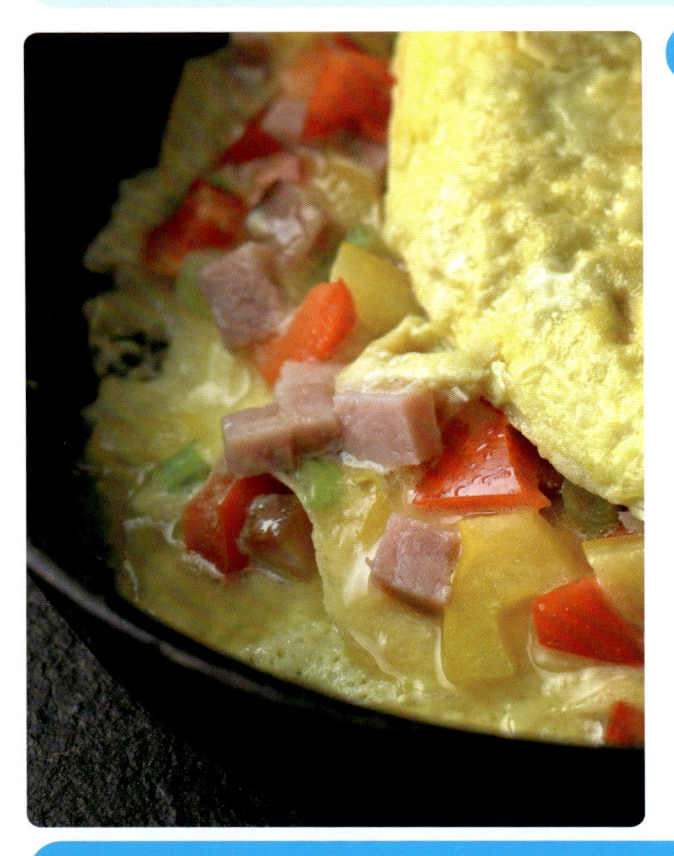

Ingredients   **Servings: 1**

Egg Scramble:
- 1 cup egg whites
- 1 egg
- 2 slices low-fat ham
- 1 slice American cheese
- 1/4 cup sweet onion (fresh/frozen)
- 1/4 cup bell pepper (fresh/frozen)
- 1 tsp onion powder
- 1/2 tsp black pepper
- 1/4 tsp salt

Optional Sides

- Salad (2 cups greens, 1 tbsp olive oil, 2 tbsp balsamic - 307c, 4P, 11C, 27F)
- Protein shake (2 cups almond milk, 1 scoop Dummy Supps - 200c, 28P, 5C, 7F)
- Toast & Jam (1 slice 647 bread, 1 tbsp SF jam- 50c, 2P, 30C, 1F)
- Salsa (2 tbsp - 10c, 0P, 2C, 0F)
- Hot sauce (1 tsp - 1c, 0P, 0C, 0F)
- Avocado (1/2 whole -120c, 2P, 6C, 11F)

Instructions

1. Chop onions and bell peppers.
2. Heat a non-stick skillet over medium heat with cooking spray.
3. Sauté onions and bell peppers for 2-3 minutes until softened.
4. Chop ham, add to skillet, and cook for 1-2 minutes.
5. Lower heat to low, add eggs, and scramble for 4-5 minutes, stirring occasionally.
6. Add seasonings and cheese, cook for 1 minute until melted.

BREAKFAST RECIPES

BUFFALO CHICKEN SCRAMBLE

Calories: 510   **Protein: 56**   **Carbs: 7**   **Fats: 28**

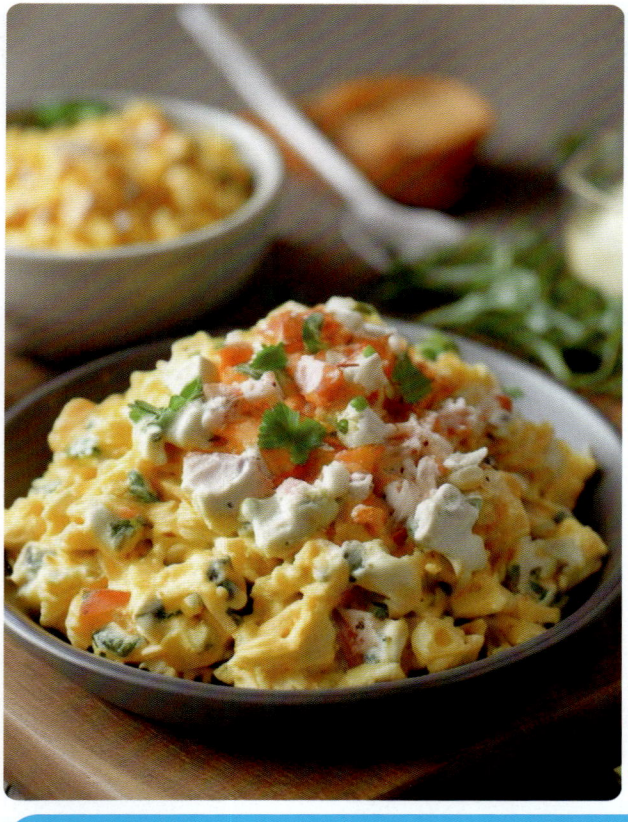

Ingredients   Servings: 1

Egg Scramble:
- 1 cup egg whites
- 1 egg
- 1/2 cup shredded chicken
- 1/4 cup red onion (fresh/frozen)
- 1/4 cup crumbled blue cheese
- 1 tsp garlic powder
- 1 tsp onion powder
- 1/2 tsp black pepper
- 1/4 tsp salt

Optional Sides
- Salad (2 cups greens, 1 tbsp olive oil, 2 tbsp balsamic - 307c, 4P, 11C, 27F)
- Protein shake (2 cups almond milk, 1 scoop Dummy Supps - 200c, 28P, 5C, 7F)
- Toast & Jam (1 slice 647 bread, 1 tbsp SF jam- 50c, 2P, 30C, 1F)
- Salsa (2 tbsp - 10c, 0P, 2C, 0F)
- Hot sauce (1 tsp - 1c, 0P, 0C, 0F)
- Avocado (1/2 whole -120c, 2P, 6C, 11F)

Instructions
1. Chop onion.
2. Heat a non-stick skillet over medium heat with cooking spray.
3. Sauté onion for 2-3 minutes until softened.
4. Add shredded chicken and cook for 1-2 minutes to warm through.
5. Lower heat to low, add eggs, and scramble for 4-5 minutes, stirring occasionally.
6. Add seasonings and blue cheese, cook for 1 minute until melted.

BREAKFAST RECIPES

STEAK & EGGS

Calories: 540 **Protein: 37** **Carbs: 1** **Fats: 27**

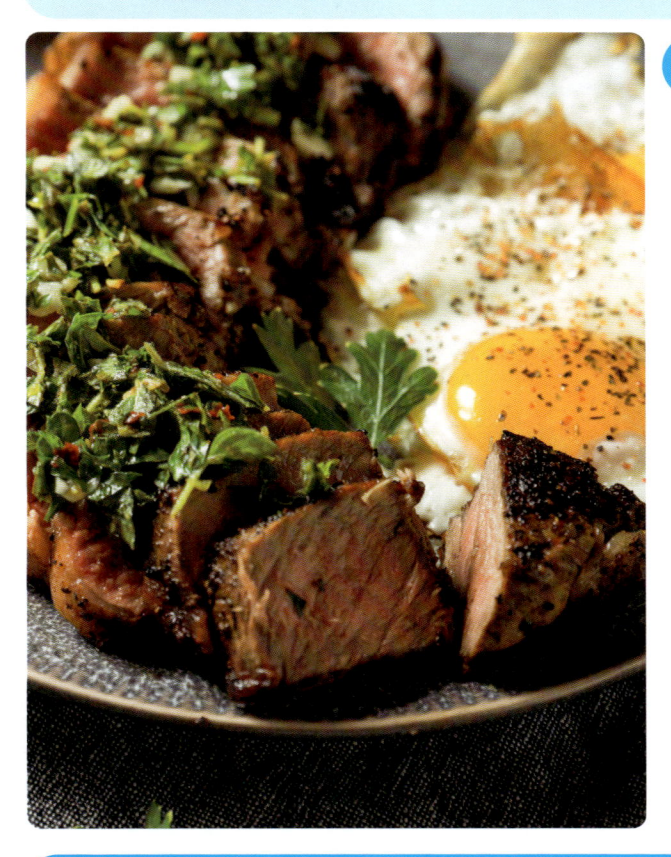

Ingredients **Servings: 1**

Steak & Eggs:
- 2 eggs
- 4 ounces steak (ribeye, sirloin, filet)
- 1 tbsp olive oil
- 1 tsp garlic powder
- 1 tsp onion powder
- 1/2 tsp black pepper
- 1/4 tsp salt

Optional Sides

- Salad (2 cups greens, 1 tbsp olive oil, 2 tbsp balsamic - 307c, 4P, 11C, 27F)
- Protein shake (2 cups almond milk, 1 scoop Dummy Supps - 200c, 28P, 5C, 7F)
- Toast & Jam (1 slice 647 bread, 1 tbsp SF jam- 50c, 2P, 30C, 1F)
- Salsa (2 tbsp - 10c, 0P, 2C, 0F)
- Hot sauce (1 tsp - 1c, 0P, 0C, 0F)
- Avocado (1/2 whole -120c, 2P, 6C, 11F)

Instructions

1. Heat a skillet over medium-high heat with 1 tbsp olive oil.
2. Season steak with garlic powder, onion powder, black pepper, and salt.
3. Cook steak for 3-4 minutes per side (or to desired doneness), then remove and rest.
4. Lower heat to medium, add eggs to the skillet, and cook 2-3 minutes until set.
5. Slice steak and serve with eggs.

BREAKFAST RECIPES

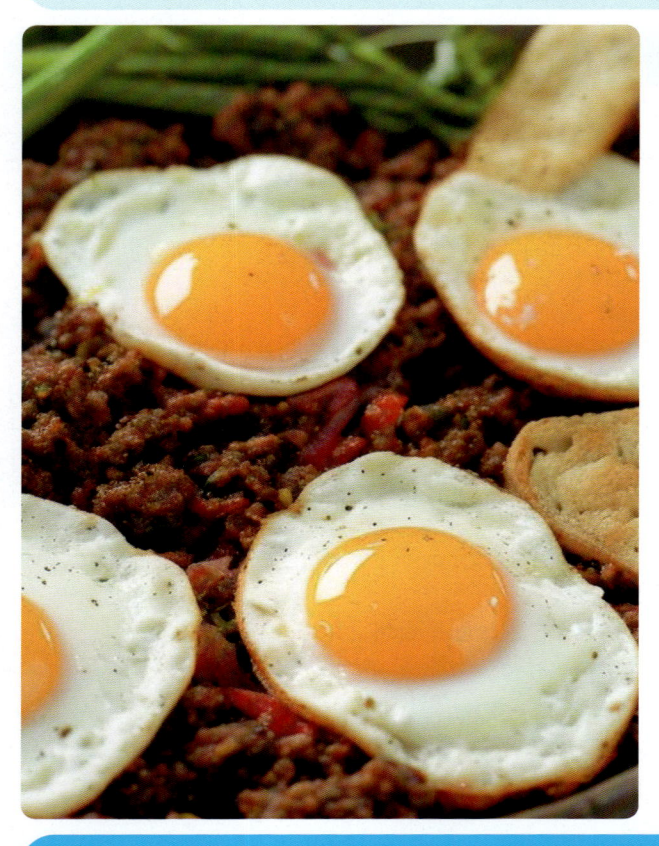

BEEF & EGGS

Calories: 410 **Protein: 50** **Carbs: 7** **Fats: 20**

Ingredients **Servings: 1**

Beef & Eggs:
- 2 eggs
- 1/2 cup lean ground beef
- 1/4 cup shredded cheese
- 1 tsp garlic powder
- 1 tsp onion powder
- 1/2 tsp black pepper
- 1/4 tsp salt

Optional Sides

- Salad (2 cups greens, 1 tbsp olive oil, 2 tbsp balsamic - 307c, 4P, 11C, 27F)
- Protein shake (2 cups almond milk, 1 scoop Dummy Supps - 200c, 28P, 5C, 7F)
- Toast & Jam (1 slice 647 bread, 1 tbsp SF jam- 50c, 2P, 30C, 1F)
- Salsa (2 tbsp - 10c, 0P, 2C, 0F)
- Hot sauce (1 tsp - 1c, 0P, 0C, 0F)
- Avocado (1/2 whole -120c, 2P, 6C, 11F)

Instructions

1. Heat a non-stick skillet over medium heat with cooking spray, cook ground beef for 4-5 minutes, breaking it up as it browns.
2. Add garlic powder, onion powder, black pepper, and salt, cook for 1 minute.
3. Remove beef, wipe skillet, and add more cooking spray.
4. Crack eggs into skillet, cook for 2-3 minutes until whites are set.
5. Top beef with shredded cheese, let melt for 1 minute.
6. Serve beef with fried eggs on top.

BREAKFAST RECIPES

POWER SCRAMBLES

DAILY MEAL PREP IDEAS

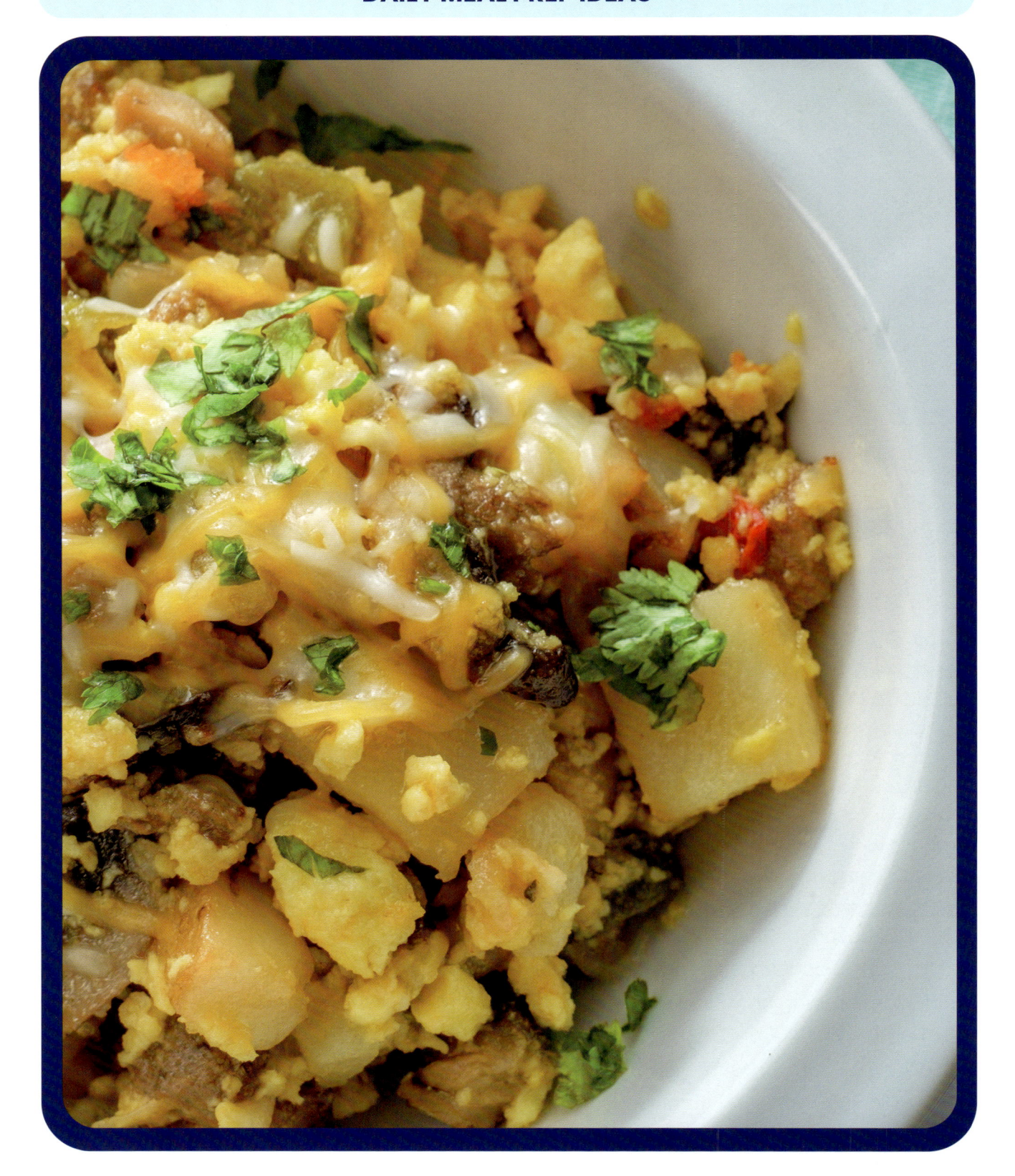

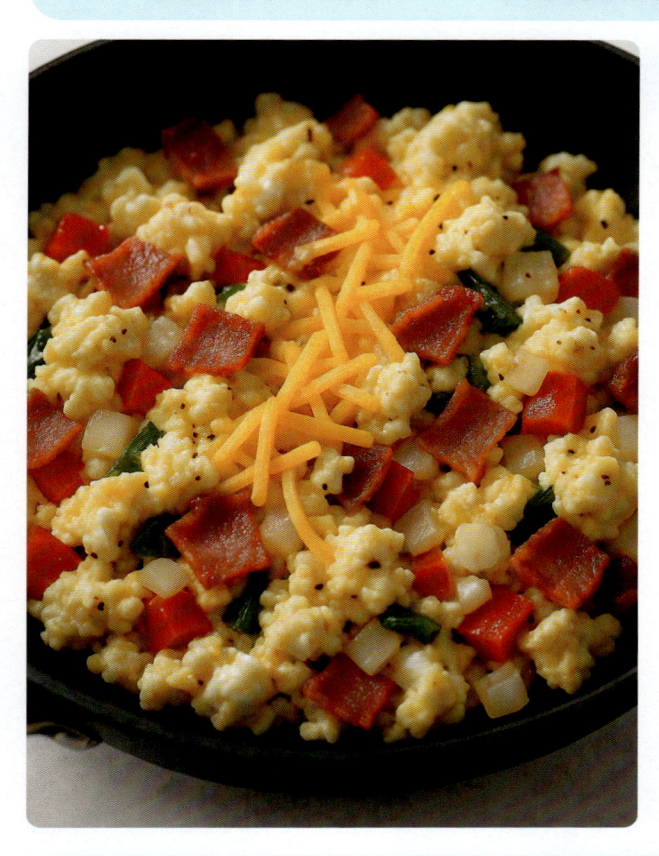

POWER SCRAMBLES

BACON & CHEESE

Calories: 380 **Protein: 52** **Carbs: 10** **Fats: 12**

Ingredients **Servings: 1**

Power Scramble:
- 1 egg
- 1/2 cup egg whites
- 1/4 cup low-fat cottage cheese
- 2 slices turkey bacon
- 1/4 cup bell pepper
- 1/4 cup white onion
- 1/4 cup shredded cheese
- 1 tsp garlic powder
- 1 tsp onion powder
- 1/2 tsp black pepper
- 1/4 tsp salt

Optional Sides

- Salad (2 cups greens, 1 tbsp olive oil, 2 tbsp balsamic - 307c, 4P, 11C, 27F)
- Protein shake (2 cups almond milk, 1 scoop Dummy Supps - 200c, 28P, 5C, 7F)
- Toast & Jam (1 slice 647 bread, 1 tbsp SF jam- 50c, 2P, 30C, 1F)
- Salsa (2 tbsp - 10c, 0P, 2C, 0F)
- Hot sauce (1 tsp - 1c, 0P, 0C, 0F)
- Avocado (1/2 whole - 120c, 2P, 6C, 11F)

Instructions

1. Preheat oven to 400°F.
2. Dice turkey bacon, bell peppers, and onions.
3. In a large mixing bowl, add egg, egg whites, cottage cheese, turkey bacon, peppers, onions, shredded cheese, and seasonings. Whisk until well combined.
4. Spray a glass/oven-safe container with cooking spray and pour in the mixture.
5. Bake at 400°F for 35-45 minutes until eggs are fully set.

POWER SCRAMBLES

SAUSAGE & CHEESE

Calories: 400 **Protein: 53** **Carbs: 11** **Fats: 13**

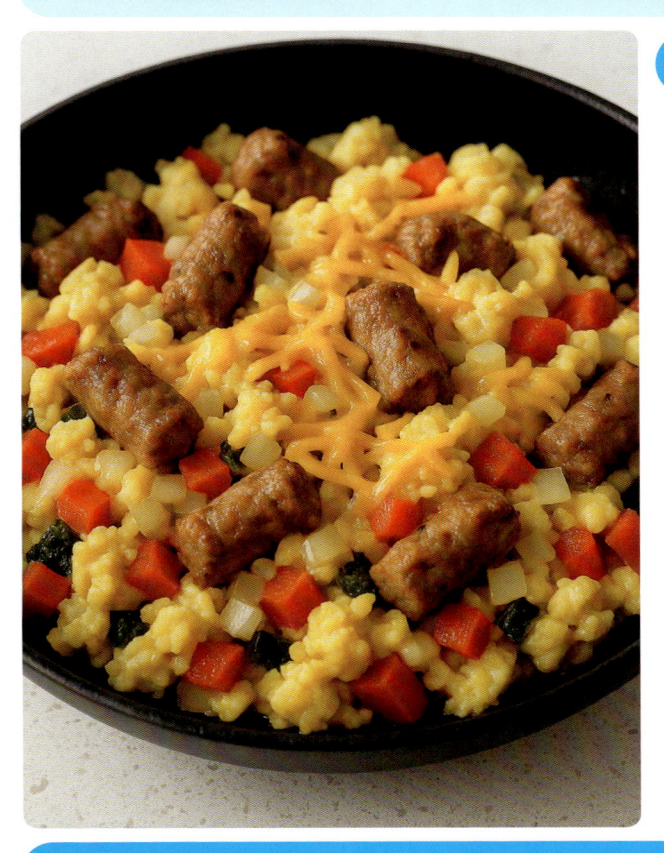

Ingredients **Servings: 1**

Power Scramble:
- 1 egg
- 1/2 cup egg whites
- 1/4 cup low-fat cottage cheese
- 4 frozen Jones Dairy turkey sausage links
- 1/4 cup bell pepper
- 1/4 cup white onion
- 1/4 cup shredded cheese
- 1 tsp garlic powder
- 1 tsp onion powder
- 1/2 tsp black pepper
- 1/4 tsp salt

Optional Sides

- Salad (2 cups greens, 1 tbsp olive oil, 2 tbsp balsamic - 307c, 4P, 11C, 27F)
- Protein shake (2 cups almond milk, 1 scoop Dummy Supps - 200c, 28P, 5C, 7F)
- Toast & Jam (1 slice 647 bread, 1 tbsp SF jam - 50c, 2P, 30C, 1F)
- Salsa (2 tbsp - 10c, 0P, 2C, 0F)
- Hot sauce (1 tsp - 1c, 0P, 0C, 0F)
- Avocado (1/2 whole - 120c, 2P, 6C, 11F)

Instructions

1. Preheat oven to 400°F.
2. Dice bell peppers and onions. Microwave turkey sausage for 45-60 seconds, then chop.
3. In a large mixing bowl, add egg, egg whites, cottage cheese, turkey sausage, bell peppers, onions, shredded cheese, and seasonings. Whisk until well combined.
4. Spray a glass/oven-safe container with cooking spray and pour in the mixture.
5. Bake at 400°F for 35-45 minutes until eggs are fully set.

POWER SCRAMBLES

WESTERN

Calories: 451   **Protein: 58**   **Carbs: 10**   **Fats: 19**

Ingredients   Servings: 1

Power Scramble:
- 1 egg
- 1/2 cup egg whites
- 1/4 cup low-fat cottage cheese
- 4 ounces uncured ham
- 1/4 cup bell pepper
- 1/4 cup white onion
- 1/4 cup shredded cheese
- 1 tsp garlic powder
- 1 tsp onion powder
- 1/2 tsp black pepper
- 1/4 tsp salt

Optional Sides

- Salad (2 cups greens, 1 tbsp olive oil, 2 tbsp balsamic - 307c, 4P, 11C, 27F)
- Protein shake (2 cups almond milk, 1 scoop Dummy Supps - 200c, 28P, 5C, 7F)
- Toast & Jam (1 slice 647 bread, 1 tbsp SF jam - 50c, 2P, 30C, 1F)
- Salsa (2 tbsp - 10c, 0P, 2C, 0F)
- Hot sauce (1 tsp - 1c, 0P, 0C, 0F)
- Avocado (1/2 whole - 120c, 2P, 6C, 11F)

Instructions

1. Preheat oven to 400°F.
2. Dice ham, bell peppers, and onions.
3. In a large mixing bowl, add egg, egg whites, cottage cheese, ham, bell peppers, onions, shredded cheese, and seasonings. Whisk until well combined.
4. Spray a glass/oven-safe container with cooking spray and pour in the mixture.
5. Bake at 400°F for 35-45 minutes until eggs are fully set.

POWER SCRAMBLES

SOUTHWESTERN

Calories: 610 **Protein: 62** **Carbs: 12**

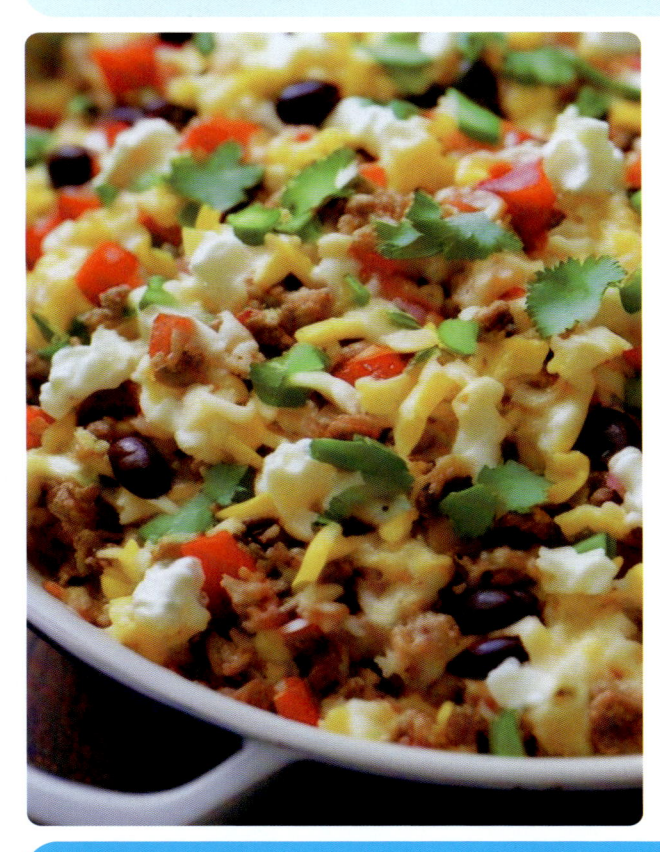

Ingredients

Power Scramble:
- 1 egg
- 1/2 cup egg whites
- 1/4 cup low-fat cottage cheese
- 1/2 cup lean ground beef
- 1/4 cup bell pepper
- 1/4 cup white onion
- 1/4 cup Mexican shredded cheese
- 2 tbsp black beans
- 1/2 jalapeno pepper
- 1 tbsp green chiles
- 2 tsp taco seasoning
- 2 tbsp cilantro

Optional Sides

- Salad (2 cups greens, 1 tbsp olive oil, 2 tbsp balsamic - 307c, 4P, 11C, 27F)
- Protein shake (2 cups almond milk, 1 scoop Dummy Supps - 200c, 28P, 5C, 7F)
- Toast & Jam (1 slice 647 bread, 1 tbsp SF jam - 50c, 2P, 30C, 1F)
- Salsa (2 tbsp - 10c, 0P, 2C, 0F)
- Hot sauce (1 tsp - 1c, 0P, 0C, 0F)
- Avocado (1/2 whole - 120c, 2P, 6C, 11F)

Instructions

1. Preheat oven to 400°F.
2. Dice bell pepper, onion, jalapeño, and cilantro.
3. Heat a non-stick skillet over medium heat with cooking spray, cook ground beef for 4-5 minutes, breaking it up as it browns. Add taco seasoning, cook for 1 minute, then remove from heat.
4. In a large mixing bowl, add egg, egg whites, cottage cheese, cooked ground beef, bell peppers, onions, black beans, jalapeño, green chiles, shredded cheese, cilantro, and seasonings. Whisk until well combined.
5. Spray a glass/oven-safe container with cooking spray and pour in the mixture.
6. Bake at 400°F for 35-45 minutes until eggs are fully set.

POWER SCRAMBLES

BUFFALO CHICKEN

Calories: 610 **Protein: 63** **Carbs: 14** **Fats: 29**

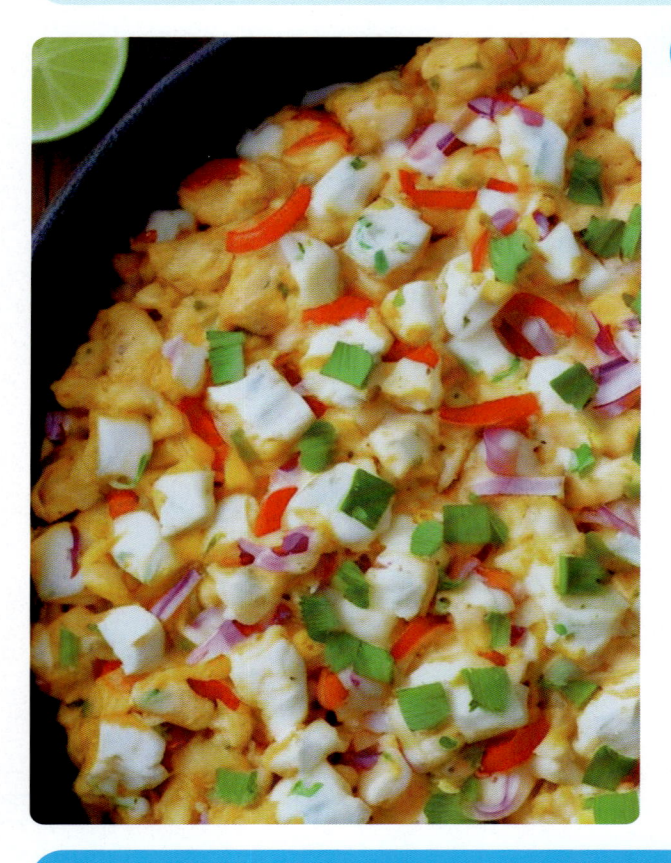

Ingredients **Servings: 1**

Power Scramble:
- 1 egg
- 1/2 cup egg whites
- 1/4 cup low-fat cottage cheese
- 1/2 cup shredded chicken
- 1/4 cup crumbled blue cheese
- 2 tbsp red hot
- 1/4 cup bell pepper
- 1/4 cup yellow onion
- 1 tsp garlic powder
- 1 tsp onion powder
- 1/2 tsp black pepper
- 1/4 tsp salt

Optional Sides
- Salad (2 cups greens, 1 tbsp olive oil, 2 tbsp balsamic - 307c, 4P, 11C, 27F)
- Protein shake (2 cups almond milk, 1 scoop Dummy Supps - 200c, 28P, 5C, 7F)
- Toast & Jam (1 slice 647 bread, 1 tbsp SF jam- 50c, 2P, 30C, 1F)
- Salsa (2 tbsp - 10c, 0P, 2C, 0F)
- Hot sauce (1 tsp - 1c, 0P, 0C, 0F)
- Avocado (1/2 whole - 120c, 2P, 6C, 11F)

Instructions
1. Preheat oven to 400°F.
2. Dice bell pepper and yellow onion.
3. In a large mixing bowl, add egg, egg whites, cottage cheese, shredded chicken, blue cheese, red hot, bell pepper, onion, garlic powder, onion powder, black pepper, and salt. Whisk until well combined.
4. Spray a glass/oven-safe container with cooking spray and pour in the mixture.
5. Bake at 400°F for 35-45 minutes until eggs are fully set.

POWER SCRAMBLES

PHILLY CHEESESTEAK

Calories: 590 **Protein: 69** **Carbs: 12** **Fats: 29**

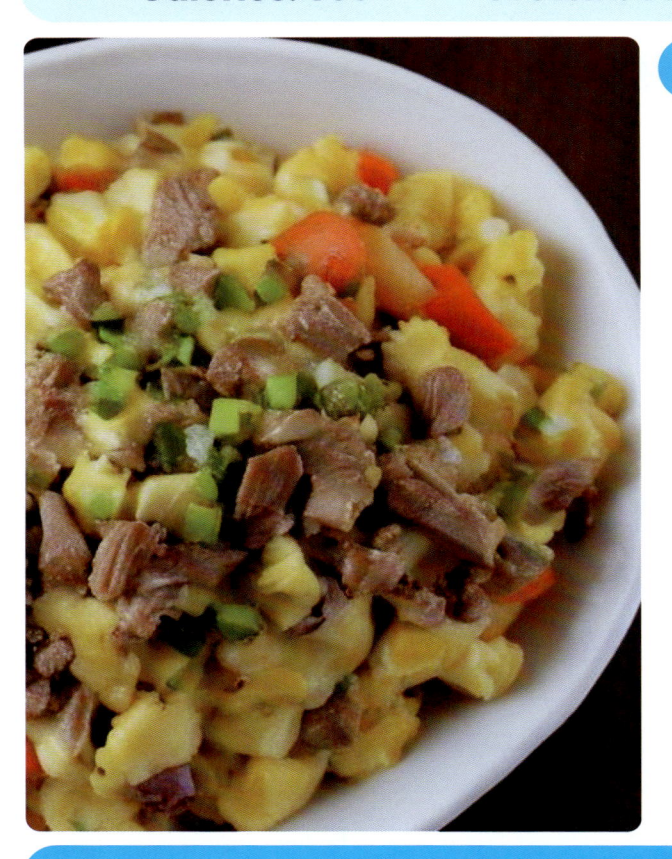

Ingredients **Servings: 1**

Power Scramble:
- 1 egg
- 1/2 cup egg whites
- 1/4 cup low-fat cottage cheese
- 1/2 cup shredded beef
- 1/4 cup shredded cheddar cheese
- 1/4 cup bell pepper
- 1/4 cup yellow onion
- 1 tsp garlic powder
- 1 tsp onion powder
- 1/2 tsp black pepper
- 1/4 tsp salt

Optional Sides
- Salad (2 cups greens, 1 tbsp olive oil, 2 tbsp balsamic - 307c, 4P, 11C, 27F)
- Protein shake (2 cups almond milk, 1 scoop Dummy Supps - 200c, 28P, 5C, 7F)
- Toast & Jam (1 slice 647 bread, 1 tbsp SF jam- 50c, 2P, 30C, 1F)
- Salsa (2 tbsp - 10c, 0P, 2C, 0F)
- Hot sauce (1 tsp - 1c, 0P, 0C, 0F)
- Avocado (1/2 whole - 120c, 2P, 6C, 11F)

Instructions
1. Preheat oven to 400°F.
2. Dice bell pepper and yellow onion.
3. In a large mixing bowl, add egg, egg whites, cottage cheese, shredded beef, cheddar cheese, bell pepper, onion, garlic powder, onion powder, black pepper, and salt. Whisk until well combined.
4. Spray a glass/oven-safe container with cooking spray and pour in the mixture.
5. Bake at 400°F for 35-45 minutes until eggs are fully set.

POWER SCRAMBLES

LOADED BEEF & EGG BAKE

Calories: 630 **Protein: 59** **Carbs: 29** **Fats: 25**

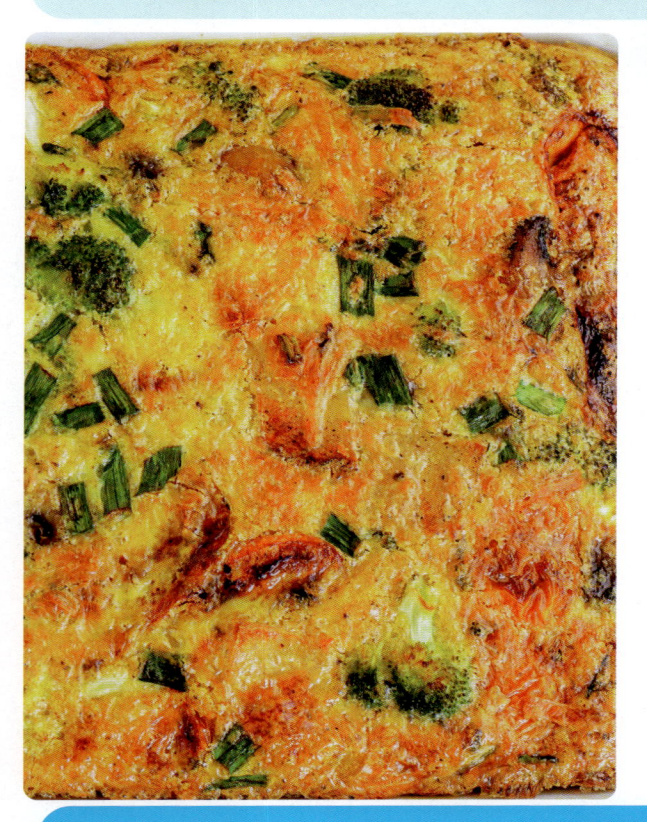

Ingredients — Servings: 6

Power Scramble:
- 1 lb lean ground beef
- 3 cups egg whites
- 3 cups low fat cottage cheese
- 6 eggs
- 2 bell peppers
- 1 red onion
- 2 cups shredded cheese
- 1 (10 ounce) bag shredded hash browns
- 1 tbsp garlic powder
- 1 tsp onion powder
- 1 tsp black pepper
- 1 tsp paprika
- 1/2 tsp salt

Optional Sides
- Salad (2 cups greens, 1 tbsp olive oil, 2 tbsp balsamic - 307c, 4P, 11C, 27F)
- Protein shake (2 cups almond milk, 1 scoop Dummy Supps - 200c, 28P, 5C, 7F)
- Toast & Jam (1 slice 647 bread, 1 tbsp SF jam- 50c, 2P, 30C, 1F)
- Salsa (2 tbsp - 10c, 0P, 2C, 0F)
- Hot sauce (1 tsp - 1c, 0P, 0C, 0F)
- Avocado (1/2 whole - 120c, 2P, 6C, 11F)

Instructions
1. Preheat oven to 400°F.
2. Dice bell peppers and red onion.
3. Heat a non-stick skillet over medium-high heat with cooking spray, cook ground beef for 8-10 minutes until fully cooked.
4. In a large mixing bowl, add eggs, egg whites, cottage cheese, cooked beef, diced peppers and onions, shredded cheese, garlic powder, onion powder, black pepper, paprika, and salt. Mix until well combined.
5. Spray a large baking dish with cooking spray and pour in the mixture.
6. Spread shredded hash browns evenly over the top.
7. Bake for 40-50 minutes or until eggs are fully set.
8. Cut into 6 even pieces.

POWER SCRAMBLES

BACON EGG & CHEESE TOTS

Calories: 600 **Protein: 55** **Carbs: 36**

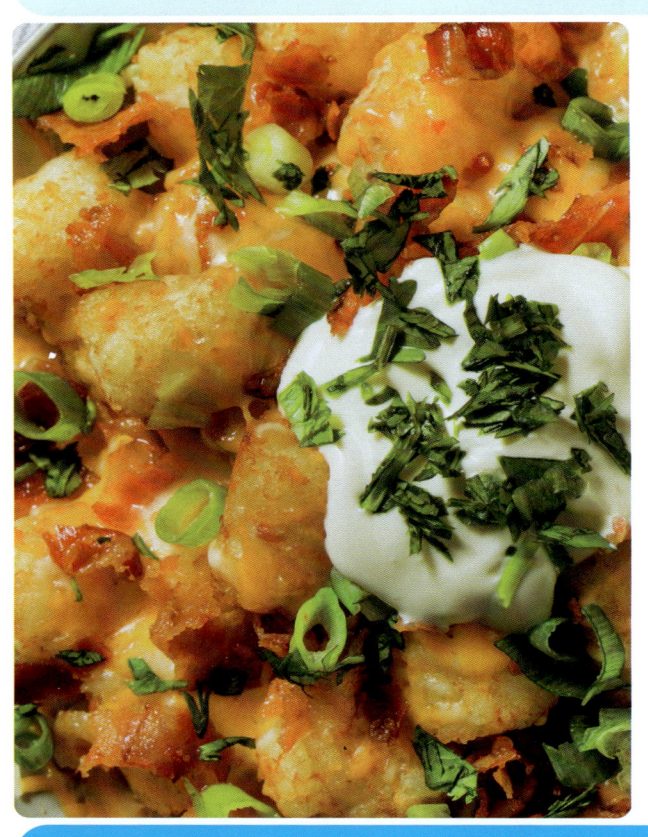

Ingredients **Servings: 6**

Power Scramble:
- 1 (20 oz. Alexia) bag tater tots
- 12 slices turkey bacon
- 6 eggs
- 3 cups egg whites
- 3 cups low fat cottage cheese
- 2 bell peppers
- 1 red onion
- 2 cups shredded cheese
- 1 tbsp garlic powder
- 1 tsp onion powder
- 1 tsp black pepper
- 1 tsp paprika
- 1/2 tsp salt

Optional Sides

- Salad (2 cups greens, 1 tbsp olive oil, 2 tbsp balsamic - 307c, 4P, 11C, 27F)
- Protein shake (2 cups almond milk, 1 scoop Dummy Supps - 200c, 28P, 5C, 7F)
- Toast & Jam (1 slice 647 bread, 1 tbsp SF jam- 50c, 2P, 30C, 1F)
- Salsa (2 tbsp - 10c, 0P, 2C, 0F)
- Hot sauce (1 tsp - 1c, 0P, 0C, 0F)
- Avocado (1/2 whole - 120c, 2P, 6C, 11F)

Instructions

1. Preheat oven to 400°F.
2. Dice bell peppers and red onion.
3. Cook turkey bacon in a non-stick skillet over medium heat for 3-4 minutes per side, then chop.
4. In a large mixing bowl, add eggs, egg whites, cottage cheese, diced peppers and onions, chopped turkey bacon, shredded cheese, garlic powder, onion powder, black pepper, paprika, and salt. Mix until well combined.
5. Spray a large baking dish with cooking spray and pour in the mixture.
6. Evenly layer tater tots on top.
7. Bake for 40-50 minutes or until eggs are fully set and tater tots are golden.
8. Cut into 6 even pieces.

POWER SCRAMBLES

SAUSAGE EGG & CHEESE TOTS

Calories: 640 **Protein: 59** **Carbs: 34**

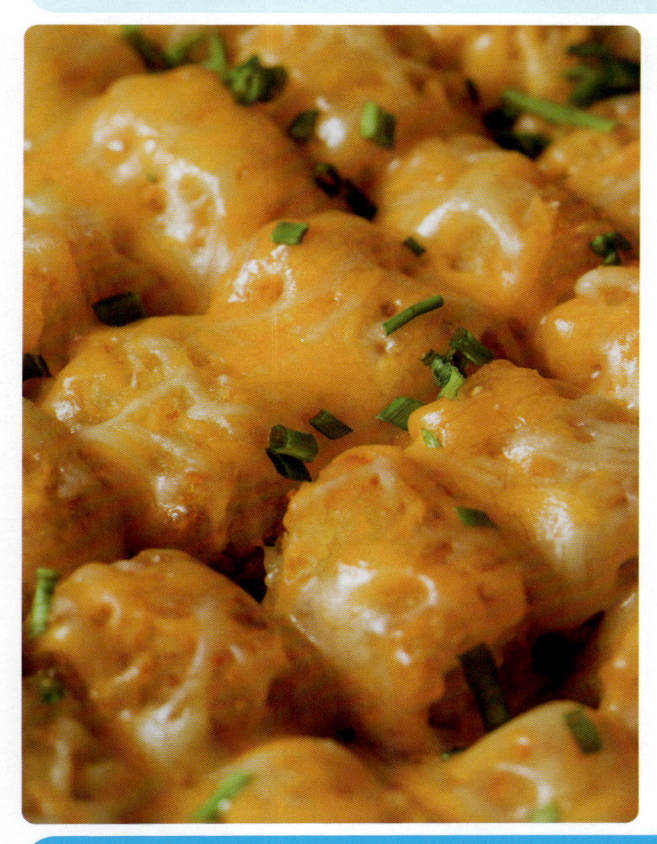

Ingredients — Servings: 6

Power Scramble:
- 1 (20 oz.) bag Alexia tater tots
- 1 (1 lb container) ground turkey sausage
- 6 eggs
- 3 cups egg whites
- 3 cups low fat cottage cheese
- 2 bell peppers
- 1 red onion
- 2 cups shredded cheese
- 1 tbsp garlic powder
- 1 tsp onion powder
- 1 tsp black pepper
- 1 tsp paprika
- 1/2 tsp salt

Optional Sides
- Salad (2 cups greens, 1 tbsp olive oil, 2 tbsp balsamic - 307c, 4P, 11C, 27F)
- Protein shake (2 cups almond milk, 1 scoop Dummy Supps - 200c, 28P, 5C, 7F)
- Toast & Jam (1 slice 647 bread, 1 tbsp SF jam - 50c, 2P, 30C, 1F)
- Salsa (2 tbsp - 10c, 0P, 2C, 0F)
- Hot sauce (1 tsp - 1c, 0P, 0C, 0F)
- Avocado (1/2 whole - 120c, 2P, 6C, 11F)

Instructions
1. Preheat oven to 400°F.
2. Dice bell peppers and red onion.
3. Heat a non-stick skillet over medium-high heat with cooking spray, cook ground turkey sausage for 8-10 minutes, breaking it up as it browns. Set aside.
4. In a large mixing bowl, add eggs, egg whites, cottage cheese, cooked turkey sausage, diced bell peppers, red onion, shredded cheese, garlic powder, onion powder, black pepper, paprika, and salt. Mix until well combined.
5. Spray a large baking dish with cooking spray and pour in the mixture.
6. Evenly layer tater tots on top.
7. Bake for 40-50 minutes or until eggs are fully set and tater tots are golden brown.

BREAKFAST SANDWICHES

BREAKFAST SANDWICHES

DAILY MEAL PREP IDEAS

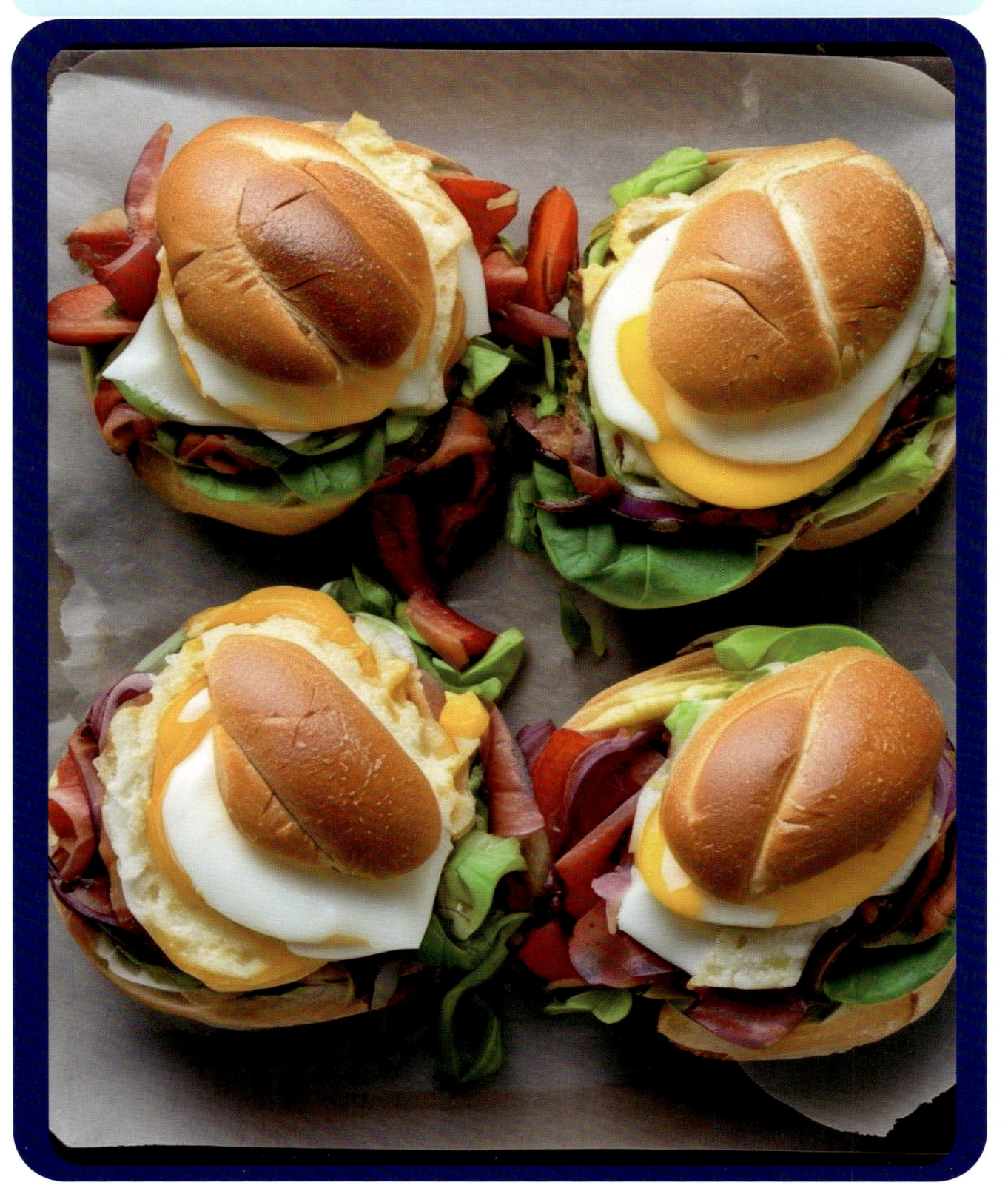

BREAKFAST SANDWICHES

BACON EGG & CHEESE MUFFIN

Calories: 440 **Protein: 43** **Carbs: 28** **Fats: 18**

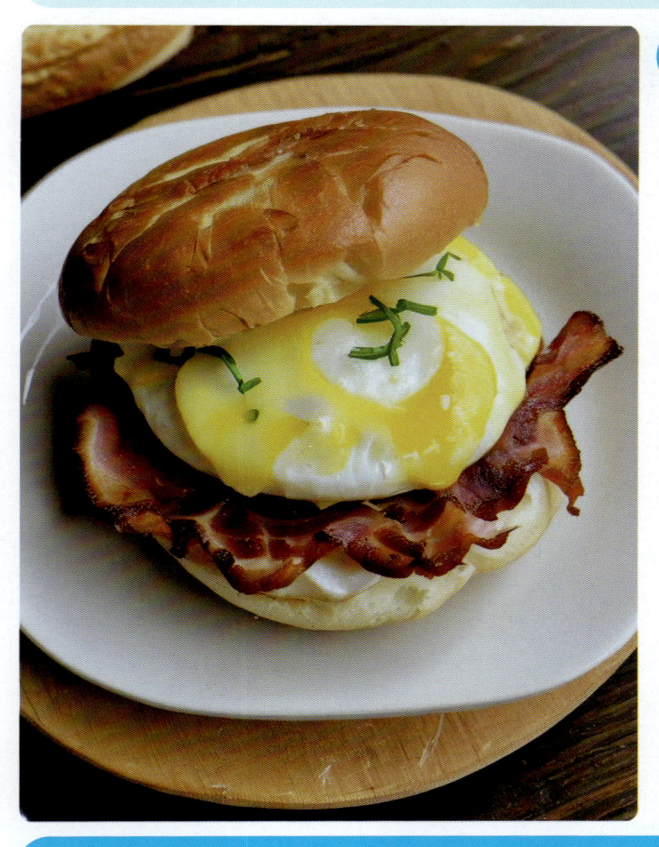

Ingredients Servings: 1

Breakfast Sandwich:
- 1 low carb 647 english muffin
- 1 egg
- 1/2 cup egg whites
- 2 slices uncured turkey bacon
- 1/4 cup shredded cheese
- 1 tsp garlic powder
- 1 tsp onion powder
- 1/2 tsp black pepper
- 1/4 tsp salt

Optional Sides
- Cilantro Lime Rice (1/3 cup non-fat greek yogurt, 3 tbsp cilantro, 1 tbsp lime juice - 50C, 7P, 3C, 1F)
- Protein shake (2 cups almond milk, 1 scoop Dummy Supps - 200c, 28P, 5C, 7F)
- Salsa (2 tbsp - 10c, 0P, 2C, 0F)
- Hot sauce (1 tsp - 1c, 0P, 0C, 0F)
- Avocado (1/2 whole - 120c, 2P, 6C, 11F)

Instructions
1. Toast English muffin until golden brown.
2. Heat a non-stick skillet over medium heat with cooking spray, cook turkey bacon for 3-4 minutes per side, then set aside.
3. Lower heat to low, add eggs, and scramble for 4-5 minutes, stirring occasionally.
4. Add seasonings and shredded cheese, cook for 1 minute until melted.
5. Assemble sandwich by layering eggs, turkey bacon, and cheese between the English muffin halves.

BREAKFAST SANDWICHES

SAUSAGE MUFFIN

Calories: 430 **Protein: 41** **Carbs: 30** **Fats: 20**

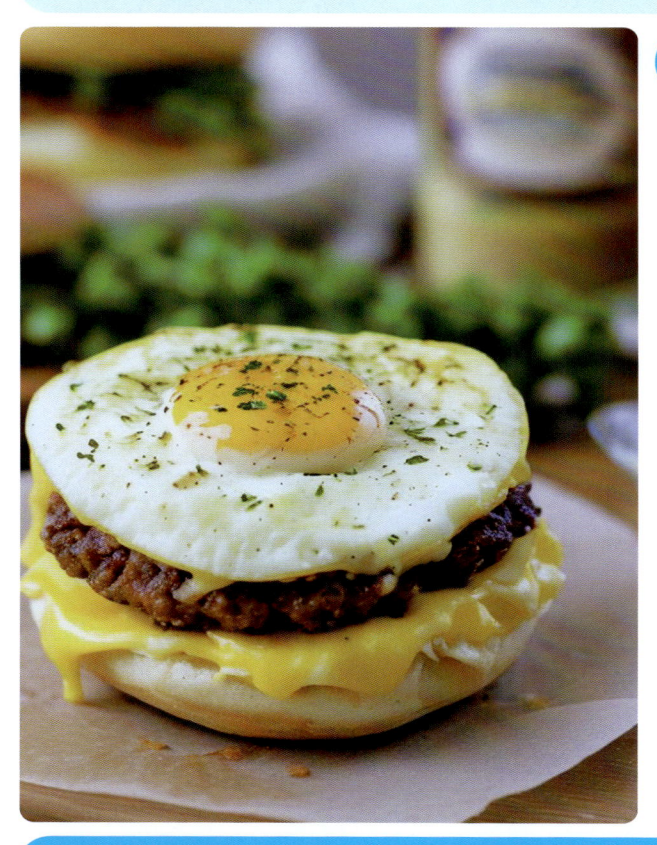

Ingredients — Servings: 1

Breakfast Sandwich:
- 1 low carb 647 english muffin
- 1 egg
- 1/2 cup egg whites
- 4 frozen Jones Dairy turkey sausage links
- 1/4 cup shredded cheese
- 1 tsp garlic powder
- 1 tsp onion powder
- 1/2 tsp black pepper
- 1/4 tsp salt

Optional Sides
- Cilantro Lime Rice (1/3 cup non-fat greek yogurt, 3 tbsp cilantro, 1 tbsp lime juice - 50C, 7P, 3C, 1F)
- Protein shake (2 cups almond milk, 1 scoop Dummy Supps - 200c, 23P, 5C, 7F)
- Salsa (2 tbsp - 10c, 0P, 2C, 0F)
- Hot sauce (1 tsp - 1c, 0P, 0C, 0F)
- Avocado (1/2 whole - 120c, 2P, 6C, 11F)

Instructions
1. Toast English muffin until golden brown.
2. Microwave turkey sausage patties for 45-60 seconds, then set aside.
3. Heat a non-stick skillet over medium heat with cooking spray, add eggs, and scramble for 4-5 minutes, stirring occasionally.
4. Add seasonings and shredded cheese, cook for 1 minute until melted.
5. Assemble sandwich by layering eggs, sausage patties, and cheese between the English muffin halves.

BREAKFAST SANDWICHES

CANADIAN EGG & CHEESE MUFFIN

Calories: 410 **Protein: 42** **Carbs: 29** **Fats: 18**

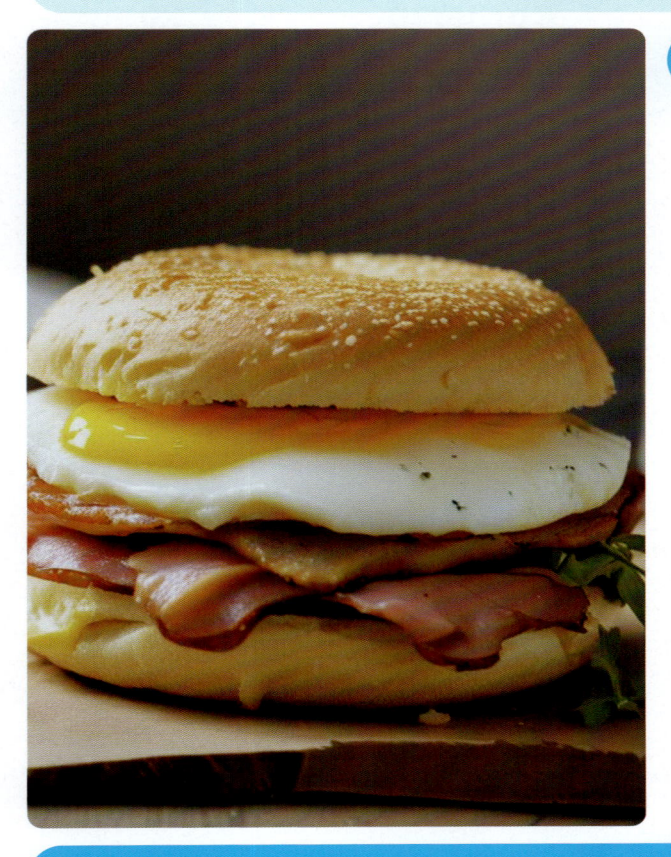

Ingredients Servings: 1

Breakfast Sandwich:
- 1 low carb 647 english muffin
- 1 egg
- 1/2 cup egg whites
- 3 slices canadian bacon
- 1/4 cup shredded cheese
- 1 tsp garlic powder
- 1 tsp onion powder
- 1/2 tsp black pepper
- 1/4 tsp salt

Optional Sides
- Cilantro Lime Rice (1/3 cup non-fat greek yogurt, 3 tbsp cilantro, 1 tbsp lime juice - 50C, 7P, 3C, 1F)
- Protein shake (2 cups almond milk, 1 scoop Dummy Supps - 200c, 28P, 5C, 7F)
- Salsa (2 tbsp - 10c, 0P, 2C, 0F)
- Hot sauce (1 tsp - 1c, 0P, 0C, 0F)
- Avocado (1/2 whole - 120c, 2P, 6C, 11F)

Instructions
1. Toast English muffin until golden brown.
2. Heat a non-stick skillet over medium heat with cooking spray, cook Canadian bacon for 1-2 minutes per side, then set aside.
3. Lower heat to low, add eggs, and scramble for 4-5 minutes, stirring occasionally.
4. Add seasonings and shredded cheese, cook for 1 minute until melted.
5. Assemble sandwich by layering eggs, Canadian bacon, and cheese between the English muffin halves.

BREAKFAST SANDWICHES

MEAT LOVERS MUFFIN

Calories: 490 **Protein: 53** **Carbs: 30** **Fats: 23**

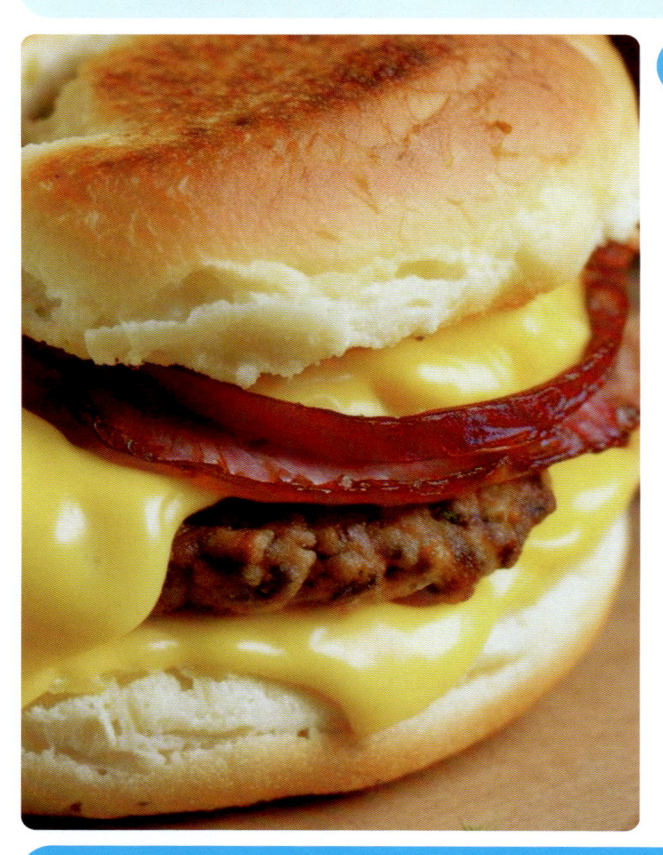

Ingredients **Servings: 1**

Breakfast Sandwich:
- 1 low carb 647 english muffin
- 1 egg
- 1/2 cup egg whites
- 2 slices uncured turkey bacon
- 4 frozen Jones Dairy turkey sausage links
- 1/4 cup shredded cheese
- 1 tsp garlic powder
- 1 tsp onion powder
- 1/2 tsp black pepper
- 1/4 tsp salt

Optional Sides

- Cilantro Lime Rice (1/3 cup non-fat greek yogurt, 3 tbsp cilantro, 1 tbsp lime juice - 50C, 7P, 3C, 1F)
- Protein shake (2 cups almond milk, 1 scoop Dummy Supps - 200c, 23P, 5C, 7F)
- Salsa (2 tbsp - 10c, 0P, 2C, 0F)
- Hot sauce (1 tsp - 1c, 0P, 0C, 0F)
- Avocado (1/2 whole - 120c, 2P, 6C, 11F)

Instructions

1. Toast the English muffin until golden brown.
2. Microwave turkey sausage links for 45-60 seconds, then set aside.
3. Heat a non-stick skillet over medium heat with cooking spray, cock turkey bacon for 3-4 minutes per side, then set aside.
4. Lower heat to low, add eggs and egg whites, and scramble for 4-5 minutes, stirring occasionally.
5. Add seasonings and shredded cheese, cook for 1 minute until cheese is melted.
6. Assemble sandwich by layering eggs, turkey bacon, sausage, and cheese between the English muffin halves.

BREAKFAST SANDWICHES

LOADED MUFFIN

Calories: 530 **Protein: 54** **Carbs: 38** **Fats: 23**

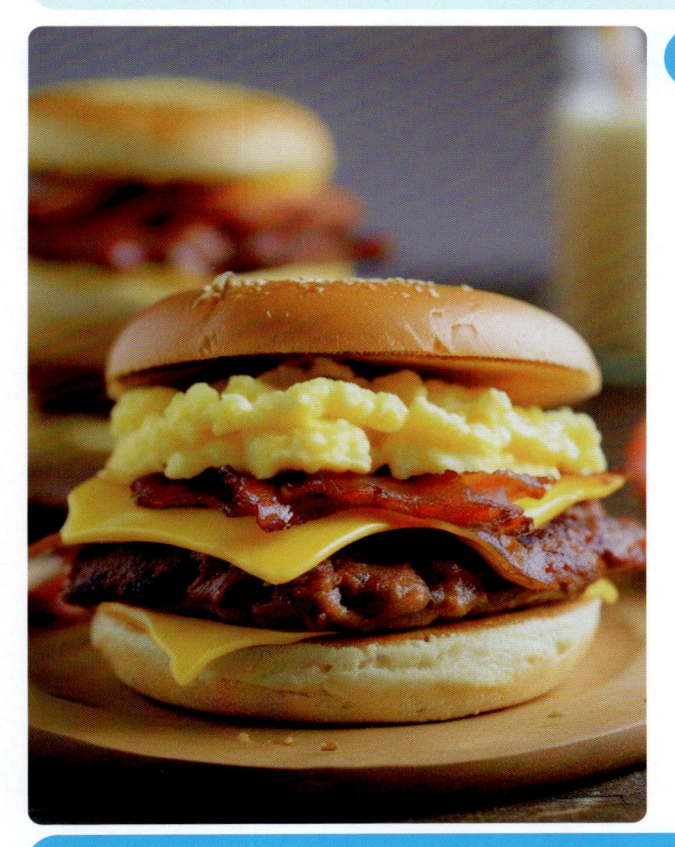

Ingredients — Servings: 1

Breakfast Sandwich:
- 1 low carb 647 english muffin
- 1 egg
- 1/2 cup egg whites
- 2 slices uncured turkey bacon
- 4 frozen Jones Dairy turkey sausage links
- 1/2 cup shredded hash browns
- 1/4 cup shredded cheese
- 1 tsp garlic powder
- 1 tsp onion powder
- 1/2 tsp black pepper
- 1/4 tsp salt

Optional Sides
- Cilantro Lime Rice (1/3 cup non-fat greek yogurt, 3 tbsp cilantro, 1 tbsp lime juice - 50C, 7P, 3C, 1F)
- Protein shake (2 cups almond milk, 1 scoop Dummy Supps - 200c, 28P, 5C, 7F)
- Salsa (2 tbsp - 10c, 0P, 2C, 0F)
- Hot sauce (1 tsp - 1c, 0P, 0C, 0F)
- Avocado (1/2 whole - 120c, 2P, 6C, 11F)

Instructions
1. Toast the English muffin until golden brown.
2. Microwave turkey sausage links for 45-60 seconds, then set aside.
3. Heat a non-stick skillet over medium heat with cooking spray, cook turkey bacon for 3-4 minutes per side, then set aside.
4. In the same skillet, cook shredded hash browns for 4-5 minutes, stirring occasionally, until golden brown. Set aside.
5. Lower heat to low, add eggs and egg whites, and scramble for 4-5 minutes, stirring occasionally.
6. Add seasonings and shredded cheese, cook for 1 minute until melted.
7. Assemble sandwich by layering eggs, turkey bacon, sausage, hash browns, and cheese between the English muffin halves.

BREAKFAST SANDWICHES

BACON EGG & CHEESE BAGEL

Calories: 440 **Protein: 42** **Carbs: 28** **Fats: 18**

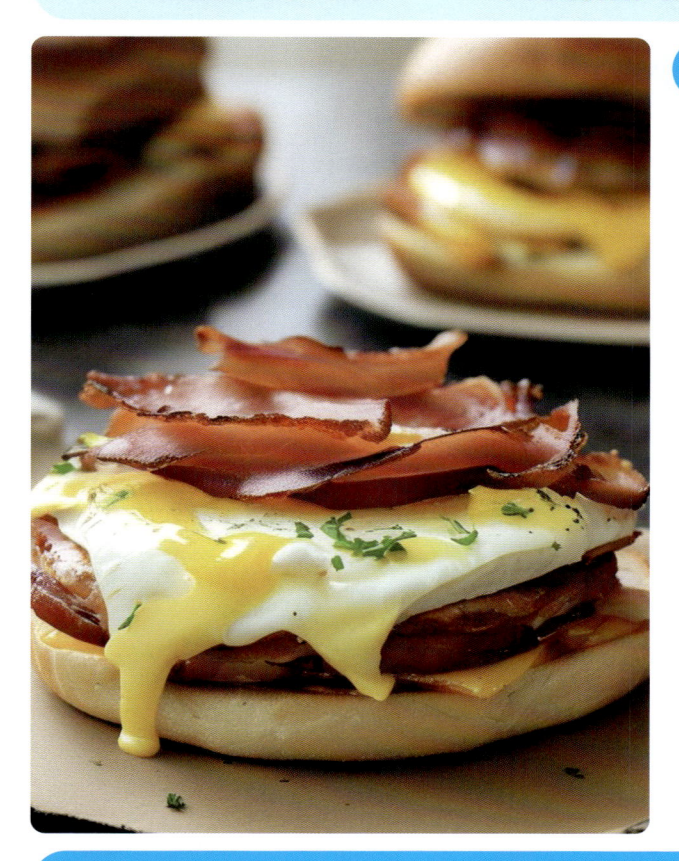

Ingredients — Servings: 1

Breakfast Sandwich:
- 1 low calorie bagel thin
- 1 egg
- 1/2 cup egg whites
- 2 slices uncured turkey bacon
- 1/4 cup shredded cheese
- 1 tsp garlic powder
- 1 tsp onion powder
- 1/2 tsp black pepper
- 1/4 tsp salt

Optional Sides
- Cilantro Lime Rice (1/3 cup non-fat greek yogurt, 3 tbsp cilantro, 1 tbsp lime juice - 50C, 7P, 3C, 1F)
- Protein shake (2 cups almond milk, 1 scoop Dummy Supps - 200c, 28P, 5C, 7F)
- Salsa (2 tbsp - 10c, 0P, 2C, 0F)
- Hot sauce (1 tsp - 1c, 0P, 0C, 0F)
- Avocado (1/2 whole - 120c, 2P, 6C, 11F)

Instructions
1. Toast bagel thin until golden brown.
2. Heat a non-stick skillet over medium heat with cooking spray, cook turkey bacon for 3-4 minutes per side, then set aside.
3. Lower heat to low, add eggs, and scramble for 4-5 minutes, stirring occasionally.
4. Add seasonings and cheese, cook for 1 minute until melted.
5. Assemble sandwich by layering eggs, turkey bacon, and cheese between the bagel thin halves.

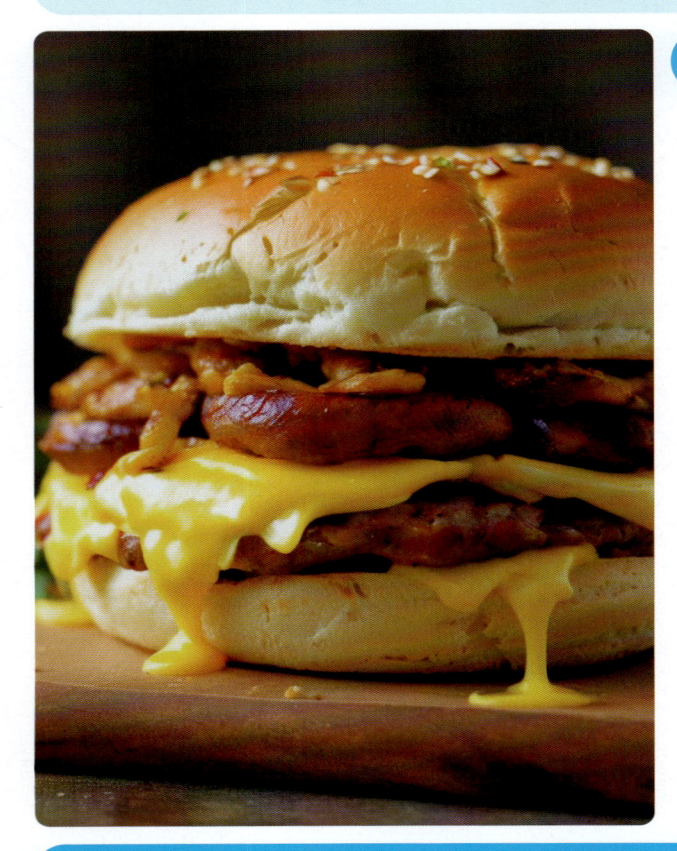

BREAKFAST SANDWICHES

SAUSAGE EGG & CHEESE BAGEL

Calories: 450 **Protein: 40** **Carbs: 31** **Fats: 20**

Ingredients **Servings: 1**

Breakfast Sandwich:
- 1 low calorie bagel thin
- 1 egg
- 1/2 cup egg whites
- 4 frozen Jones Dairy turkey sausage links
- 1/4 cup shredded cheese
- 1 tsp garlic powder
- 1 tsp onion powder
- 1/2 tsp black pepper
- 1/4 tsp salt

Optional Sides
- Cilantro Lime Rice (1/3 cup non-fat greek yogurt, 3 tbsp cilantro, 1 tbsp lime juice - 50C, 7P, 3C, 1F)
- Protein shake (2 cups almond milk, 1 scoop Dummy Supps - 200c, 28P, 5C, 7F)
- Salsa (2 tbsp - 10c, 0P, 2C, 0F)
- Hot sauce (1 tsp - 1c, 0P, 0C, 0F)
- Avocado (1/2 whole - 120c, 2P, 6C, 11F)

Instructions
1. Toast bagel thin until golden brown.
2. Microwave turkey sausage links for 45-60 seconds, then set aside.
3. Heat a non-stick skillet over medium heat with cooking spray, add eggs, and scramble for 4-5 minutes, stirring occasionally.
4. Add seasonings and cheese, cook for 1 minute until melted.
5. Assemble sandwich by layering eggs, turkey sausage, and cheese between the bagel thin halves.

BREAKFAST SANDWICHES

CANADIAN BACON EGG AND CHEESE BAGEL

Calories: 430 **Protein: 41** **Carbs: 30** **Fats: 18**

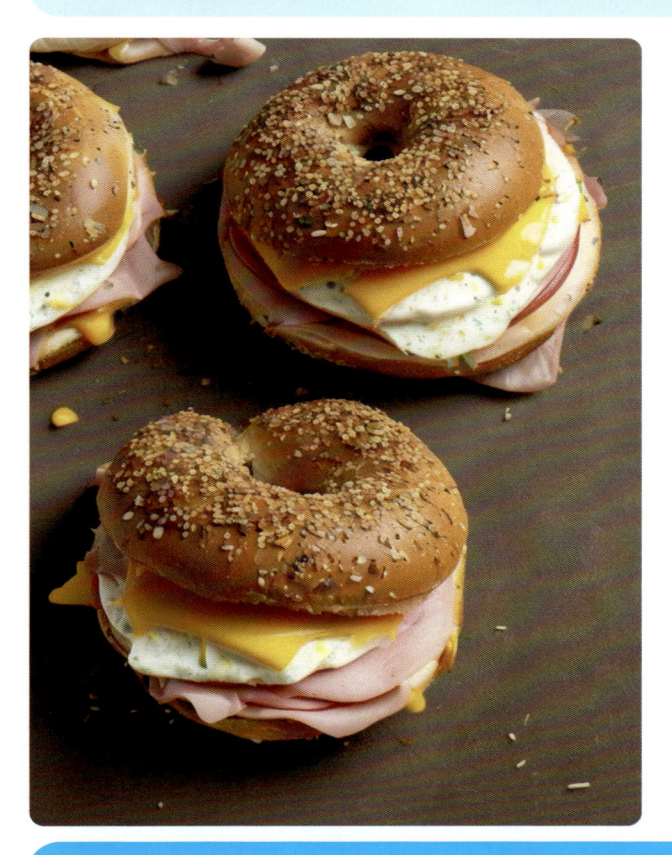

Ingredients **Servings: 1**

Breakfast Sandwich:

- 1 low calorie bagel thin
- 1 egg
- 1/2 cup egg whites
- 3 slices canadian bacon
- 1/4 cup shredded cheese
- 1 tsp garlic powder
- 1 tsp onion powder
- 1/2 tsp black pepper
- 1/4 tsp salt

Optional Sides

- Cilantro Lime Rice (1/3 cup non-fat greek yogurt, 3 tbsp cilantro, 1 tbsp lime juice - 50C, 7P, 3C, 1F)
- Protein shake (2 cups almond milk, 1 scoop Dummy Supps - 200c, 28P, 5C, 7F)
- Salsa (2 tbsp - 10c, 0P, 2C, 0F)
- Hot sauce (1 tsp - 1c, 0P, 0C, 0F)
- Avocado (1/2 whole - 120c, 2P, 6C, 11F)

Instructions

1. Toast bagel thin until golden brown.
2. Heat a non-stick skillet over medium heat with cooking spray, cook Canadian bacon for 1-2 minutes per side, then set aside.
3. Lower heat to low, add eggs, and scramble for 4-5 minutes, stirring occasionally.
4. Add seasonings and shredded cheese, cook for 1 minute until melted.
5. Assemble sandwich by layering eggs, Canadian bacon, and cheese between the bagel thin halves.

BREAKFAST SANDWICHES

MEAT LOVERS BAGEL

Calories: 520 **Protein: 52** **Carbs: 31** **Fats: 23**

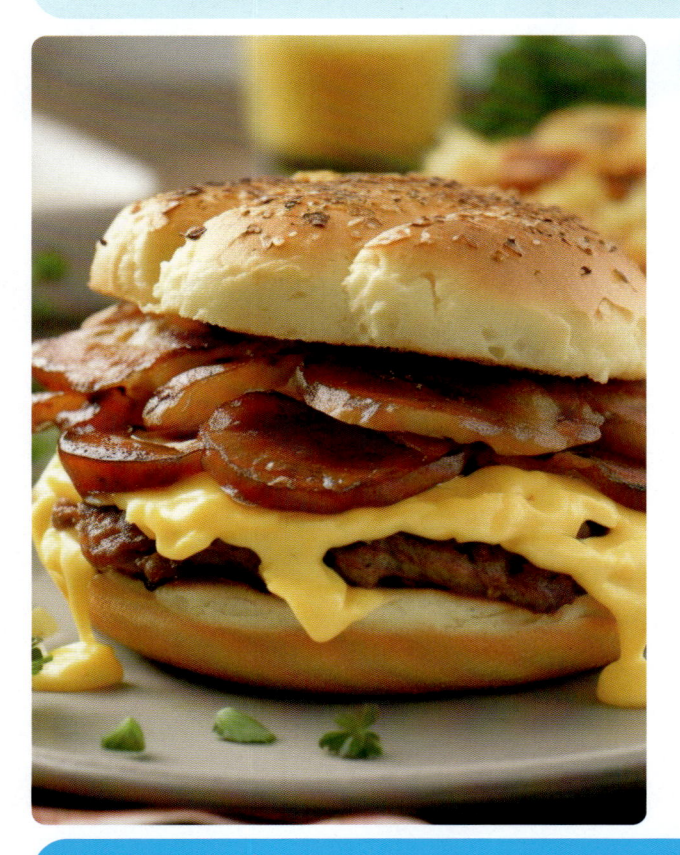

Ingredients Servings: 1

Breakfast Sandwich:
- 1 low calorie bagel thin
- 1 egg
- 1/2 cup egg whites
- 2 slices uncured turkey bacon
- 4 frozen Jones Dairy turkey sausage links
- 1/4 cup shredded cheese
- 1 tsp garlic powder
- 1 tsp onion powder
- 1/2 tsp black pepper
- 1/4 tsp salt

Optional Sides
- Cilantro Lime Rice (1/3 cup non-fat greek yogurt, 3 tbsp cilantro, 1 tbsp lime juice - 50C, 7P, 3C, 1F)
- Protein shake (2 cups almond milk, 1 scoop Dummy Supps - 200c, 28P, 5C, 7F)
- Salsa (2 tbsp - 10c, 0P, 2C, 0F)
- Hot sauce (1 tsp - 1c, 0P, 0C, 0F)
- Avocado (1/2 whole - 120c, 2P, 6C, 11F)

Instructions
1. Toast bagel thin until golden brown.
2. Microwave turkey sausage links for 45-60 seconds, then set aside.
3. Heat a non-stick skillet over medium heat with cooking spray, cook turkey bacon for 3-4 minutes per side, then set aside.
4. Lower heat to low, add eggs, and scramble for 4-5 minutes, stirring occasionally.
5. Add seasonings and shredded cheese, cook for 1 minute until melted.
6. Assemble sandwich by layering eggs, turkey bacon, sausage, and cheese between the bagel thin halves.

BREAKFAST SANDWICHES

LOADED BAGEL

Calories: 550   **Protein: 53**   **Carbs: 39**   **Fats: 23**

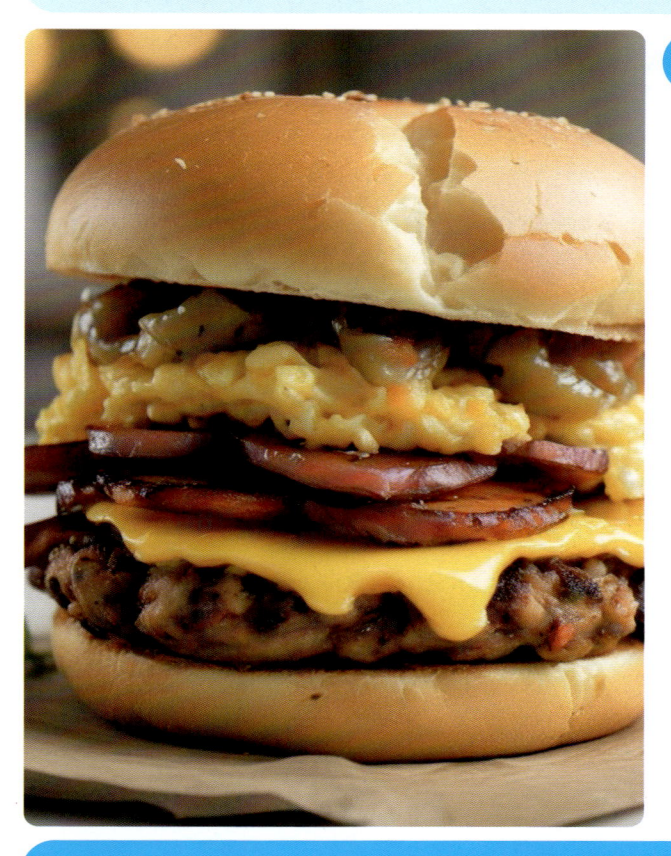

Ingredients — Servings: 1

Breakfast Sandwich:
- 1 low calorie bagel thin
- 1 egg
- 1/2 cup egg whites
- 2 slices uncured turkey bacon
- 4 frozen Jones Dairy turkey sausage links
- 1/2 cup shredded hash browns
- 1/4 cup shredded cheese
- 1 tsp garlic powder
- 1 tsp onion powder
- 1/2 tsp black pepper
- 1/4 tsp salt

Optional Sides
- Cilantro Lime Rice (1/3 cup non-fat greek yogurt, 3 tbsp cilantro, 1 tbsp lime juice - 50C, 7P, 3C, 1F)
- Protein shake (2 cups almond milk, 1 scoop Dummy Supps - 200c, 28P, 5C, 7F)
- Salsa (2 tbsp - 10c, 0P, 2C, 0F)
- Hot sauce (1 tsp - 1c, 0P, 0C, 0F)
- Avocado (1/2 whole - 120c, 2P, 6C, 11F)

Instructions
1. Toast bagel thin until golden brown.
2. Microwave turkey sausage links for 45-60 seconds, then set aside.
3. Heat a non-stick skillet over medium heat with cooking spray, cook turkey bacon for 3-4 minutes per side, then set aside.
4. In the same skillet, cook shredded hash browns for 4-5 minutes, stirring occasionally, until golden brown. Set aside.
5. Lower heat to low, add eggs, and scramble for 4-5 minutes, stirring occasionally.
6. Add seasonings and shredded cheese, cook for 1 minute until melted.
7. Assemble sandwich by layering eggs, turkey bacon, sausage, hash browns, and cheese between the bagel thin halves.

BREAKFAST SANDWICHES

SIMPLE EGG SANDWICH

Calories: 390 **Protein: 43** **Carbs: 30** **Fats: 15**

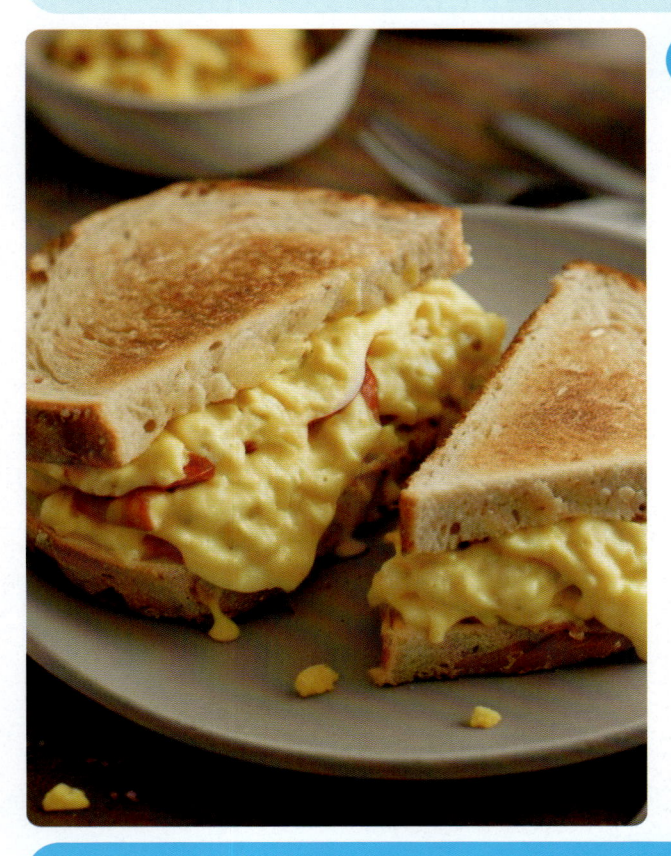

Ingredients — Servings: 1

Breakfast Sandwich:
- 2 pieces 647 bread
- 1 egg
- 1 cup egg whites
- 1/4 cup shredded cheese
- 1 tsp garlic powder
- 1 tsp onion powder
- 1/2 tsp black pepper
- 1/4 tsp salt

Optional Sides
- Cilantro Lime Rice (1/3 cup non-fat greek yogurt, 3 tbsp cilantro, 1 tbsp lime juice - 50C, 7P, 3C, 1F)
- Protein shake (2 cups almond milk, 1 scoop Dummy Supps - 200c, 28P, 5C, 7F)
- Salsa (2 tbsp - 10c, 0P, 2C, 0F)
- Hot sauce (1 tsp - 1c, 0P, 0C, 0F)
- Avocado (1/2 whole - 120c, 2P, 6C, 11F)

Instructions
1. Toast bread until golden brown.
2. Heat a non-stick skillet over medium heat with cooking spray.
3. Lower heat to low, add eggs and egg whites, and scramble for 4-5 minutes, stirring occasionally.
4. Add seasonings and shredded cheese, cook for 1 minute until melted.
5. Assemble sandwich by placing scrambled eggs between toasted bread slices.

BREAKFAST WRAPS/BURRITOS

BREAKFAST WRAPS/BURRITOS

DAILY MEAL PREP IDEAS

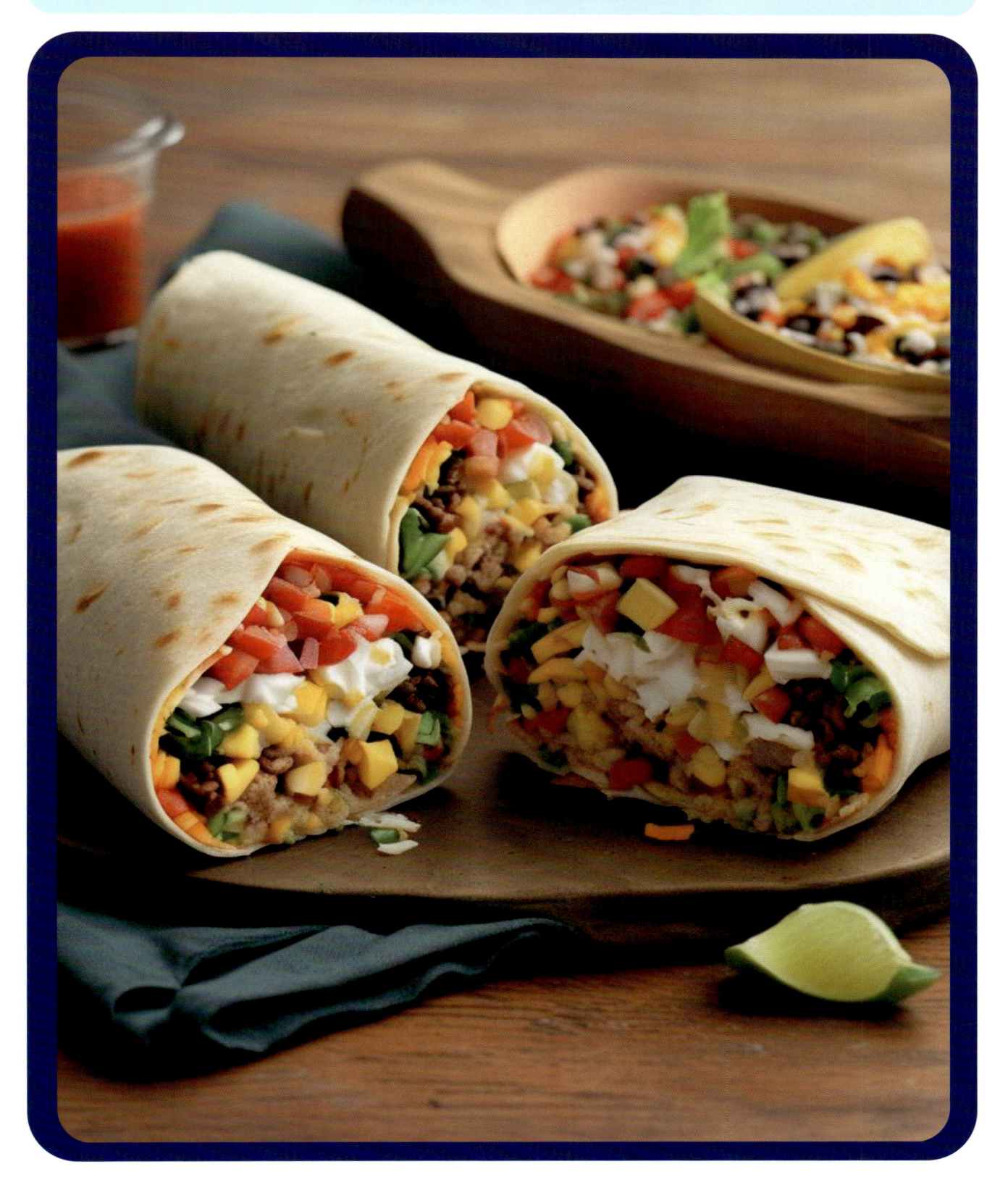

BREAKFAST WRAPS/BURRITOS

BACON EGG & CHEESE BURRITO

Calories: 400 **Protein: 43** **Carbs: 8** **Fats: 20**

Ingredients **Servings: 1**

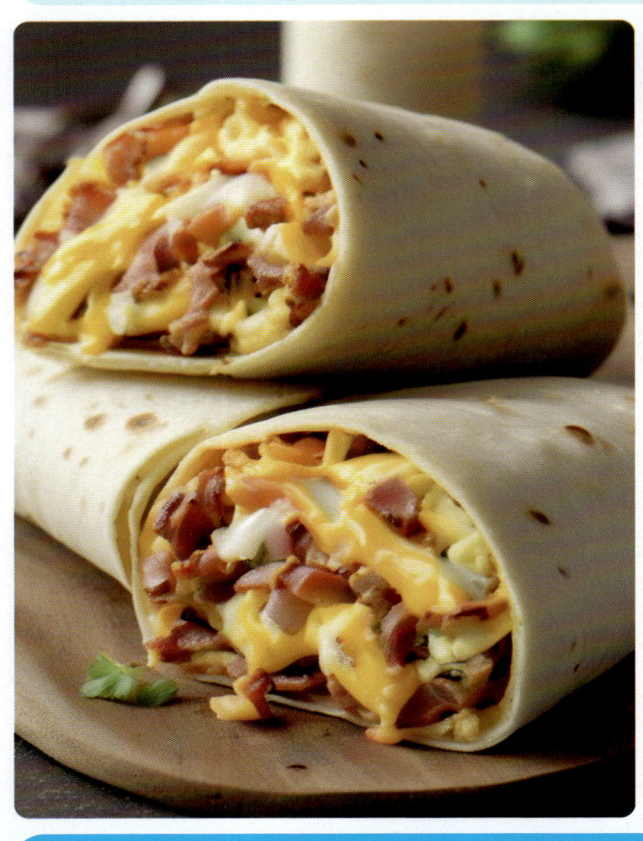

Breakfast Burrito:
- 1 (12 oz.) Mission low carb tortilla
- 1 egg
- 1/2 cup egg whites
- 2 slices turkey bacon
- 1/4 cup shredded cheese
- 1 tsp garlic powder
- 1 tsp onion powder
- 1/2 tsp black pepper
- 1/4 tsp salt

Optional Sides
- Cilantro Lime Rice (1/3 cup non-fat greek yogurt, 3 tbsp cilantro, 1 tbsp lime juice - 50C, 7P, 3C, 1F)
- Protein shake (2 cups almond milk, 1 scoop Dummy Supps - 200c, 28P, 5C, 7F)
- Salsa (2 tbsp - 10c, 0P, 2C, 0F)
- Hot sauce (1 tsp - 1c, 0P, 0C, 0F)
- Avocado (1/2 whole - 120c, 2P, 6C, 11F)

Instructions
1. Heat a non-stick skillet over medium heat with cooking spray, cook turkey bacon for 3-4 minutes per side, then chop.
2. Lower heat to low, add eggs and egg whites, and scramble for 4-5 minutes, stirring occasionally.
3. Add seasonings and shredded cheese, cook for 1 minute until melted.
4. Warm tortilla in a dry skillet or microwave for 15-20 seconds.
5. Assemble burrito by adding scrambled eggs, turkey bacon, and cheese to the tortilla.
6. Wrap tightly, folding in the sides, then rolling from the bottom up.

BREAKFAST WRAPS/BURRITOS

SAUSAGE EGG & CHEESE BURRITO

Calories: 420 **Protein: 41** **Carbs: 10** **Fats: 22**

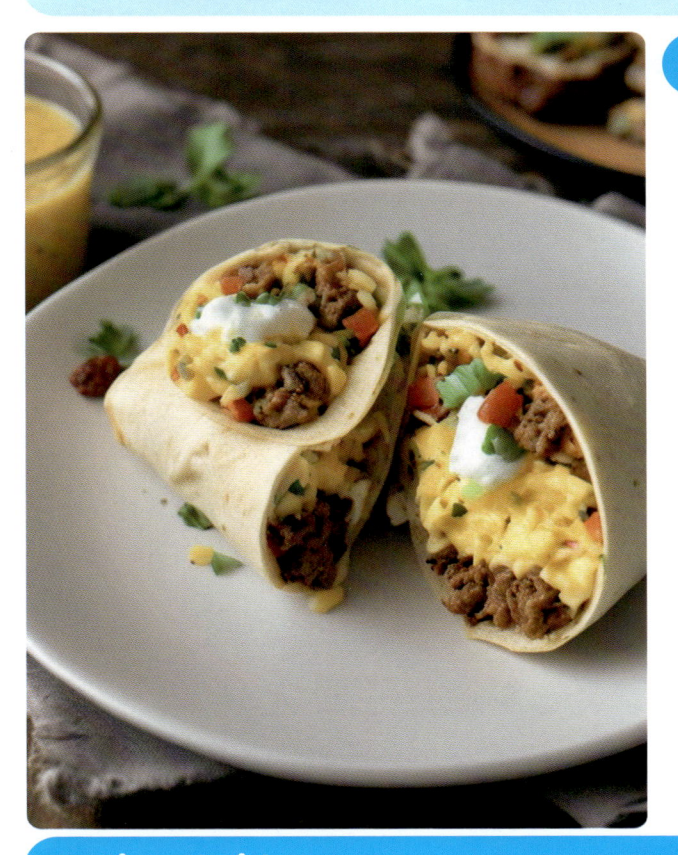

Ingredients   Servings: 1

Breakfast Burrito:
- 1 (12 oz.) Mission low carb tortilla
- 1 egg
- 1/2 cup egg whites
- 4 Jones Dairy frozen turkey sausage links
- 1/4 cup shredded cheese
- 1 tsp garlic powder
- 1 tsp onion powder
- 1/2 tsp black pepper
- 1/4 tsp salt

Optional Sides

- Cilantro Lime Rice (1/3 cup non-fat greek yogurt, 3 tbsp cilantro, 1 tbsp lime juice - 50C, 7P, 3C, 1F)
- Protein shake (2 cups almond milk, 1 scoop Dummy Supps - 200c, 28P, 5C, 7F)
- Salsa (2 tbsp - 10c, 0P, 2C, 0F)
- Hot sauce (1 tsp - 1c, 0P, 0C, 0F)
- Avocado (1/2 whole - 120c, 2P, 6C, 11F)

Instructions

1. Microwave turkey sausage links for 45-60 seconds, then chop.
2. Heat a non-stick skillet over medium heat with cooking spray.
3. Lower heat to low, add eggs and egg whites, and scramble for 4-5 minutes, stirring occasionally.
4. Add seasonings and shredded cheese, cook for 1 minute until melted.
5. Warm tortilla in a dry skillet or microwave for 15-20 seconds.
6. Assemble burrito by layering scrambled eggs, turkey sausage, and cheese in the tortilla.
7. Wrap tightly, folding in the sides, then rolling from the bottom up.

BREAKFAST WRAPS/BURRITOS

MEAT LOVERS BURRITO

Calories: 480 **Protein: 53** **Carbs: 10** **Fats: 25**

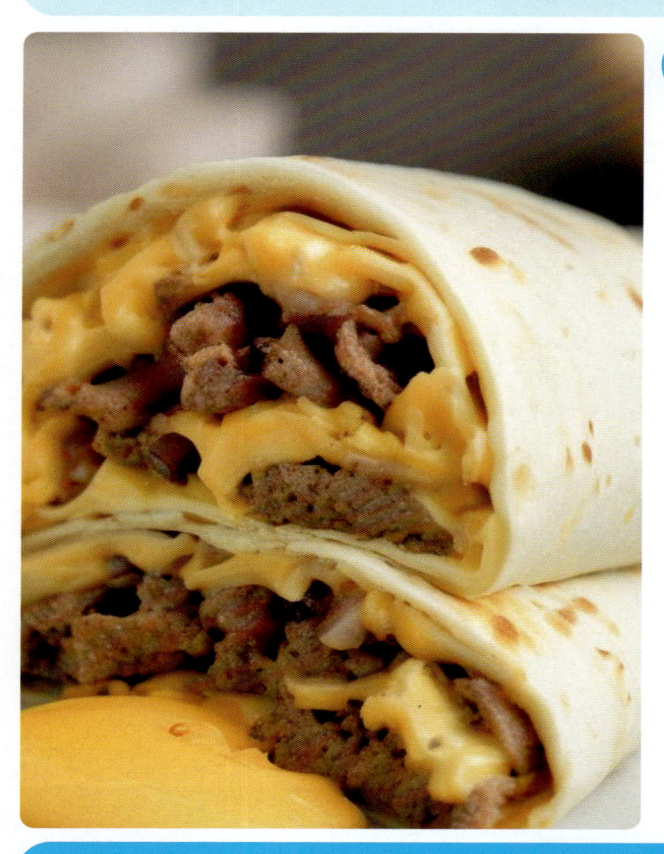

Ingredients Servings: 1

Breakfast Burrito:
- 1 (12 oz.) Mission low carb tortilla
- 1 egg
- 1/2 cup egg whites
- 2 slices turkey bacon
- 4 Jones Dairy frozen turkey sausage links
- 1/4 cup shredded cheese
- 1 tsp garlic powder
- 1 tsp onion powder
- 1/2 tsp black pepper
- 1/4 tsp salt

Optional Sides

- Cilantro Lime Rice (1/3 cup non-fat greek yogurt, 3 tbsp cilantro, 1 tbsp lime juice - 50C, 7P, 3C, 1F)
- Protein shake (2 cups almond milk, 1 scoop Dummy Supps - 200c, 28P, 5C, 7F)
- Salsa (2 tbsp - 10c, 0P, 2C, 0F)
- Hot sauce (1 tsp - 1c, 0P, 0C, 0F)
- Avocado (1/2 whole - 120c, 2P, 6C, 11F)

Instructions

1. Heat a non-stick skillet over medium heat with cooking spray, cook turkey bacon for 3-4 minutes per side, then chop.
2. Microwave turkey sausage links for 45-60 seconds, then chop.
3. Lower heat to low, add eggs and egg whites, and scramble for 4-5 minutes, stirring occasionally.
4. Add seasonings and shredded cheese, cook for 1 minute until melted.
5. Warm tortilla in a dry skillet or microwave for 15-20 seconds.
6. Assemble burrito by layering scrambled eggs, turkey bacon, sausage, and cheese in the tortilla.
7. Wrap tightly, folding in the sides, then rolling from the bottom up.

BREAKFAST WRAPS/BURRITOS

LOADED BURRITO

Calories: 510   **Protein: 54**   **Carbs: 18**   **Fats: 25**

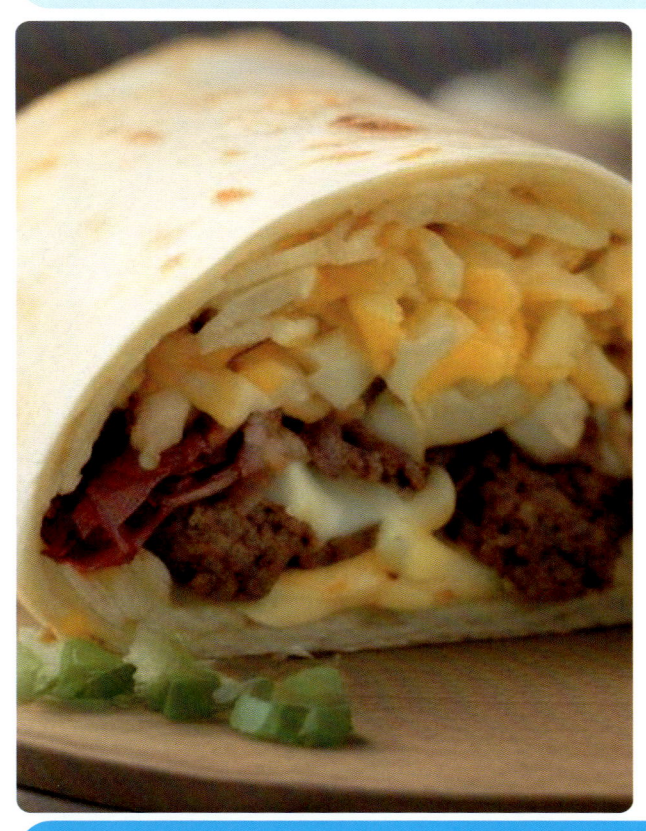

Ingredients   **Servings: 1**

Breakfast Burrito:
- 1 (12 oz.) Mission low carb tortilla
- 1 egg
- 1/2 cup egg whites
- 2 slices turkey bacon
- 4 Jones Dairy frozen turkey sausage links
- 1/2 cup shredded hash browns
- 1/4 cup shredded cheese
- 1 tsp garlic powder
- 1 tsp onion powder
- 1/2 tsp black pepper
- 1/4 tsp salt

Optional Sides

- Cilantro Lime Rice (1/3 cup non-fat greek yogurt, 3 tbsp cilantro, 1 tbsp lime juice - 50C, 7P, 3C, 1F)
- Protein shake (2 cups almond milk, 1 scoop Dummy Supps - 200c, 23P, 5C, 7F)
- Salsa (2 tbsp - 10c, 0P, 2C, 0F)
- Hot sauce (1 tsp - 1c, 0P, 0C, 0F)
- Avocado (1/2 whole - 120c, 2P, 6C, 11F)

Instructions

1. Heat a non-stick skillet over medium heat with cooking spray, cook turkey bacon for 3-4 minutes per side, then chop.
2. Microwave turkey sausage links for 45-60 seconds, then chop.
3. In the same skillet, cook shredded hash browns for 4-5 minutes, stirring occasionally, until golden brown. Set aside.
4. Lower heat to low, add eggs and egg whites, and scramble for 4-5 minutes, stirring occasionally.
5. Add seasonings and shredded cheese, cook for 1 minute until melted.
6. Warm tortilla in a dry skillet or microwave for 15-20 seconds.
7. Assemble burrito by layering scrambled eggs, turkey bacon, sausage, hash browns, and cheese in the tortilla.
8. Wrap tightly, folding in the sides, then rolling from the bottom up.

BREAKFAST WRAPS/BURRITOS

SOUTHWEST BURRITO

Calories: 520 **Protein: 55** **Carbs: 12** **Fats: 26**

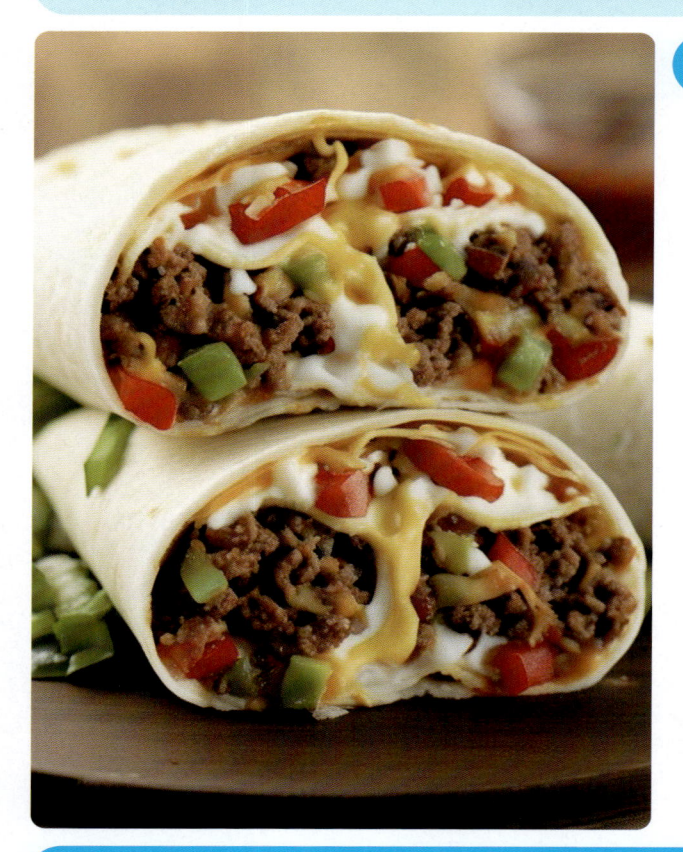

Ingredients **Servings: 1**

Breakfast Burrito:
- 1 (12 oz.) Mission low carb tortilla
- 1 egg
- 1/2 cup egg whites
- 1/2 cup bell pepper (fresh/frozen)
- 1/2 cup sweet onion (fresh/frozen)
- 1/2 cup ground beef
- 1/4 cup pepper jack shredded cheese
- 2 tbsp diced green chilies
- 2 tsp taco seasoning

Optional Sides

- Cilantro Lime Rice (1/3 cup non-fat greek yogurt, 3 tbsp cilantro, 1 tbsp lime juice - 50C, 7P, 3C, 1F)
- Protein shake (2 cups almond milk, 1 scoop Dummy Supps - 200c, 28P, 5C, 7F)
- Salsa (2 tbsp - 10c, 0P, 2C, 0F)
- Hot sauce (1 tsp - 1c, 0P, 0C, 0F)
- Avocado (1/2 whole - 120c, 2P, 6C, 11F)

Instructions

1. Chop bell pepper, sweet onion, and jalapeño peppers.
2. Heat a non-stick skillet over medium heat with cooking spray, cook ground beef for 4-5 minutes, breaking it up as it browns.
3. Add chopped bell pepper, onion, green chilies, jalapeños, and taco seasoning, cook for 2-3 minutes, then set aside.
4. Lower heat to low, add eggs and egg whites, and scramble for 4-5 minutes, stirring occasionally.
5. Add shredded pepper jack cheese, cook for 1 minute until melted.

BREAKFAST WRAPS/BURRITOS

BEEF BREAKFAST BURRITO

Calories: 570 **Protein: 56** **Carbs: 24** **Fats: 27**

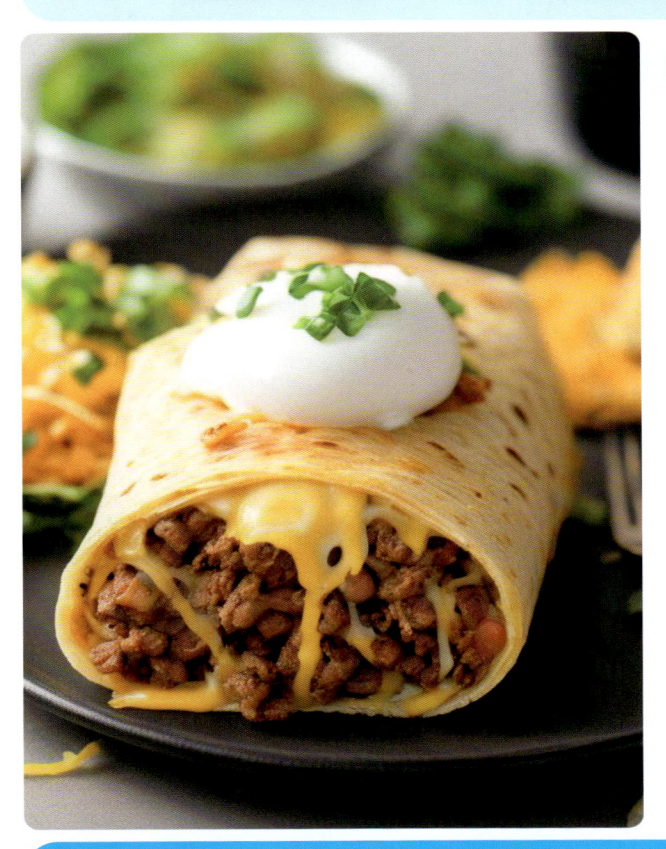

Ingredients **Servings: 1**

Breakfast Burrito:
- 1 (12 oz.) Mission low carb tortilla
- 1 egg
- 1/2 cup egg whites
- 1 cup lean ground beef
- 1/4 cup shredded cheese
- 1 cup shredded hash browns
- 2 tbsp diced green chilies
- 2 tsp taco seasoning

Optional Sides
- Cilantro Lime Rice (1/3 cup non-fat greek yogurt, 3 tbsp cilantro, 1 tbsp lime juice - 50C, 7P, 3C, 1F)
- Protein shake (2 cups almond milk, 1 scoop Dummy Supps - 200c, 28P, 5C, 7F)
- Salsa (2 tbsp - 10c, 0P, 2C, 0F)
- Hot sauce (1 tsp - 1c, 0P, 0C, 0F)
- Avocado (1/2 whole - 120c, 2P, 6C, 11F)

Instructions
1. Air fry or bake hash browns in the oven at 400°F for 5-7 minutes or until desired crispiness.
2. Add ground beef to pan with cooking spray on medium-high heat with taco seasoning.
3. Cook for 4-5 minutes until completely cooked then remove.
4. Add eggs, egg whites, and beef to the pan with cooking spray on medium high heat and scramble until eggs are completely cooked.
5. Warm the tortilla in the microwave for 10-15 seconds.
6. Place the scramble on the tortilla with shredded cheese and wrap.

BREAKFAST WRAPS/BURRITOS

BACON WAKE UP WRAP

Calories: 330 **Protein: 28** **Carbs: 22** **Fats: 20**

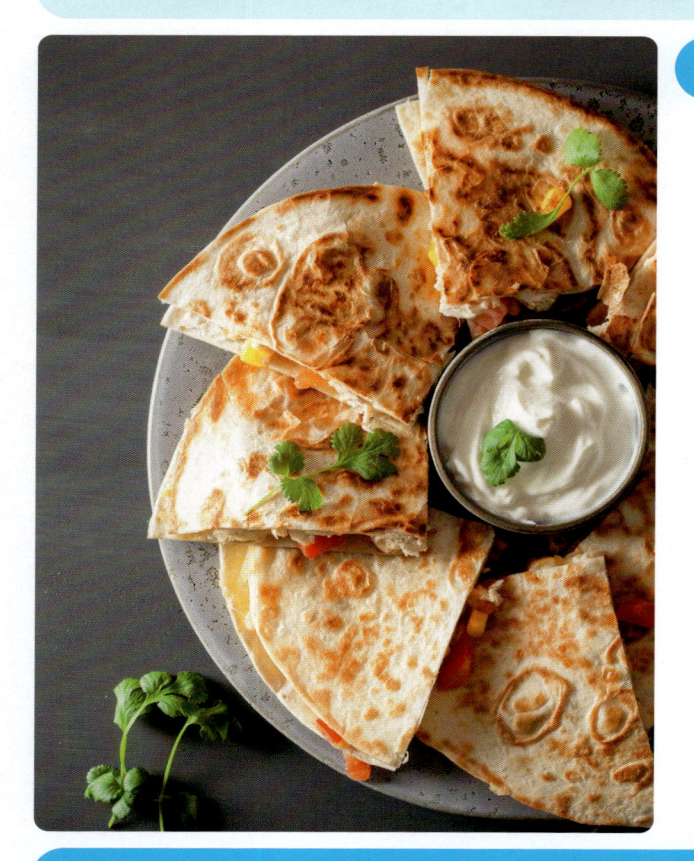

Ingredients **Servings: 8**

Breakfast Wrap:
- 6 whole eggs
- 2 cups egg whites
- 8 (12 oz.) Mission low carb tortillas
- 2 cups shredded cheese
- 12 slices turkey bacon
- 2 tablespoons diced green chilies
- 1 tbsp garlic powder
- 1 tsp onion powder
- 1 tsp paprika
- 1/2 tsp black pepper
- 1/4 tsp salt

Optional Sides

- Cilantro Lime Rice (1/3 cup non-fat greek yogurt, 3 tbsp cilantro, 1 tbsp lime juice - 50C, 7P, 3C, 1F)
- Protein shake (2 cups almond milk, 1 scoop Dummy Supps - 200c, 28P, 5C, 7F)
- Salsa (2 tbsp - 10c, 0P, 2C, 0F)
- Hot sauce (1 tsp - 1c, 0P, 0C, 0F)
- Avocado (1/2 whole - 120c, 2P, 6C, 11F)

Instructions

1. In a large mixing bowl, combine eggs, egg whites, green chilies, garlic powder, onion powder, paprika, black pepper, and salt. Mix until smooth.
2. Spray a baking sheet with cooking spray, pour egg mixture evenly, and bake for 8-10 minutes until set.
3. Heat a large pan over medium-high heat with cooking spray, cook turkey bacon for 3-4 minutes per side until crispy, then dice into small pieces.
4. Clean the pan and spray with cooking spray.
5. Assemble wraps: In the pan, place a tortilla, add 2 tbsp cheese, a layer of egg, 2 tbsp diced turkey bacon, and 2 tbsp cheese.
6. Fold tortilla over itself, pressing lightly, and cook for 4-5 minutes per side until golden brown.

BREAKFAST WRAPS/BURRITOS

SAUSAGE WAKE UP WRAP

Calories: 370 **Protein: 32** **Carbs: 22** **Fats: 23**

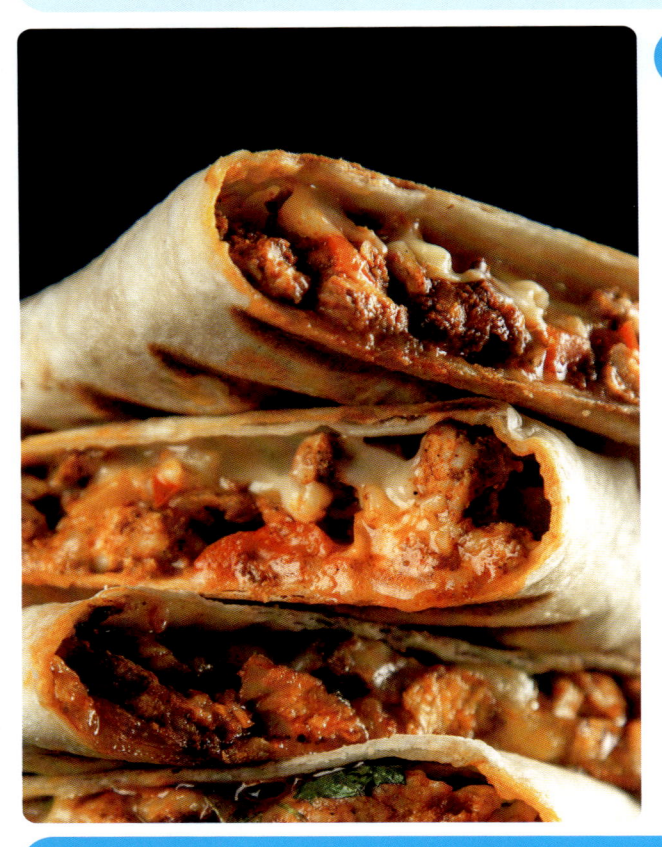

Ingredients **Servings: 8**

Breakfast Wrap:
- 6 whole eggs
- 2 cups egg whites
- 8 (12 oz.) Mission low carb tortillas
- 2 cups shredded cheese
- 1 (bag 24 links) Jones Dairy turkey sausage
- 1 tbsp garlic powder
- 1 tsp onion powder
- 1 tsp paprika
- 1/2 tsp black pepper
- 1/4 tsp salt

Optional Sides

- Cilantro Lime Rice (1/3 cup non-fat greek yogurt, 3 tbsp cilantro, 1 tbsp lime juice - 50C, 7P, 3C, 1F)
- Protein shake (2 cups almond milk, 1 scoop Dummy Supps - 200c, 23P, 5C, 7F)
- Salsa (2 tbsp - 10c, 0P, 2C, 0F)
- Hot sauce (1 tsp - 1c, 0P, 0C, 0F)
- Avocado (1/2 whole - 120c, 2P, 6C, 11F)

Instructions

1. In a large mixing bowl, combine eggs, egg whites, garlic powder, onion powder, paprika, black pepper, and salt. Whisk until smooth.
2. Spray a baking sheet with cooking spray, pour egg mixture evenly, and bake for 8-10 minutes until set.
3. Microwave turkey sausage links for 45-60 seconds, then chop into small pieces.
4. Heat a large pan over medium-high heat with cooking spray, cook chopped sausage for 2-3 minutes until lightly browned.
5. Clean the pan and spray with cooking spray.
6. Assemble wraps: In the pan, place a tortilla, add 2 tbsp cheese, a layer of egg, 2 tbsp chopped turkey sausage, and 2 tbsp cheese.
7. Fold tortilla over itself, pressing lightly, and cook for 4-5 minutes per side until golden brown.

BREAKFAST WRAPS/BURRITOS

LOADED WAKE UP WRAP

Calories: 420 **Protein: 35** **Carbs: 26** **Fats: 25**

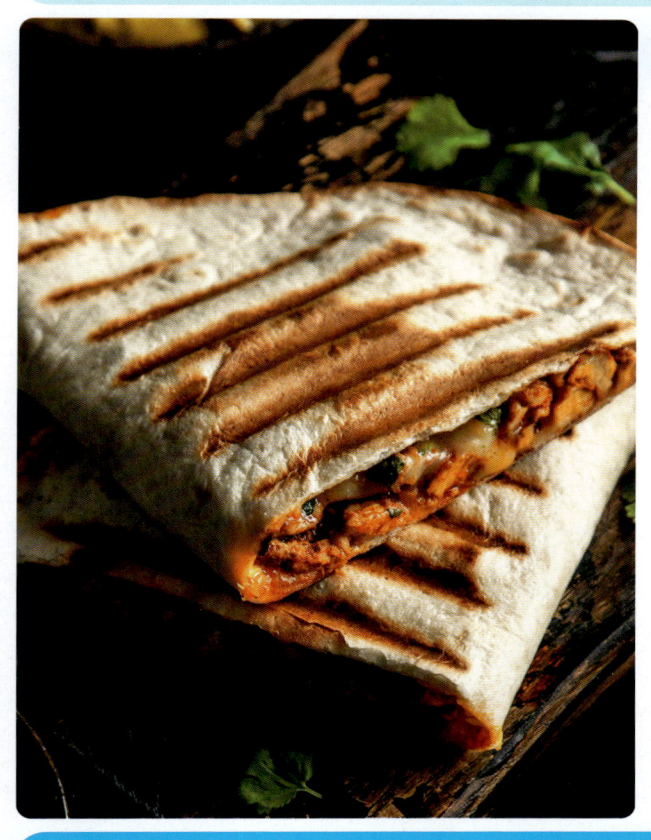

Ingredients Servings: 8

Breakfast Wrap:
- 6 whole eggs
- 3 cups egg whites
- 8 (12 oz.) Mission low carb tortillas
- 1 cup shredded cheese
- 1/2 (bag 12 links) Jones Dairy turkey sausage
- 6 slices turkey bacon
- 2 cups shredded hash browns
- 1 tbsp garlic powder
- 1 tsp onion powder
- 1 tsp paprika
- 1/2 tsp black pepper
- 1/4 tsp salt

Optional Sides

- Cilantro Lime Rice (1/3 cup non-fat greek yogurt, 3 tbsp cilantro, 1 tbsp lime juice - 50C, 7P, 3C, 1F)
- Protein shake (2 cups almond milk, 1 scoop Dummy Supps - 200c, 28P, 5C, 7F)
- Salsa (2 tbsp - 10c, 0P, 2C, 0F)
- Hot sauce (1 tsp - 1c, 0P, 0C, 0F)
- Avocado (1/2 whole - 120c, 2P, 6C, 11F)

Instructions

1. In a large mixing bowl, combine eggs, egg whites, garlic powder, onion powder, paprika, black pepper, and salt. Whisk until smooth.
2. Spray a baking sheet with cooking spray, pour egg mixture evenly, and bake for 8-10 minutes until set.
3. Microwave turkey sausage links for 45-60 seconds, then chop.
4. Heat a large pan over medium-high heat with cooking spray, cook chopped turkey sausage for 2-3 minutes until lightly browned. Set aside.
5. In the same pan, cook turkey bacon for 3-4 minutes per side, then chop.
6. In the same pan, cook shredded hash browns for 4-5 minutes, stirring occasionally, until golden brown. Set aside.
7. Clean the pan and spray with cooking spray.
8. Assemble wraps: In the pan, place a tortilla, add 2 tbsp cheese, a layer of egg, 2 tbsp chopped turkey sausage, 2 tbsp chopped bacon, 2 tbsp hash browns, and 2 tbsp cheese.
9. Fold tortilla over itself, pressing lightly, and cook for 4-5 minutes per side until golden brown.

BREAKFAST RECIPES

EGG BITES

DAILY MEAL PREP IDEAS

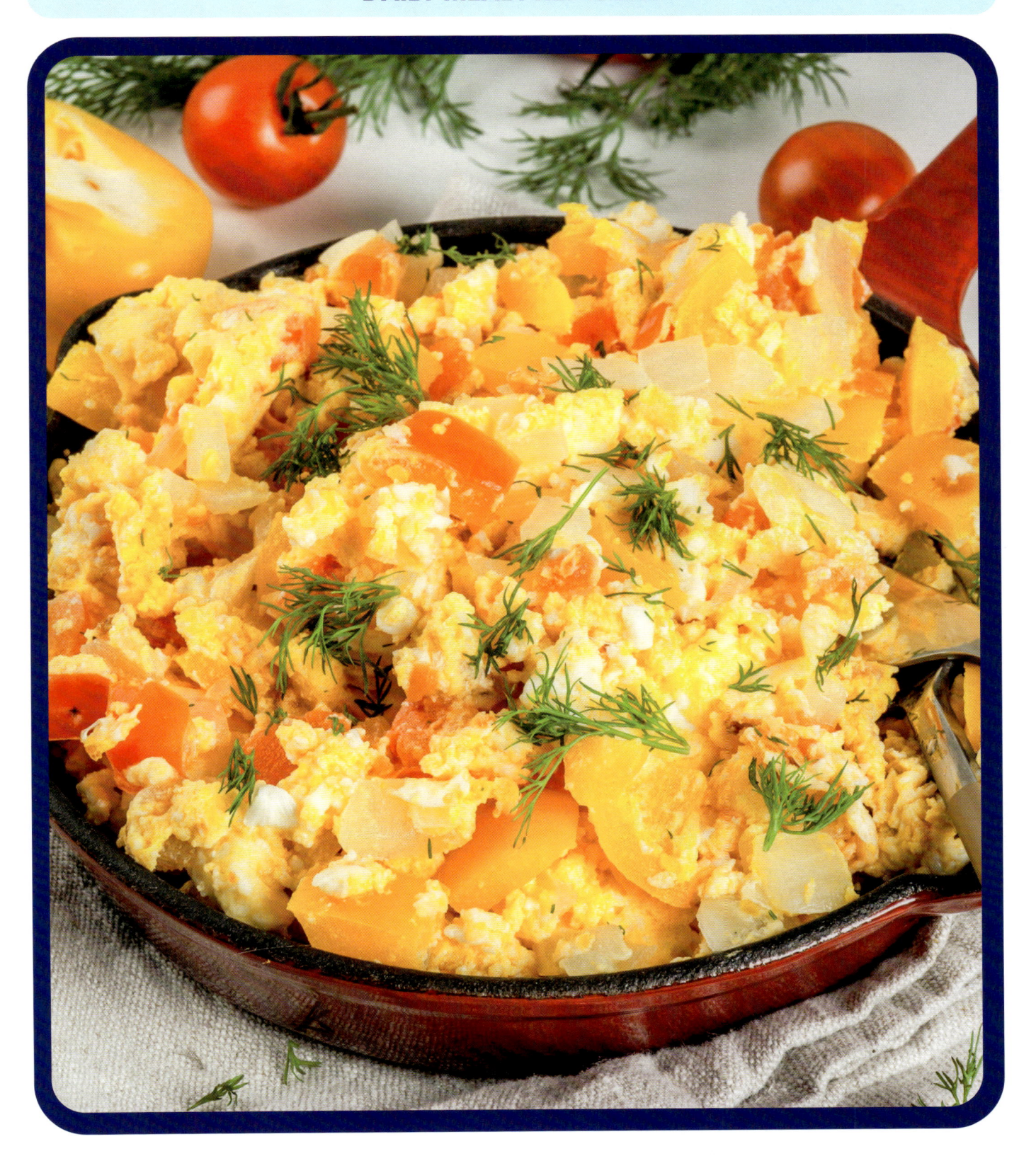

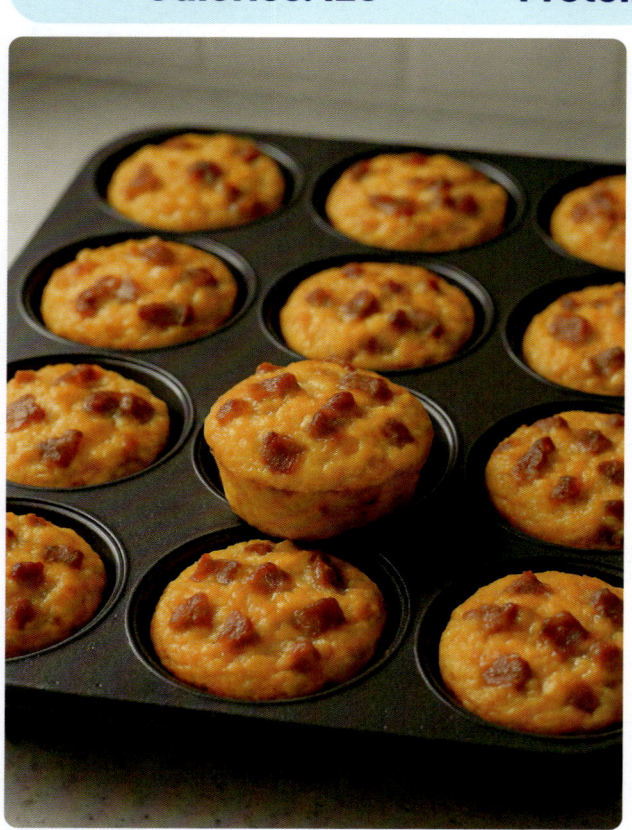

BREAKFAST RECIPES

BACON EGG & CHEESE MUFFIN

Calories: 120 **Protein: 16** **Carbs: 2** **Fats: 6**

Ingredients **Servings: 12**

Egg Muffins:
- 1 cup egg whites
- 6 whole eggs
- 1/2 cup cheddar shredded cheese
- 1 1/4 cup low fat cottage cheese
- 12 slices turkey bacon
- 1/2 tsp garlic salt
- 1/2 tsp black pepper
- 1/2 tsp onion powder

Optional Sides
- Salad (2 cups greens, 1 tbsp olive oil, 2 tbsp balsamic - 307c, 4P, 11C, 27F)
- Protein shake (2 cups almond milk, 1 scoop Dummy Supps - 200c, 28P, 5C, 7F)
- Salsa (2 tbsp - 10c, 0P, 2C, 0F)
- Hot sauce (1 tsp - 1c, 0P, 0C, 0F)
- Avocado (1/2 whole -120c, 2P, 6C, 11F)

Instructions
1. Preheat oven to 300°F. Place a brownie tray filled with water on the bottom rack for humidity.
2. Grease a muffin tin (preferably silicone).
3. Cook bacon in pan on medium high heat for 5 minutes each side. Chop into small pieces.
4. Blend eggs, cottage cheese, shredded cheese, and seasonings until just smooth.
5. Pour the mixture halfway into each muffin cup.
6. Add chopped sausage into each cup (or mix in before pouring).
7. Bake for 35–37 minutes until fully set.
8. Cool slightly and enjoy. Store extras in the fridge or freezer.

BREAKFAST RECIPES

SAUSAGE EGG & CHEESE MUFFIN

Calories: 160   **Protein: 52**   **Carbs: 2**   **Fats: 10**

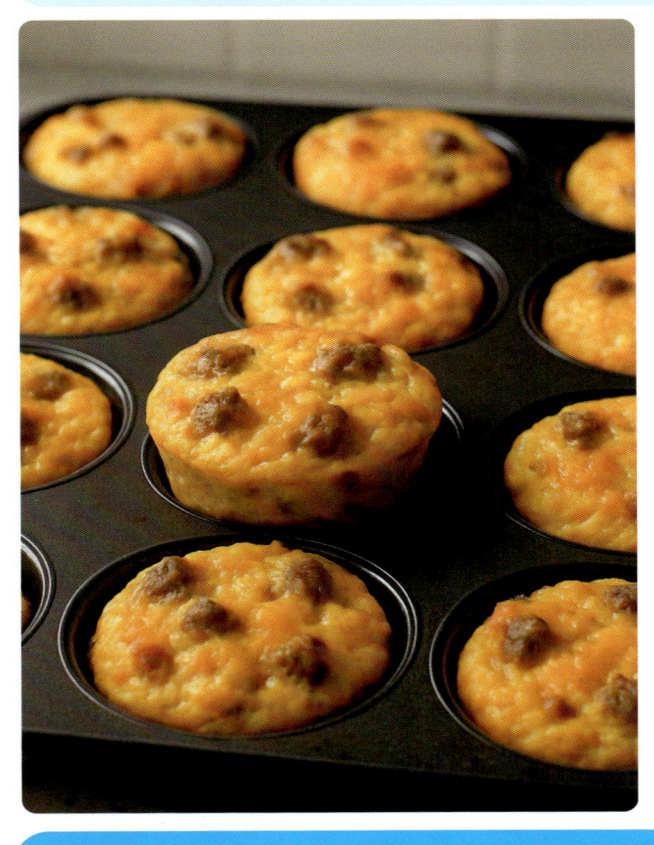

Ingredients   **Servings: 12**

Egg Muffins:
- 1 cup egg whites
- 6 whole eggs
- 1/2 cup cheddar shredded cheese
- 1 1/4 cup low fat cottage cheese
- 28 links Jones Dairy Farm chicken sausage
- 1/2 tsp garlic salt
- 1/2 tsp black pepper
- 1/2 tsp onion powder

Optional Sides

- Salad (2 cups greens, 1 tbsp olive oil, 2 tbsp balsamic - 307c, 4P, 11C, 27F)
- Protein shake (2 cups almond milk, 1 scoop Dummy Supps - 200c, 28P, 5C, 7F)
- Salsa (2 tbsp - 10c, 0P, 2C, 0F)
- Hot sauce (1 tsp - 1c, 0P, 0C, 0F)
- Avocado (1/2 whole -120c, 2P, 6C, 11F)

Instructions

1. Preheat oven to 300°F. Place a tray of water on the bottom rack for steam.
2. Grease a muffin tin (silicone preferred).
3. Microwave the chicken sausage for ~2 minutes or until heated through. Then chop into small pieces.
4. Blend eggs, egg whites, cottage cheese, cheddar cheese, and seasonings until smooth.
5. Pour the egg mixture halfway into each muffin cup.
6. Add chopped sausage evenly to each cup.
7. Bake for 35–37 minutes, until fully set.
8. Cool slightly and enjoy. Store extras in fridge or freezer.

BREAKFAST RECIPES

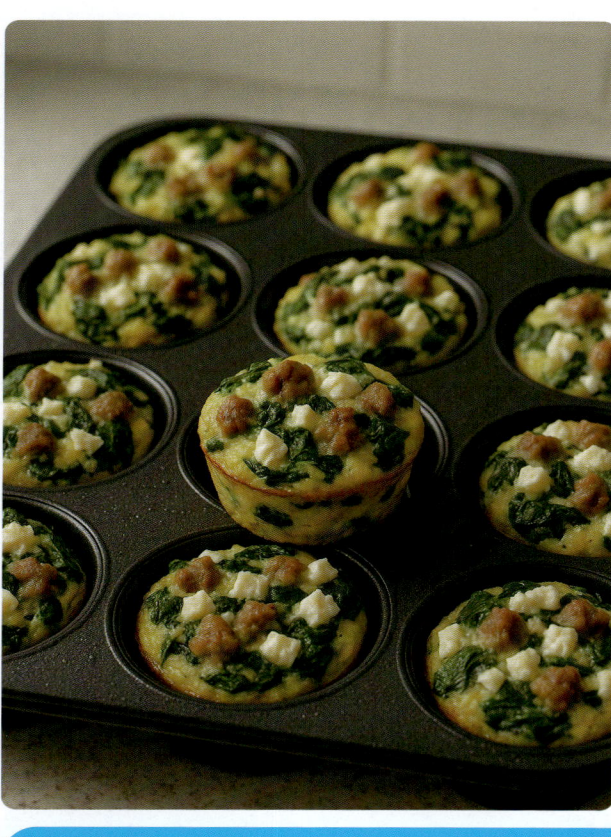

GREEK EGG MUFFIN

Calories: 150 **Protein: 16** **Carbs: 2** **Fats: 9**

Ingredients **Servings: 12**

Egg Muffins:
- 1 cup egg whites
- 6 whole eggs
- 1/2 cup lowfat feta cheese
- 1 1/4 cup low fat cottage cheese
- 28 links Jones Dairy Farm chicken sausage
- 2 cups spinach
- 1/2 tsp garlic salt
- 1/2 tsp black pepper
- 1/2 tsp onion powder

Optional Sides

- Salad (2 cups greens, 1 tbsp olive oil, 2 tbsp balsamic - 307c, 4P, 11C, 27F)
- Protein shake (2 cups almond milk, 1 scoop Dummy Supps - 200c, 28P, 5C, 7F)
- Salsa (2 tbsp - 10c, 0P, 2C, 0F)
- Hot sauce (1 tsp - 1c, 0P, 0C, 0F)
- Avocado (1/2 whole -120c, 2P, 6C, 11F)

Instructions

1. Preheat oven to 300°F. Place a tray of water on the bottom rack for steam.
2. Grease a muffin tin (silicone preferred).
3. Microwave the sausage for ~2 minutes or until heated through. Then chop into small pieces.
4. Blend eggs, egg whites, cottage cheese, and seasonings until smooth.
5. Pour the egg mixture halfway into each muffin cup.
6. Chop spinach.
7. Add chopped sausage, feta, and spinach evenly to each cup.
8. Bake for 35–37 minutes, until fully set.
9. Cool slightly and enjoy. Store extras in fridge or freezer.

BREAKFAST RECIPES

WESTERN OMELET EGG MUFFINS

Calories: 120 **Protein: 14** **Carbs: 3** **Fats: 5**

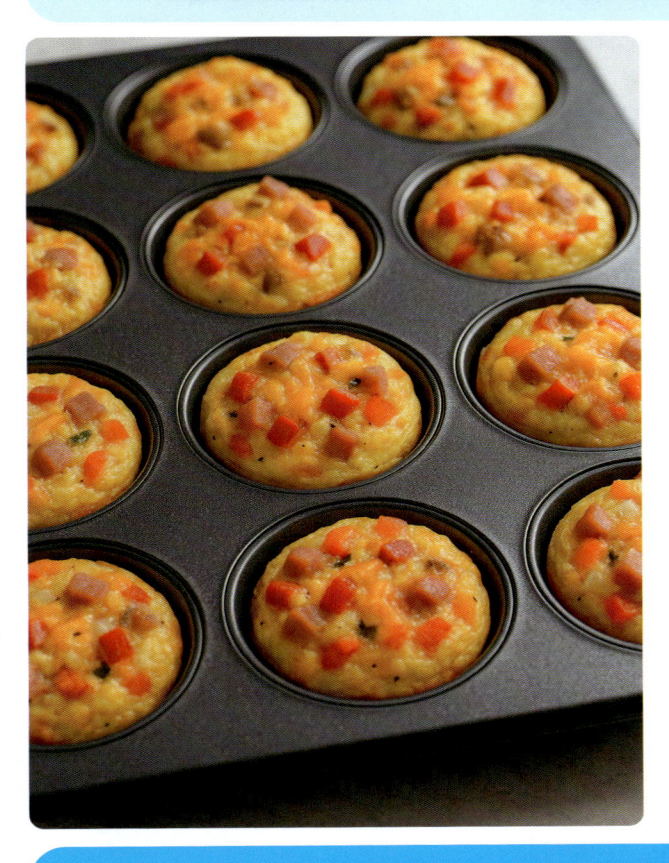

Ingredients **Servings: 12**

Egg Muffins:
- 1 cup egg whites
- 6 whole eggs
- 1/2 cup shredded cheddar cheese
- 1 1/4 cup low-fat cottage cheese
- 12 (2 oz.) slices uncured cooked ham
- 1/2 cup diced red bell pepper
- 1/2 cup diced yellow onion
- 1/2 tsp garlic salt
- 1/2 tsp black pepper
- 1/2 tsp onion powder

Optional Sides
- Salad (2 cups greens, 1 tbsp olive oil, 2 tbsp balsamic - 307c, 4P, 11C, 27F)
- Protein shake (2 cups almond milk, 1 scoop Dummy Supps - 200c, 28P, 5C, 7F)
- Salsa (2 tbsp - 10c, 0P, 2C, 0F)
- Hot sauce (1 tsp - 1c, 0P, 0C, 0F)
- Avocado (1/2 whole -120c, 2P, 6C, 11F)

Instructions
1. Preheat oven to 300°F. Place a tray of water on the bottom rack for steam.
2. Grease a muffin tin (silicone preferred).
3. Dice ham, peppers, and onions. Microwave ham for ~1 minute if needed.
4. Blend eggs, egg whites, cottage cheese, cheddar cheese, and seasonings until smooth (don't over-blend).
5. Pour the egg mixture halfway into each muffin cup.
6. Add diced ham, peppers, and onions evenly into each cup.
7. Bake for 35–37 minutes, until fully set.
8. Cool slightly and enjoy. Store extras in fridge or freezer.

BREAKFAST RECIPES

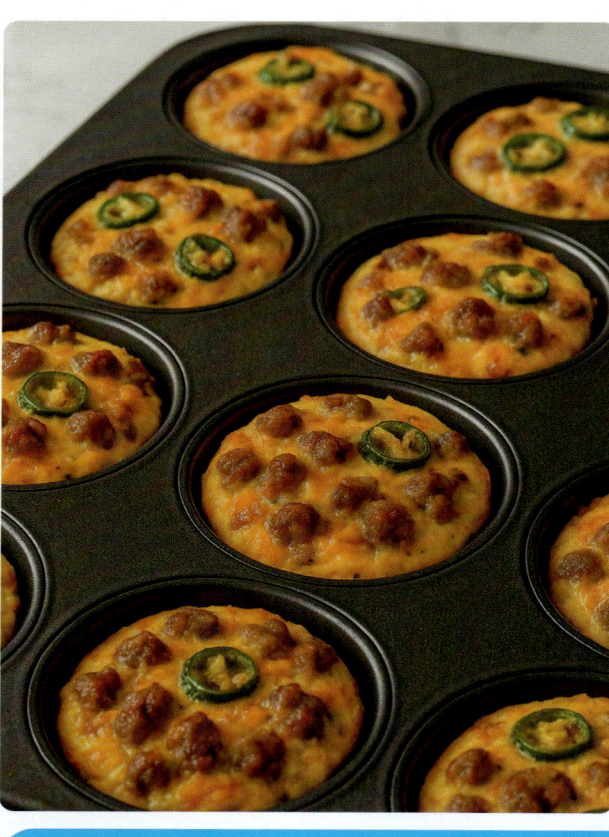

MEXICAN EGG MUFFINS

Calories: 160 **Protein: 16** **Carbs: 3** **Fats: 10**

Ingredients   Servings: 12

Egg Muffins:
- 1 cup egg whites
- 6 whole eggs
- 1/2 cup shredded Mexican cheese blend
- 1 1/4 cup low-fat cottage cheese
- 28 links Jones Dairy Farm chicken sausage
- 4 tbsp diced jalapeños (fresh or jarred)
- 1/2 tsp cumin
- 1/2 tsp garlic salt
- 1/2 tsp black pepper

Optional Sides

- Salad (2 cups greens, 1 tbsp olive oil, 2 tbsp balsamic - 307c, 4P, 11C, 27F)
- Protein shake (2 cups almond milk, 1 scoop Dummy Supps - 200c, 28P, 5C, 7F)
- Salsa (2 tbsp - 10c, 0P, 2C, 0F)
- Hot sauce (1 tsp - 1c, 0P, 0C, 0F)
- Avocado (1/2 whole -120c, 2P, 6C, 11F)

Instructions

1. Preheat oven to 300ºF. Place a tray of water on the bottom rack for steam.
2. Grease a muffin tin (silicone preferred).
3. Microwave the sausage ~2 minutes, then chop into small pieces.
4. Blend eggs, egg whites, cottage cheese, shredded cheese, and seasonings until smooth.
5. Pour egg mixture halfway into muffin cups.
6. Add chopped sausage and diced jalapeños evenly.
7. Bake 35–37 minutes, until set.
8. Cool slightly and enjoy. Store extras in fridge or freezer.

BREAKFAST RECIPES

MEAT LOVERS EGG MUFFINS

Calories: 210   **Protein: 23**   **Carbs: 3**   **Fats: 12**

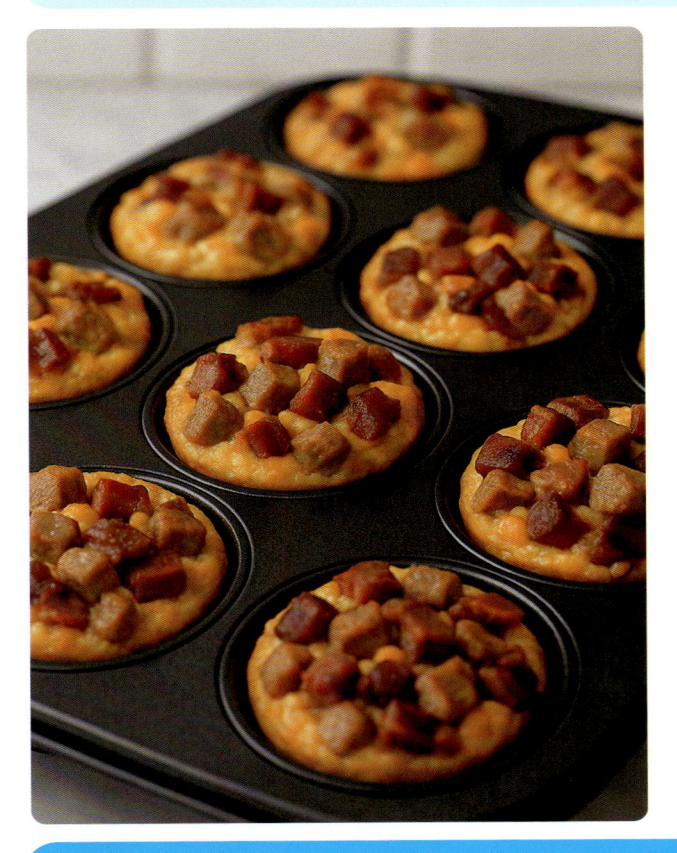

Ingredients   **Servings: 12**

Egg Muffins:
- 1 cup egg whites
- 6 whole eggs
- 1/2 cup shredded cheddar cheese
- 1 1/4 cup low-fat cottage cheese
- 28 links chicken sausage
- 6 slices cooked turkey bacon
- 6 (2 oz.) slices uncured ham
- 1/2 tsp garlic salt
- 1/2 tsp black pepper
- 1/2 tsp onion powder

Optional Sides
- Salad (2 cups greens, 1 tbsp olive oil, 2 tbsp balsamic - 307c, 4P, 11C, 27F)
- Protein shake (2 cups almond milk, 1 scoop Dummy Supps - 200c, 28P, 5C, 7F)
- Salsa (2 tbsp - 10c, 0P, 2C, 0F)
- Hot sauce (1 tsp - 1c, 0P, 0C, 0F)
- Avocado (1/2 whole -120c, 2P, 6C, 11F)

Instructions
1. Preheat oven to 300°F. Place a tray of water on the bottom rack.
2. Grease a muffin tin (silicone preferred).
3. Cook bacon in pan on medium high heat for 5 minutes each side. Chop into small pieces.
4. Microwave sausage and ham if needed, then chop all meats.
5. Blend eggs, egg whites, cottage cheese, cheddar cheese, and seasonings.
6. Pour egg mixture halfway into each muffin cup.
7. Add sausage, bacon, and ham evenly.
8. Bake for 35–37 minutes.
9. Cool slightly and enjoy. Store in fridge or freezer.

BREAKFAST RECIPES

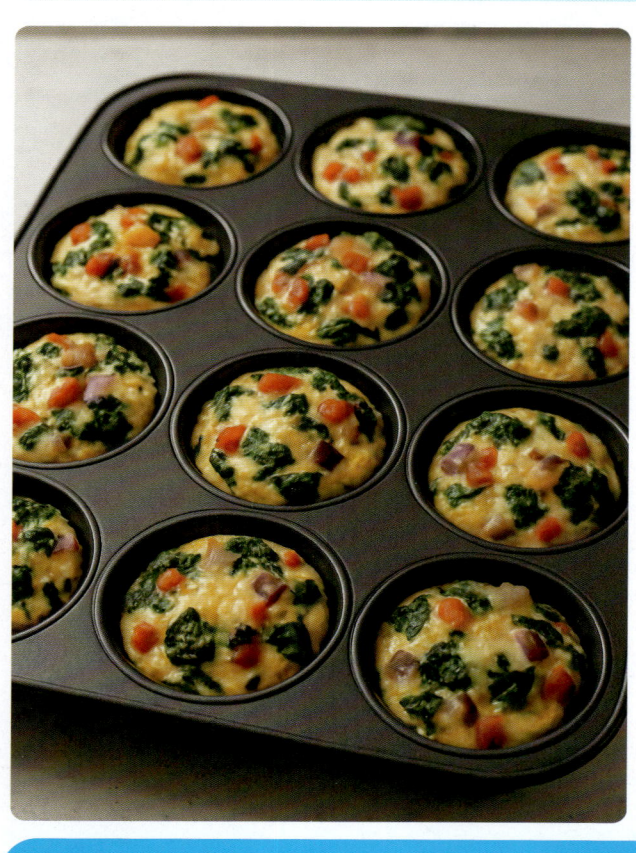

VEGGIE EGG MUFFINS

Calories: 90 **Protein: 9** **Carbs: 3** **Fats: 4**

Ingredients   Servings: 12

Egg Muffins:
- 1 cup egg whites
- 6 whole eggs
- ½ cup shredded mozzarella or cheddar
- 1 1/4 cup low-fat cottage cheese
- 1 cup chopped spinach
- 1/2 cup diced bell pepper
- 1/2 cup chopped red onion
- 1/2 cup mushrooms
- 1/2 tsp garlic salt
- 1/2 tsp black pepper

Optional Sides

- Salad (2 cups greens, 1 tbsp olive oil, 2 tbsp balsamic - 307c, 4P, 11C, 27F)
- Protein shake (2 cups almond milk, 1 scoop Dummy Supps - 200c, 28P, 5C, 7F)
- Salsa (2 tbsp - 10c, 0P, 2C, 0F)
- Hot sauce (1 tsp - 1c, 0P, 0C, 0F)
- Avocado (1/2 whole -120c, 2P, 6C, 11F)

Instructions

1. Preheat oven to 300°F. Place a tray of water on the bottom rack.
2. Grease a muffin tin (silicone preferred).
3. Chop all veggies (lightly sauté mushrooms and onions if preferred).
4. Blend eggs, egg whites, cottage cheese, shredded cheese, and seasonings until smooth.
5. Pour egg mixture halfway into muffin cups.
6. Add chopped veggies evenly.
7. Bake for 35–37 minutes.
8. Cool slightly and enjoy. Store extras in fridge or freezer.

BREAKFAST RECIPES

PEPPERONI PIZZA EGG MUFFINS

Calories: 100   **Protein: 12**   **Carbs: 22**   **Fats: 6**

Ingredients   **Servings: 12**

Egg Muffins:
- 1 cup egg whites
- 6 whole eggs
- 1 1/4 cup low-fat cottage cheese
- 1 cup shredded mozzarella cheese
- 30 slices turkey pepperoni
- 1/2 tsp Italian seasoning
- 1/2 tsp garlic powder
- 1/2 tsp onion powder

Optional Sides

- Salad (2 cups greens, 1 tbsp olive oil, 2 tbsp balsamic - 307c, 4P, 11C, 27F)
- Protein shake (2 cups almond milk, 1 scoop Dummy Supps - 200c, 28P, 5C, 7F)
- Salsa (2 tbsp - 10c, 0P, 2C, 0F)
- Hot sauce (1 tsp - 1c, 0P, 0C, 0F)
- Avocado (1/2 whole -120c, 2P, 6C, 11F)

Instructions

1. Preheat oven to 300°F. Place a tray of water on the bottom rack for steam.
2. Grease a muffin tin (silicone preferred).
3. Microwave turkey pepperoni for ~30 seconds if needed, then chop.
4. Blend egg whites, eggs, cottage cheese, mozzarella, and seasonings until smooth.
5. Pour mixture halfway into each muffin cup.
6. Add chopped pepperoni evenly into each cup.
7. Bake 35–37 minutes, until fully set.
8. Cool slightly and enjoy. Store extras in fridge or freezer.

BREAKFAST RECIPES

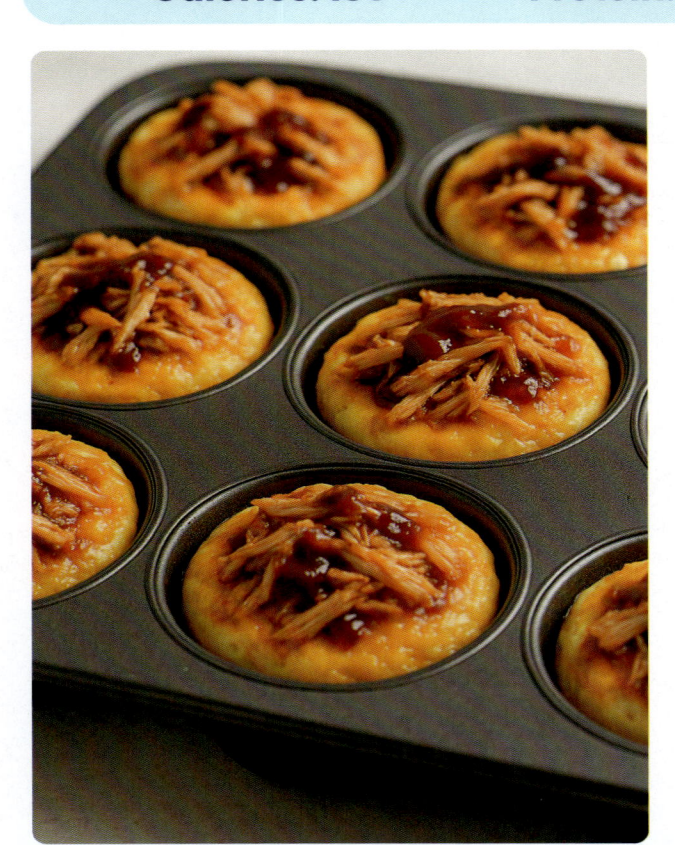

BBQ CHICKEN & CHEDDAR EGG MUFFINS

Calories: 130 **Protein: 14** **Carbs: 4** **Fats: 6**

Ingredients   Servings: 12

Egg Muffins:
- 1 cup egg whites
- 6 whole eggs
- 1 1/4 cup low-fat cottage cheese
- 1/2 cup shredded cheddar cheese
- 2 cups cooked shredded chicken breast
- 12 tbsp G Hughes BBQ sauce
- 1/2 tsp garlic salt
- 1/2 tsp smoked paprika
- 1/2 tsp black pepper

Optional Sides

- Salad (2 cups greens, 1 tbsp olive oil, 2 tbsp balsamic - 307c, 4P, 11C, 27F)
- Protein shake (2 cups almond milk, 1 scoop Dummy Supps - 200c, 28P, 5C, 7F)
- Salsa (2 tbsp - 10c, 0P, 2C, 0F)
- Hot sauce (1 tsp - 1c, 0P, 0C, 0F)
- Avocado (1/2 whole -120c, 2P, 6C, 11F)

Instructions

1. Preheat oven to 300°F. Place a tray of water on the bottom rack for steam.
2. Grease a muffin tin (silicone preferred).
3. Shred or chop cooked chicken, then toss with BBQ sauce.
4. Blend eggs, egg whites, cottage cheese, cheddar cheese, and seasonings until smooth.
5. Pour mixture halfway into each muffin cup.
6. Add BBQ chicken evenly into each cup.
7. Bake for 35–37 minutes, until fully set.
8. Cool slightly and enjoy. Store extras in fridge or freezer.

OATMEAL

OATMEAL

DAILY MEAL PREP IDEAS

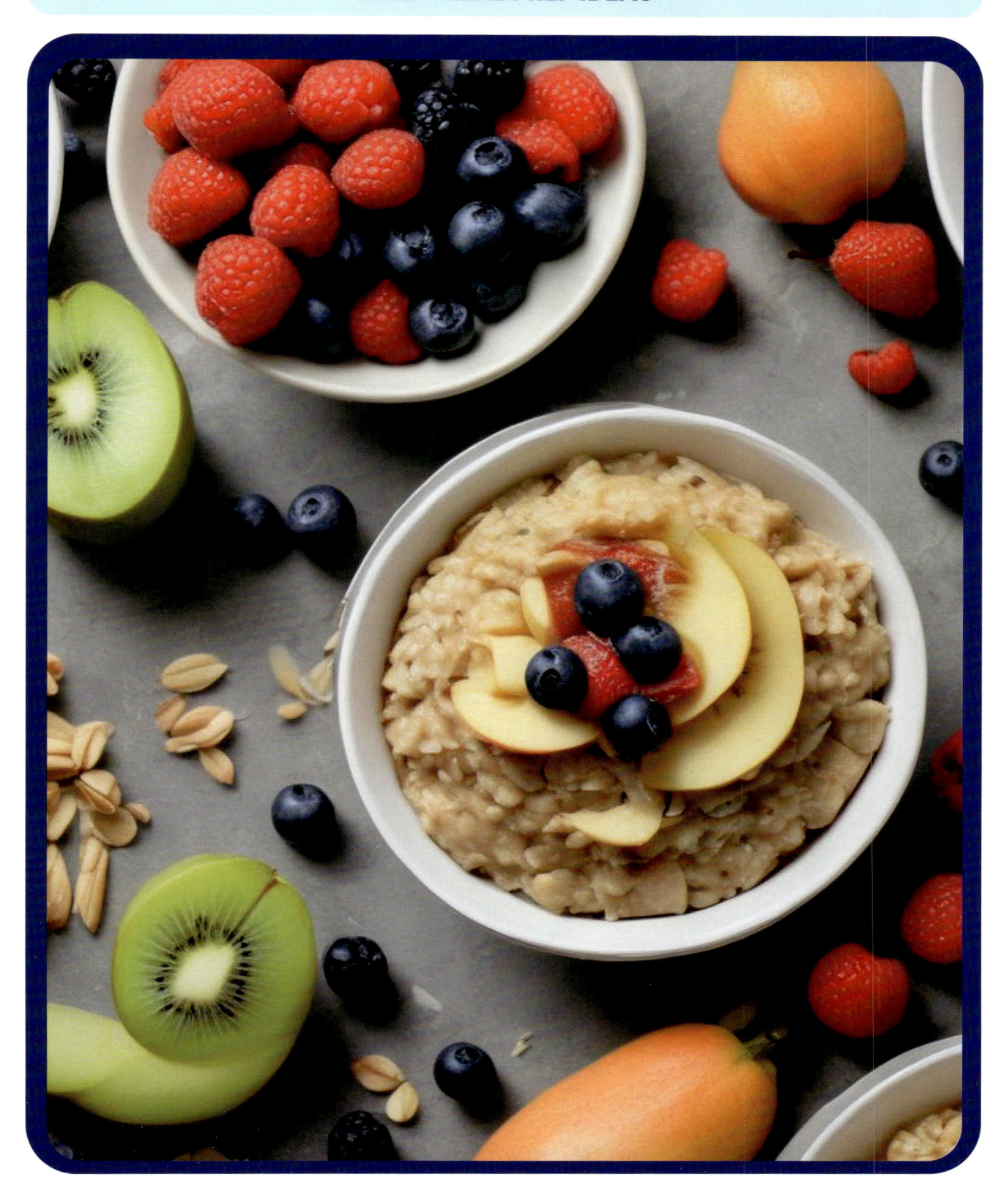

OATMEAL

CLASSIC CINNAMON

Calories: 340 **Protein: 30** **Carbs: 44** **Fat: 11**

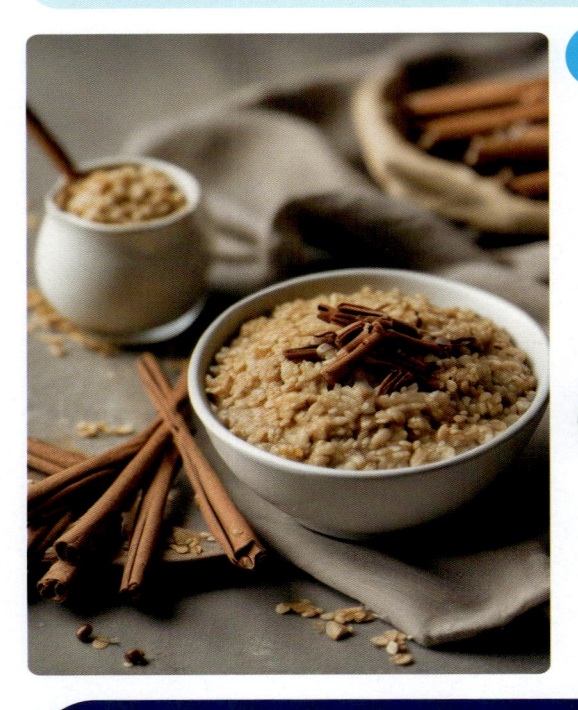

Ingredients — Servings: 1

- 1/2 cup quick oats
- 3/4 cup water
- 1 scoop Dummy Supps vanilla whey
- 2 tbsp unsweetened almond milk
- 1/2 tsp vanilla extract
- 1 tsp cinnamon
- 1/4 tsp salt
- 1 tbsp maple syrup
- 2 tbsp almond milk

Instructions

1. Add oats and water to a microwave-safe bowl. Microwave for 1-2 minutes until oats are softened.
2. Stir in protein powder, almond milk, vanilla extract, and cinnamon until smooth.
3. Drizzle maple syrup and salt on top and mix well.

CHOCOLATE PEANUT BUTTER

Calories: 440 **Protein: 39** **Carbs: 47** **Fat: 12**

Ingredients — Servings: 1

- 1/2 cup quick oats
- 3/4 cup water
- 1 scoop Dummy Supps chocolate PB whey
- 2 tbsp unsweetened almond milk
- 1/2 banana
- 1/2 tsp vanilla extract
- 1/4 tsp salt
- 1 tbsp chocolate espresso Dummy Butter
- 2 tbsp almond milk

Instructions

1. Slice banana.
2. Add oats and water to a microwave-safe bowl. Microwave for 1-2 minutes until oats are softened.
3. Stir in protein powder, almond milk, vanilla extract, and sliced banana until smooth.
4. Top with Chocolate Espresso Dummy Butter, salt, and mix slightly.

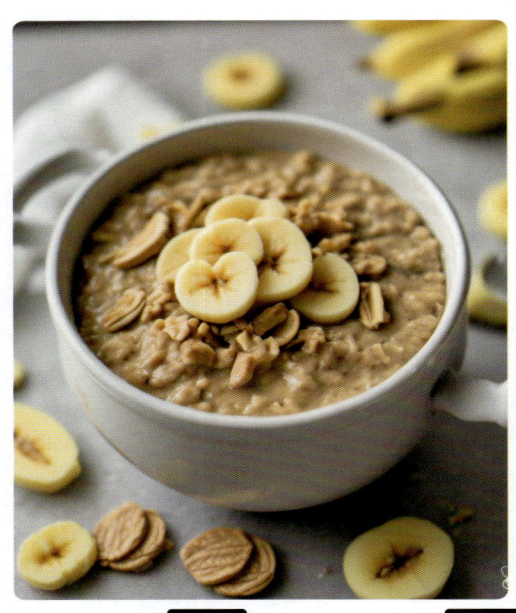

Dummy Supps Whey Protein — SCAN ME

Dummy Butter Peanut Butter — SCAN ME

OATMEAL

VANILLA BLUEBERRY

Calories: 325 **Protein: 30** **Carbs: 42** **Fat: 5**

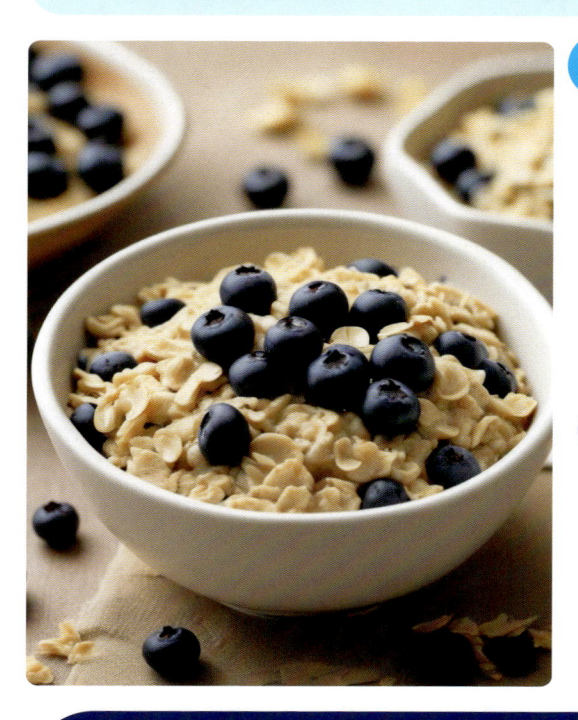

Ingredients — Servings: 1

- 1/2 cup quick oats
- 3/4 cup water
- 1 scoop Dummy Supps vanilla whey
- 2 tbsp unsweetened almond milk
- 1/2 tsp vanilla extract
- 1/4 tsp salt
- 1 cup fresh/frozen blueberries
- 2 tbsp almond milk

Instructions

1. Add oats and water to a microwave-safe bowl. Microwave for 1-2 minutes until oats are softened.
2. Stir in protein powder, almond milk, vanilla extract, and salt until smooth.
3. Fold in blueberries and mix gently.

BANANAS FOSTER

Calories: 400 **Protein: 30** **Carbs: 57** **Fat: 4**

Ingredients — Servings: 1

- 1/2 cup quick oats
- 3/4 cup water
- 1 scoop Dummy Supps chocolate PB whey
- 2 tbsp unsweetened almond milk
- 1/2 banana
- 1/2 tsp vanilla extract
- 1/4 tsp salt
- 1 tbsp chocolate espresso Dummy Butter
- 2 tbsp almond milk

Instructions

1. Add oats and water to a microwave-safe bowl. Microwave for 1-2 minutes until oats are softened.
2. Stir in protein powder, almond milk, vanilla extract, cinnamon, and nutmeg until smooth.
3. Slice banana into thin rounds.
4. Heat a small pan over medium heat, add sliced banana and maple syrup. Cook for 1-2 minutes, stirring occasionally, until caramelized.
5. Top oatmeal with caramelized bananas.

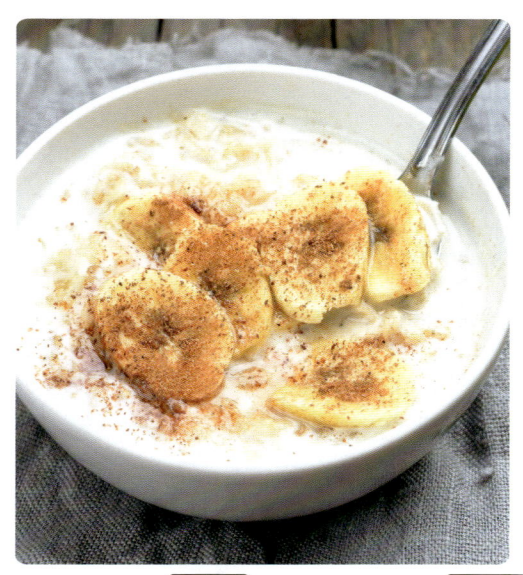

Dummy Supps Whey Protein — SCAN ME

Dummy Butter Peanut Butter — SCAN ME

OATMEAL

APPLE CRISP

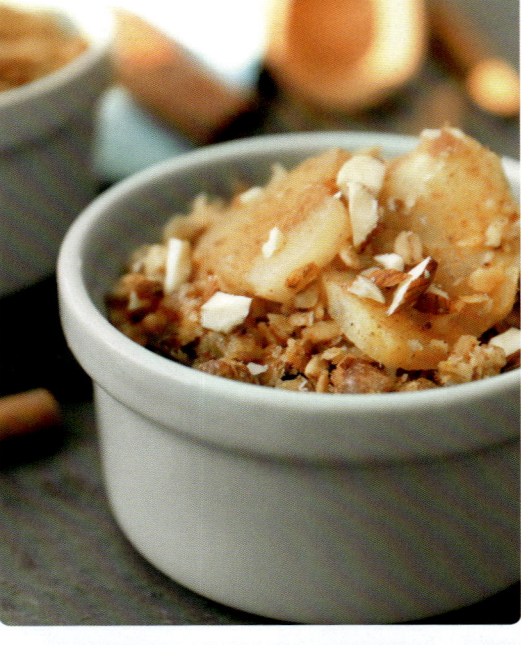

Calories: 440 **Protein: 30** **Carbs: 58** **Fat: 4**

Ingredients — Servings: 1

- 1/2 cup quick oats
- 3/4 cup water
- 1 scoop Dummy Supps vanilla whey
- 2 tbsp unsweetened almond milk
- 1/2 whole apple
- 1 tbsp maple syrup
- 1/2 tsp vanilla extract
- 1 tbsp cinnamon
- 1 tsp nutmeg
- 2 tbsp almond milk

Instructions

1. Dice apple into small pieces.
2. Add oats and water to a microwave-safe bowl. Microwave for 1-2 minutes until oats are softened.
3. Stir in protein powder, almond milk, vanilla extract, cinnamon, and nutmeg until smooth.
4. Heat a small pan over medium heat, add diced apple and maple syrup. Cook for 2-3 minutes, stirring occasionally, until apples are soft and caramelized.
5. Top oatmeal with warm maple cinnamon apples.

CHOCOLATE ALMOND OATMEAL

Calories: 420 **Protein: 41** **Carbs: 38** **Fat: 16**

Ingredients — Servings: 1

- 1/2 cup quick oats
- 3/4 cup water
- 1 scoop Dummy Supps chocolate whey
- 2 tbsp unsweetened almond milk
- 1 tbsp cocoa powder
- 1 tbsp chopped almonds
- 1/4 tsp salt
- 1 tbsp chocolate espresso Dummy Butter
- 2 tbsp almond milk

Instructions

1. Add oats and water to a microwave-safe bowl. Microwave for 1-2 minutes until oats are softened.
2. Stir in protein powder, almond milk, cocoa powder, and salt until smooth.
3. Top with chopped almonds and Dummy Butter Chocolate Espresso Peanut Butter.

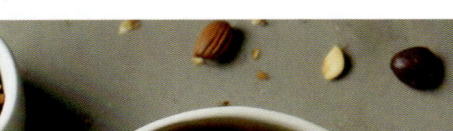

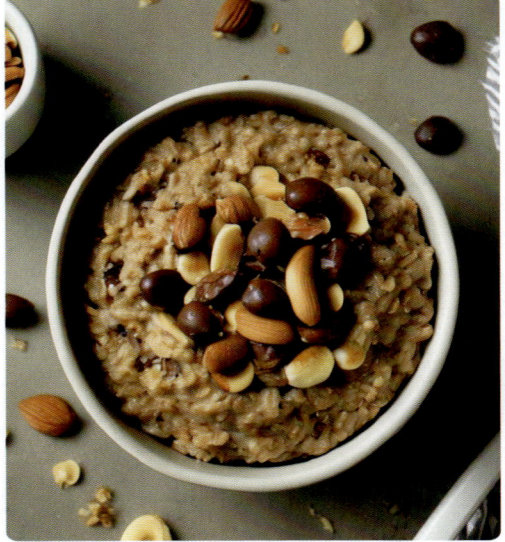

Dummy Supps Whey Protein **Dummy Butter Peanut Butter**

OATMEAL

BERRY BLAST OATMEAL

Calories: 470   **Protein: 40**   **Carbs: 60**   **Fat: 12**

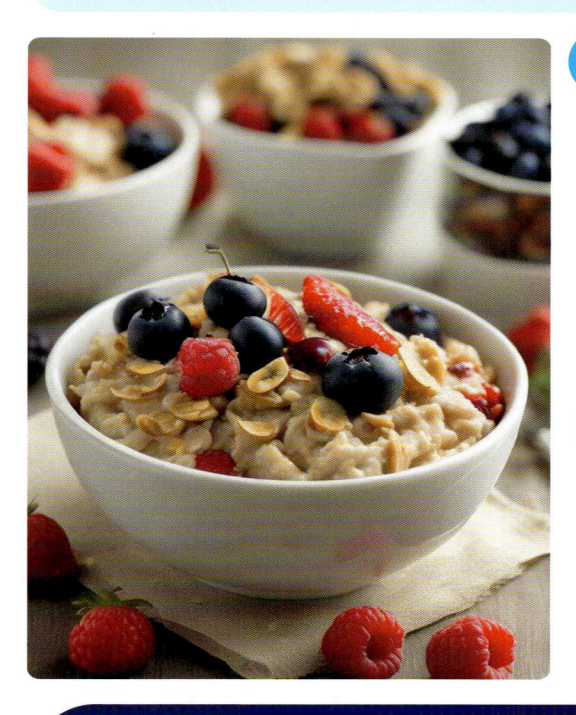

Ingredients — Servings: 1

- 1/2 cup quick oats
- 3/4 cup water
- 1 scoop Dummy Supps berry whey
- 2 tbsp unsweetened almond milk
- 1/2 cup mixed berries
- 1/2 tsp vanilla extract
- 1 tbsp honey
- 1/4 tsp salt
- 1 tbsp PB&J Dummy Butter
- 2 tbsp almond milk

Instructions

1. Add oats and water to a microwave-safe bowl. Microwave for 1-2 minutes until oats are softened.
2. Stir in protein powder, almond milk, vanilla extract, honey, and salt until smooth.
3. Fold in mixed berries and mix gently.
4. Top with Dummy Butter PB&J.

CHOCOLATE BROWNIE OATMEAL

Calories: 450   **Protein: 41**   **Carbs: 45**   **Fat: 17**

Ingredients — Servings: 1

- 1/2 cup oats
- 3/4 cup water
- 1 scoop Dummy Supps Chocolate Whey
- 1 tbsp unsweetened cocoa powder
- 1 tsp monk fruit sweetener
- 1/2 tsp vanilla extract
- 1/4 tsp salt
- 2 tbsp Lily's chocolate chips
- 2 tbsp almond milk

Instructions

1. Add oats and water to a microwave-safe bowl. Microwave for 1-2 minutes until oats are softened.
2. Stir in Dummy Supps Chocolate Whey, cocoa powder, monk fruit sweetener, and vanilla extract until smooth.
3. Fold in Lily's chocolate chips and mix gently.
4. Top with salt.

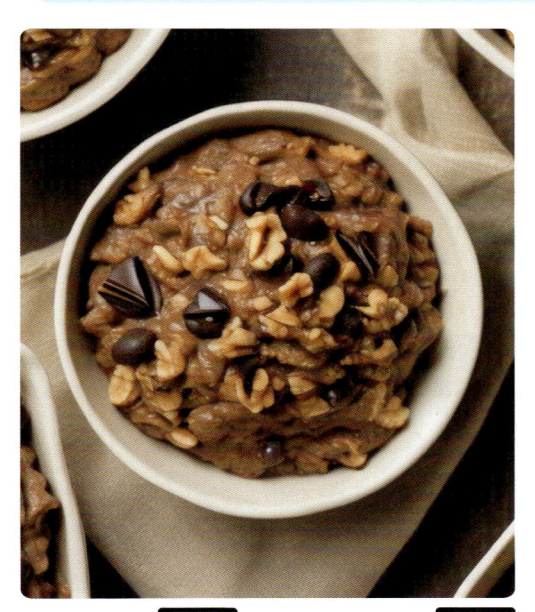

Dummy Supps Whey Protein — SCAN ME

Dummy Butter Peanut Butter — SCAN ME

OATMEAL

PUMPKIN SPICE OATMEAL

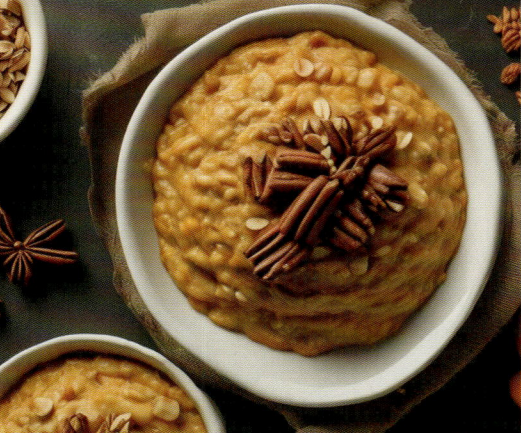

Calories: 500   **Protein: 41**   **Carbs: 52**   **Fat: 20**

Ingredients   Servings: 1

- 1/2 cup quick oats
- 3/4 cup water
- 1 scoop Dummy Supps vanilla whey
- 2 tbsp unsweetened almond milk
- 2 tbsp pumpkin puree
- 1/2 tsp pumpkin spice
- 2 tbsp Lilly's chocolate chips
- 1 tbsp chocolate espresso Dummy Butter
- 2 tbsp almond milk

Instructions

1. Add oats and water to a microwave-safe bowl. Microwave for 1-2 minutes until oats are softened.
2. Stir in protein powder, almond milk, pumpkin puree, and pumpkin spice until smooth.
3. Fold in Lilly's chocolate chips and mix gently.
4. Top with Chocolate Espresso Dummy Butter.

COCONUT CHOCOLATE OATMEAL

Calories: 480   **Protein: 40**   **Carbs: 46**   **Fat: 19**

Ingredients   Servings: 1

- 1/2 cup quick oats
- 3/4 cup water
- 1 scoop Dummy Supps chocolate whey
- 2 tbsp unsweetened almond milk
- 1 tbsp shredded coconut
- 1/2 tsp vanilla extract
- 2 tbsp Lilly's chocolate chips
- 1 tbsp chocolate espresso Dummy Butter
- 2 tbsp almond milk

Instructions

1. Add oats and water to a microwave-safe bowl. Microwave for 1-2 minutes until oats are softened.
2. Stir in protein powder, almond milk, shredded coconut, and vanilla extract until smooth.
3. Fold in Lilly's chocolate chips and mix gently.
4. Top with Chocolate Espresso Dummy Butter.

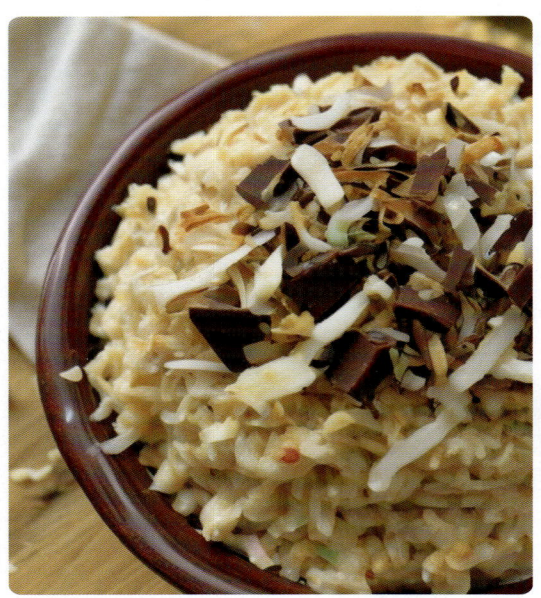

Dummy Supps Whey Protein

Dummy Butter Peanut Butter

OVERNIGHT OATS

OVERNIGHT OATS

DAILY MEAL PREP IDEAS

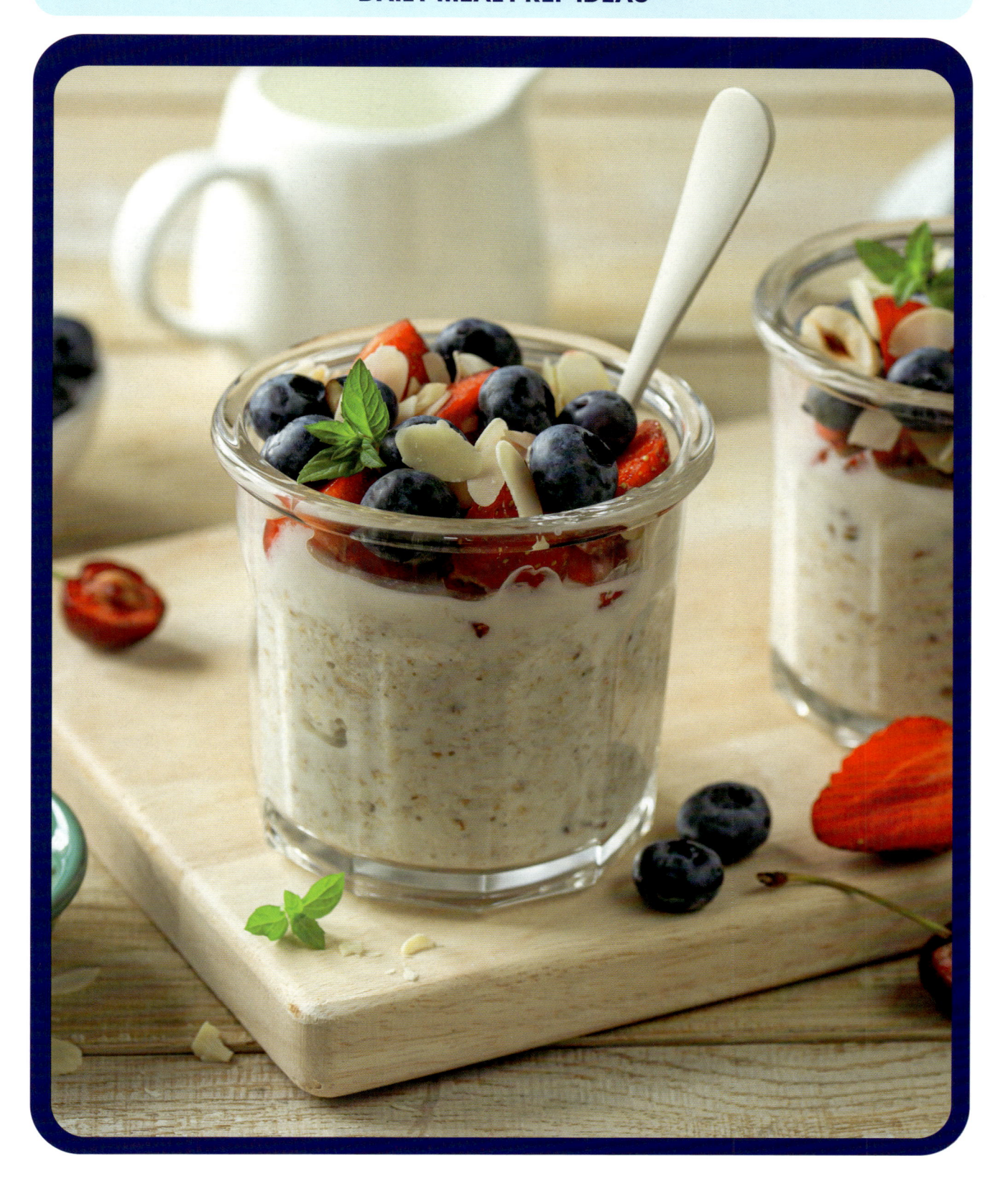

OVERNIGHT OATS

CINNAMON ROLL DELIGHT

Calories: 530 **Protein: 42** **Carbs: 52** **Fat: 22**

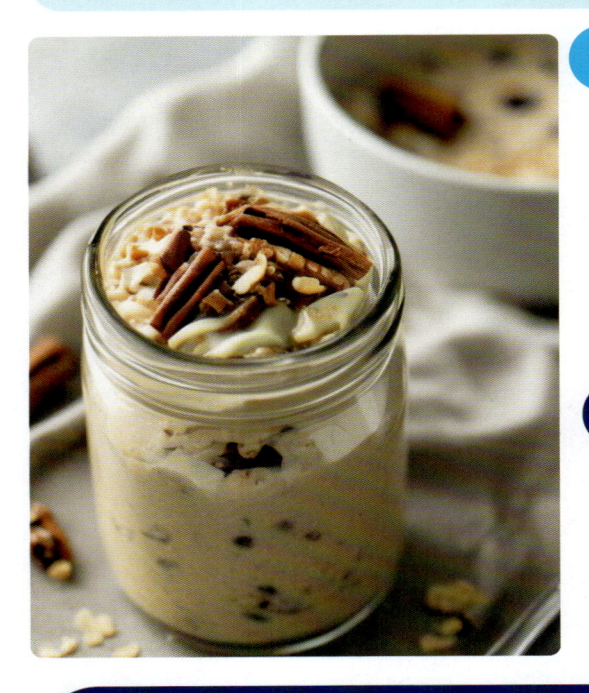

Ingredients — Servings: 1

- 1/2 cup quick oats
- 3/4 cup unsweetened almond milk
- 1 scoop Dummy Supps Cinnamon Roll Whey
- 2 tbsp whipped cream cheese
- 1/2 tsp cinnamon
- 1 tbsp chopped walnuts
- 1 tbsp Chocolate Espresso Dummy Butter
- 1 tbsp maple syrup

Instructions

1. In a jar, combine oats, almond milk, protein powder, cream cheese, cinnamon, maple syrup, and walnuts. Stir well until smooth.
2. Seal the jar and refrigerate for 30 minutes or overnight.
3. Before serving, stir again and top with Chocolate Espresso Dummy Butter.

SALTED CARAMEL CRUNCH

Calories: 420 **Protein: 41** **Carbs: 36** **Fat: 17**

Ingredients — Servings: 1

- 1/2 cup quick oats
- 3/4 cup unsweetened almond milk
- 1 scoop Dummy Supps Salted Caramel Whey
- 2 tbsp chopped walnuts
- 1 tbsp Chocolate Espresso Dummy Butter
- 1/4 tsp salt

Instructions

1. In a jar, combine oats, almond milk, protein powder, chopped pecans, and salt. Stir well until smooth.
2. Seal the jar and refrigerate for 30 minutes or overnight.
3. Before serving, stir again and top with Chocolate Espresso Dummy Butter.

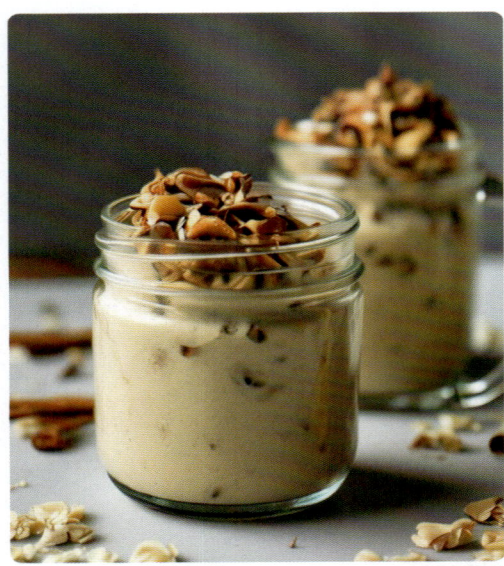

Dummy Supps Whey Protein [SCAN ME]

Dummy Butter Peanut Butter [SCAN ME]

OVERNIGHT OATS

PEANUT BUTTER BANANA

Calories: 450 **Protein: 38** **Carbs: 48** **Fat: 14**

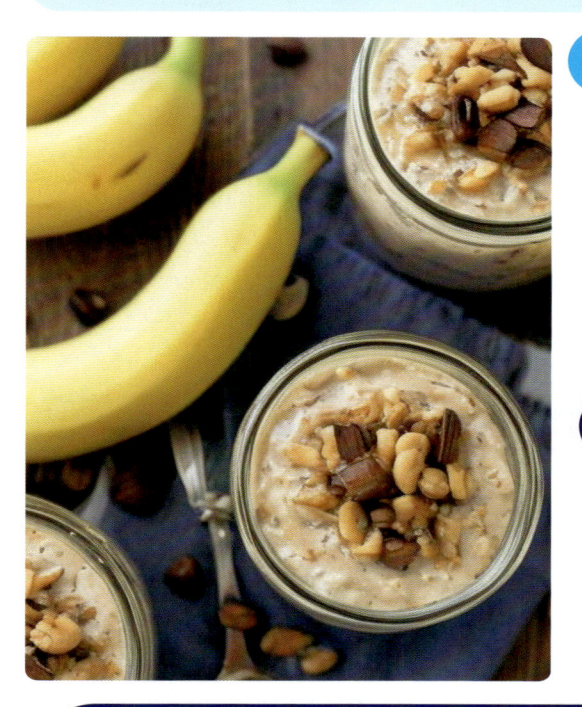

Ingredients — Servings: 1

- 1/2 cup quick oats
- 3/4 cup unsweetened almond milk
- 1 scoop Dummy Supps Chocolate Peanut Butter Whey
- 1/2 banana
- 1 tbsp natural peanut butter
- 1/2 tsp cinnamon

Instructions

1. In a jar, mash the banana until smooth.
2. Add oats, almond milk, protein powder, and cinnamon. Stir well until combined.
3. Seal the jar and refrigerate for 30 minutes or overnight.
4. Before serving, stir again and top with natural peanut butter.

MOCHA CHIP

Calories: 470 **Protein: 42** **Carbs: 46** **Fat: 19**

Ingredients — Servings: 1

- 1/2 cup quick oats
- 3/4 cup unsweetened almond milk
- 1 scoop Dummy Supps Chocolate Espresso Whey
- 1 tsp instant coffee
- 1 tbsp cocoa powder
- 1 tbsp Chocolate Espresso Dummy Butter
- 1 tbsp Lilly's chocolate chips

Instructions

1. In a jar, combine oats, almond milk, protein powder, instant coffee, and cocoa powder. Stir well until smooth.
2. Seal the jar and refrigerate for 30 minutes or overnight.
3. Before serving, stir again and top with Chocolate Espresso Dummy Butter and Lilly's chocolate chips.

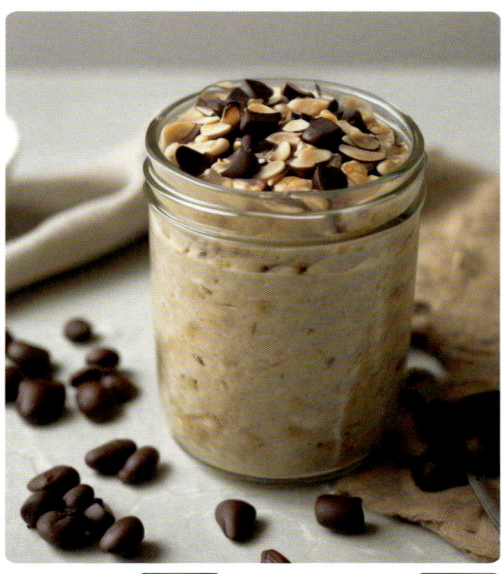

Dummy Supps Whey Protein [SCAN ME]

Dummy Butter Peanut Butter [SCAN ME]

OVERNIGHT OATS

CHOCOLATE COCONUT

Calories: 500 **Protein: 41** **Carbs: 47** **Fat: 21**

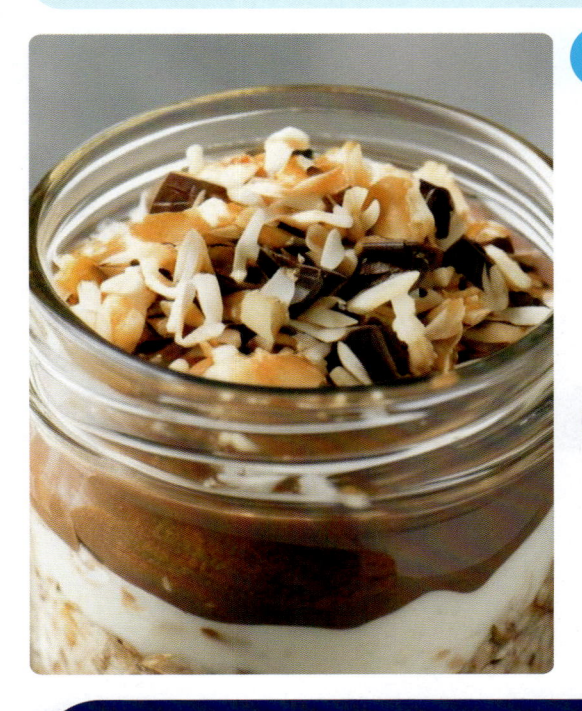

Ingredients — Servings: 1

- 1/2 cup quick oats
- 3/4 cup unsweetened almond milk
- 1 scoop Dummy Supps Chocolate Whey
- 1 tbsp shredded coconut
- 1/2 tsp vanilla extract
- 1 tbsp Chocolate Espresso Dummy Butter
- 1 tbsp Lily's chocolate chips

Instructions

1. In a jar, combine oats, almond milk, protein powder, shredded coconut, and vanilla extract. Stir well until smooth.
2. Seal the jar and refrigerate for 30 minutes or overnight.
3. Before serving, stir again and top with Chocolate Espresso Dummy Butter and Lily's chocolate chips.

BERRY BLISS

Calories: 440 **Protein: 41** **Carbs: 44** **Fat: 14**

Ingredients — Servings: 1

- 1/2 cup quick oats
- 3/4 cup unsweetened almond milk
- 1 scoop Dummy Supps Berry Whey
- 1/2 cup mixed berries
- 1/2 tsp vanilla extract
- 1 tbsp PB&J Dummy Butter

Instructions

1. In a jar, combine oats, almond milk, protein powder, mixed berries, and vanilla extract. Stir well until smooth.
2. Seal the jar and refrigerate for 30 minutes or overnight.
3. Before serving, stir again and top with PB&J Dummy Butter.

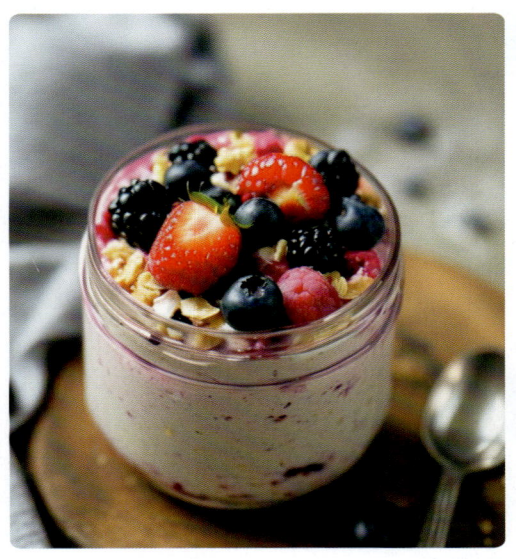

Dummy Supps Whey Protein **Dummy Butter Peanut Butter**

OVERNIGHT OATS

APPLE PIE OATS

Calories: 480   **Protein: 41**   **Carbs: 50**   **Fat: 17**

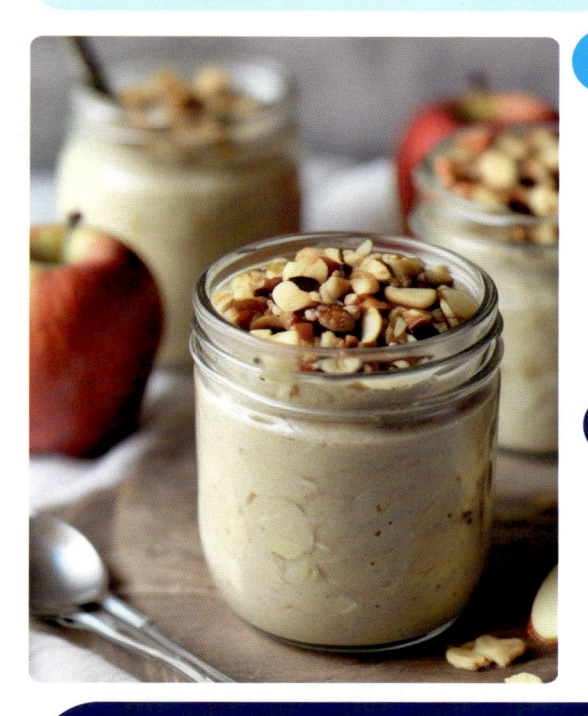

Ingredients   Servings: 1

- 1/2 cup quick oats
- 3/4 cup unsweetened almond milk
- 1 scoop Dummy Supps Cinnamon Roll Whey
- 1/2 small apple
- 1/2 tsp cinnamon
- 1 tbsp chopped walnuts
- 1/4 tsp salt
- 1/2 tsp vanilla extract

Instructions

1. Dice the apple into small pieces.
2. In a jar, combine oats, almond milk, protein powder, cinnamon, and diced apple. Stir well until smooth.
3. Seal the jar and refrigerate for 30 minutes or overnight.
4. Before serving, stir again and top with chopped walnuts.

CHOCOLATE CARAMEL DREAM

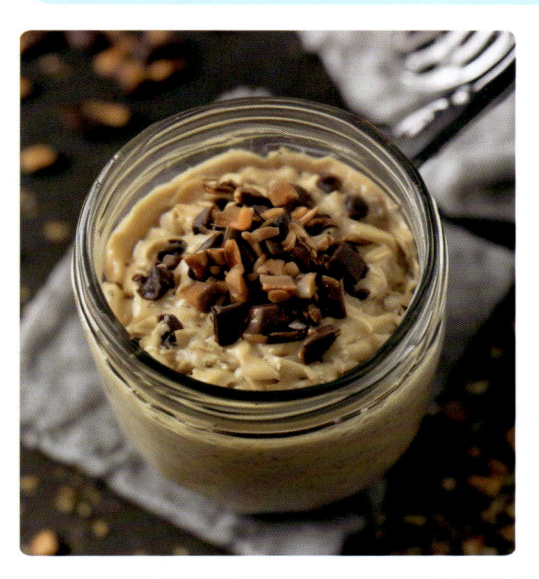

Calories: 430   **Protein: 41**   **Carbs: 39**   **Fat: 18**

Ingredients   Servings: 1

- 1/2 cup quick oats
- 3/4 cup unsweetened almond milk
- 1/2 scoop Dummy Supps Salted Caramel Whey + ½ scoop Chocolate Whey
- 1 tbsp cocoa powder
- 1 tbsp chopped walnuts
- 1 tbsp Chocolate Espresso Dummy Butter

Instructions

1. In a jar, combine oats, almond milk, protein powder, and cocoa powder. Stir well until smooth.
2. Seal the jar and refrigerate for 30 minutes or overnight.
3. Before serving, stir again and top with chopped walnuts and Chocolate Espresso Dummy Butter.

Dummy Supps Whey Protein   **Dummy Butter Peanut Butter**

OVERNIGHT OATS

PB&J OVERNIGHT OATS

Calories: 450   **Protein: 41**   **Carbs: 42**   **Fat: 17**

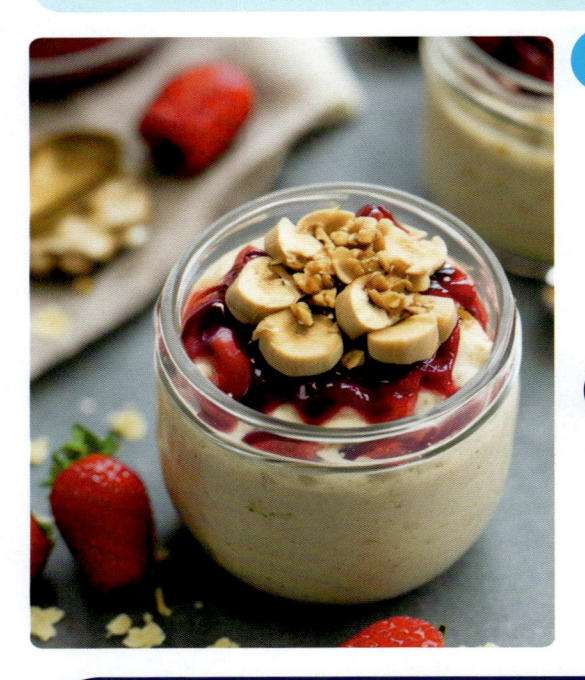

Ingredients   Servings: 1

- 1/2 cup quick oats
- 3/4 cup unsweetened almond milk
- 1 scoop Dummy Supps Berry Whey
- 1/2 cup diced strawberries
- 1/2 tsp vanilla extract
- 1 tbsp chopped walnuts
- 1 tbsp PB&J Dummy Butter

Instructions

1. In a jar, combine oats, almond milk, protein powder, diced strawberries, and vanilla extract. Stir well until smooth.
2. Seal the jar and refrigerate for 30 minutes or overnight.
3. Before serving, stir again and top with PB&J Dummy Butter.

MAPLE PECAN CRUNCH

Calories: 480   **Protein: 41**   **Carbs: 50**   **Fat: 17**

Ingredients   Servings: 1

- 1/2 cup quick oats
- 3/4 cup unsweetened almond milk
- 1 scoop Dummy Supps Cinnamon Roll Whey
- 1 tbsp maple syrup
- 1 tbsp chopped pecans
- 1/2 tsp cinnamon

Instructions

1. In a jar, combine oats, almond milk, protein powder, maple syrup, and cinnamon. Stir well until smooth.
2. Seal the jar and refrigerate for 30 minutes or overnight.
3. Before serving, stir again and top with chopped pecans.

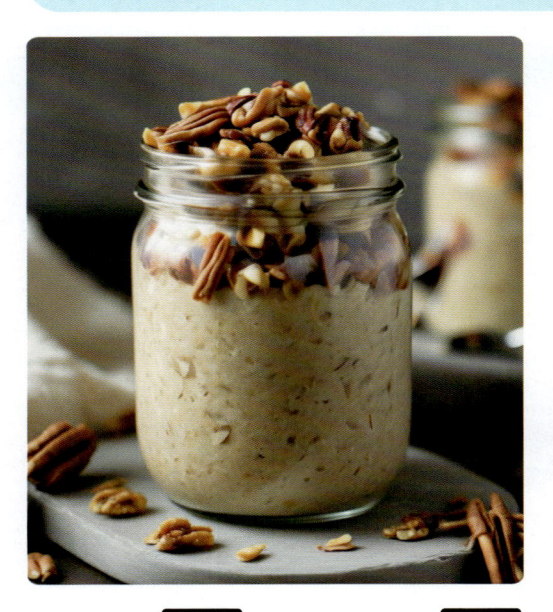

Dummy Supps Whey Protein   Dummy Butter Peanut Butter

OVERNIGHT OATS

ESPRESSO DELIGHT

Calories: 460 **Protein: 41** **Carbs: 43** **Fat: 18**

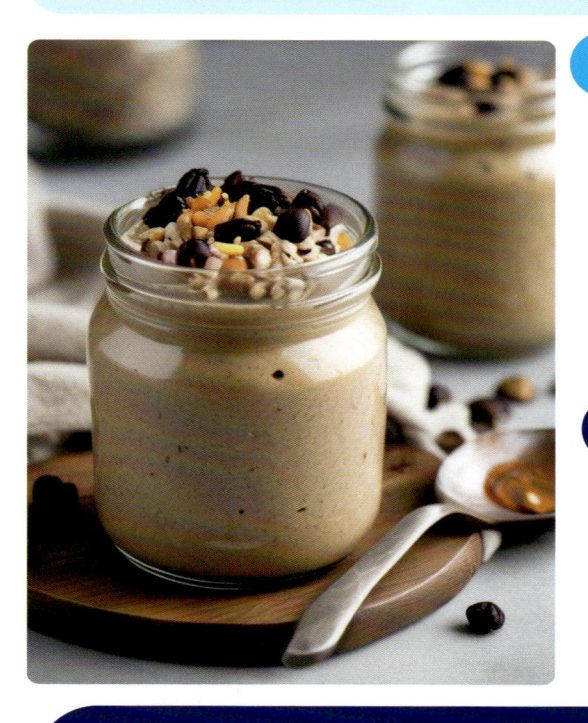

Ingredients — Servings: 1

- 1/2 cup quick oats
- 3/4 cup unsweetened almond milk
- 1 scoop Dummy Supps Chocolate Espresso Whey
- 1 tsp instant coffee
- 2 tbsp Lilly's chocolate chips
- 1 tbsp Chocolate Espresso Dummy Butter

Instructions

1. In a jar, combine oats, almond milk, protein powder, and instant coffee. Stir well until smooth.
2. Seal the jar and refrigerate for 30 minutes or overnight.
3. Before serving, stir again and top with Lily's chocolate chips and Chocolate Espresso Dummy Butter.

CHOCOLATE PEANUT BUTTER EXPLOSION

Calories: 510 **Protein: 43** **Carbs: 45** **Fat: 23**

Ingredients — Servings: 1

- 1/2 cup quick oats
- 3/4 cup unsweetened almond milk
- 1 scoop Dummy Supps Chocolate Peanut Butter Whey
- 1 tbsp natural peanut butter
- 2 tbsp Lily's chocolate chips
- 1 tbsp peanuts

Instructions

1. In a jar, combine oats, almond milk, and protein powder. Stir well until smooth.
2. Seal the jar and refrigerate for 30 minutes or overnight.
3. Before serving, stir again and top with natural peanut butter, Lily's chocolate chips, and peanuts.

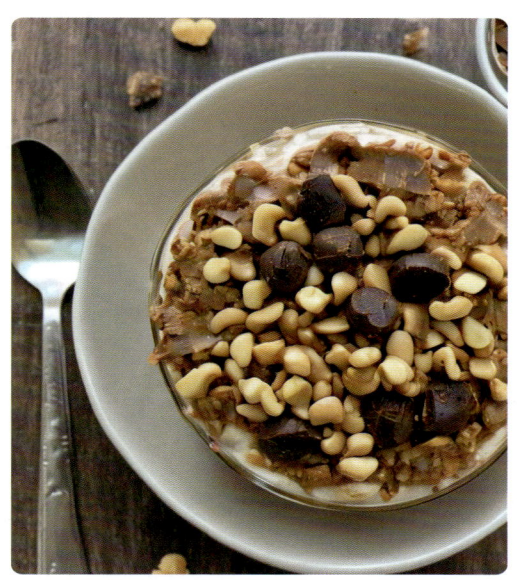

Dummy Supps Whey Protein — SCAN ME

Dummy Butter Peanut Butter — SCAN ME

OVERNIGHT OATS

VANILLA STRAWBERRY OVERNIGHT OATS

Calories: 490 **Protein: 43** **Carbs: 49** **Fat: 18**

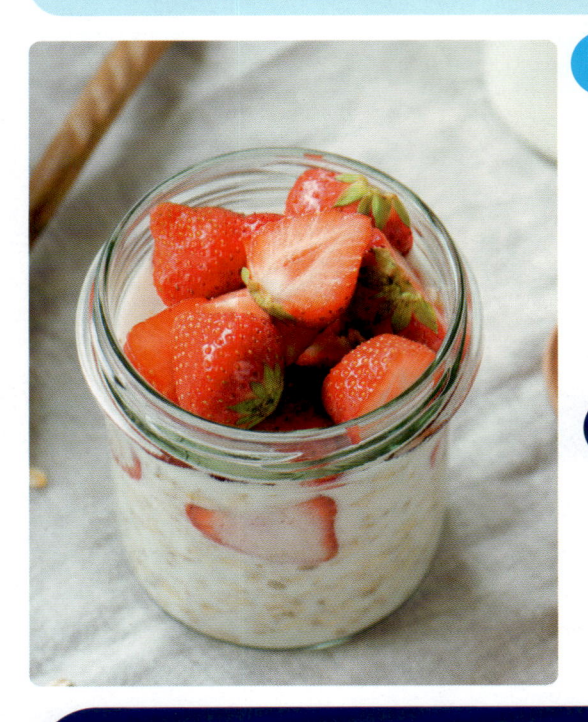

Ingredients Servings: 1

- 1/2 cup quick oats
- 3/4 cup unsweetened almond milk
- 1 scoop Dummy Supps vanilla whey
- 1/2 cup strawberries
- 1/2 tsp vanilla extract
- 1 tbsp Lilly's white chocolate chips
- 1/4 tsp salt
- 1 tbsp PB&J Dummy Butter

Instructions

1. In a jar, combine oats, almond milk, protein powder, diced strawberries, vanilla extract, and salt. Stir well until smooth.
2. Seal the jar and refrigerate for 30 minutes or overnight.
3. Before serving, stir again and top with Lily's white chocolate chips and PB&J Dummy Butter.

CHOCOLATE STRAWBERRY OVERNIGHT OATS

Calories: 500 **Protein: 43** **Carbs: 52** **Fat: 19**

Ingredients Servings: 1

- c3/4 cup unsweetened almond milk
- 1 scoop Dummy Supps chocolate whey
- 1/2 cup strawberries
- 1 tbsp cocoa powder
- 1/2 tsp vanilla extract
- 1/4 tsp salt
- 1 tbsp Lilly's chocolate chips
- 1 tbsp PB&J Dummy Butter

Instructions

1. In a jar, combine oats, almond milk, protein powder, cocoa powder, vanilla extract, salt, and diced strawberries. Stir well until smooth.
2. Seal the jar and refrigerate for 30 minutes or overnight.
3. Before serving, stir again and top with PB&J Dummy Butter.

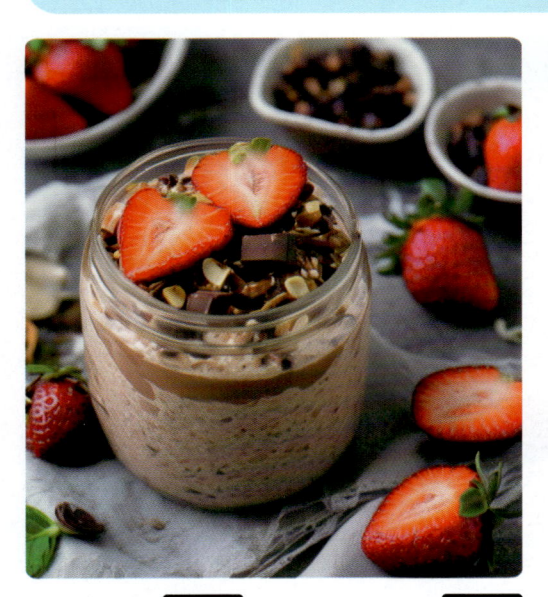

Dummy Supps Whey Protein

Dummy Butter Peanut Butter

OVERNIGHT OATS

RASPBERRY VANILLA OVERNIGHT OATS

Calories: 490 **Protein: 43** **Carbs: 48** **Fat: 18**

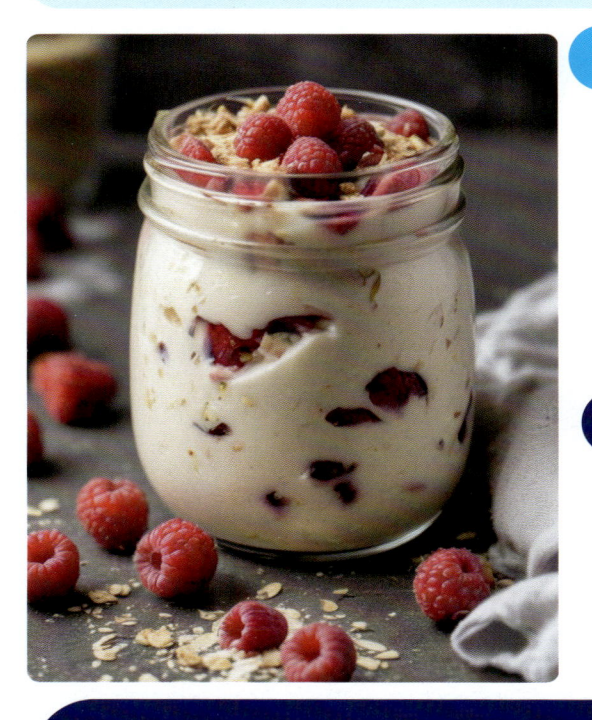

Ingredients Servings: 1

- 1/2 cup quick oats
- 3/4 cup unsweetened almond milk
- 1 scoop Dummy Supps Vanilla Whey
- 1/2 cup fresh or frozen raspberries
- 1/2 tsp vanilla extract
- 1 tbsp Lily's white chocolate chips
- 1 tbsp PB&J Dummy Butter

Instructions

1. In a jar, combine oats, almond milk, protein powder, raspberries, and vanilla extract. Stir well until smooth.
2. Seal the jar and refrigerate for 30 minutes or overnight.
3. Before serving, stir again and top with Lily's white chocolate chips and PB&J Dummy Butter.

CHOCOLATE RASPBERRY OVERNIGHT OATS

Calories: 500 **Protein: 43** **Carbs: 50** **Fat: 19**

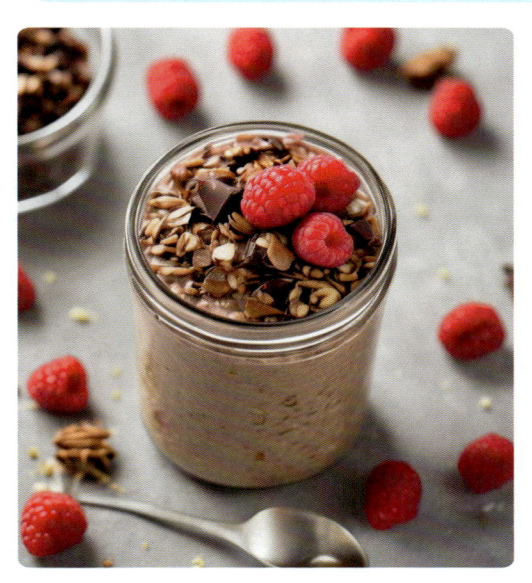

Ingredients Servings: 1

- 1/2 cup quick oats
- 3/4 cup unsweetened almond milk
- 1 scoop Dummy Supps Chocolate Whey
- 1/4 cup raspberries
- 1 tbsp cocoa powder
- 1 tbsp Lily's chocolate chips
- 1 tbsp Dummy Butter Chocolate Espresso

Instructions

1. In a jar, combine oats, almond milk, protein powder, cocoa powder, and raspberries. Stir well until smooth.
2. Seal the jar and refrigerate for 30 minutes or overnight.
3. Before serving, stir again and top with Lily's chocolate chips and Dummy Butter Chocolate Espresso.

Dummy Supps Whey Protein [SCAN ME]

Dummy Butter Peanut Butter [SCAN ME]

OTHER BREAKFASTS

OTHER BREAKFASTS

DAILY MEAL PREP IDEAS

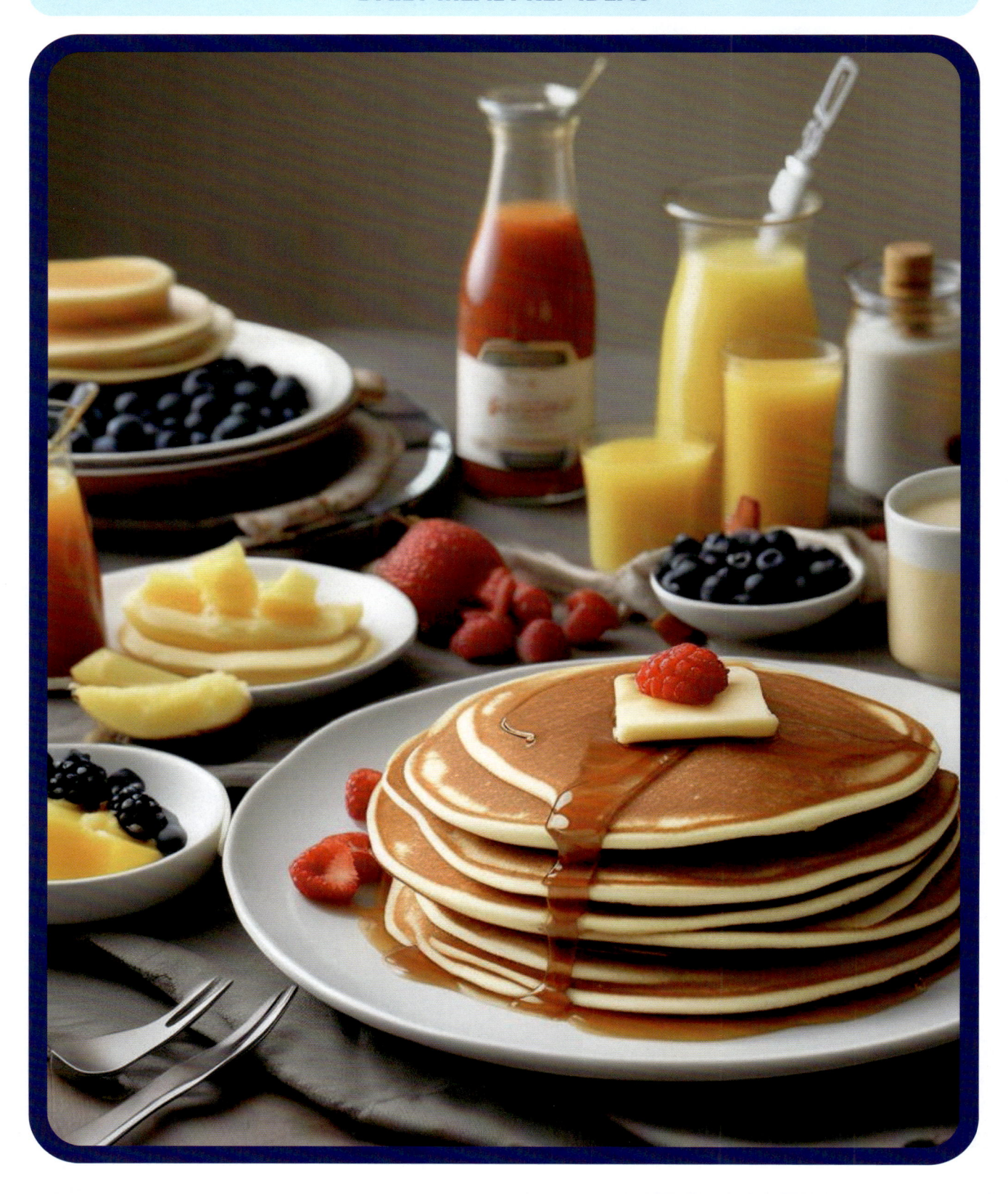

OTHER BREAKFASTS

PARFAIT & SHAKE

Calories: 540   **Protein: 44**   **Carbs: 42**   **Fats: 24**

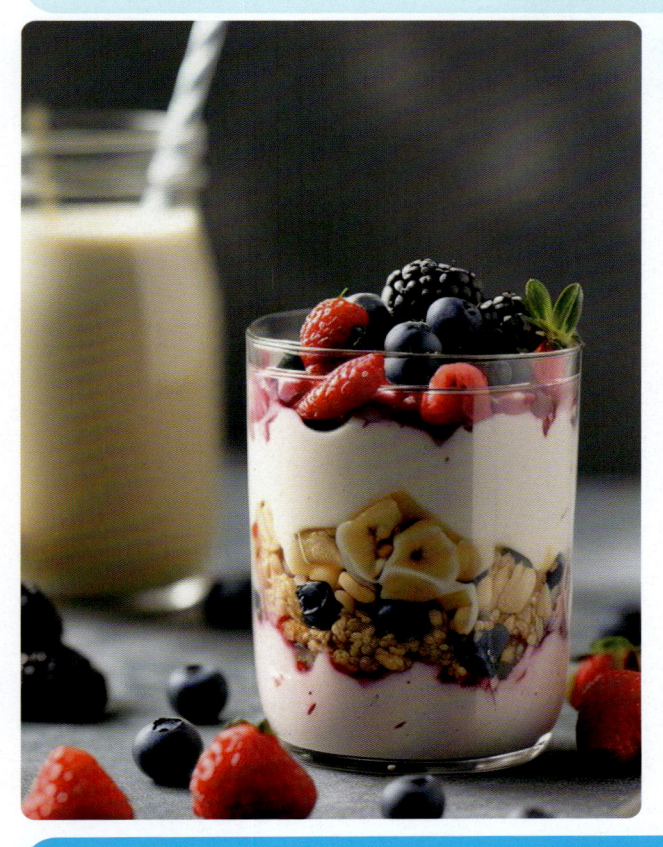

Ingredients   **Servings: 1**

Parfait & Shake:

- 3/4 cup nonfat plain greek yogurt (FAGE lactose free, Chobani, Oikos)
- 1 cup mixed berries (strawberries, blueberries, raspberries, blackberries)
- 2 tbsp PB&J Dummy Butter
- 1 scoop Dummy Supps whey
- 2 cups unsweetened almond milk

Optional Sides

- Salad (2 cups greens, 1 tbsp olive oil, 2 tbsp balsamic - 307c, 4P, 11C, 27F)
- Lilly's dark chips (1 serving - 60c, 1P, 5C, 5F)
- Powdered PB (2 tbsp - 50c, 5P, 5C, 2F)
- Honey (2 tbsp, 128c, 0P, 80C, 0F)

Instructions

1. In a bowl or jar, layer Greek yogurt, mixed berries, and PB&J Dummy Butter.
2. In a shaker, combine whey protein and almond milk, then shake until well mixed.
3. Serve the parfait chilled with the protein shake on the side.

Dummy Supps Whey Protein

Dummy Butter Peanut Butter

OTHER BREAKFASTS

BLUEBERRY FRENCH TOAST CASSEROLE

Calories: 360 **Protein: 36** **Carbs: 37** **Fats: 12**

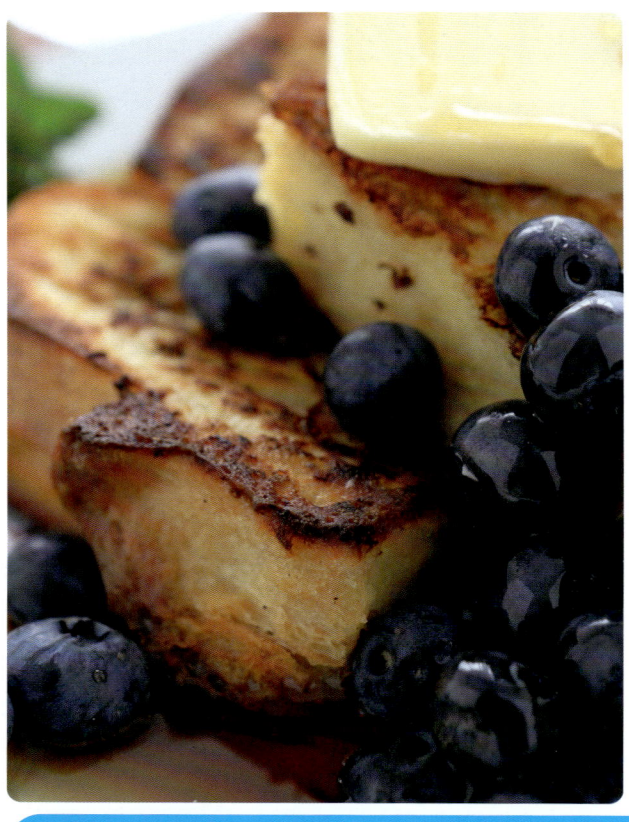

Ingredients **Servings: 9**

Cassorole:
- 12 slices 647 low-carb bread
- 6 eggs
- 3 cup egg whites
- 2 cups unsweetened almond milk
- 1 cup nonfat plain greek yogurt
- 5 scoops Dummy Supps vanilla whey protein
- 1 cup whipped cream cheese
- 2 tbsp vanilla extract
- 4 cups fresh blueberries
- 2 tbsp cinnamon
- 2 tbsp sugar free maple syrup (per portion)

Frosting:
- 1/2 cup whipped cream cheese
- 1/4 cup nonfat plain greek yogurt
- 2 tbsp monk fruit/stevia sweetener
- 1 scoop Dummy Supps vanilla whey
- 2 tbsp unsweetened almond milk

Dummy Supps Whey Protein

Instructions

1. Preheat oven to 350ºF and lightly coat a baking dish with cooking spray.
2. Cut bread into cubes and spread evenly in the baking dish.
3. In a large bowl, whisk together eggs, egg whites, almond milk, Greek yogurt, protein powder, whipped cream cheese, vanilla extract, and cinnamon until smooth.
4. Pour the mixture evenly over the bread, ensuring all pieces are coated.
5. Gently fold in blueberries.
6. Let sit for 10 minutes to absorb, then bake for 50-60 minutes until golden brown and set.
7. In a bowl, whisk together whipped cream cheese, Greek yogurt, sweetener, protein powder, and almond milk until smooth. Spread over the warm French toast bake before serving or serve on the side.
8. Drizzle each portion with sugar-free maple syrup.

OTHER BREAKFASTS

PEACH COBBLER FRENCH TOAST BAKE

Calories: 360 **Protein: 36** **Carbs: 33** **Fats: 12**

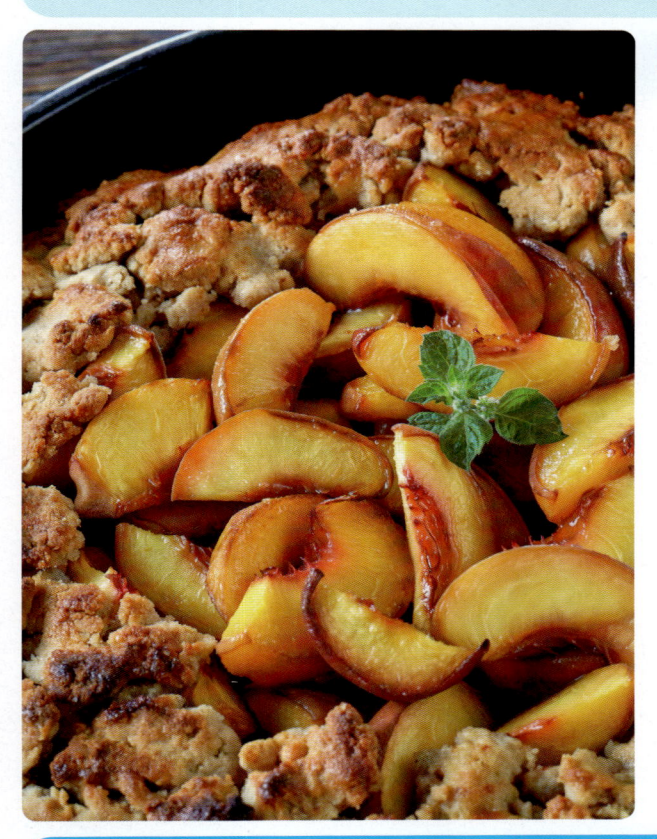

Ingredients   Servings: 9

Cassorole:
- 12 slices 647 low-carb bread
- 6 eggs
- 3 cup egg whites
- 2 cups unsweetened almond milk
- 1 cup nonfat plain greek yogurt
- 5 scoops Dummy Supps vanilla whey protein
- 1 cup whipped cream cheese
- 1 tbsp vanilla extract
- 2 (15 ounce) cans unsweetened sliced peaches
- 2 tbsp cinnamon
- 2 tbsp sugar free maple syrup (per portion)

Frosting:
- 1/2 cup whipped cream cheese
- 1/4 cup nonfat plain greek yogurt
- 2 tbsp monk fruit/stevia sweetener
- 1 scoop Dummy Supps vanilla whey
- 2 tbsp unsweetened almond milk

Dummy Supps Whey Protein

Instructions

1. Preheat oven to 350°F and lightly coat a baking dish with cooking spray.
2. Cut bread into cubes and spread evenly in the baking dish.
3. In a large bowl, whisk together eggs, egg whites, almond milk, Greek yogurt, protein powder, whipped cream cheese, vanilla extract, and cinnamon until smooth.
4. Drain peaches and gently fold them into the mixture.
5. Pour the mixture evenly over the bread, ensuring all pieces are coated.
6. Let sit for 10 minutes to absorb, then bake for 50-60 minutes until golden brown and set.
7. In a bowl, whisk together whipped cream cheese, Greek yogurt, sweetener, protein powder, and almond milk until smooth. Spread over the warm French toast bake before serving or serve on the side.
8. Drizzle each portion with sugar-free maple syrup.

OTHER BREAKFASTS

APPLE COBBLER FRENCH TOAST BAKE

Calories: 330 **Protein: 36** **Carbs: 27** **Fats: 12**

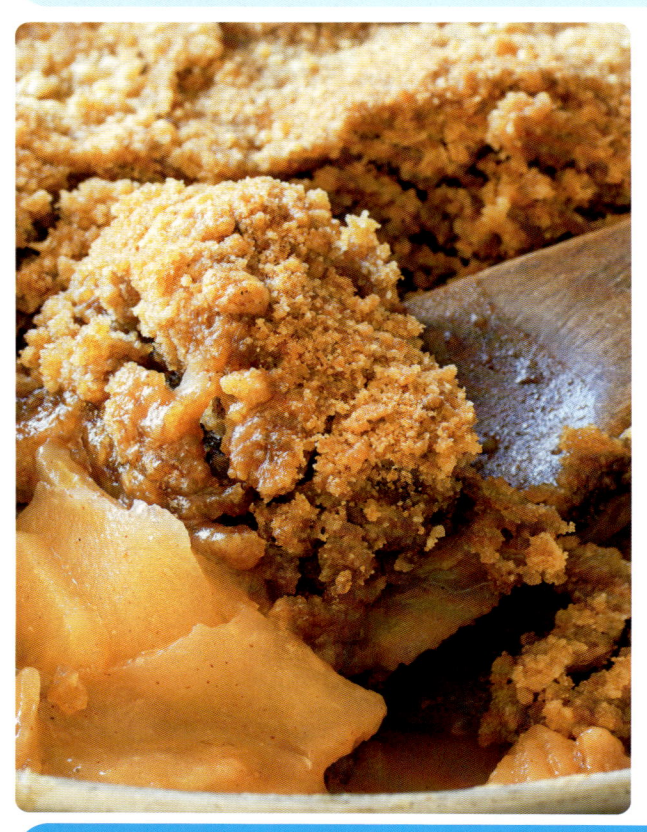

Ingredients **Servings: 9**

Cassorole:
- 12 slices 647 low-carb bread
- 6 eggs
- 3 cup egg whites
- 2 cups unsweetened almond milk
- 1 cup nonfat plain greek yogurt
- 5 scoops Dummy Supps vanilla whey protein
- 1 cup whipped cream cheese
- 2 (15 ounce) cans unsweetened apples
- 1 tbsp vanilla extract
- 2 tbsp cinnamon
- 2 tbsp sugar free maple syrup (per portion)

Frosting:
- 1/2 cup whipped cream cheese
- 1/4 cup nonfat plain greek yogurt
- 2 tbsp monk fruit/stevia sweetener
- 1 scoop Dummy Supps vanilla whey
- 2 tbsp unsweetened almond milk

Dummy Supps Whey Protein

Instructions

1. Preheat oven to 350°F and lightly coat a baking dish with cooking spray.
2. Cut bread into cubes and spread evenly in the baking dish.
3. In a large bowl, whisk together eggs, egg whites, almond milk, Greek yogurt, protein powder, whipped cream cheese, vanilla extract, and cinnamon until smooth.
4. Drain apples and gently fold them into the mixture.
5. Pour the mixture evenly over the bread, ensuring all pieces are coated.
6. Let sit for 10 minutes to absorb, then bake for 50-60 minutes until golden brown and set.
7. In a bowl, whisk together whipped cream cheese, Greek yogurt, sweetener, protein powder, and almond milk until smooth. Spread over the warm French toast bake before serving or serve on the side.
8. Drizzle each portion with sugar-free maple syrup.

OTHER BREAKFASTS

PB CHOCOLATE FRENCH TOAST BAKE

Calories: 440 **Protein: 40** **Carbs: 30** **Fats: 21**

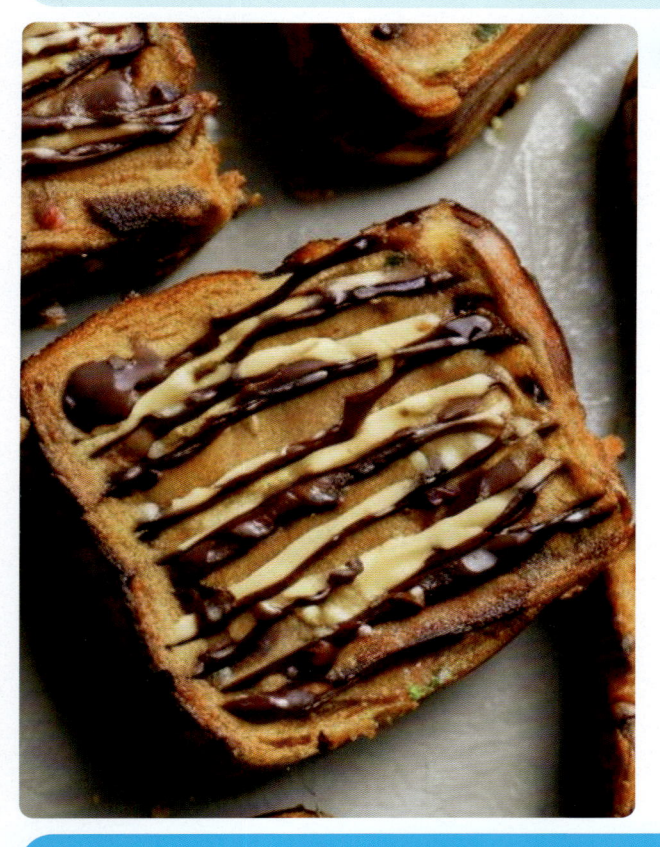

Ingredients Servings: 9

Cassorole:
- 12 slices 647 low-carb bread
- 6 eggs
- 3 cup egg whites
- 2 cups unsweetened almond milk
- 1 cup nonfat plain greek yogurt
- 5 scoops Dummy Supps Chocolate Peanut Butter whey
- 1 cup whipped cream cheese
- 1/2 cup Chocolate Espresso Dummy Butter/Peanut Butter
- 1 tbsp vanilla extract
- 2 tbsp cinnamon
- 2 tbsp sugar free maple syrup (per portion)

Frosting:
- 1/2 cup whipped cream cheese
- 1/4 cup nonfat plain greek yogurt
- 2 tbsp monk fruit/stevia sweetener
- 1 scoop Dummy Supps vanilla whey
- 2 tbsp unsweetened almond milk
- 2 tbsp Chocolate Espresso Dummy Butter

Dummy Supps Whey Protein — SCAN ME

Instructions

1. Preheat oven to 350ºF and lightly coat a baking dish with cooking spray.
2. Cut bread into cubes and spread evenly in the baking dish.
3. In a large bowl, whisk together eggs, egg whites, almond milk, Greek yogurt, protein powder, vanilla extract, cinnamon, and ¼ cup Dummy Butter Peanut Butter until smooth.
4. Pour the mixture evenly over the bread, ensuring all pieces are coated.
5. Let sit for 10 minutes to absorb, then bake for 50-60 minutes until golden brown and set.
6. In a bowl, whisk together whipped cream cheese, Greek yogurt, sweetener, protein powder, almond milk, and 2 tbsp Dummy Butter Peanut Butter until smooth.
7. Spread frosting over the warm French toast bake before serving or serve on the side.
8. Drizzle each portion with sugar-free maple syrup and the remaining ¼ cup Dummy Butter Peanut Butter.

OTHER BREAKFASTS

PROTEIN PANCAKES

Calories: 527 **Protein: 64** **Carbs: 46** **Fats: 7**

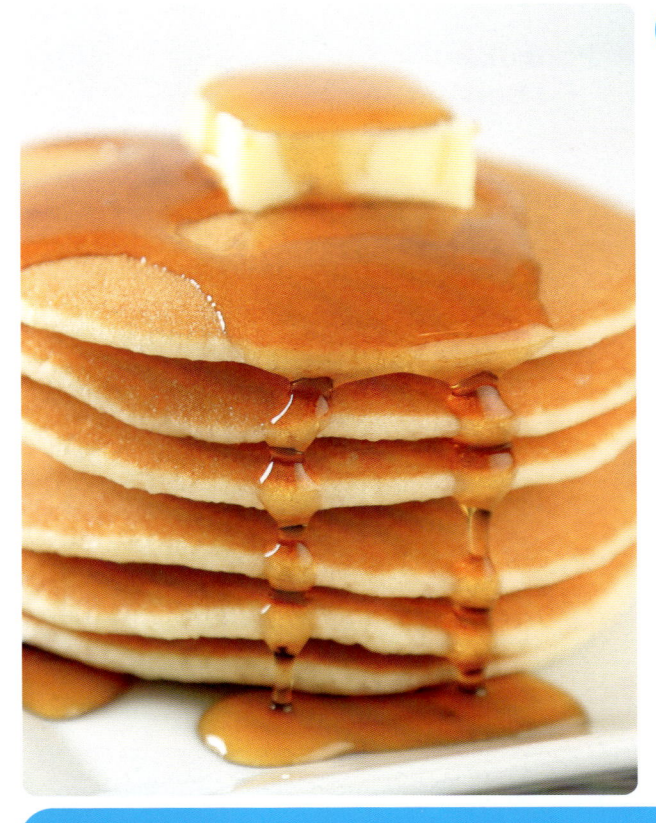

Ingredients **Servings: 1**

Pancakes:
- 1 banana
- 1 egg
- 2 tbsp unsweetened almond flour
- 1/4 cup nonfat plain Greek yogurt
- 2 scoops Dummy Supps Vanilla Whey
- 1 tsp vanilla extract
- 1/4 tsp baking powder
- 1/4 tsp salt

Optional Sides

- Salad (2 cups greens, 1 tbsp olive oil, 2 tbsp balsamic - 307c, 4P, 11C, 27F)
- Protein shake (2 cups almond milk, 1 scoop Dummy Supps - 200c, 28P, 5C, 7F)
- Butter (1 tsp - 32c, 0P, 0C, 4F)
- Sugar-free maple syrup (2 tbsp - 5c, 0P, 3C, 0F)

Dummy Supps Whey Protein

Instructions

1. Mash the banana in a bowl until smooth.
2. Add egg, almond flour, Greek yogurt, protein powder, vanilla extract, baking powder, and salt. Stir until fully combined.
3. Heat a non-stick skillet over low heat and coat with cooking spray.
4. Pour batter onto the skillet in small circles and cook for 3-4 minutes until bubbles form on the surface.
5. Flip and cook for another 2-3 minutes until golden brown.

OTHER BREAKFASTS

CHOCOLATE CHIP PROTEIN PANCAKES

Calories: 590 **Protein: 65** **Carbs: 46** **Fats: 18**

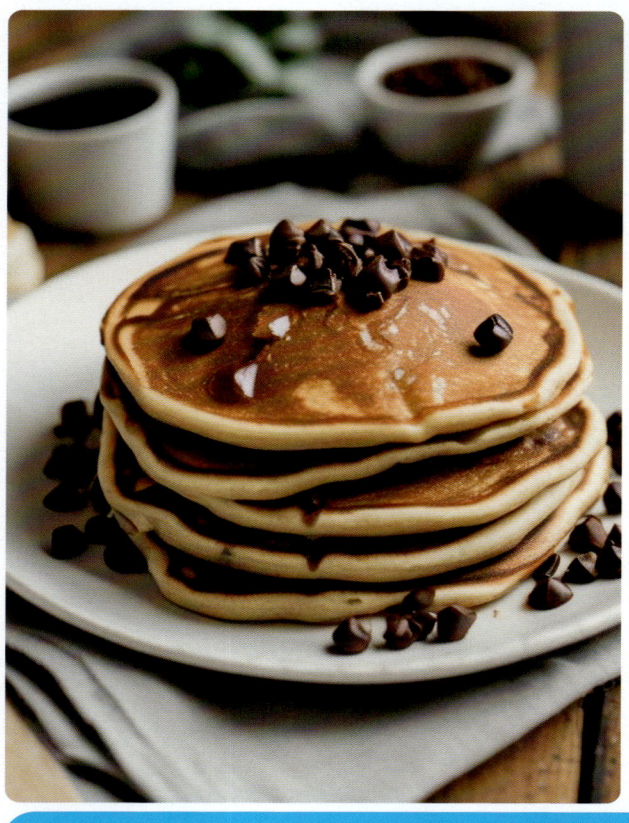

Ingredients Servings: 1

Pancakes:
- 1 banana
- 1 egg
- 2 tbsp unsweetened almond milk
- 1/4 cup nonfat plain Greek yogurt
- 2 scoops Dummy Supps Vanilla Whey
- 2 tbsp Lilly's dark chocolate chips
- 1 tsp vanilla extract
- 1/4 tsp baking powder
- 1/4 tsp salt
- 2 tbsp almond flour

Optional Sides
- Salad (2 cups greens, 1 tbsp olive oil, 2 tbsp balsamic - 307c, 4P, 11C, 27F)
- Protein shake (2 cups almond milk, 1 scoop Dummy Supps - 200c, 28P, 5C, 7F)
- Butter (1 tsp - 32c, 0P, 0C, 4F)
- Sugar-free maple syrup (2 tbsp - 5c, 0P, 3C, 0F)

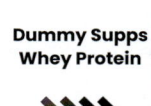

Dummy Supps Whey Protein — SCAN ME

Instructions
1. Mash the banana in a bowl until smooth.
2. Add egg, almond milk, Greek yogurt, almond flour, protein powder, vanilla extract, baking powder, and salt. Stir until fully combined.
3. Fold in Lily's dark chocolate chips.
4. Heat a non-stick skillet over low heat and coat with cooking spray.
5. Pour batter onto the skillet in small circles and cook for 3-4 minutes until bubbles form on the surface.
6. Flip and cook for another 2-3 minutes until golden brown.

OTHER BREAKFASTS

CHOCOLATE PB BANANA PANCAKES

Calories: 590   **Protein: 65**   **Carbs: 46**   **Fats: 18**

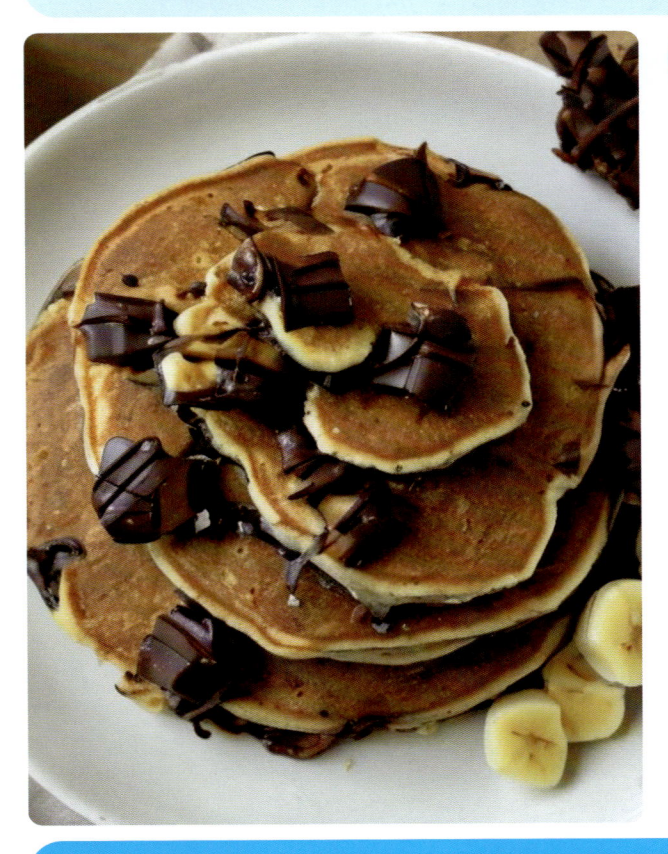

Ingredients   **Servings: 1**

Pancakes:
- 1 banana
- 1 egg
- 2 tbsp almond milk
- 1/4 cup nonfat plain greek yogurt
- 2 scoops Dummy Supps Chocolate Whey
- 1 tsp vanilla extract
- 1/4 tsp baking powder
- 1/4 tsp salt
- 2 tbsp almond flour

Optional Sides

- Salad (2 cups greens, 1 tbsp olive oil, 2 tbsp balsamic - 307c, 4P, 11C, 27F)
- Protein shake (2 cups almond milk, 1 scoop Dummy Supps - 200c, 28P, 5C, 7F)
- Butter (1 tsp - 32c, 0P, 0C, 4F)
- Sugar-free maple syrup (2 tbsp - 5c, 0P, 3C, 0F)

Dummy Supps Whey Protein — SCAN ME

Instructions

1. Mash the banana in a bowl until smooth.
2. Add egg, almond milk, Greek yogurt, almond flour, protein powder, vanilla extract, baking powder, and salt. Stir until fully combined.
3. Heat a non-stick skillet over low heat and coat with cooking spray.
4. Pour batter onto the skillet in small circles and cook for 3-4 minutes until bubbles form on the surface.
5. Flip and cook for another 2-3 minutes until golden brown and fully set.

OTHER BREAKFASTS

BLUEBERRY PANCAKES

Calories: 570 **Protein: 65** **Carbs: 45** **Fats: 14**

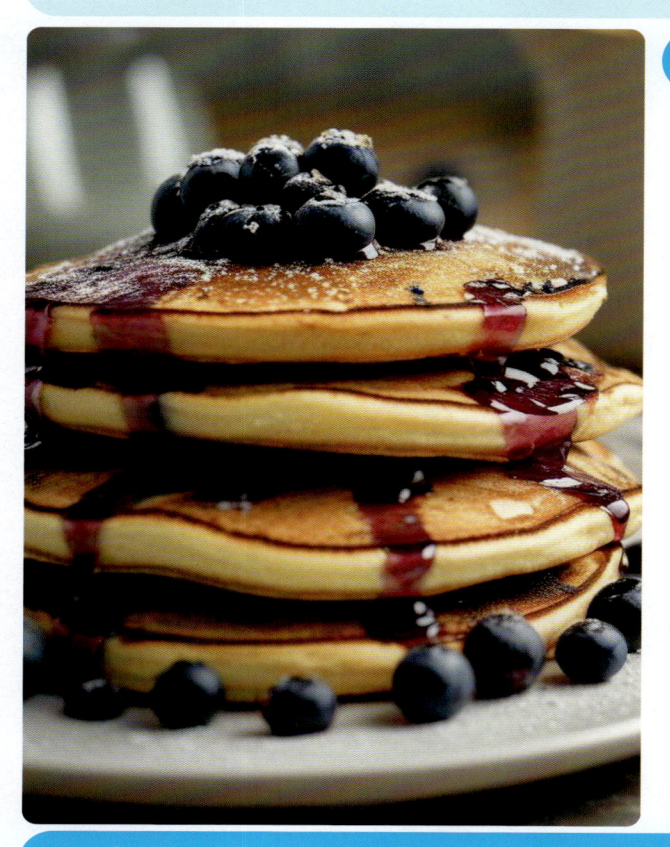

Ingredients **Servings: 1**

Pancakes:
- 1 banana
- 1 egg
- 2 tbsp unsweetened almond milk
- 1/4 cup nonfat plain Greek yogurt
- 2 scoops Dummy Supps Berry/Vanilla Whey
- 1 cup fresh or frozen blueberries
- 1 tsp vanilla extract
- 1/4 tsp baking powder
- 1/4 tsp salt
- 2 tbsp almond flour

Optional Sides
- Salad (2 cups greens, 1 tbsp olive oil, 2 tbsp balsamic - 307c, 4P, 11C, 27F)
- Protein shake (2 cups almond milk, 1 scoop Dummy Supps - 200c, 28P, 5C, 7F)
- Butter (1 tsp - 32c, 0P, 0C, 4F)
- Sugar-free maple syrup (2 tbsp - 5c, 0P, 3C, 0F)

Dummy Supps Whey Protein [QR code]

Instructions
1. In a bowl, mash the banana until smooth.
2. Add egg, almond milk, Greek yogurt, almond flour, protein powder, vanilla extract, baking powder, and salt. Stir until fully combined.
3. Gently fold in blueberries.
4. Heat a non-stick skillet over low heat and coat with cooking spray.
5. Pour batter onto the skillet in small circles and cook for 3-4 minutes until bubbles form on the surface.
6. Flip and cook for another 2-3 minutes until golden brown.

OTHER BREAKFASTS

CHOCOLATE ESPRESSO PANCAKES

Calories: 590   **Protein: 65**   **Carbs: 46**   **Fats: 18**

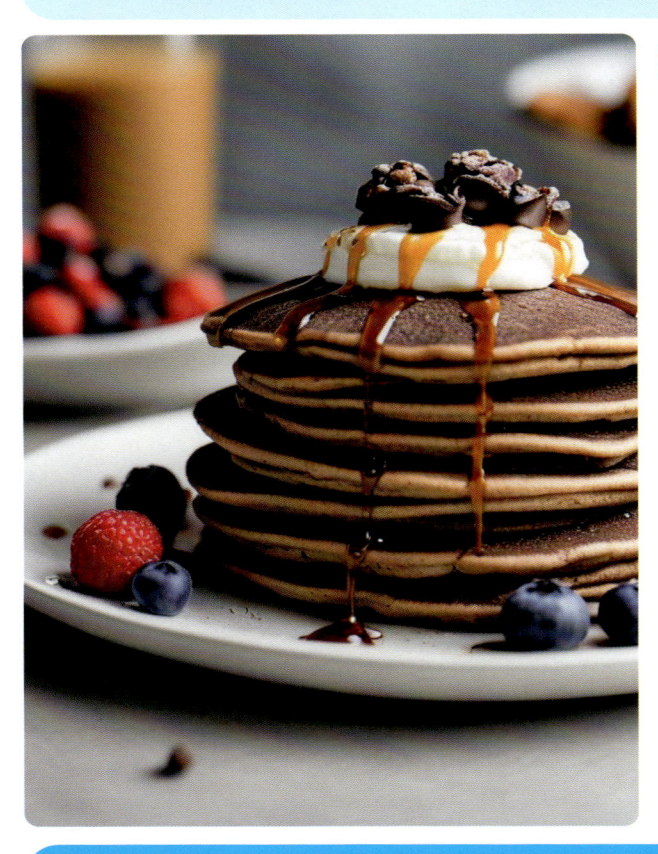

Ingredients   Servings: 1

Pancakes:
- 1 banana
- 1 egg
- 2 tbsp unsweetened almond milk
- 1/4 cup nonfat plain Greek yogurt
- 2 scoops Dummy Supps Chocolate Whey
- 2 tbsp Lilly's Dark Chocolate Chips
- 1 tsp instant coffee
- 1 tsp vanilla extract
- 1/4 tsp baking powder
- 1/4 tsp salt
- 2 tbsp almond flour

Optional Sides
- Salad (2 cups greens, 1 tbsp olive oil, 2 tbsp balsamic - 307c, 4P, 11C, 27F)
- Protein shake (2 cups almond milk, 1 scoop Dummy Supps - 200c, 28P, 5C, 7F)
- Butter (1 tsp - 32c, 0P, 0C, 4F)
- Sugar-free maple syrup (2 tbsp - 5c, 0P, 3C, 0F)

Dummy Supps Whey Protein

Instructions
1. In a bowl, mash the banana until smooth.
2. Add egg, almond milk, Greek yogurt, almond flour, protein powder, instant coffee, vanilla extract, baking powder, and salt. Stir until fully combined.
3. Fold in Lily's dark chocolate chips.
4. Heat a non-stick skillet over low heat and coat with cooking spray.
5. Pour batter onto the skillet in small circles and cook for 3-4 minutes until bubbles form on the surface.
6. Flip and cook for another 2-3 minutes until golden brown.

OTHER BREAKFASTS

SALTED CARAMEL PANCAKES

Calories: 590 **Protein: 65** **Carbs: 46** **Fats: 18**

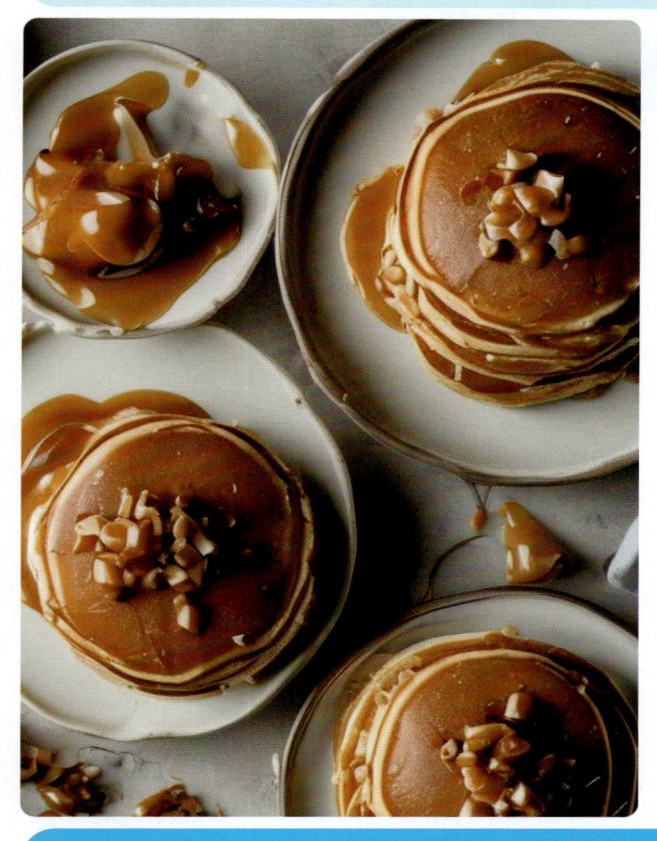

Ingredients — Servings: 1

Pancakes:
- 1 banana
- 1 egg
- 2 tbsp unsweetened almond milk
- 1/4 cup nonfat plain Greek yogurt
- 2 scoops Dummy Supps Salted Caramel Whey
- 2 tbsp Lilly's Salted Caramel Chips
- 1 tsp vanilla extract
- 1/4 tsp baking powder
- 1/4 tsp salt
- 2 tbsp almond flour

Optional Sides
- Salad (2 cups greens, 1 tbsp olive oil, 2 tbsp balsamic - 307c, 4P, 11C, 27F)
- Protein shake (2 cups almond milk, 1 scoop Dummy Supps - 200c, 28P, 5C, 7F)
- Butter (1 tsp - 32c, 0P, 0C, 4F)
- Sugar-free maple syrup (2 tbsp - 5c, 0P, 3C, 0F)

Dummy Supps Whey Protein

Instructions
1. Mash the banana in a bowl until smooth.
2. Add egg, almond milk, Greek yogurt, almond flour, protein powder, vanilla extract, baking powder, and salt. Stir until fully combined.
3. Fold in Lily's Salted Caramel Chips.
4. Heat a non-stick skillet over low heat and coat with cooking spray.
5. Pour batter onto the skillet in small circles and cook for 3-4 minutes until bubbles form on the surface.
6. Flip and cook for another 2-3 minutes until golden brown.

OTHER BREAKFASTS

CINNAMON ROLL PANCAKES

Calories: 580   **Protein: 65**   **Carbs: 40**   **Fats: 19**

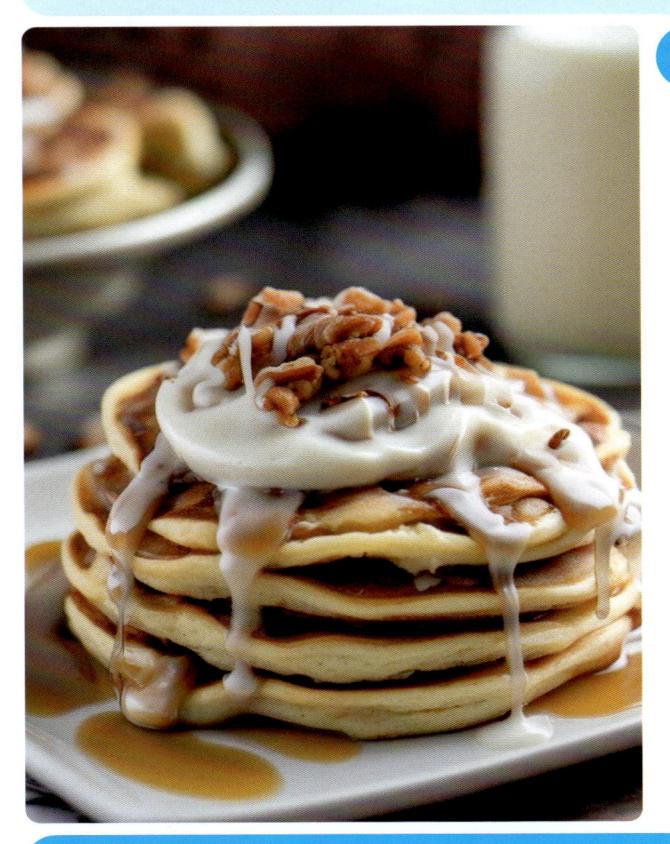

Ingredients   Servings: 1

Pancakes:
- 1 banana
- 1 egg
- ¼ cup nonfat plain Greek yogurt
- 2 scoops Dummy Supps Vanilla Whey
- 1 tsp vanilla extract
- 1/4 tsp baking powder
- 1/4 tsp salt
- 1/2 tsp cinnamon
- 1/4 cup whipped cream cheese
- 1/4 tsp monk fruit/stevia sweetener
- 1 tbsp unsweetened almond milk
- 2 tbsp almond flour

Optional Sides
- Salad (2 cups greens, 1 tbsp olive oil, 2 tbsp balsamic - 307c, 4P, 11C, 27F)
- Protein shake (2 cups almond milk, 1 scoop Dummy Supps - 200c, 28P, 5C, 7F)
- Butter (1 tsp - 32c, 0P, 0C, 4F)
- Sugar-free maple syrup (2 tbsp - 5c, 0P, 3C, 0F)

Dummy Supps Whey Protein

Instructions
1. Mash the banana in a bowl until smooth.
2. Add egg, Greek yogurt, almond flour, protein powder, vanilla extract, baking powder, salt, and cinnamon. Stir until fully combined.
3. Heat a non-stick skillet over low heat and coat with cooking spray.
4. Pour batter onto the skillet in small circles and cook for 3-4 minutes until bubbles form on the surface.
5. Flip and cook for another 2-3 minutes until golden brown.
6. In a separate bowl, whisk together whipped cream cheese, sweetener, and almond milk until smooth.
7. Spread frosting over pancakes before serving.

OTHER BREAKFASTS

PROTEIN WAFFLES

Calories: 400   **Protein: 45**   **Carbs: 29**   **Fats: 10**

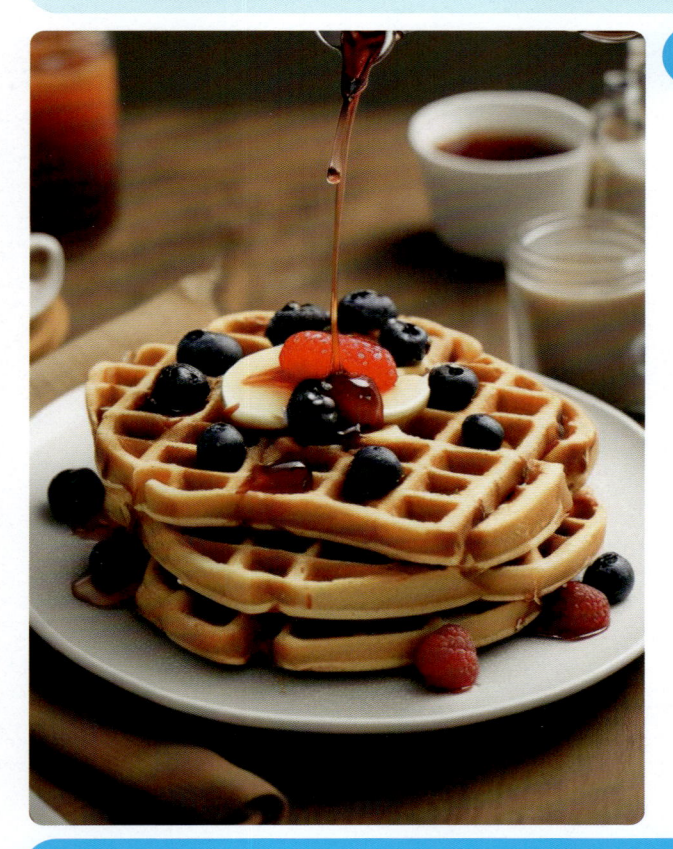

Ingredients   Servings: 1

Waffles:
- 1/2 cup nonfat plain greek yogurt
- 1 egg
- 1/4 cup oat flour
- 1 scoop Dummy Supps Vanilla whey protein
- 1 tbsp vanilla extract
- 1/4 tsp baking powder
- 1/4 tsp salt

Optional Sides
- Salad (2 cups greens, 1 tbsp olive oil, 2 tbsp balsamic - 307c, 4P, 11C, 27F)
- Protein shake (2 cups almond milk, 1 scoop Dummy Supps - 200c, 28P, 5C, 7F)
- Butter (1 tsp - 32c, 0P, 0C, 4F)
- Sugar-free maple syrup (2 tbsp - 5c, 0P, 3C, 0F)

Dummy Supps Whey Protein SCAN ME

Instructions
1. Preheat waffle iron and lightly coat with cooking spray.
2. In a bowl, whisk together Greek yogurt, egg, and vanilla extract until smooth.
3. In a separate bowl, mix oat flour, whey protein, baking powder, baking soda, and salt.
4. Combine dry ingredients into wet ingredients and mix until a smooth batter forms. Let it sit for 5 minutes to allow the flour to absorb liquid.
5. Pour batter into the waffle iron and cook on medium-low heat until golden brown and crisp (about 4-6 minutes depending on waffle iron).

OTHER BREAKFASTS

CHOCOLATE CHIP PROTEIN WAFFLES

Calories: 460 **Protein: 46** **Carbs: 37** **Fats: 14**

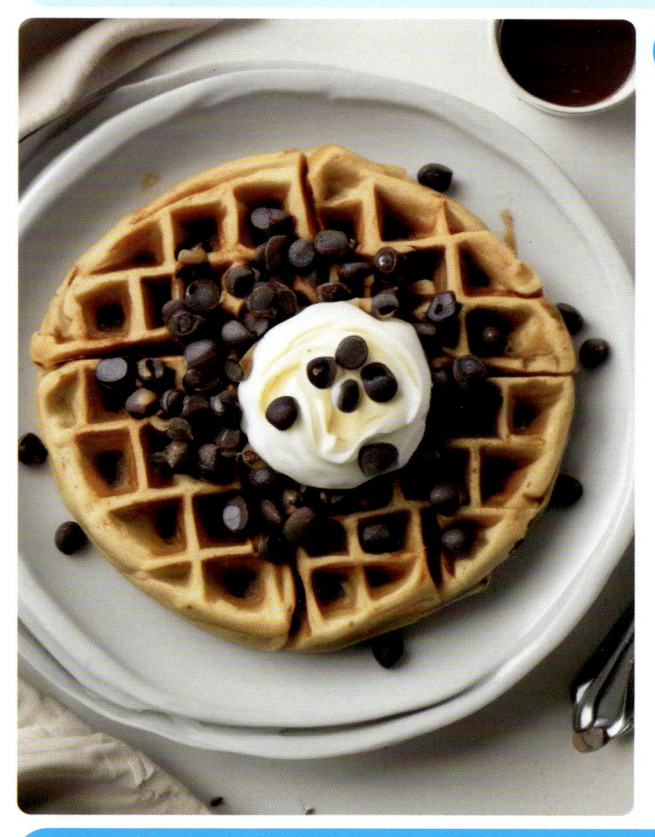

Ingredients **Servings: 1**

Waffles:
- 1/2 cup nonfat plain greek yogurt
- 1 egg
- 1/4 cup oat flour
- 1 scoop Dummy Supps Vanilla whey protein
- 1 tbsp vanilla extract
- 2 tbsp Lilly's dark chocolate chips
- 1/4 tsp baking powder
- 1/4 tsp salt

Optional Sides
- Salad (2 cups greens, 1 tbsp olive oil, 2 tbsp balsamic - 307c, 4P, 11C, 27F)
- Protein shake (2 cups almond milk, 1 scoop Dummy Supps - 200c, 28P, 5C, 7F)
- Butter (1 tsp - 32c, 0P, 0C, 4F)
- Sugar-free maple syrup (2 tbsp - 5c, 0P, 3C, 0F)

Dummy Supps Whey Protein

Instructions
1. Preheat waffle iron and lightly coat with cooking spray.
2. In a bowl, whisk together Greek yogurt, egg, and vanilla extract until smooth.
3. In a separate bowl, mix oat flour, whey protein, baking powder, baking soda, and salt.
4. Combine dry ingredients into wet ingredients and mix until a smooth batter forms. Let it sit for 5 minutes to allow the flour to absorb liquid.
5. Fold in Lily's dark chocolate chips.
6. Pour batter into the waffle iron and cook on medium-low heat until golden brown and crisp (about 4-6 minutes depending on waffle iron).

OTHER BREAKFASTS

CHOCOLATE PEANUT BUTTER WAFFLES

Calories: 600 **Protein: 54** **Carbs: 42** **Fats: 26**

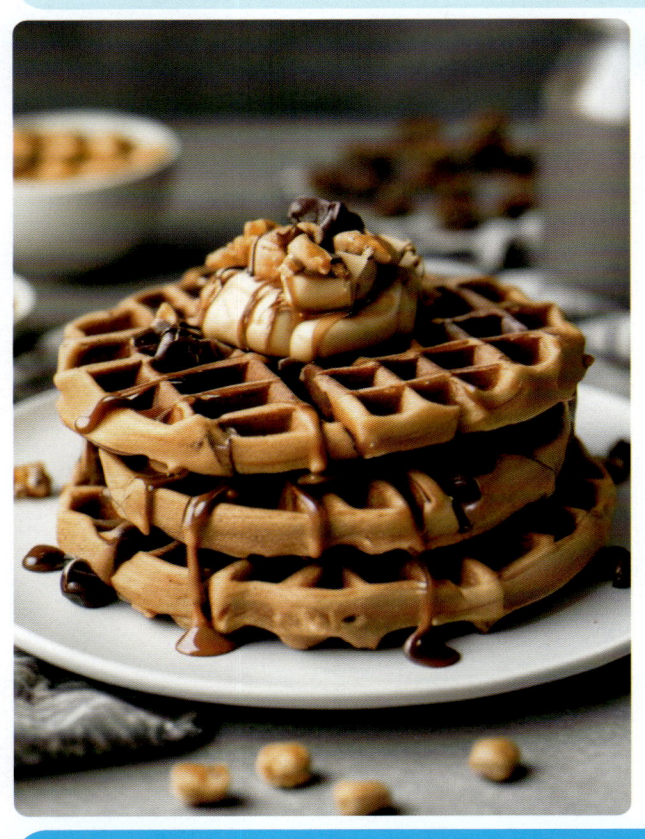

Ingredients Servings: 1

Waffles:
- 1/2 cup nonfat plain Greek yogurt
- 1 egg
- 1/4 cup oat flour
- 1 scoop Dummy Supps Chocolate Peanut Butter Whey
- 1 tbsp vanilla extract
- 2 tbsp Lilly's peanut butter chips
- 1 tbsp Dummy Butter Peanut Butter
- 1/4 tsp baking powder
- 1/4 tsp salt

Optional Sides
- Salad (2 cups greens, 1 tbsp olive oil, 2 tbsp balsamic - 307c, 4P, 11C, 27F)
- Protein shake (2 cups almond milk, 1 scoop Dummy Supps - 200c, 28P, 5C, 7F)
- Butter (1 tsp - 32c, 0P, 0C, 4F)
- Sugar-free maple syrup (2 tbsp - 5c, 0P, 3C, 0F)

Dummy Supps Whey Protein

Instructions
1. Preheat waffle iron and lightly coat with cooking spray.
2. In a bowl, whisk together Greek yogurt, egg, vanilla extract, and Dummy Butter Peanut Butter until smooth.
3. In a separate bowl, mix oat flour, whey protein, baking powder, baking soda, and salt.
4. Combine dry ingredients into wet ingredients and mix until a smooth batter forms. Let sit for 5 minutes.
5. Pour batter into the waffle iron and cook on medium-low heat for 4-6 minutes until golden brown and crisp.

OTHER BREAKFASTS

CINNAMON ROLL WAFFLES

Calories: 580   **Protein: 48**   **Carbs: 45**   **Fats: 23**

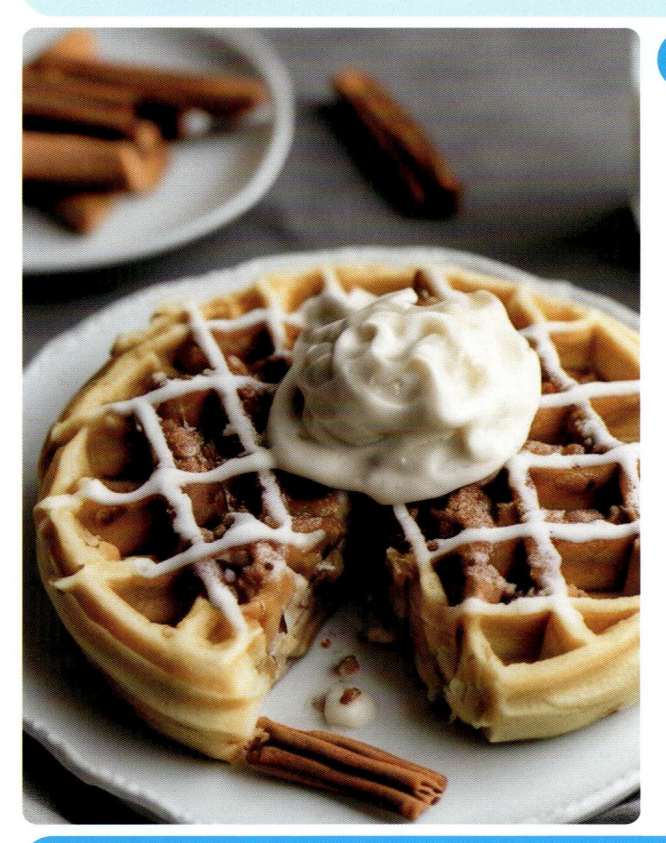

Ingredients — Servings: 1

Waffles:
- 1/2 cup nonfat plain Greek yogurt
- 1 egg
- 1/4 cup oat flour
- 1 scoop Dummy Supps Vanilla Whey
- 2 tbsp Lilly's chocolate cinnamon chips
- 1 tbsp vanilla extract
- 1/2 tsp cinnamon
- 1/4 tsp baking powder
- 1/4 tsp salt
- 1/4 cup whipped cream cheese
- 1 tsp monk fruit/stevia sweetener
- 1 tbsp unsweetened almond milk

Optional Sides

- Salad (2 cups greens, 1 tbsp olive oil, 2 tbsp balsamic - 307c, 4P, 11C, 27F)
- Protein shake (2 cups almond milk, 1 scoop Dummy Supps - 200c, 28P, 5C, 7F)
- Butter (1 tsp - 32c, 0P, 0C, 4F)
- Sugar-free maple syrup (2 tbsp - 5c, 0P, 3C, 0F)

Dummy Supps Whey Protein — SCAN ME

Instructions

1. Preheat waffle iron and lightly coat with cooking spray.
2. In a bowl, whisk together Greek yogurt, egg, and vanilla extract until smooth.
3. In a separate bowl, mix oat flour, whey protein, cinnamon, baking powder, baking soda, and salt.
4. Combine dry ingredients into wet ingredients and mix until a smooth batter forms. Let sit for 5 minutes.
5. Fold in Lily's chocolate cinnamon chips.
6. Pour batter into the waffle iron and cook on medium-low heat for 4-6 minutes until golden brown and crisp.
7. In a small bowl, whisk together whipped cream cheese, sweetener, and almond milk until smooth.
8. Spread frosting over warm waffles before serving.

OTHER BREAKFASTS

SALTED CARAMEL WAFFLES

Calories: 460 **Protein: 46** **Carbs: 37** **Fats: 14**

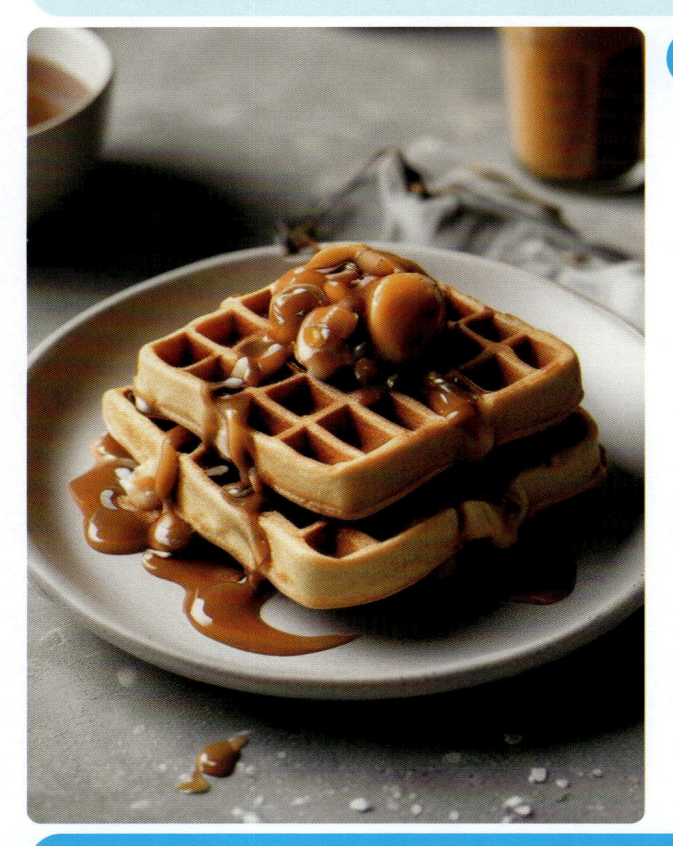

Ingredients   Servings: 1

Waffles:
- 1/2 cup nonfat plain Greek yogurt
- 1 egg
- 1/4 cup oat flour
- 1 scoop Dummy Supps Salted Caramel Whey
- 2 tbsp Lilly's Salted Caramel Chips
- 1 tbsp vanilla extract
- 1/4 tsp baking powder
- 1/4 tsp salt

Optional Sides

- Salad (2 cups greens, 1 tbsp olive oil, 2 tbsp balsamic - 307c, 4P, 11C, 27F)
- Protein shake (2 cups almond milk, 1 scoop Dummy Supps - 200c, 28P, 5C, 7F)
- Butter (1 tsp - 32c, 0P, 0C, 4F)
- Sugar-free maple syrup (2 tbsp - 5c, 0P, 3C, 0F)

Dummy Supps Whey Protein

Instructions

1. Preheat waffle iron and lightly coat with cooking spray.
2. In a bowl, whisk together Greek yogurt, egg, and vanilla extract until smooth.
3. In a separate bowl, mix oat flour, whey protein, cinnamon, baking powder, baking soda, and salt.
4. Combine dry ingredients into wet ingredients and mix until a smooth batter forms. Let sit for 5 minutes.
5. Fold in Lily's chocolate cinnamon chips.
6. Pour batter into the waffle iron and cook on medium-low heat for 4-6 minutes until golden brown and crisp.
7. In a small bowl, whisk together whipped cream cheese, sweetener, and almond milk until smooth.
8. Spread frosting over warm waffles before serving.

OTHER BREAKFASTS

CHOCOLATE ESPRESSO WAFFLES

Calories: 470 **Protein: 45** **Carbs: 45** **Fats: 23**

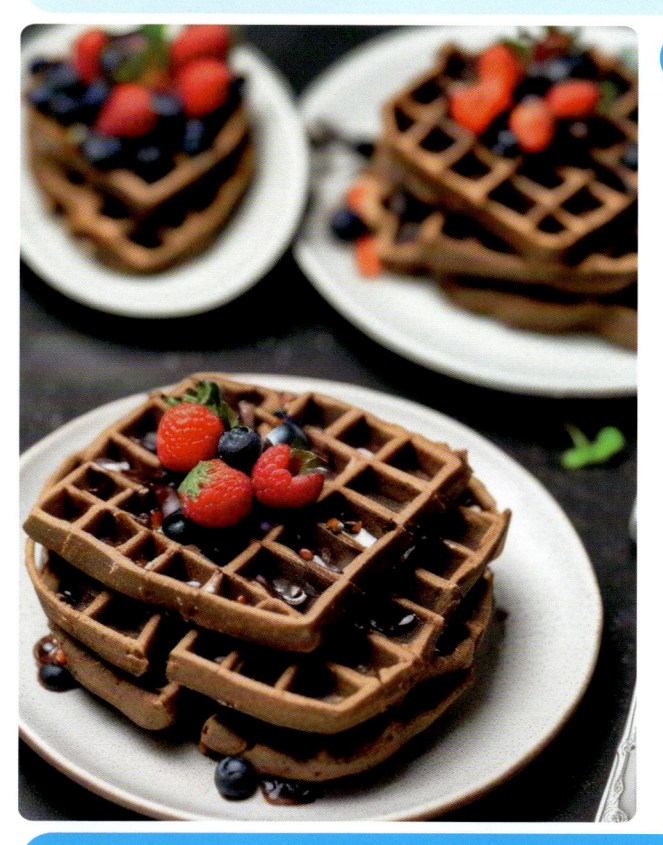

Ingredients Servings: 1

Waffles:
- 1/2 cup nonfat plain Greek yogurt
- 1 egg
- 1/4 cup oat flour
- 1 scoop Dummy Supps Chocolate Whey
- 2 tbsp Lilly's Dark Chocolate Chips
- 1 tbsp vanilla extract
- 1 tsp instant coffee
- 1 tbsp cocoa powder
- 1/4 tsp baking powder
- 1/4 tsp salt

Optional Sides
- Salad (2 cups greens, 1 tbsp olive oil, 2 tbsp balsamic - 307c, 4P, 11C, 27F)
- Protein shake (2 cups almond milk, 1 scoop Dummy Supps - 200c, 28P, 5C, 7F)
- Butter (1 tsp - 32c, 0P, 0C, 4F)
- Sugar-free maple syrup (2 tbsp - 5c, 0P, 3C, 0F)

Dummy Supps Whey Protein

Instructions
1. Preheat waffle iron and lightly coat with cooking spray.
2. In a bowl, whisk together Greek yogurt, egg, vanilla extract, and instant coffee until smooth.
3. In a separate bowl, mix oat flour, whey protein, cocoa powder, baking powder, baking soda, and salt.
4. Combine dry ingredients into wet ingredients and mix until a smooth batter forms. Let sit for 5 minutes.
5. Fold in Lily's Dark Chocolate Chips.
6. Pour batter into the waffle iron and cook on medium-low heat for 4-6 minutes until golden brown and crisp.

OTHER BREAKFASTS

PUMPKIN SPICE WAFFLES

Calories: 430 **Protein: 46** **Carbs: 34** **Fats: 10**

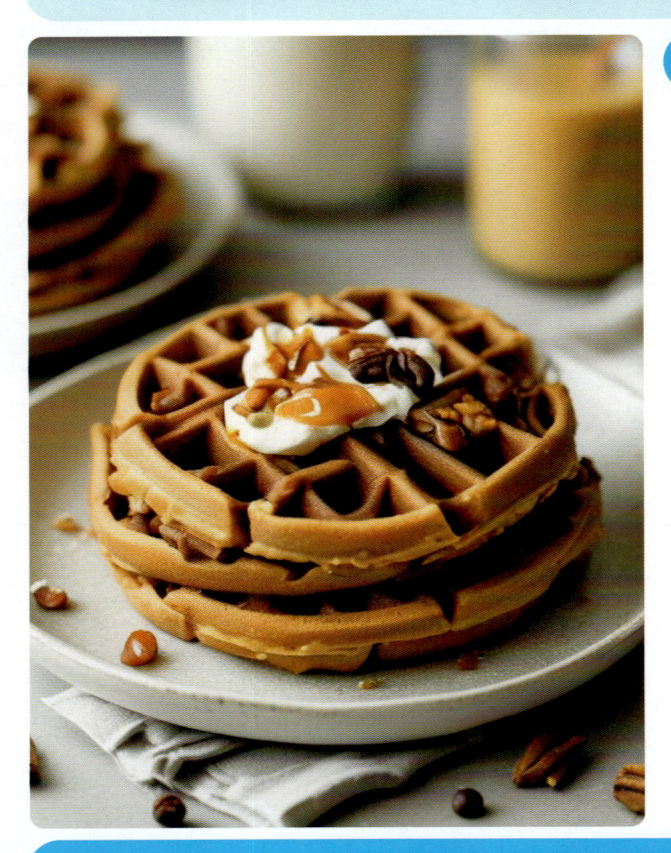

Ingredients Servings: 1

Waffles:
- 1/2 cup nonfat plain Greek yogurt
- 1 egg
- 1/4 cup oat flour
- 1 scoop Dummy Supps Vanilla Whey Protein
- 1/4 cup pumpkin puree
- 1 tbsp vanilla extract
- 1 tbsp almond milk
- 1/4 tsp baking powder
- 1/4 tsp salt
- 1 tsp pumpkin spice
- 1/2 tsp cinnamon

Optional Sides
- Salad (2 cups greens, 1 tbsp olive oil, 2 tbsp balsamic - 307c, 4P, 11C, 27F)
- Protein shake (2 cups almond milk, 1 scoop Dummy Supps - 200c, 28P, 5C, 7F)
- Lilly's dark chips (1 serving - 60c, 1P, 5C, 5F)
- Butter (1 tsp - 32c, 0P, 0C, 4F)
- Sugar-free maple syrup (2 tbsp - 5c, 0P, 3C, 0F)

Dummy Supps Whey Protein

Instructions
1. Preheat waffle iron and lightly coat with cooking spray.
2. In a bowl, whisk together Greek yogurt, egg, pumpkin puree, almond milk, and vanilla extract until smooth.
3. In a separate bowl, mix oat flour, whey protein, baking powder, baking soda, pumpkin spice, cinnamon, and salt.
4. Combine dry ingredients into wet ingredients and mix until a smooth batter forms. Let sit for 5 minutes.
5. Pour batter into the waffle iron and cook on medium-low heat for 4-6 minutes until golden brown and crisp.

OTHER BREAKFASTS

SAUSAGE MUFFINS

Calories: 480 **Protein: 49** **Carbs: 30** **Fats: 17**

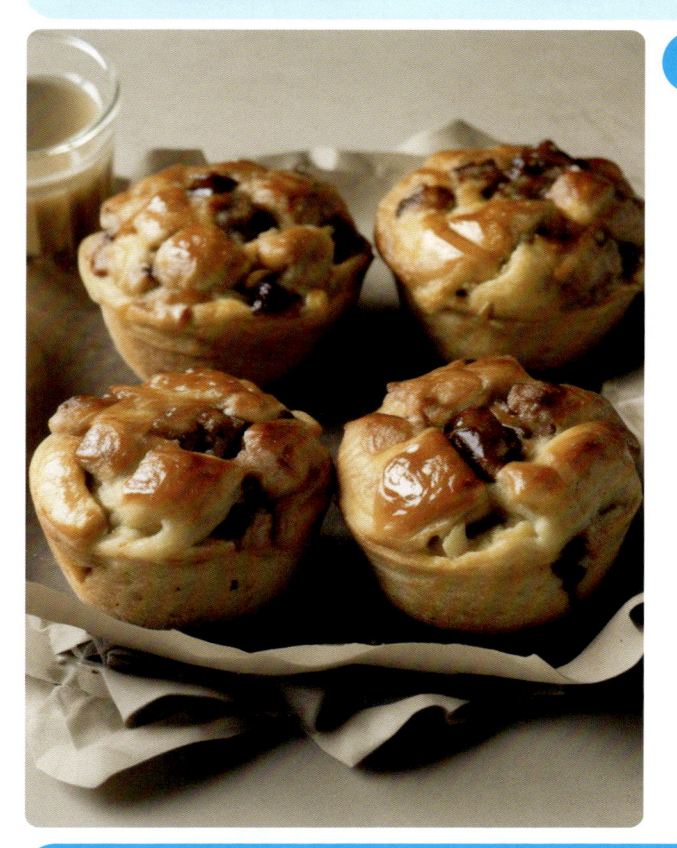

Ingredients **Servings: 6**

Muffins:

- 2 lb turkey sausage
- 2 cups Kodiak protein pancake mix
- 1 cup egg whites
- 1 cup sharp cheddar cheese
- 1/4 cup maple syrup
- 1 tsp garlic powder
- 1/2 tsp black pepper
- 1/2 tsp smoked paprika

Optional Sides

- Salad (2 cups greens, 1 tbsp olive oil, 2 tbsp balsamic - 307c, 4P, 11C, 27F)
- Protein shake (2 cups almond milk, 1 scoop Dummy Supps - 200c, 28P, 5C, 7F)
- Sugar-free maple syrup (2 tbsp, 5c, 0P, 3C, 0F)

Instructions

1. Preheat oven to 400° F
2. Cook turkey sausage in a pan with cooking spray on medium-high heat for 8-10 minutes until completely cooked.
3. Spray a large muffin tin with cooking spray.
4. In a large mixing bowl, combine protein pancake mix, egg whites, sharp cheddar cheese, maple syrup, and mix well.
5. Add cooked sausage to the batter.
6. Pour the mixture into the muffin tins.
7. Bake for 20 minutes until golden and completely cooked.

OTHER BREAKFASTS

PROTEIN BAGELS

Calories: 225   **Protein: 16**   **Carbs: 34**   **Fats: 1**

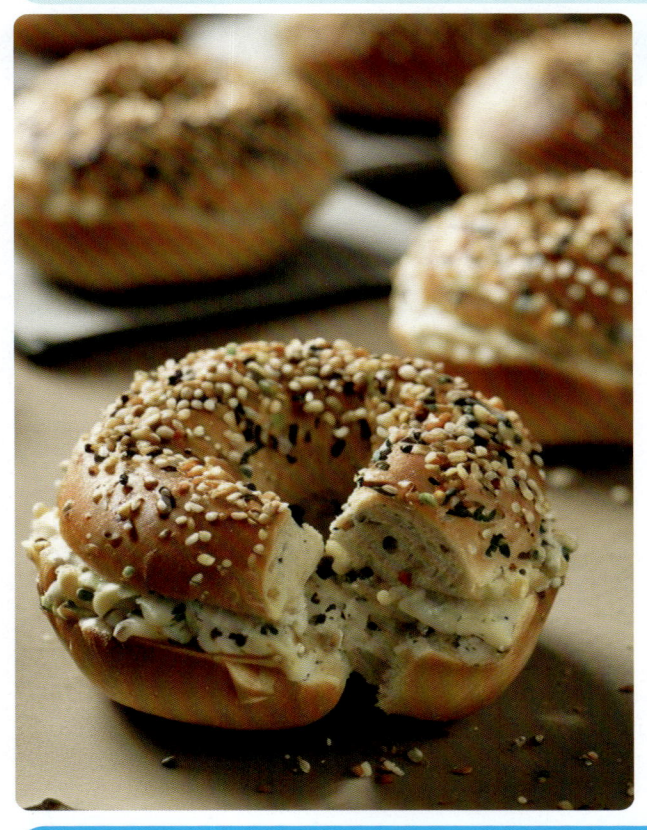

Ingredients   Servings: 1

Bagels:
- 1 1/2 cup all purpose flour
- 1 1/2 cup nonfat plain greek yogurt
- 4 tbsp egg whites
- 2 tsp baking powder
- 1/2 tsp baking powder
- 1/2 tsp salt
- 2 tbsp everything but the bagel seasoning

Optional Sides
- Whipped cream cheese (2 tbsp, 50c, 1P, 2C, 5F)
- Sugar free jelly (2 tbsp, 48c, 0P, 12C, 0F)
- Butter (1 tsp - 32c, 0P, 0C, 4F)

Instructions
1. Preheat oven to 375°F.
2. In a large mixing bowl, combine flour, Greek yogurt, egg whites, baking powder, baking soda, and salt. Mix until a dough forms.
3. Transfer dough to a lightly floured surface and knead for 2-3 minutes until smooth.
4. Divide dough into 4-6 equal portions, roll each into a log, and shape into bagels.
5. Place bagels on a parchment-lined baking sheet.
6. Brush each bagel with egg whites and sprinkle with Everything but the Bagel seasoning.
7. Bake for 25 minutes until golden brown.
8. Let cool for a few minutes before serving.

INDIVIDUAL MEAL PREP

SINGLE SERVING PREPS

DAILY MEAL PREP IDEAS

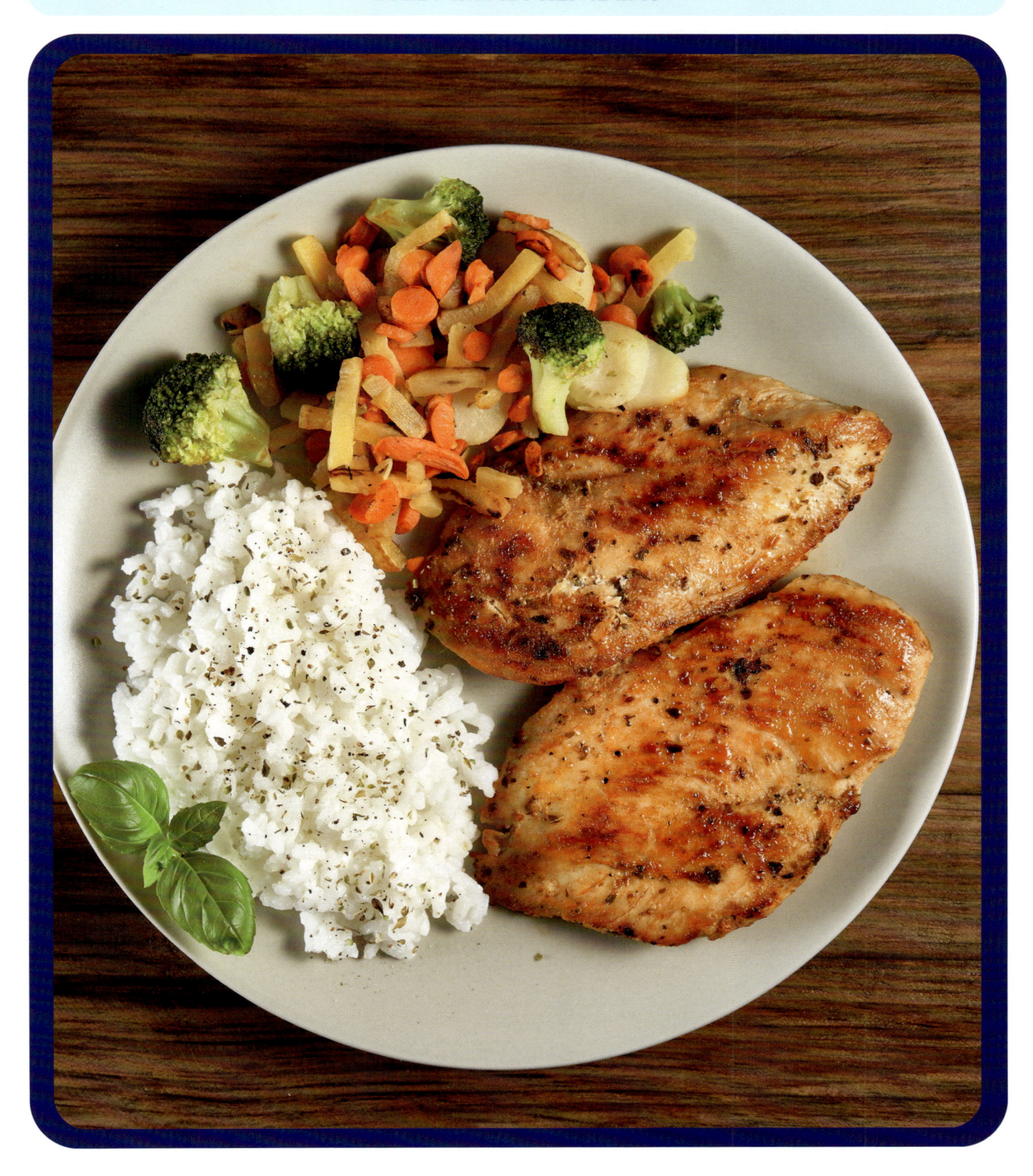

INDIVIDUAL MEAL PREP

CHICKEN PARMESAN

Calories: 510 **Protein: 65** **Carbs: 22** **Fat: 13**

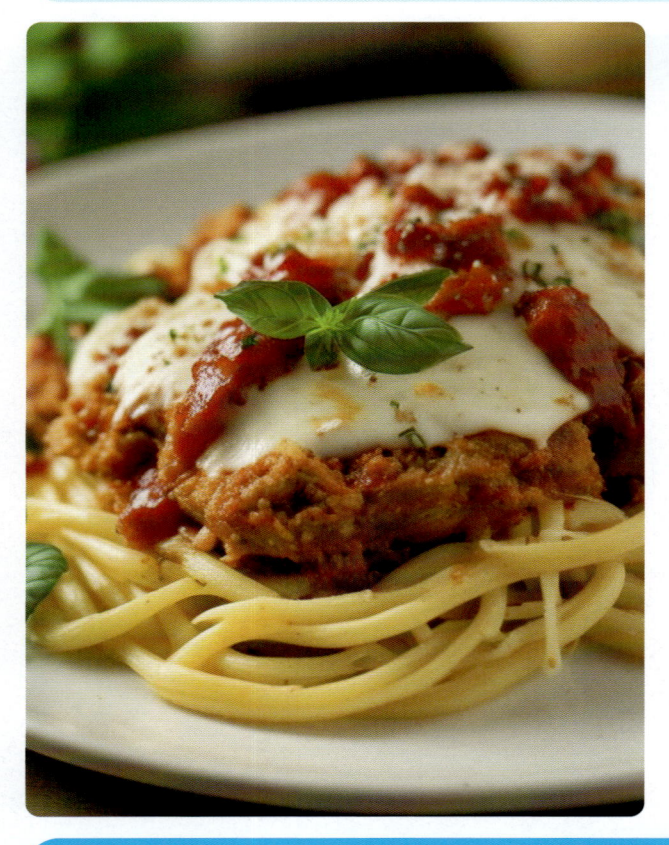

Ingredients   Servings: 1

Chicken Parmesan:
- 1 (6 oz.) chicken breast
- 1/4 cup egg whites
- 1/2 cup panko bread crumbs
- 1/4 cup low-fat mozzarella cheese
- 2 tbsp marinara sauce
- 1 tsp garlic powder
- 1/2 tsp onion powder
- 1 tsp Italian seasoning
- 1/2 tsp black pepper
- 1/4 tsp crushed red pepper

Optional Sides
- Protein pasta (2 oz: 190c, 10P, 38C, 1F)
- Salad (2 cups greens, 1 tbsp extra virgin olive oil, 2 tbsp balsamic - 307c, 4P, 11C, 27F)
- Protein shake (2 cups almond milk, 1 scoop Dummy Supps - 200c, 28P, 5C, 7F)

Instructions
1. Preheat air fryer or oven to 400°F.
2. Place egg whites and panko bread crumbs into separate large mixing bowls.
3. Season bread crumbs with listed seasonings.
4. Butterfly chicken breast, dredge in egg whites, then coat in bread crumbs.
5. Air fry/bake chicken for 10 minutes at 400°F.
6. Flip the chicken and top with mozzarella cheese and marinara sauce.
7. Cook for an additional 8-10 minutes until the cheese is melted and the chicken is completely cooked.

INDIVIDUAL MEAL PREP

CHICKEN ALFREDO

Calories: 590 **Protein: 66** **Carbs: 39** **Fat: 18**

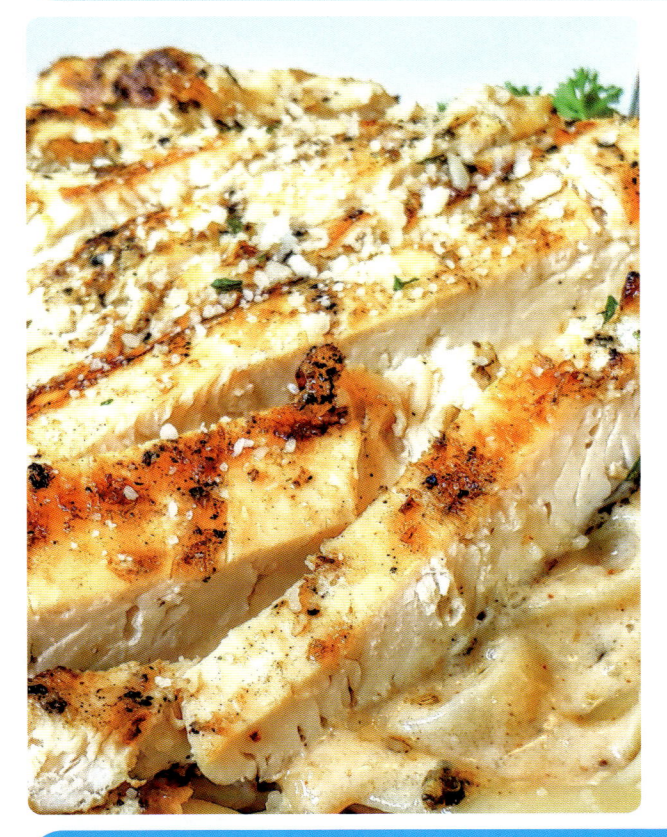

Ingredients — Servings: 1

Chicken:
- 1 (6 oz.) chicken breast
- 1/4 cup egg whites
- 1/2 cup panko bread crumbs
- 1 tsp garlic powder
- 1 tsp onion powder
- 1 tsp Italian seasoning
- 1/2 tsp black pepper
- 1/4 tsp salt

Alfredo Sauce:
- 1/2 cup low-fat cottage cheese
- 2 tbsp minced garlic
- 2 tbsp parmesan cheese
- 1/4 cup low-fat mozzarella cheese
- 1 tsp Italian seasoning
- 1/2 tsp black pepper

Optional Sides

- Protein pasta (2 oz: 190c, 10P, 38C, 1F)
- Salad (2 cups greens, 1 tbsp extra virgin olive oil, 2 tbsp balsamic - 307c, 4P, 11C, 27F)
- Protein shake (2 cups almond milk, 1 scoop Dummy Supps - 200c, 28P, 5C, 7F)

Instructions

1. Preheat air fryer or oven to 400°F.
2. Place egg whites and panko bread crumbs into separate large mixing bowls.
3. Season bread crumbs with listed seasonings.
4. Butterfly chicken breast, dredge in egg whites, then coat in bread crumbs.
5. Air fry/bake chicken for 10 minutes at 400°F then flip and cook for additional 8-10 minutes.
6. Blend cottage cheese, garlic, parmesan, mozzarella, Italian seasoning, and pepper until smooth.
7. Dice chicken and add sauce.

INDIVIDUAL MEAL PREP

CHICKEN MILANESE

Calories: 600 **Protein: 66** **Carbs: 39** **Fat: 18**

Ingredients **Servings: 1**

Chicken:
- 1 (6 oz.) chicken breast
- 1/4 cup egg whites
- 1/2 cup panko bread crumbs
- 1 tsp garlic powder
- 1 tsp onion powder
- 1 tsp Italian seasoning
- 1/2 tsp black pepper
- 1/4 tsp salt

Arugula Salad:
- 2 cups arugula
- 2 tbsp lemon juice
- 2 tbsp asiago cheese
- 1/2 tsp black pepper
- 2 tbsp balsamic glaze
- 2 tbsp diced cherry tomato

Optional Sides
- Protein pasta (2 oz: 190c, 10P, 38C, 1F)
- Salad (2 cups greens, 1 tbsp extra virgin olive oil, 2 tbsp balsamic - 307c, 4P, 11C, 27F)
- Protein shake (2 cups almond milk, 1 scoop Dummy Supps - 200c, 28P, 5C, 7F)

Instructions
1. Preheat air fryer or oven to 400°F.
2. Place egg whites and panko bread crumbs into separate large mixing bowls.
3. Season bread crumbs with listed seasonings.
4. Butterfly chicken breast, dredge in egg whites, then coat in bread crumbs.
5. Air fry/bake chicken for 10 minutes at 400°F then flip and cook for additional 10 minutes.
6. Combine arugula salad ingredients into small bowl and mix well.
7. Add arugula salad to plate, top with chicken, and drizzle balsamic glaze on top.

INDIVIDUAL MEAL PREP

CHICKEN BRUSCHETTA

Calories: 550 **Protein: 59** **Carbs: 40** **Fat: 15**

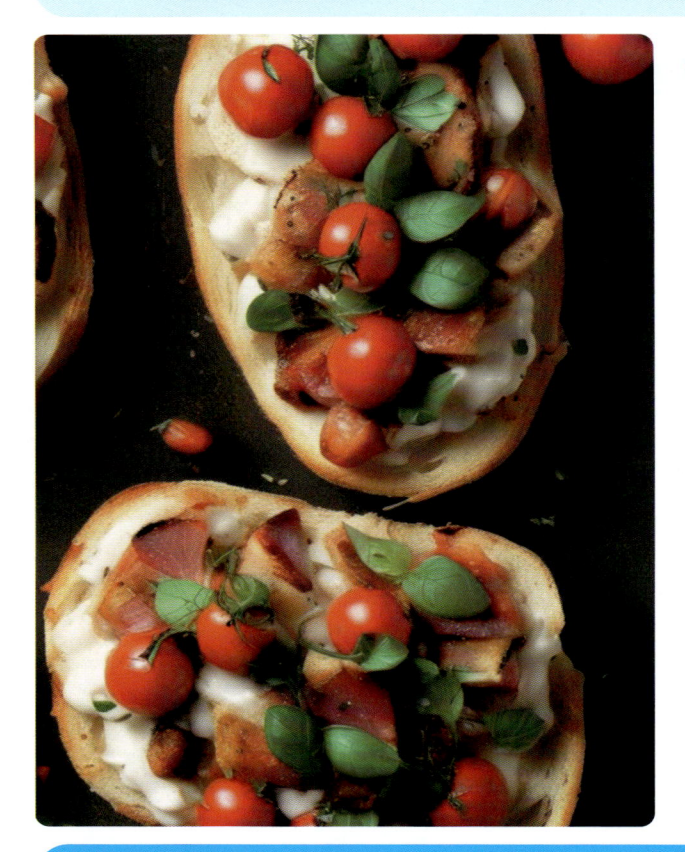

Ingredients — Servings: 1

Chicken:
- 1 (6 oz.) chicken breast
- 1/4 cup egg whites
- 1/2 cup panko bread crumbs
- 1 tsp garlic powder
- 1 tsp onion powder
- 1 tsp Italian seasoning
- 1/2 tsp black pepper
- 1/4 tsp salt

Bruschetta:
- 2 roma tomatoes
- 2 (2 oz.) slices fresh mozzarella cheese
- 2 tbsp balsamic glaze
- 1/2 tsp black pepper
- 1/4 tsp salt

Optional Sides
- Protein pasta (2 oz: 190c, 10P, 38C, 1F)
- Salad (2 cups greens, 1 tbsp extra virgin olive oil, 2 tbsp balsamic - 307c, 4P, 11C, 27F)
- Protein shake (2 cups almond milk, 1 scoop Dummy Supps - 200c, 28P, 5C, 7F)

Instructions
1. Slice tomatoes and mozzarella cheese.
2. Preheat air fryer or oven to 400°F.
3. Place egg whites and panko bread crumbs into separate large mixing bowls.
4. Season bread crumbs with listed seasonings.
5. Butterfly chicken breast, dredge in egg whites, then coat in bread crumbs.
6. Air fry/bake chicken for 10 minutes at 400°F then flip and cook for additional 10 minutes.
7. On top of chicken add sliced tomatoes, mozzarella cheese, balsamic glaze, salt, and pepper.

INDIVIDUAL MEAL PREP

CHICKEN TENDERS

Calories: 380   **Protein: 57**   **Carbs: 25**   **Fat: 7**

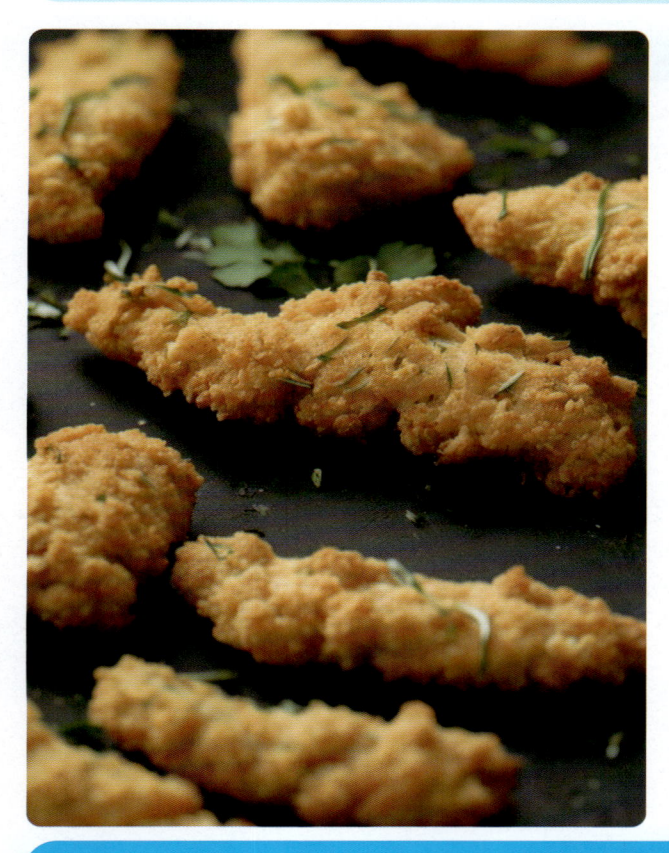

Ingredients   Servings: 1

Chicken:
- 1 (6 oz.) chicken breast
- 1/4 cup egg whites
- 1/2 cup panko bread crumbs
- 2 tbsp dijon mustard
- 1 tsp garlic powder
- 1 tsp onion powder
- 1/2 tsp black pepper
- 1/4 tsp salt

Protein Ranch:
- 1/2 cup nonfat plain greek yogurt
- 1 tbsp ranch seasoning
- 1 tsp lime juice

Optional Sides
- Salad (2 cups greens, 1 tbsp extra virgin olive oil, 2 tbsp balsamic - 307c, 4P, 11C, 27F)
- Protein shake (2 cups almond milk, 1 scoop Dummy Supps - 190c, 26P, 9C, 6F)
- G Hughes sugar free ketchup (2 tbsp - 10c, 0P, 2C, 0F)
- Alexia sweet potato fries (12 fries - 140c, 1P, 24C, 5F)

Instructions
1. Preheat air fryer or oven to 400°F.
2. Place egg whites and panko bread crumbs into separate large mixing bowls.
3. Mix dijon mustard in egg whites.
4. Season bread crumbs with listed seasonings.
5. Slice chicken breast into strips, dredge in egg whites, then coat in bread crumbs.
6. Air fry/bake chicken for 12-15 minutes at 400°F until cooked.
7. Add protein ranch ingredients to bowl and mix well.

INDIVIDUAL MEAL PREP

SWEET AND SPICY BITES

Calories: 380 **Protein: 57** **Carbs: 25** **Fat: 7**

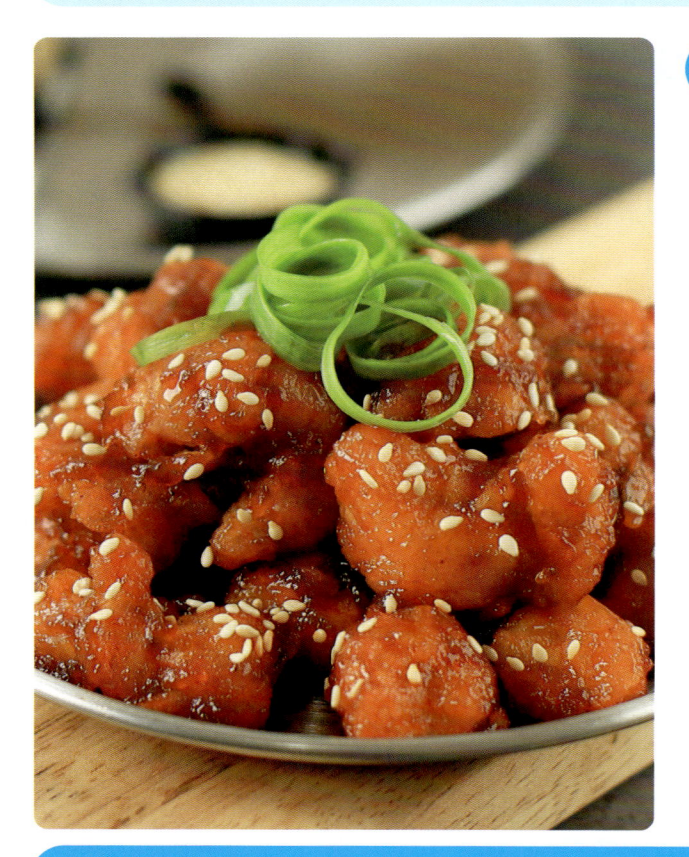

Ingredients Servings: 1

Chicken:
- 1 (6 oz.) chicken breast
- 1/4 cup egg whites
- 1/2 cup panko bread crumbs
- 1 tsp garlic powder
- 1 tsp onion powder
- 1/2 tsp black pepper
- 1/4 tsp salt
- 2 tbsp green onions

Sweet & Spicy Sauce:
- 2 tbsp honey
- 2 tbsp soy sauce
- 1 tbsp sriracha
- 1 tsp minced garlic
- 1 tsp minced ginger

Optional Sides
- Salad (2 cups greens, 1 tbsp extra virgin olive oil, 2 tbsp balsamic - 307c, 4P, 11C, 27F)
- Protein shake (2 cups almond milk, 1 scoop Dummy Supps - 190c, 26P, 9C, 6F)
- Cooked rice (1/2 cup - 150c, 0P, 20C, 0F)

Instructions
1. Dice chicken breast into bite sized pieces.
2. Preheat air fryer or oven to 400°F.
3. Place egg whites and panko bread crumbs into separate large mixing bowls.
4. Season bread crumbs with listed seasonings.
5. Dredge chicken in egg whites, then coat in bread crumbs.
6. Air fry/bake chicken for 10-12 minutes at 400°F until completely cooked.
7. To a small pan on low heat add sweet and spicy sauce ingredients,stir and let simmer for 5 minutes. Add sauce to chicken.
8. Garnish with green onions.

INDIVIDUAL MEAL PREP

CHICKEN PROTEIN PASTA

Calories: 540 **Protein: 65** **Carbs: 50** **Fat: 12**

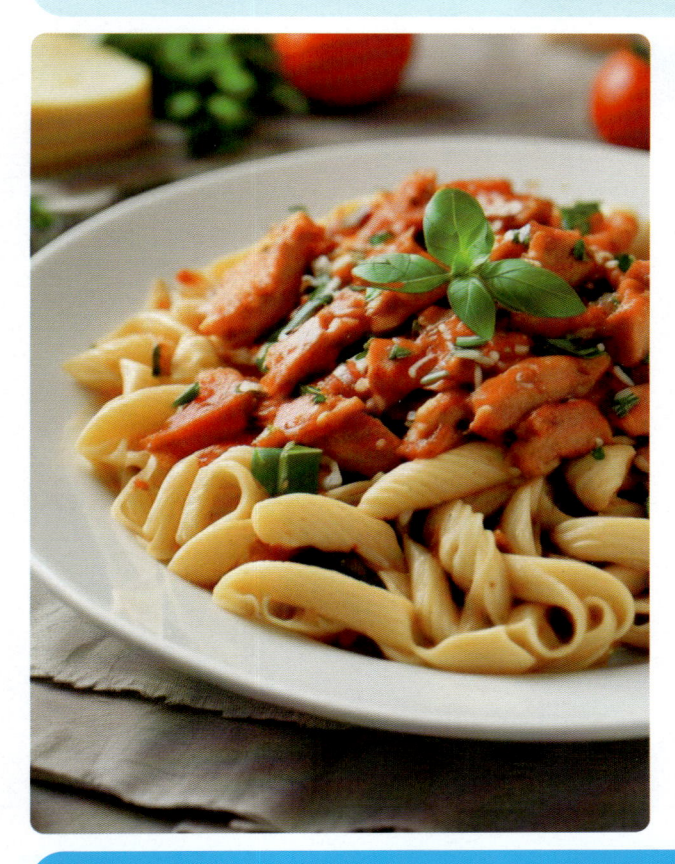

Ingredients **Servings: 1**

Pasta:
- 1 (6 oz.) chicken breast
- 1/2 cup cooked protein pasta
- 1 tbsp minced garlic
- 1 cup marinara sauce
- 2 tbsp parmesan cheese
- 1 tsp garlic powder
- 1 tsp onion powder
- 1 tsp Italian seasoning
- 1/2 tsp black pepper
- 1/4 tsp salt

Optional Sides
- Salad (2 cups greens, 1 tbsp extra virgin olive oil, 2 tbsp balsamic - 307c, 4P, 11C, 27F)
- Protein shake (2 cups almond milk, 1 scoop Dummy Supps - 190c, 26P, 9C, 6F)

Instructions
1. Dice chicken into bite-sized pieces.
2. Season chicken with listed seasonings.
3. Heat a pan with cooking spray on medium-high. Add minced garlic and chicken.
4. Cook for 8-10 minutes until fully cooked.
5. Boil pasta for 9-11 minutes. Drain.
6. Add cooked pasta, chicken, marinara sauce, and parmesan cheese to the pan.
7. Stir on low heat for 5 minutes.

INDIVIDUAL MEAL PREP

CHICKEN BACON RANCH BOWL

Calories: 530 **Protein: 61** **Carbs: 32** **Fat: 10**

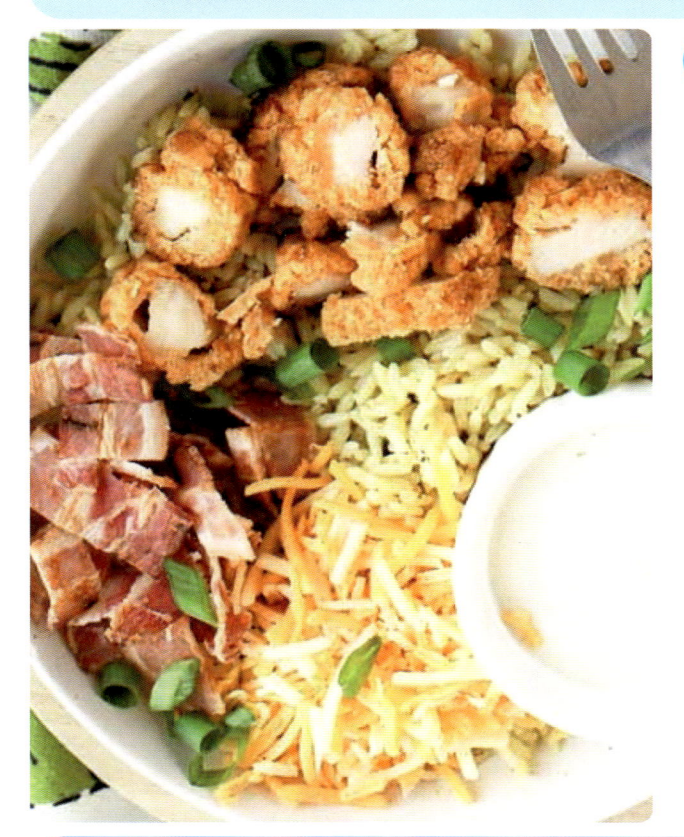

Ingredients Servings: 1

Bowl:
- 1 (6 oz.) chicken breast
- 1/2 cup cooked rice
- 1 tbsp minced garlic
- 2 slices turkey bacon
- 2 tbsp parmesan cheese
- 1 tsp garlic powder
- 1 tsp onion powder
- 1/2 tsp black pepper
- 1/4 tsp salt

Protein Ranch:
- 1/4 cup nonfat plain greek yogurt
- 2 tsp ranch seasoning
- 2 tsp lime juice

Optional Sides

- Salad (2 cups greens, 1 tbsp extra virgin olive oil, 2 tbsp balsamic - 307c, 4P, 11C, 27F)
- Protein shake (2 cups almond milk, 1 scoop Dummy Supps - 190c, 26P, 9C, 6F)

Instructions

1. Dice chicken into bite-sized pieces.
2. Season chicken with listed seasonings.
3. Heat a pan with cooking spray on medium-high. Add minced garlic and chicken.
4. Cook for 8-10 minutes until fully cooked.
5. Cook turkey bacon in the same pan until crispy, then chop into small pieces.
6. Add 1/2 cup water and 1/4 cup rice in pot, bring to boil on high heat, turn to low, cover, and cook for 5-7 minutes or microwave rice.
7. In a small bowl, mix ingredients for the protein ranch.
8. Combine cooked rice, chicken, turkey bacon, and parmesan cheese to the pan. Stir on low heat for 3-5 minutes.
9. Top with protein ranch.

INDIVIDUAL MEAL PREP

SOUTHWEST CHICKEN BOWL

Calories: 570 **Protein: 60** **Carbs: 34** **Fat: 21**

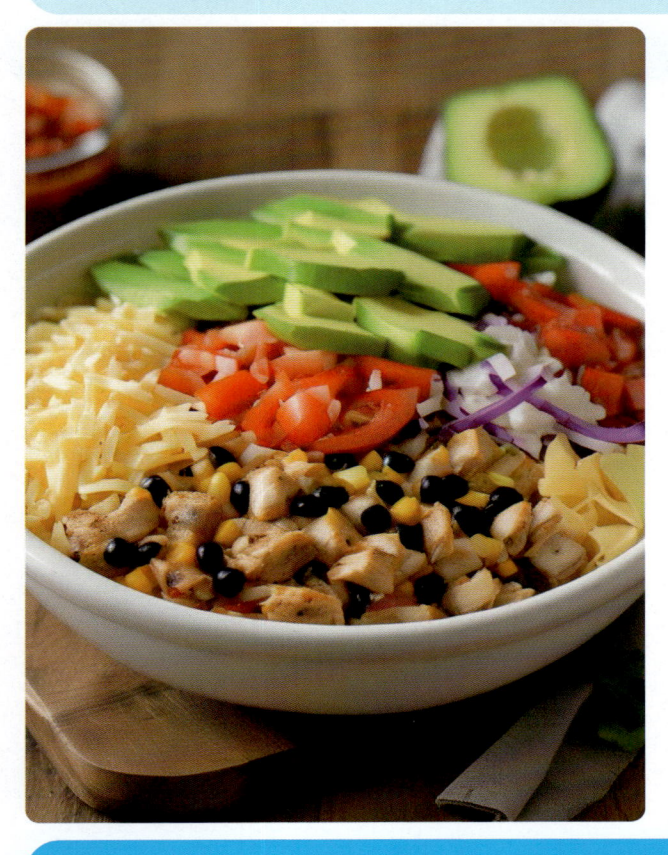

Ingredients **Servings: 1**

Southwest Bowl:
- 1 (6 oz.) chicken breast
- 1/2 cup cooked rice
- 2 tbsp green chilies
- 2 tbsp tomatoes
- 1/4 red onion
- 1/2 bell pepper
- 2 tbsp black beans
- 2 tbsp mexican cheese
- 1 tsp garlic powder
- 1 tsp onion powder
- 1/2 tsp black pepper
- 1/4 tsp salt

Optional Sides

- Salad (2 cups greens, 1 tbsp extra virgin olive oil, 2 tbsp balsamic - 307c, 4P, 11C, 27F)
- Protein shake (2 cups almond milk, 1 scoop Dummy Supps - 190c, 26P, 9C, 6F)
- Salsa (2 tbsp - 10c, 0P, 2C, 0F)
- Hot sauce (1 tsp - 1c, 0P, 0C, 0F)
- Avocado (1/2 whole - 120c, 2P, 6C, 11F)

Instructions

1. Slice peppers and onions. Dice tomatoes. Dice chicken into bite-sized pieces.
2. Heat a pan with cooking spray on medium-high. Add peppers, onions, chicken, green chilies, and listed seasonings.
3. Cook for 8-10 minutes until fully cooked.
4. Add 1/2 cup water and 1/4 cup rice in pot, bring to boil on high heat, turn to low, cover, and cook for 5-7 minutes or microwave rice.
5. To meal prep container combine rice, chicken, sauteed vegetables, diced tomatoes, black beans, and shredded cheese.

INDIVIDUAL MEAL PREP

GREEK CHICKEN BOWL

Calories: 600   **Protein: 65**   **Carbs: 31**   **Fat: 20**

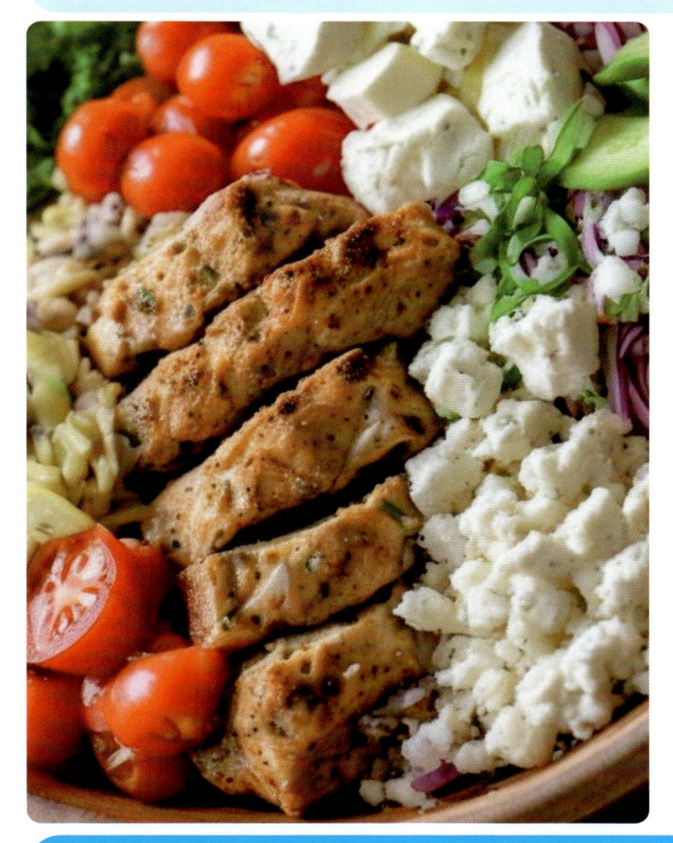

Ingredients   Servings: 1

Bowl:
- 1 (6 oz.) chicken breast
- 1/2 cup cooked rice
- 2 tbsp cup cucumber
- 2 tbsp cherry tomatoes
- 2 tbsp red onion
- 2 tbsp banana peppers
- 1/4 cup feta cheese
- 1 tsp garlic powder
- 1 tsp onion powder
- 1/4 tsp salt
- 1/2 black pepper

Tzatziki:
- 1/2 cup nonfat plain greek yogurt
- 2 tbsp cucumber
- 2 tsp lemon juice
- 1/4 tsp salt
- 1/2 tsp black pepper
- 1 tsp dill

Optional Sides

- Salad (2 cups greens, 1 tbsp extra virgin olive oil, 2 tbsp balsamic - 307c, 4P, 11C, 27F)
- Protein shake (2 cups almond milk, 1 scoop Dummy Supps - 190c, 26P, 9C, 6F)
- Avocado (1/2 whole - 120c, 2P, 6C, 11F)

Instructions

1. Dice cucumber, tomatoes, and onions. Dice chicken into bite-sized pieces.
2. Heat a pan with cooking spray on medium-high. Add chicken and listed seasonings.
3. Cook for 8-10 minutes until fully cooked.
4. Add 1/2 cup water and 1/4 cup rice in pot, bring to boil on high heat, turn to low, cover, and cook for 5-7 minutes or microwave rice.
5. To bowl, add tzatziki ingredients and mix well.
6. To meal prep container combine rice, chicken, spinach, diced vegetables, banana peppers, feta cheese, and top with tzatziki.

INDIVIDUAL MEAL PREP

CLASSIC CHICKEN & RICE

Calories: 530 **Protein: 59** **Carbs: 33** **Fat: 17**

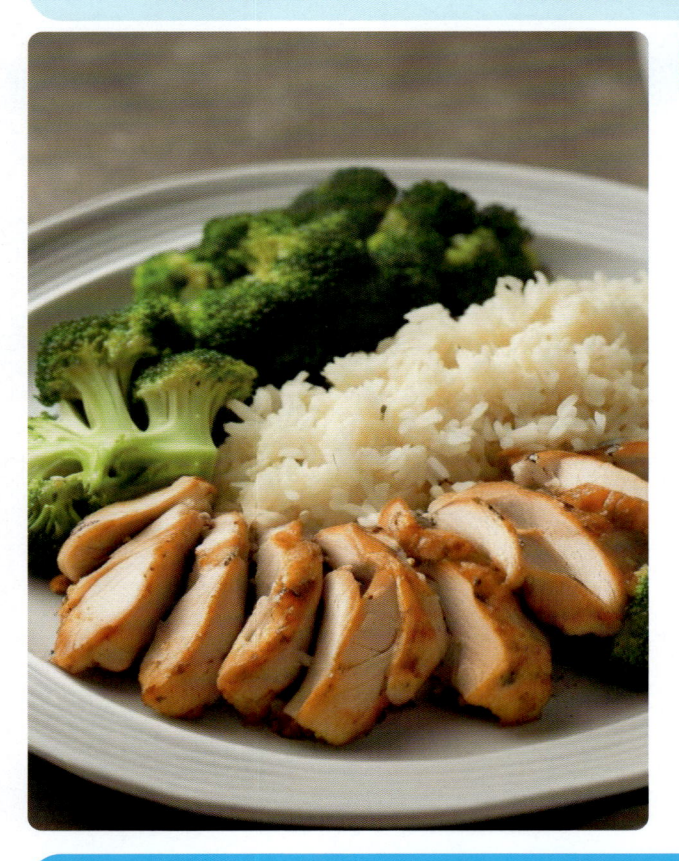

Ingredients Servings: 1

Chicken and Rice:

- 1 (6 oz.) chicken breast
- 1/2 cup cooked rice
- 1 tbsp extra virgin olive oil
- 2 cups frozen broccoli
- 1 tbsp lemon juice
- 1 tsp garlic powder
- 1 tsp onion powder
- 1/4 tsp salt
- 1/2 tsp black pepper

Optional Sides

- Salad (2 cups greens, 1 tbsp extra virgin olive oil, 2 tbsp balsamic - 307c, 4P, 11C, 27F)
- Protein shake (2 cups almond milk, 1 scoop Dummy Supps - 190c, 26P, 9C, 6F)
- Avocado (1/2 whole - 120c, 2P, 6C, 11F)

Instructions

1. Preheat oven to 400°F.
2. Butterfly the chicken breast and season with listed seasonings.
3. Place chicken on a baking sheet and bake for 15-18 minutes, or until the internal temperature reaches 165°F.
4. Place frozen broccoli in a microwave-safe bowl with 2 tbsp water, cover, and microwave for 3-4 minutes until tender. Drain excess water and season with lemon juice, salt, and black pepper.
5. Add ½ cup water and ¼ cup rice in a pot, bring to a boil on high heat, turn to low, cover, and cook for 5-7 minutes or microwave rice.
6. Serve butterflied lemon garlic chicken over rice with steamed broccoli on the side.

INDIVIDUAL MEAL PREP

LEMON PEPPER CHICKEN & RICE

Calories: 540 **Protein: 33** **Carbs: 59** **Fat: 17**

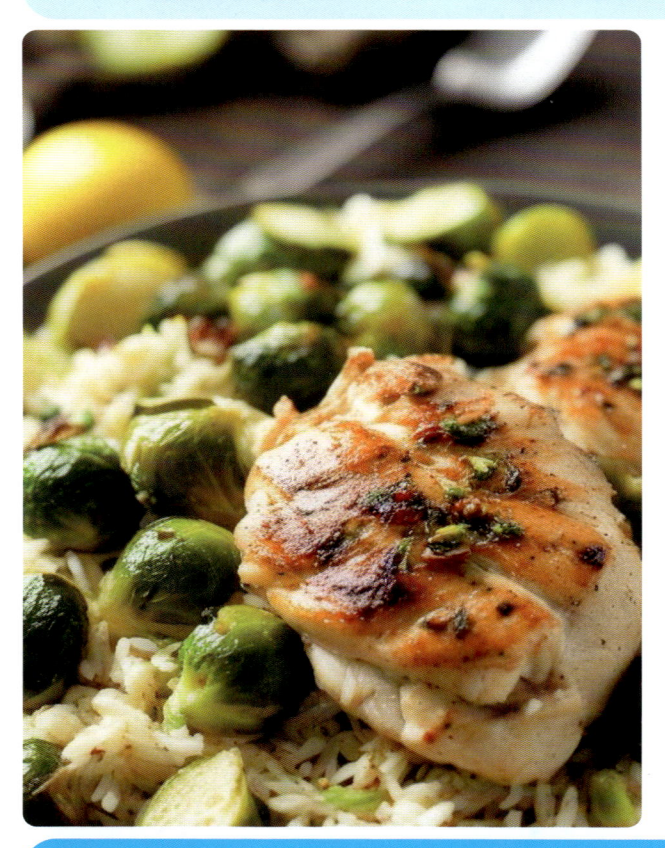

Ingredients Servings: 1

Chicken and Rice:

- 1 (6 oz.) chicken breast
- 1/2 cup cooked rice
- 1 tbsp extra virgin olive oil
- 2 cups roasted Brussels sprouts
- 2 tbsp BBQ sauce
- 1 tsp garlic powder
- 1 tsp onion powder
- 1/2 tsp black pepper
- 1/4 tsp salt

Optional Sides

- Salad (2 cups greens, 1 tbsp extra virgin olive oil, 2 tbsp balsamic - 307c, 4P, 11C, 27F)
- Protein shake (2 cups almond milk, 1 scoop Dummy Supps - 190c, 26P, 9C, 6F)
- Avocado (1/2 whole - 120c, 2P, 6C, 11F)

Instructions

1. Preheat oven to 400°F.
2. Butterfly chicken and season with olive oil, garlic powder, black pepper, salt, and lemon zest.
3. Place chicken on a baking sheet and bake for 15-18 minutes until the internal temperature reaches 165°F.
4. Slice brussel sprouts in half and toss in bowl with cooking spray, salt, and black pepper and spread them on a baking sheet. Roast for 20-25 minutes until tender and crispy.
5. Add ½ cup water and ¼ cup rice in a pot, bring to boil on high heat, turn to low, cover, and cook for 5-7 minutes or microwave rice.
6. Drizzle cooked chicken with lemon juice before serving.
7. Serve chicken over rice with broccoli on the side.

INDIVIDUAL MEAL PREP

BBQ CHICKEN & RICE

Calories: 560 **Protein: 60** **Carbs: 42** **Fat: 17**

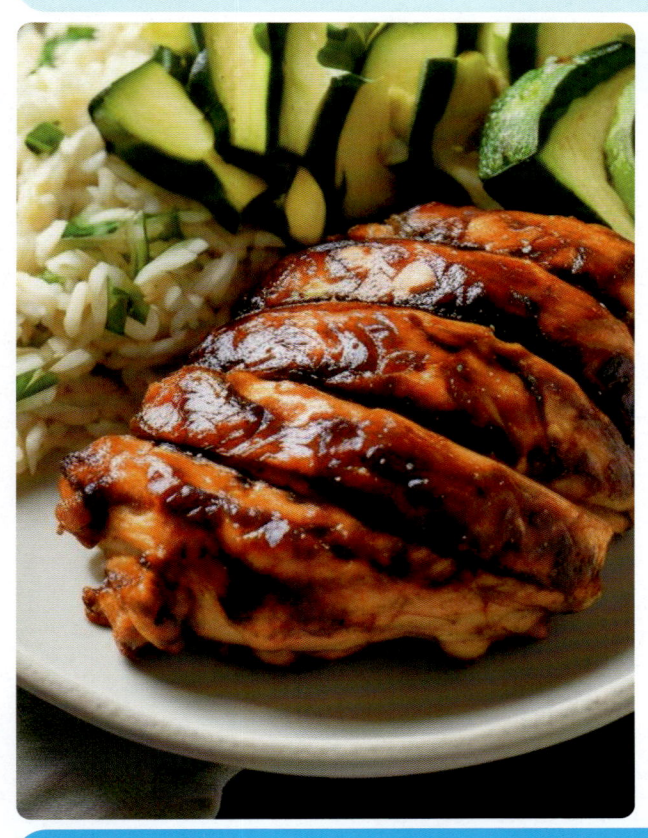

Ingredients   Servings: 1

Chicken and Rice:
- 1 (6 oz.) chicken breast
- 1/2 cup cooked rice
- 1 tbsp extra virgin olive oil
- 2 cups frozen zucchini
- 1/2 tsp garlic powder
- 1/2 tsp onion powder
- 1/4 tsp salt
- 1/4 tsp black pepper
- 4 tbsp G Hughes BBQ sauce

Optional Sides

- Salad (2 cups greens, 1 tbsp extra virgin olive oil, 2 tbsp balsamic - 307c, 4P, 11C, 27F)
- Protein shake (2 cups almond milk, 1 scoop Dummy Supps - 190c, 26P, 9C, 6F)
- Avocado (1/2 whole - 120c, 2P, 6C, 11F)

Instructions

1. Preheat oven to 400°F.
2. Butterfly the chicken breast and rub with olive oil, garlic powder, onion powder, salt, and black pepper.
3. Place chicken on a baking sheet and bake for 15-18 minutes, or until the internal temperature reaches 165°F.
4. Remove from the oven and brush with G Hughes BBQ sauce. Let rest for 2-3 minutes before serving.
5. Heat a pan over medium heat with cooking spray. Add frozen zucchini and sauté for 4-5 minutes, stirring occasionally, until tender. Season with salt and black pepper.
6. Add ½ cup water and ¼ cup rice in a pot, bring to a boil on high heat, turn to low, cover, and cook for 5-7 minutes or microwave rice.
7. Serve BBQ chicken over rice with sautéed zucchini on the side.

INDIVIDUAL MEAL PREP

CHIPOTLE-STYLE CHICKEN & RICE

Calories: 530 **Protein: 56** **Carbs: 36** **Fat: 16**

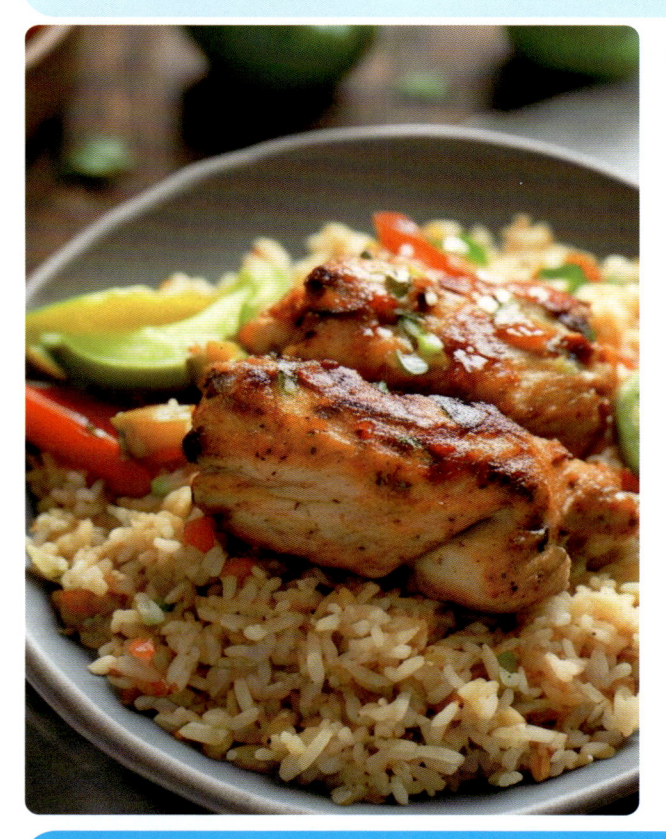

Ingredients Servings: 1

Chicken and Rice:
- 1 (6 oz.) chicken breast
- 1/2 cup cooked rice
- 1 tbsp extra virgin olive oil
- 1 tbsp cilantro
- 1/2 lime juice
- 2 cups frozen peppers and onions
- 1/2 tsp cumin
- 1/2 tsp chili powder
- 1/2 tsp smoked paprika
- 1/2 tsp garlic powder
- 1/4 tsp salt
- 1/4 tsp black pepper

Optional Sides
- Salad (2 cups greens, 1 tbsp extra virgin olive oil, 2 tbsp balsamic - 307c, 4P, 11C, 27F)
- Protein shake (2 cups almond milk, 1 scoop Dummy Supps - 190c, 26P, 9C, 6F)
- Salsa (2 tbsp - 10c, 0P, 2C, 0F)
- Hot sauce (1 tsp - 1c, 0P, 0C, 0F)
- Avocado (1/2 whole - 120c, 2P, 6C, 11F)

Instructions
1. Dice chicken.
2. Heat a pan over medium heat and coat with cooking spray.
3. Add frozen peppers and onions, season with salt and black pepper, and cook for 3-4 minutes until softened.
4. Add diced chicken to the pan, season with cumin, chili powder, smoked paprika, and garlic powder, and cook for 8-10 minutes, stirring occasionally, until fully cooked.
5. Add ½ cup water and ¼ cup rice in a pot, bring to a boil on high heat, turn to low, cover, and cook for 5-7 minutes or microwave rice.
6. Stir fresh cilantro and lime juice into cooked rice.
7. Serve seasoned chicken and sautéed peppers and onions over cilantro-lime rice.

INDIVIDUAL MEAL PREP

CAJUN CHICKEN & RICE

Calories: 530   **Protein: 56**   **Carbs: 36**   **Fat: 16**

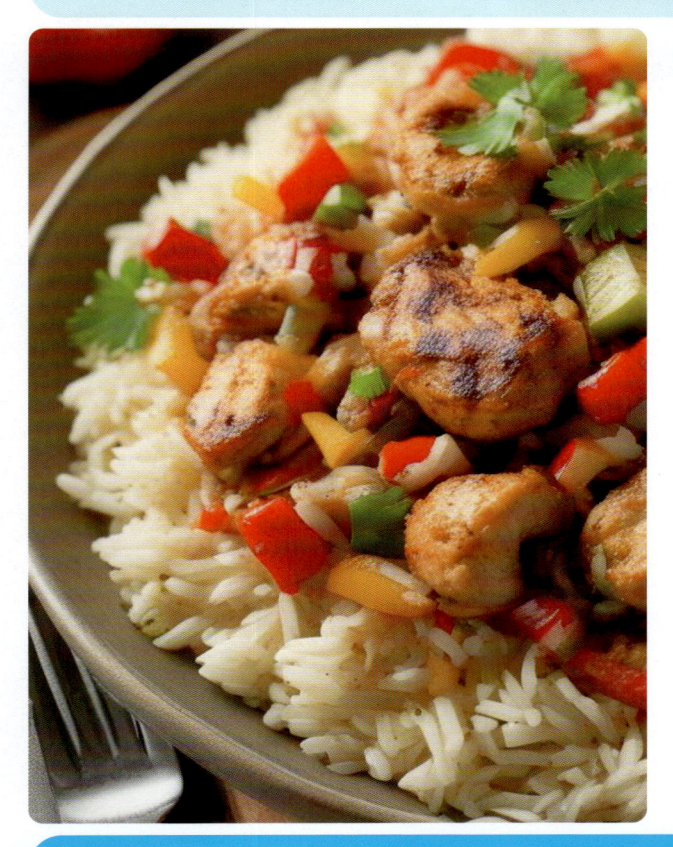

Ingredients   **Servings: 1**

Chicken and Rice:
- 1 (6 oz.) chicken breast
- 1/2 cup cooked rice
- 1 tbsp extra virgin olive oil
- 2 cups frozen peppers and onions
- 1 tsp Cajun seasoning
- 1/2 tsp garlic powder
- 1/2 tsp smoked paprika
- 1/4 tsp salt
- 1/4 tsp black pepper

Optional Sides
- Salad (2 cups greens, 1 tbsp extra virgin olive oil, 2 tbsp balsamic - 307c, 4P, 11C, 27F)
- Protein shake (2 cups almond milk, 1 scoop Dummy Supps - 190c, 26P, 9C, 6F)
- Avocado (1/2 whole - 120c, 2P, 6C, 11F)

Instructions
1. Dice chicken.
2. Heat a pan over medium heat and coat with cooking spray.
3. Add frozen bell peppers and onions, season with salt and black pepper, and cook for 3-4 minutes until softened.
4. Add diced chicken to the pan, season with Cajun seasoning, garlic powder, and smoked paprika, and cook for 8-10 minutes, stirring occasionally, until fully cooked.
5. Add ½ cup water and ¼ cup rice in a pot, bring to a boil on high heat, turn to low, cover, and cook for 5-7 minutes or microwave rice.
6. Serve seasoned chicken and sautéed peppers and onions over rice.

INDIVIDUAL MEAL PREP

HONEY GARLIC CHICKEN & RICE

Calories: 630 **Protein: 61** **Carbs: 52** **Fat: 20**

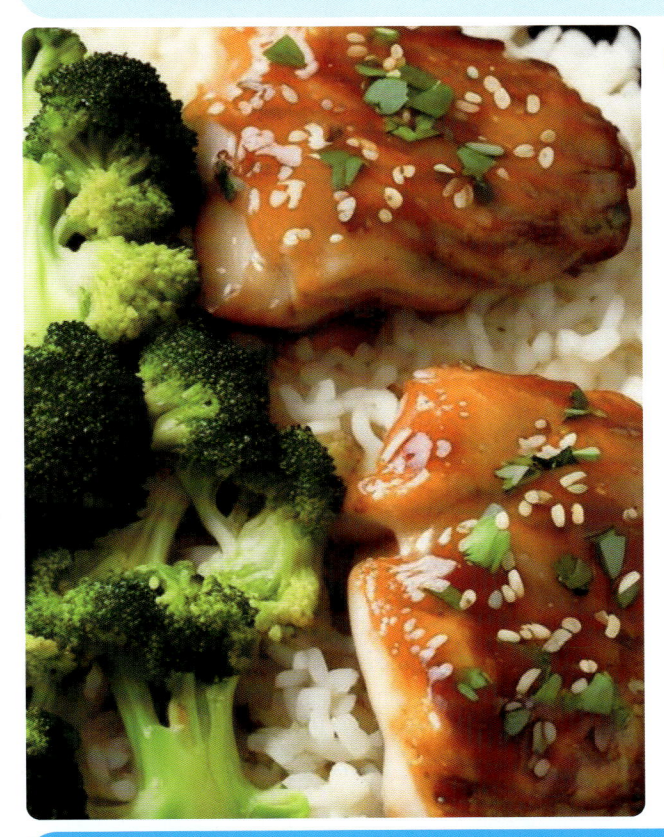

Ingredients **Servings: 1**

Chicken and Rice:
- 1 (6 oz.) chicken breast
- 1/2 cup cooked rice
- 1 tbsp extra virgin olive oil
- 2 cups frozen broccoli
- 1 tbsp honey
- 1 tbsp soy sauce
- 1 tsp garlic powder
- 1/2 tsp black pepper
- 1/2 tsp salt
- 1 tsp sesame seeds

Optional Sides
- Salad (2 cups greens, 1 tbsp extra virgin olive oil, 2 tbsp balsamic - 307c, 4P, 11C, 27F)
- Protein shake (2 cups almond milk, 1 scoop Dummy Supps - 190c, 26P, 9C, 6F)
- Avocado (1/2 whole - 120c, 2P, 6C, 11F)

Instructions
1. Heat a pan over medium heat and 1/2 tbsp olive oil.
2. Dice the chicken breast into bite-sized pieces and season with garlic powder, black pepper, and salt.
3. Add the diced chicken to the pan and cook for 8-10 minutes, stirring occasionally, until golden brown and fully cooked.
4. Push the chicken to one side of the pan and add frozen broccoli. Cook for 3-4 minutes until heated through.
5. In a small bowl, mix honey and soy sauce until combined.
6. Pour the sauce over the chicken and broccoli, stirring to coat evenly. Cook for 1-2 minutes until well combined.
7. Serve over cooked rice and garnish with sesame seeds.

INDIVIDUAL MEAL PREP

GARLIC BUTTER CHICKEN & RICE

Calories: 630 **Protein: 61** **Carbs: 52** **Fat: 20**

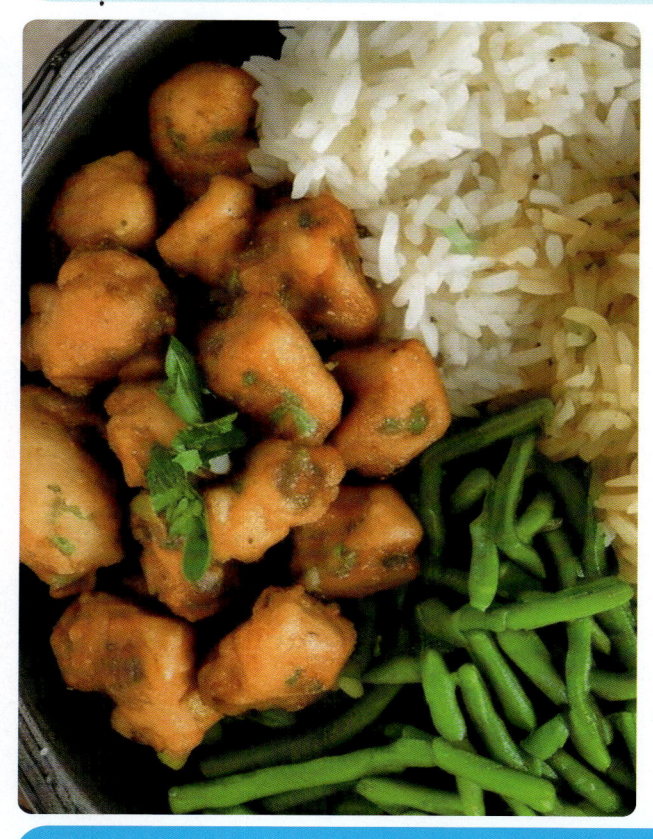

Ingredients **Servings: 1**

Chicken and Rice:
- 1 (6 oz.) chicken breast
- 1/2 cup cooked rice
- 2 cups fresh or frozen green beans
- 2 tbsp minced garlic
- 1 tbsp butter
- 1 tsp garlic powder
- 1/2 tsp black pepper
- 1/2 tsp paprika
- 1/4 tsp salt

Optional Sides
- Salad (2 cups greens, 1 tbsp extra virgin olive oil, 2 tbsp balsamic - 307c, 4P, 11C, 27F)
- Protein shake (2 cups almond milk, 1 scoop Dummy Supps - 190c, 26P, 9C, 6F)
- Avocado (1/2 whole - 120c, 2P, 6C, 11F)

Instructions
1. Dice chicken and trim green beans if fresh.
2. Heat a pan over medium heat with cooking spray.
3. Add minced garlic and cook for 30 seconds until fragrant.
4. Add diced chicken, season with garlic powder, paprika, salt, and black pepper, and sauté for 6-8 minutes, stirring occasionally, until almost fully cooked.
5. When the chicken is about done, add butter and stir until melted, coating the chicken evenly. Cook for 1-2 more minutes and remove.
6. In the same pan, add trimmed fresh green beans and sauté for 8-10 minutes, stirring occasionally, until tender. Season with salt and black pepper.
7. Add ½ cup water and ¼ cup rice in a pot, bring to a boil on high heat, turn to low, cover, and cook for 5-7 minutes or microwave rice.
8. Serve diced garlic butter chicken over rice with sautéed green beans on the side.

INDIVIDUAL MEAL PREP

GARLIC HERB CHICKEN & ROASTED POTATOES

Calories: 550 **Protein: 43** **Carbs: 59** **Fat: 16**

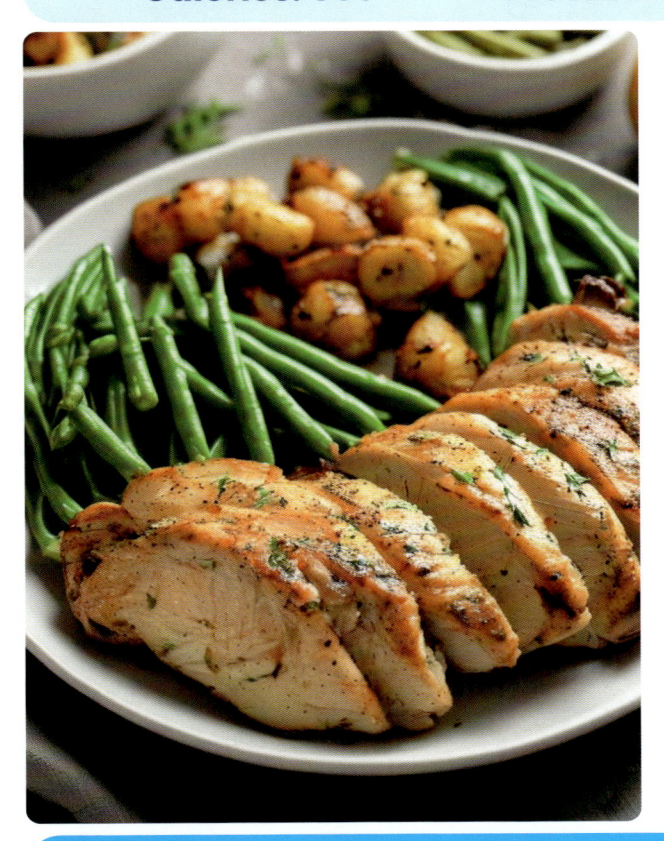

Ingredients **Servings: 1**

Chicken and Potatoes:
- 1 (6 oz.) chicken breast
- 1 (6 oz.) russet potato
- 1 tbsp extra virgin olive oil
- 2 cups fresh green beans
- 1 tbsp olive oil
- 2 tbsp minced garlic
- 2 tsp garlic powder
- 1 tsp Italian seasoning
- 1/2 tsp onion powder
- 1/2 tsp black pepper
- 1/2 tsp salt

Optional Sides

- Salad (2 cups greens, 1 tbsp extra virgin olive oil, 2 tbsp balsamic - 307c, 4P, 11C, 27F)
- Protein shake (2 cups almond milk, 1 scoop Dummy Supps - 190c, 26P, 9C, 6F)
- Avocado (1/2 whole - 120c, 2P, 6C, 11F)

Instructions

1. Preheat oven to 400°F.
2. Dice the potato into small cubes and dice the chicken into bite-sized pieces. Trim the green beans by cutting off the ends.
3. Toss diced potatoes with 1/2 tbsp olive oil, 1/4 tsp salt, and 1/4 tsp black pepper. Spread on a baking sheet and roast for 20-30 minutes, flipping halfway.
4. Lightly coat green beans with cooking spray and season with salt and black pepper. Add to the baking sheet with potatoes for the last 12-15 minutes of roasting.
5. Heat a pan over medium heat with ½ tbsp olive oil.
6. Add diced chicken and season with minced garlic, garlic powder, Italian seasoning, onion powder, salt, and black pepper. Cook for 8-10 minutes, stirring occasionally, until fully cooked and golden brown.
7. Serve garlic herb chicken over roasted potatoes with roasted green beans on the side.

INDIVIDUAL MEAL PREP

TERIYAKI CHICKEN & SWEET POTATOES

Calories: 560   **Protein: 59**   **Carbs: 40**   **Fat: 18**

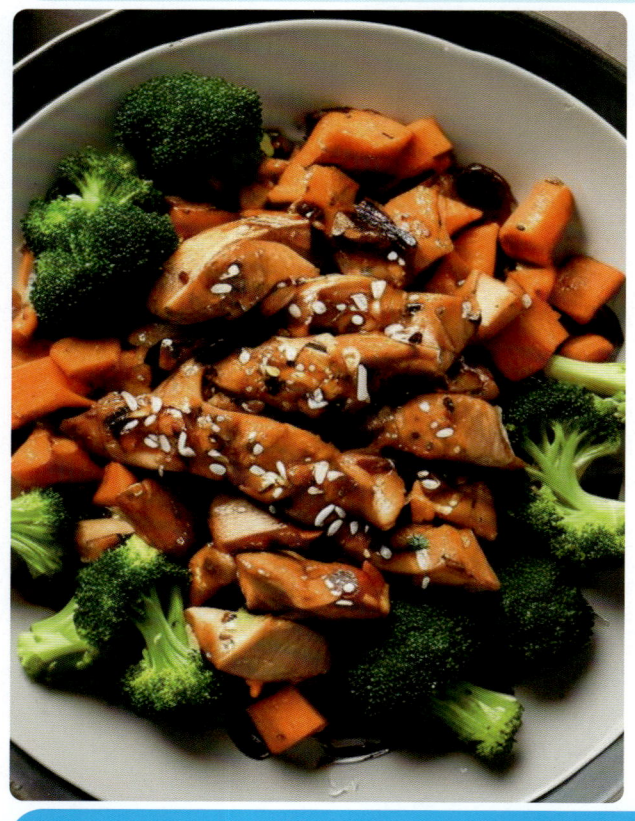

Ingredients   Servings: 1

Chicken and Potatoes:
- 1 (6 oz.) chicken breast
- 1 (6 oz.) sweet potato
- 2 cups frozen broccoli
- 4 tbsp G Hughes Sugar-Free Teriyaki Sauce
- 1 tbsp olive oil
- 1 tsp garlic powder
- 1 tsp onion powder
- 1/2 tsp black pepper
- 1/4 tsp salt
- 1 tbsp lemon juice
- 1 tsp sesame seeds

Optional Sides
- Salad (2 cups greens, 1 tbsp extra virgin olive oil, 2 tbsp balsamic - 307c, 4P, 11C, 27F)
- Protein shake (2 cups almond milk, 1 scoop Dummy Supps - 190c, 26P, 9C, 6F)
- Avocado (1/2 whole - 120c, 2P, 6C, 11F)

Instructions
1. Preheat oven to 400°F.
2. Dice the sweet potato into small cubes and dice the chicken into bite-sized pieces.
3. Toss diced sweet potatoes with ½ tbsp olive oil, salt, and black pepper. Spread on a baking sheet and roast for 20-25 minutes until tender.
4. Heat a pan over medium heat with cooking spray.
5. Add ½ tbsp olive oil, then add diced chicken. Season with garlic powder, onion powder, salt, and black pepper. Cook for 8-10 minutes, stirring occasionally, until fully cooked.
6. Stir in G Hughes Teriyaki Sauce, coating the chicken evenly. Simmer for 1-2 minutes.
7. Place frozen broccoli in a microwave-safe bowl with 2 tbsp water, cover, and microwave for 3-4 minutes until tender. Drain excess water and season with salt, black pepper and lemon juice.
8. Serve teriyaki chicken over roasted sweet potatoes with steamed broccoli on the side. Garnish with sesame seeds.

INDIVIDUAL MEAL PREP

PARMESAN CRUSTED CHICKEN & ROASTED POTATOES

Calories: 600 **Protein: 63** **Carbs: 42** **Fat: 20**

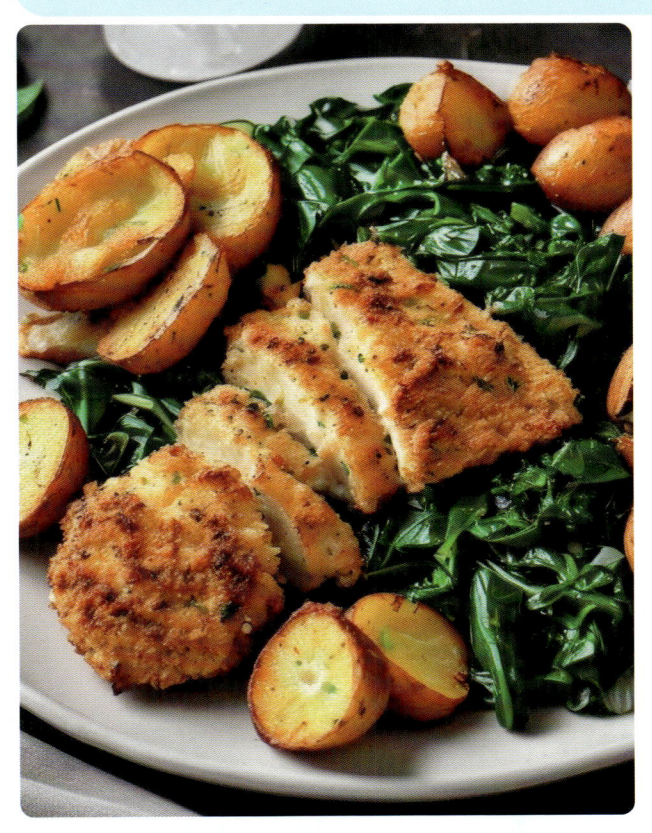

Ingredients Servings: 1

Chicken and Potatoes:
- 1 (6 oz.) chicken breast
- 1 (6 oz.) russet potato
- 1 tbsp olive oil
- 2 cups fresh spinach
- 2 tbsp minced garlic
- 2 tbsp Parmesan cheese
- 2 tbsp breadcrumbs
- 1 tsp garlic powder
- 1 tsp onion powder
- 1 tsp Italian seasoning
- 1/2 tsp salt
- 1/2 tsp black pepper

Optional Sides
- Salad (2 cups greens, 1 tbsp extra virgin olive oil, 2 tbsp balsamic - 307c, 4P, 11C, 27F)
- Protein shake (2 cups almond milk, 1 scoop Dummy Supps - 190c, 26P, 9C, 6F)

Instructions
1. Preheat oven to 400°F.
2. Dice the potato into small cubes and butterfly the chicken.
3. Toss diced potatoes with ½ tbsp olive oil, ¼ tsp salt, and ¼ tsp black pepper. Spread on a baking sheet and roast for 20-25 minutes, flipping halfway.
4. In a bowl, mix Parmesan cheese, breadcrumbs, garlic powder, onion powder, Italian seasoning, and black pepper.
5. Rub butterflied chicken with ½ tbsp olive oil, then coat both sides with the Parmesan breadcrumb mixture.
6. Heat a pan over medium heat with cooking spray. Add chicken and cook for 4-5 minutes per side, until golden brown and fully cooked.
7. In the same pan, add spinach and sauté for 2-3 minutes until wilted. Season with salt and black pepper.
8. Serve Parmesan crusted chicken over roasted potatoes with sautéed spinach on the side.

INDIVIDUAL MEAL PREP

HONEY MUSTARD CHICKEN & POTATOES

Calories: 590   **Protein: 61**   **Carbs: 44**   **Fat: 20**

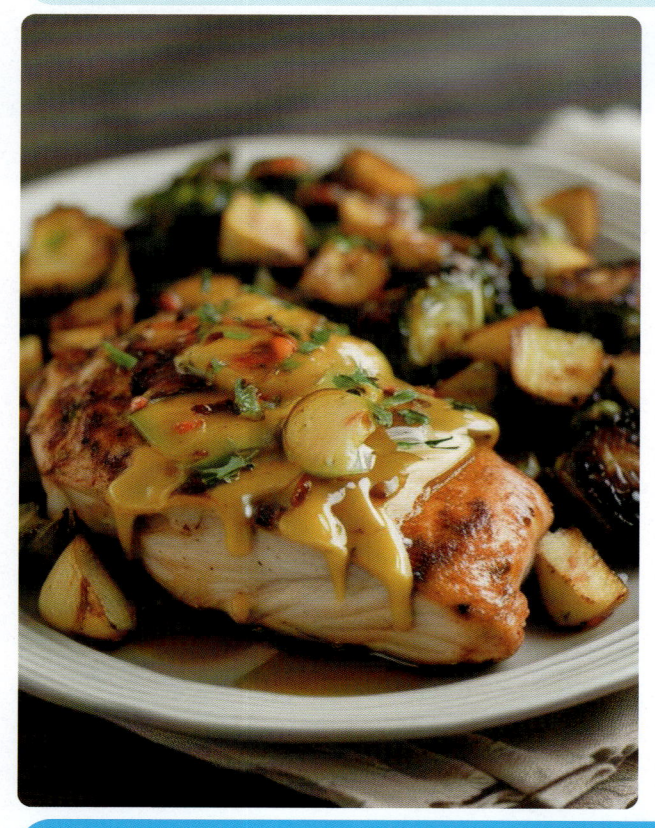

Ingredients   Servings: 1

Chicken and Potatoes:
- 1 (6 oz.) chicken breast
- 1 (6 oz.) russet potato
- 1 tbsp olive oil
- 2 cups Brussels sprouts
- 4 tbsp G Hughes Sugar-Free Honey Mustard
- 1 tsp garlic powder
- 1/2 tsp onion powder
- 1/2 tsp black pepper
- 1/4 tsp salt

Optional Sides
- Salad (2 cups greens, 1 tbsp extra virgin olive oil, 2 tbsp balsamic - 307c, 4P, 11C, 27F)
- Protein shake (2 cups almond milk, 1 scoop Dummy Supps - 190c, 26P, 9C, 6F)
- Avocado (1/2 whole - 120c, 2P, 6C, 11F)

Instructions
1. Preheat oven to 400°F.
2. Dice the potato into small cubes and trim and halve the Brussels sprouts.
3. Toss diced potatoes with ½ tbsp olive oil, ¼ tsp salt, and ¼ tsp black pepper. Spread on a baking sheet and roast for 20-25 minutes, flipping halfway.
4. Toss Brussels sprouts with cooking spray, salt, and black pepper. Add to the baking sheet with potatoes for the last 12-15 minutes of roasting.
5. Heat a pan over medium heat with ½ tbsp olive oil.
6. Dice the chicken breast and season with garlic powder, onion powder, and black pepper.
7. Add chicken to the pan and cook for 5-6 minutes per side, until golden brown and fully cooked.
8. In the last 1-2 minutes of cooking, brush the chicken with G Hughes Sugar-Free Honey Mustard, allowing it to caramelize slightly.
9. Serve honey mustard chicken with roasted potatoes and Brussels sprouts.

INDIVIDUAL MEAL PREP

BBQ CHICKEN & SWEET POTATO

Calories: 540   **Protein: 58**   **Carbs: 43**   **Fat: 16**

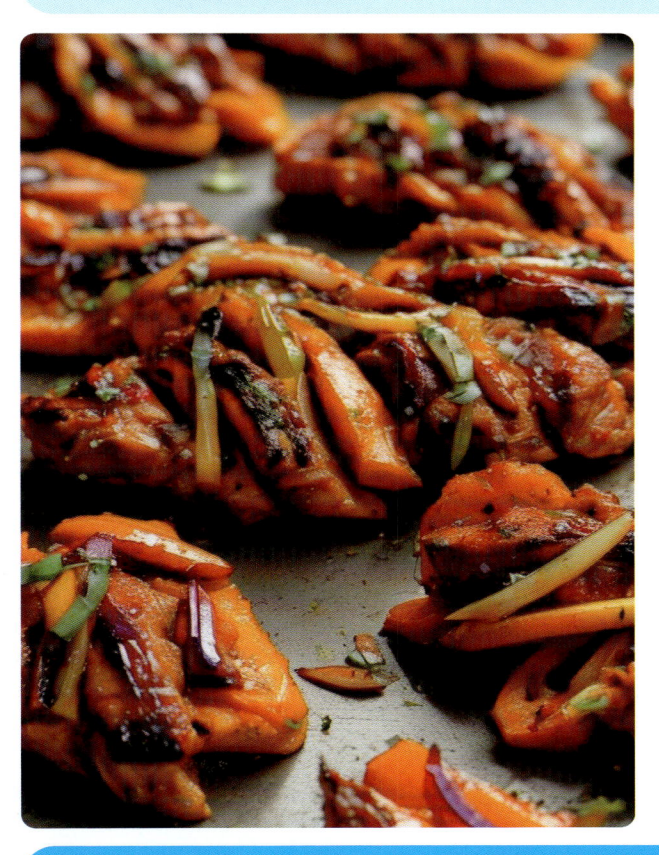

Ingredients   **Servings: 1**

Chicken and Potatoes:
- 1 (6 oz.) chicken breast
- 1 (6 oz.) sweet potato
- 1 tbsp olive oil
- 2 cups frozen bell peppers and onions
- 4 tbsp G Hughes Sugar-Free BBQ Sauce
- 1 tsp garlic powder
- 1/2 tsp smoked paprika
- 1/2 tsp black pepper
- 1/4 tsp salt

Optional Sides
- Salad (2 cups greens, 1 tbsp extra virgin olive oil, 2 tbsp balsamic - 307c, 4P, 11C, 27F)
- Protein shake (2 cups almond milk, 1 scoop Dummy Supps - 190c, 26P, 9C, 6F)
- Avocado (1/2 whole - 120c, 2P, 6C, 11F)

Instructions
1. Preheat oven to 400°F.
2. Dice the sweet potato into small cubes and toss with ½ tbsp olive oil, ¼ tsp salt, and ¼ tsp black pepper. Spread on a baking sheet and roast for 20-25 minutes, flipping halfway.
3. Heat a pan over medium heat with ½ tbsp olive oil.
4. Dice the chicken breast and season with garlic powder, smoked paprika, and black pepper.
5. Add chicken to the pan and cook for 8-10 minutes, stirring occasionally, until fully cooked and golden brown.
6. Push the chicken to one side of the pan and add the frozen bell peppers and onions. Cook for 3-4 minutes until softened.
7. Add the roasted sweet potatoes to the pan and stir to combine.
8. Pour the BBQ sauce over the mixture, tossing everything to coat evenly.

INDIVIDUAL MEAL PREP

CHICKEN BACON RANCH HASH

Calories: 650   **Protein: 65**   **Carbs: 43**   **Fat: 23**

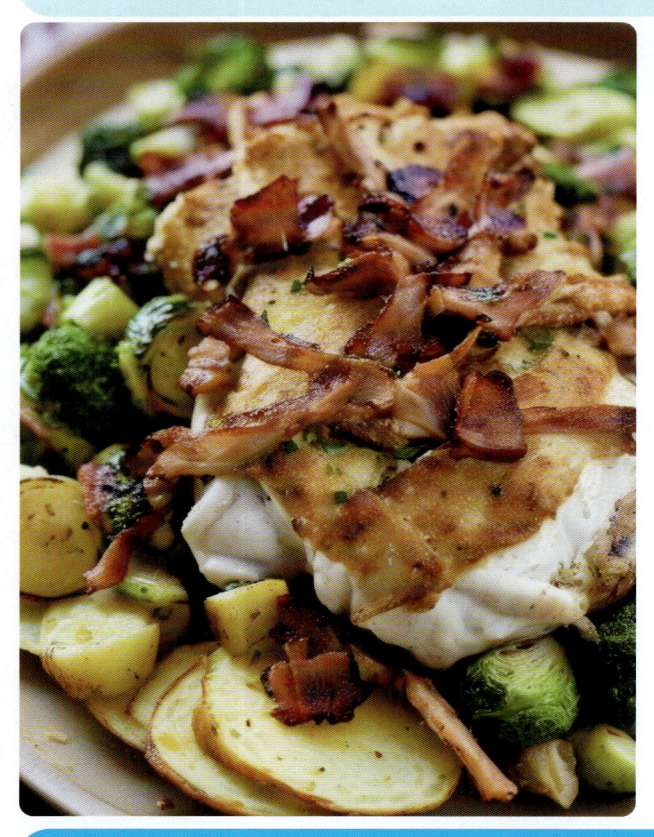

Ingredients   Servings: 1

Chicken and Potatoes:
- 1 (6 oz.) chicken breast
- 1 (6 oz.) russet potato
- 2 slices turkey bacon
- 1 tbsp olive oil
- 2 cups brussel sprouts
- 1/2 tsp garlic powder
- 1/2 tsp onion powder
- 1/2 tsp paprika
- 1/4 tsp salt
- 1/4 tsp black pepper
- ¼ cup nonfat plain greek yogurt
- 1 tbsp ranch dressing seasoning
- 1 tbsp green onions

Optional Sides
- Salad (2 cups greens, 1 tbsp extra virgin olive oil, 2 tbsp balsamic - 307c, 4P, 11C, 27F)
- Protein shake (2 cups almond milk, 1 scoop Dummy Supps - 190c, 26P, 9C, 6F)
- Avocado (1/2 whole - 120c, 2P, 6C, 11F)

Instructions
1. Preheat oven to 400°F.
2. Dice the potato into small cubes and trim and halve Brussels sprouts.
3. Toss diced potatoes with ½ tbsp olive oil, ¼ tsp salt, and ¼ tsp black pepper. Spread on a baking sheet and roast for 20-25 minutes, flipping halfway.
4. Toss Brussels sprouts with cooking spray, salt, and black pepper. Add to the baking sheet with potatoes for the last 12-15 minutes of roasting.
5. Heat a pan over medium heat with ½ tbsp olive oil.
6. Add chopped turkey bacon and cook for 3-4 minutes, until crispy. Remove and set aside.
7. In the same pan, add diced chicken and season with garlic powder, onion powder, paprika, salt, and black pepper. Cook for 4-5 minutes per side, until golden brown and fully cooked.
8. In a small bowl, mix Greek yogurt and ranch dressing seasoning until smooth.
9. Combine the roasted potatoes, Brussels sprouts, and cooked turkey bacon with the chicken in the pan. Stir and cook for 2-3 minutes to blend flavors.
10. Drizzle with the Greek yogurt ranch mixture and toss to coat evenly.

INDIVIDUAL MEAL PREP

BUFFALO CHICKEN BOWL

Calories: 470 **Protein: 53** **Carbs: 27** **Fat: 10**

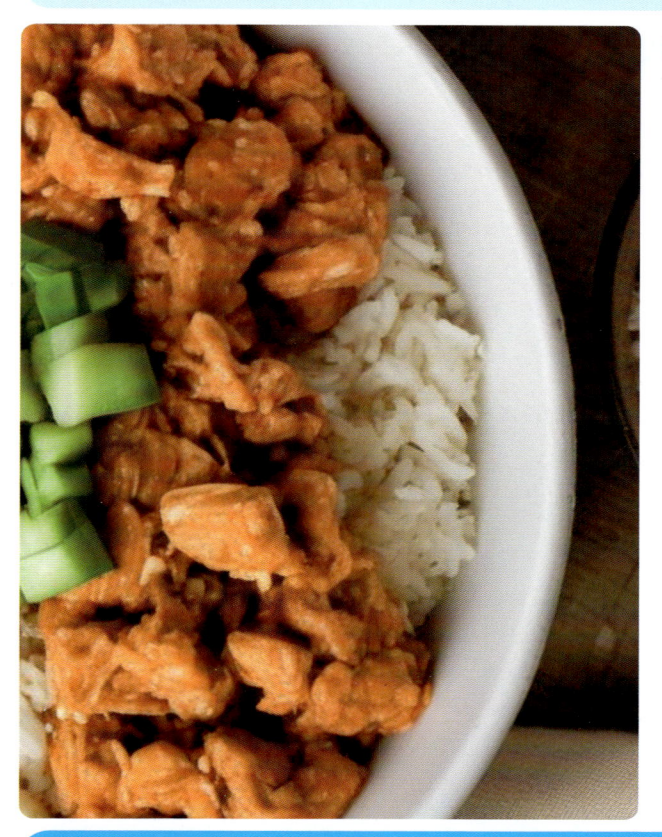

Ingredients **Servings: 1**

Bowl:
- 1 (6 oz.) chicken breast
- 1/2 cup cooked rice
- 2 tbsp ranch dressing seasoning
- 1 tsp garlic powder
- 1 tsp onion powder
- 1/2 tsp black pepper

Buffalo Sauce:
- 1/2 cup low fat cottage cheese
- 2 tbsp buffalo sauce
- 2 tbsp shredded cheddar cheese

Optional Sides
- Salad (2 cups greens, 1 tbsp extra virgin olive oil, 2 tbsp balsamic - 307c, 4P, 11C, 27F)
- Protein shake (2 cups almond milk, 1 scoop Dummy Supps - 190c, 26P, 9C, 6F)
- Avocado (1/2 whole - 120c, 2P, 6C, 11F)

Instructions
1. Dice chicken into bite-sized pieces.
2. Heat a pan with cooking spray on medium-high. Add minced garlic, chicken, and listed seasonings.
3. Cook for 8-10 minutes until fully cooked.
4. Add 1/2 cup water and 1/4 cup rice in pot, bring to boil on high heat, turn to low, cover, and cook for 5-7 minutes or microwave rice.
5. Blend cottage cheese, buffalo sauce, and shredded cheese and mix with chicken.
6. Stir on low heat for 5 minutes.
7. Combine chicken and rice.

INDIVIDUAL MEAL PREP

CHICKEN FAJITA BOWL

Calories: 530 **Protein: 55** **Carbs: 31** **Fat: 12**

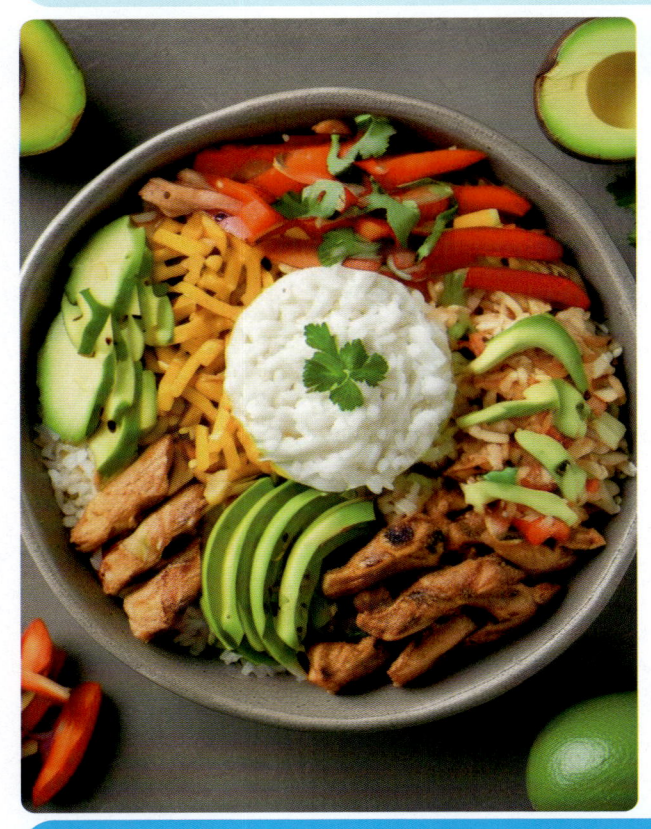

Ingredients Servings: 1

Bowl:
- 1 (6 oz.) chicken breast
- 1/2 cup cooked rice
- 2 tbsp green chilies
- 1/4 red onion
- 1/2 bell pepper
- 2 tbsp mexican cheese
- 2 tsp lime juice
- 2 tbsp taco seasoning

Optional Sides
- Salad (2 cups greens, 1 tbsp olive oil, 2 tbsp balsamic - 307c, 4P, 11C, 27F)
- Protein shake (2 cups almond milk, 1 scoop Dummy Supps - 200c, 28P, 5C, 7F)
- Salsa (2 tbsp - 10c, 0P, 2C, 0F)
- Hot sauce (1 tsp - 1c, 0P, 0C, 0F)
- Avocado (1/2 whole - 120c, 2P, 6C, 11F)

Instructions
1. Heat a pan over medium heat.
2. Dice the chicken breast into bite sized pieces.
3. Add chicken to a pan with cooking spray and listed seasonings and cook for 8-10 minutes, stirring occasionally, until fully cooked and golden brown.
4. Add diced red onion and bell pepper to the pan. Cook for 2-3 minutes until softened.
5. Stir in green chilies and remaining taco seasoning. Cook for 1 minute, allowing flavors to blend.
6. Mix in the cooked rice and stir until evenly coated. Cook for 2 minutes until heated through.
7. Remove from heat and drizzle with lime juice.
8. Top with Mexican cheese and let it melt slightly.

INDIVIDUAL MEAL PREP

TERIYAKI CHICKEN BOWL

Calories: 414   **Protein: 49**   **Carbs: 33**   **Fat: 4**

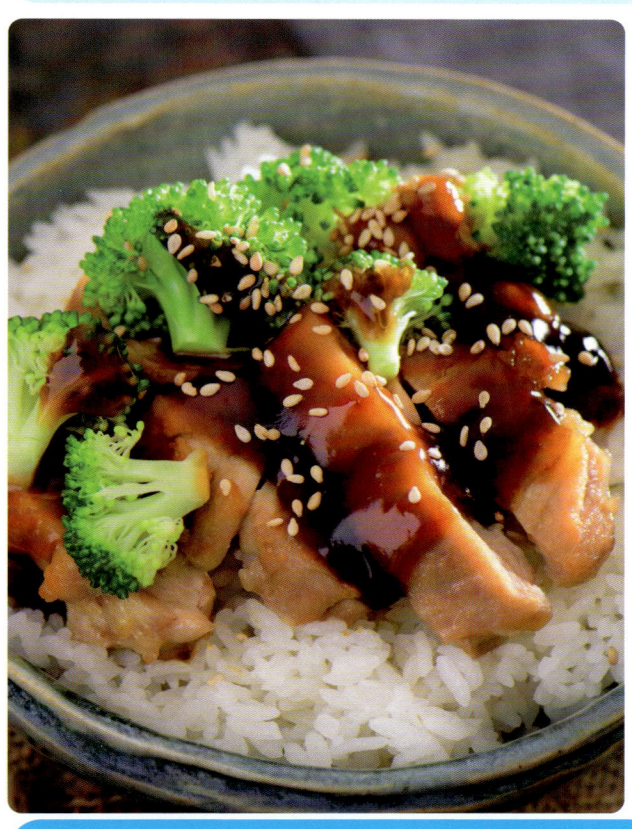

Ingredients   **Servings: 1**

Bowl:
- 1 (6 oz.) chicken breast
- 1/2 cup cooked rice
- 1/2 cup G Hughes teriyaki marinade
- 2 cups broccoli florets
- 1 tsp garlic powder
- 1 tsp onion powder
- 1/2 tsp black pepper
- 1 tbsp lemon juice
- 1 tsp sesame seeds

Optional Sides
- Salad (2 cups greens, 1 tbsp extra virgin olive oil, 2 tbsp balsamic - 307c, 4P, 11C, 27F)
- Protein shake (2 cups almond milk, 1 scoop Dummy Supps - 190c, 26P, 9C, 6F)
- Avocado (1/2 whole - 120c, 2P, 6C, 11F)

Instructions
1. Dice chicken into bite-sized pieces.
2. Heat a pan with cooking spray on medium-high. Add chicken and listed seasonings. Cook for 8-10 minutes until fully cooked.
3. Steam broccoli in a microwave or pan until tender for 5-7 minutes, drain water, season with salt, pepper, and lemon juice.
4. Add teriyaki marinade to the pan with cooked chicken and stir on low heat for 3-5 minutes.
5. Add 1/2 cup water and 1/4 cup rice in pot, bring to boil on high heat, turn to low, cover, and cook for 5-7 minutes or microwave rice.
6. Plate rice, top with teriyaki chicken, broccoli, sesame seeds and serve.

INDIVIDUAL MEAL PREP

SPICY KOREAN CHICKEN & RICE

Calories: 550 **Protein: 59** **Carbs: 41** **Fat: 16**

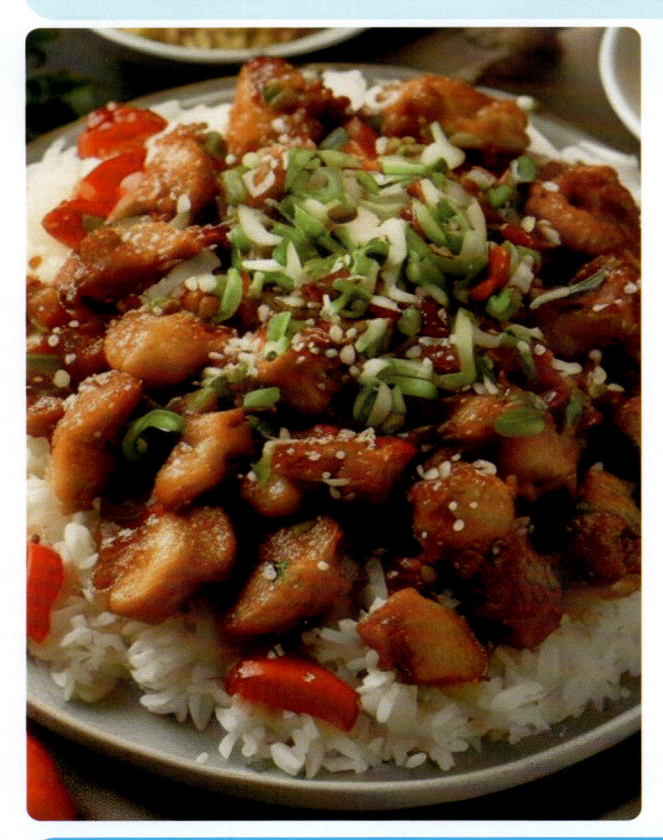

Ingredients **Servings: 1**

Chicken and Rice:
- 1 (6 oz.) chicken breast
- 1/2 cup cooked rice
- 2 cups frozen bell peppers and onions
- 1/2 tbsp gochujang (Korean chili paste)
- 1 tbsp soy sauce
- 1 tbsp sesame oil
- 1 tsp garlic powder
- ½ tsp black pepper
- ¼ tsp salt
- 1 tsp sesame seeds

Optional Sides

- Salad (2 cups greens, 1 tbsp extra virgin olive oil, 2 tbsp balsamic - 307c, 4P, 11C, 27F)
- Protein shake (2 cups almond milk, 1 scoop Dummy Supps - 190c, 26P, 9C, 6F)

Instructions

1. Heat a pan over medium heat and add ½ tbsp sesame oil.
2. Dice the chicken breast and season with garlic powder, black pepper, and salt.
3. Add chicken to the pan and cook for 8-10 minutes, stirring occasionally, until golden brown and cooked through.
4. Push the chicken to one side of the pan and add the frozen bell peppers and onions. Sauté for 3-4 minutes until softened.
5. In a small bowl, mix gochujang, soy sauce, and remaining sesame oil.
6. Pour the sauce mixture over the chicken and vegetables, stirring well to coat everything evenly. Cook for 1-2 minutes, allowing the flavors to blend.
7. Stir in the cooked rice and toss everything together. Cook for another 1-2 minutes until the rice is heated through.
8. Garnish with sesame seeds.

INDIVIDUAL MEAL PREP

BEEF PROTEIN PASTA

Calories: 640 **Protein: 52** **Carbs: 50** **Fat: 23**

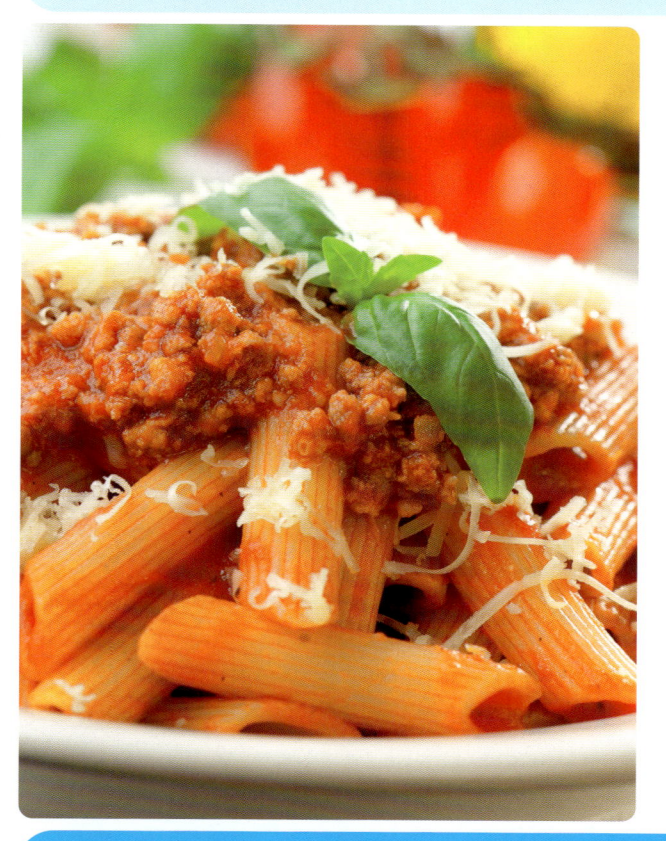

Ingredients **Servings: 1**

Pasta:
- 6 oz. or 3/4 cup lean ground beef
- 1/2 cup cooked protein pasta
- 1 tablespoon minced garlic
- 1 cup marinara sauce
- 2 tablespoons parmesan cheese
- 1 tsp garlic powder
- 1 tsp onion powder
- 1 tsp Italian seasoning
- 1/2 tsp black pepper
- 1/4 tsp salt

Optional Sides
- Salad (2 cups greens, 1 tbsp extra virgin olive oil, 2 tbsp balsamic - 307c, 4P, 11C, 27F)
- Protein shake (2 cups almond milk, 1 scoop Dummy Supps - 190c, 26P, 9C, 6F)

Instructions
1. Heat a pan with cooking spray on medium-high.
2. Add ground beef, minced garlic and listed seasonings.
3. Cook for 8-10 minutes until fully cooked.
4. Boil pasta for 9-11 minutes. Drain.
5. Combine pasta, beef, marinara, and parmesan in the pan.
6. Stir on low heat for 5 minutes.

INDIVIDUAL MEAL PREP

BEEF & RICE

Calories: 460   **Protein: 43**   **Carbs: 36**   **Fat: 16**

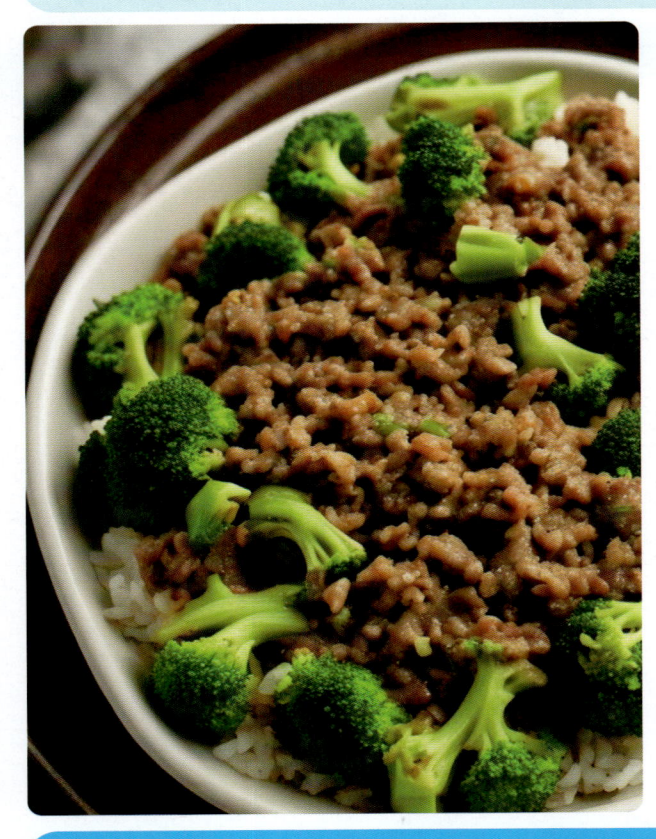

Ingredients   Servings: 1

Beef and Rice:
- 6 oz. or 3/4 cup lean ground beef
- 1/2 cup cooked rice
- 1 tablespoon minced garlic
- 2 cups mixed frozen broccoli
- 1 tsp garlic powder
- 1 tsp onion powder
- 1 tsp paprika
- 1/4 tsp salt
- 1/2 tsp black pepper

Optional Sides

- Salad (2 cups greens, 1 tbsp extra virgin olive oil, 2 tbsp balsamic - 307c, 4P, 11C, 27F)
- Protein shake (2 cups almond milk, 1 scoop Dummy Supps - 190c, 26P, 9C, 6F)
- G Hughes Sauce (2 tbsp - 10c, 0P, 5C, 0F)

Instructions

1. Place frozen broccoli in a microwave-safe bowl with 2 tbsp water, cover, and microwave for 3-4 minutes until tender. Drain excess water and season with salt and black pepper.
2. Heat a pan over medium heat and coat with cooking spray.
3. Add ground beef and minced garlic to the pan. Cook for 5-7 minutes, breaking up the meat, until fully browned.
4. Season beef with garlic powder, onion powder, salt, and black pepper. Stir to combine.
5. Add broccoli to pan with beef.
6. Add ½ cup water and ¼ cup rice in a pot, bring to a boil on high heat, turn to low, cover, and cook for 5-7 minutes or microwave rice.
7. Serve seasoned ground beef over rice.

INDIVIDUAL MEAL PREP

CLASSIC CHEESEBURGER

Calories: 560 **Protein: 48** **Carbs: 34** **Fat: 32**

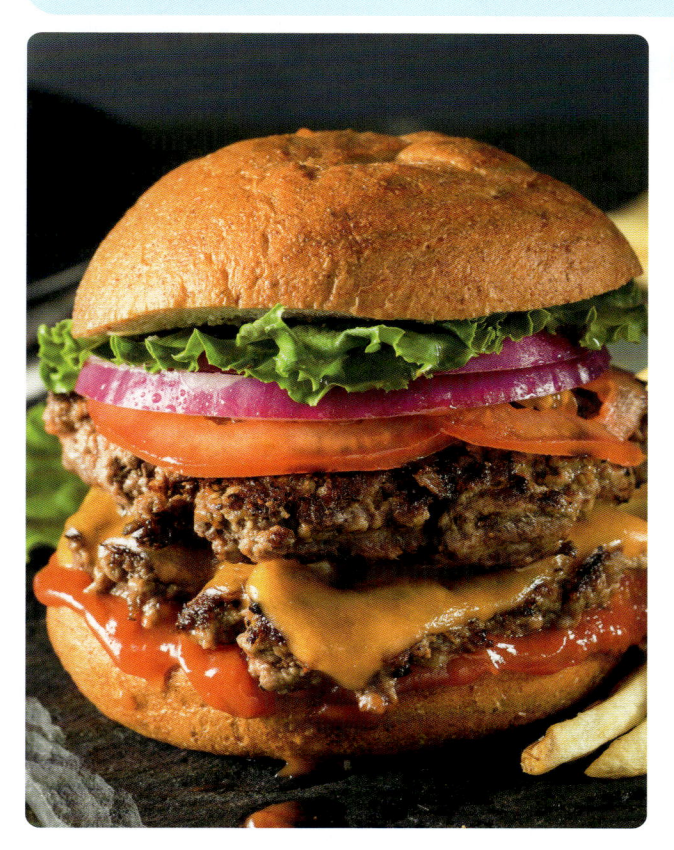

Ingredients Servings: 1

Bowl:
- 1 (6 oz. or 3/4 cup) patty lean ground beef
- 1 647 low carb bun
- 1/4 cup sweet onion
- 2 slices tomato
- 4 dill pickles
- 1 slice cheese
- 1 tsp garlic powder
- 1 tsp onion powder
- 1/2 tsp black pepper
- 1/4 tsp salt

Mac Sauce:
- 2 tbsp ketchup
- 2 tbsp lite mayo
- 2 tbsp dill relish
- 1 tsp mustard
- 1 tsp pickle juice

Optional Sides

- Salad (2 cups greens, 1 tbsp extra virgin olive oil, 2 tbsp balsamic - 307c, 4P, 11C, 27F)
- Protein Shake (2 cups almond milk, 1 scoop Dummy Supps - 190c, 26P, 9C, 6F)
- Alexia Sweet Potato Fries (12 fries - 140c, 1P, 24C, 5F)

Instructions

1. Dice onions. Slice tomato.
2. Form beef into a patty and season with listed seasonings.
3. Heat a pan with cooking spray on medium-high. Cook burger for 4-5 minutes each side or until desired internal cook.
4. To bowl, add mac sauce ingredients and mix well.
5. To bun combine beef patty, cheese, vegetables, and top with mac sauce.

INDIVIDUAL MEAL PREP

BURGER & FRIES BOWL

Calories: 620 **Protein: 44** **Carbs: 34** **Fat: 36**

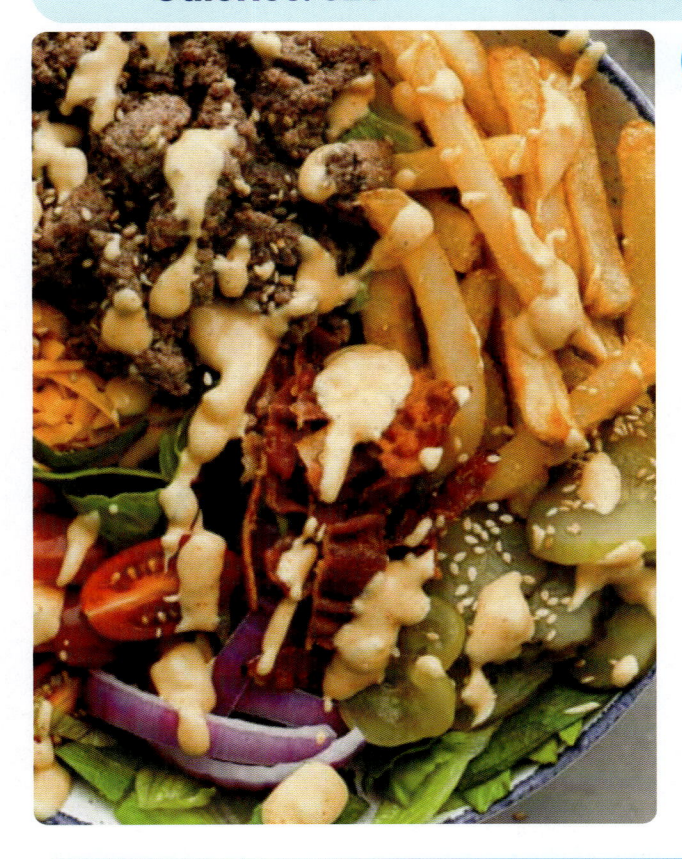

Ingredients   Servings: 1

Bowl:
- 3/4 cup ground beef
- 12 (Alexia) sweet potato french fries
- 2 tbsp sweet onion
- 2 tbsp diced tomatoes
- 2 tbsp dill pickles
- 1/4 cup shredded cheese
- 1 tsp garlic powder
- 1 tsp onion powder
- 1/4 tsp salt
- 1/2 tsp black pepper

Mac Sauce:
- 2 tbsp ketchup
- 2 tbsp lite mayo
- 2 tbsp dill relish
- 1 tsp mustard
- 1 tsp pickle juice

Optional Sides
- Salad (2 cups greens, 1 tbsp extra virgin olive oil, 2 tbsp balsamic - 307c, 4P, 11C, 27F)
- Protein shake (2 cups almond milk, 1 scoop Dummy Supps - 190c, 26P, 9C, 6F)
- Avocado (1/2 whole - 120c, 2P, 6C, 11F)

Instructions
1. Preheat oven or air fryer to 400°F.
2. Chop onions, tomatoes, and pickles.
3. Heat a pan with cooking spray on medium-high. Add ground beef and listed seasonings.
4. Cook for 8-10 minutes until fully cooked.
5. Add french fries to baking sheet in oven/air fryer for 10-12 minutes, shaking halfway.
6. To bowl, add mac sauce ingredients and mix well.
7. Combine fries, beef, cheese, diced vegetables, and top with mac sauce.

INDIVIDUAL MEAL PREP

CHEESEBURGER BOWL

Calories: 590 **Protein: 45** **Carbs: 33** **Fat: 28**

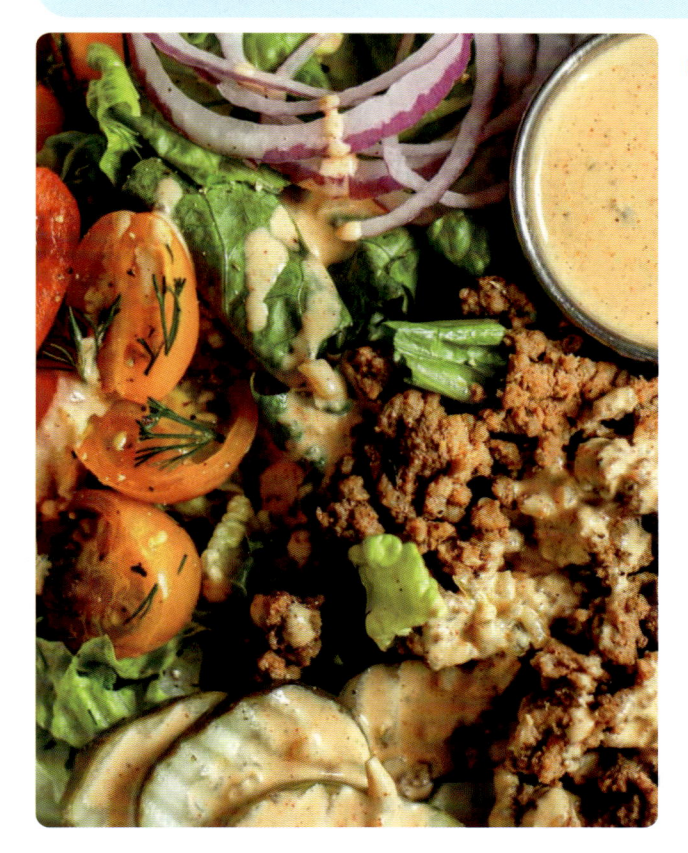

Ingredients **Servings: 1**

Bowl:
- 6 oz. or 3/4 cup lean ground beef
- 1/2 cup cooked rice
- 2 tbsp sweet onion
- 2 tbsp diced tomatoes
- 2 tbsp dill pickles
- 1/4 cup shredded cheese
- 1 tsp garlic powder
- 1 tsp onion powder
- 1/2 tsp black pepper
- 1/4 tsp salt

Mac Sauce:
- 2 tbsp G Hughes sugar free ketchup
- 2 tbsp lite mayo
- 2 tbsp dill relish
- 1 tsp mustard
- 1 tsp pickle juice

Optional Sides

- Salad (2 cups greens, 1 tbsp extra virgin olive oil, 2 tbsp balsamic - 307c, 4P, 11C, 27F)
- Protein shake (2 cups almond milk, 1 scoop Dummy Supps - 190c, 26P, 9C, 6F)
- Alexia sweet potato fries (12 fries - 140c, 1P, 24C, 5F)

Instructions

1. Chop onions, tomatoes, and pickles.
2. Heat a pan with cooking spray on medium-high. Add ground beef and listed seasonings.
3. Cook for 8-10 minutes until fully cooked.
4. Add 1/2 cup water and 1/4 cup rice in pot, bring to boil on high heat, turn to low, cover, and cook for 5-7 minutes or microwave rice.
5. To bowl, add mac sauce ingredients and mix well.
6. Combine rice, beef, cheese, diced vegetables, and top with mac sauce.

INDIVIDUAL MEAL PREP

BEEF QUESADILLA

Calories: 480 **Protein: 49** **Carbs: 24** **Fat: 18**

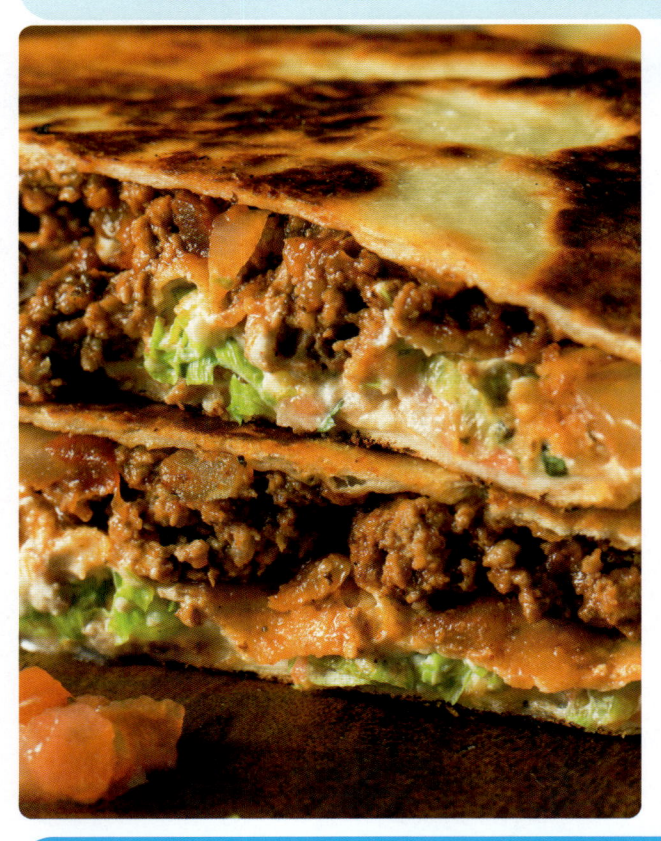

Ingredients **Servings: 1**

Quesadilla:

- 6 oz. or 3/4 cup lean ground beef
- 1 (12 oz.) low-carb tortilla
- 2 tbsp green chilis
- 1/4 cup onion
- 1/4 cup bell pepper
- 1/2 cup shredded cheese
- 2 tsp taco seasoning

Optional Sides

- Salad (2 cups greens, 1 tbsp olive oil, 2 tbsp balsamic - 307c, 4P, 11C, 27F)
- Protein shake (2 cups almond milk, 1 scoop Dummy Supps - 200c, 28P, 5C, 7F)
- Salsa (2 tbsp - 10c, 0P, 2C, 0F)
- Hot sauce (1 tsp - 1c, 0P, 0C, 0F)
- Avocado (1/2 whole - 120c, 2P, 6C, 11F)

Instructions

1. Slice peppers and onions.
2. Cook ground beef in a pan with taco seasoning and green chilis over medium-high heat for 8-10 minutes until fully cooked. Remove.
3. In the same pan, cook diced onions and bell peppers with cooking spray for 5 minutes until softened. Remove.
4. Add a tortilla to the pan with cooking spray on medium-low heat.
5. Add shredded cheese, ground beef, onions, and peppers to one half of the tortilla.
6. Fold the tortilla in half and cook for 2-3 minutes on each side until the cheese is melted and the tortilla is golden and crispy.

INDIVIDUAL MEAL PREP

TEX-MEX BEEF & POTATO SKILLET

Calories: 640 **Protein: 46** **Carbs: 39** **Fat: 36**

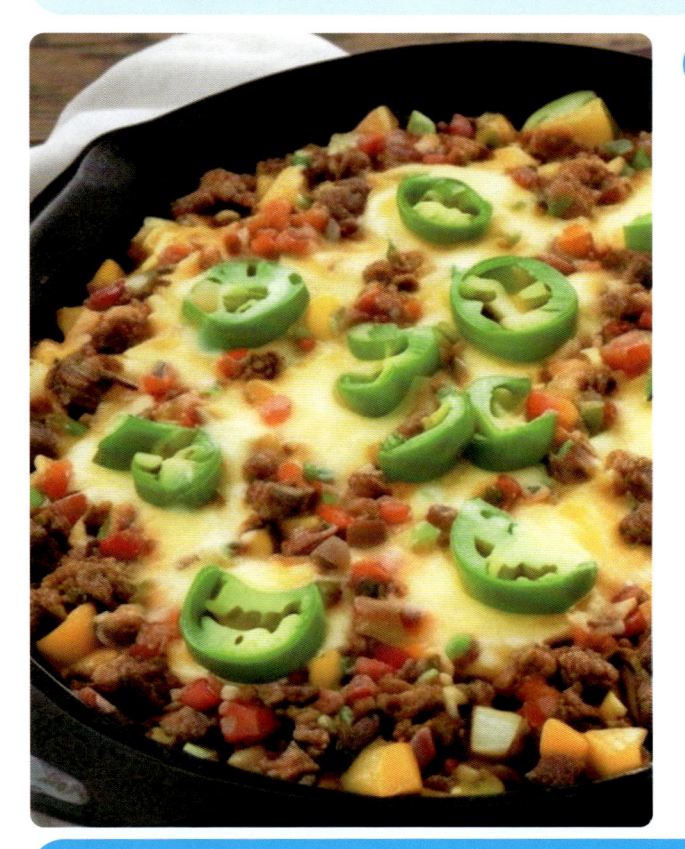

Ingredients Servings: 1

Skillet:
- 6 oz. or 3/4 cup lean ground beef
- 1 (6 oz.) russet potato
- 2 cups frozen bell peppers and onions
- 2 tbsp jalapenos
- 1 tbsp olive oil
- 1/4 cup shredded cheese
- 1 tsp chili powder
- 1/2 tsp cumin
- 1/2 tsp smoked paprika
- 1 tsp garlic powder
- 1 tsp onion powder
- 1/2 tsp salt
- 1/2 tsp black pepper
- 2 tbsp cilantro

Optional Sides
- Salad (2 cups greens, 1 tbsp extra virgin olive oil, 2 tbsp balsamic - 307c, 4P, 11C, 27F)
- Protein shake (2 cups almond milk, 1 scoop Dummy Supps - 190c, 26P, 9C, 6F)
- Avocado (1/2 whole - 120c, 2P, 6C, 11F)

Instructions
1. Dice the potato into small cubes.
2. Heat a large skillet over medium heat with cooking spray.
3. Add frozen bell peppers, onions, and jalapeños to the skillet and sauté for 4-5 minutes, stirring occasionally, until softened and any excess moisture evaporates. Remove from the skillet and set aside.
4. Add ½ tbsp olive oil to the skillet, then add diced potatoes. Season with chili powder, cumin, smoked paprika, garlic powder, onion powder, salt, and black pepper. Cook for 8-10 minutes, stirring occasionally, until golden brown and tender. Remove from the skillet and set aside with the vegetables.
5. In the same skillet, add ½ tbsp olive oil and ground beef. Cook for 5-7 minutes, breaking it up as it browns.
6. Return cooked potatoes and sautéed vegetables to the skillet and stir everything together.
7. Sprinkle shredded cheese over the mixture and let it melt for 1-2 minutes before serving.
8. Garnish with chopped cilantro before serving.

INDIVIDUAL MEAL PREP

SPICY KOREAN BEEF & RICE

Calories: 580   **Protein: 42**   **Carbs: 41**   **Fat: 29**

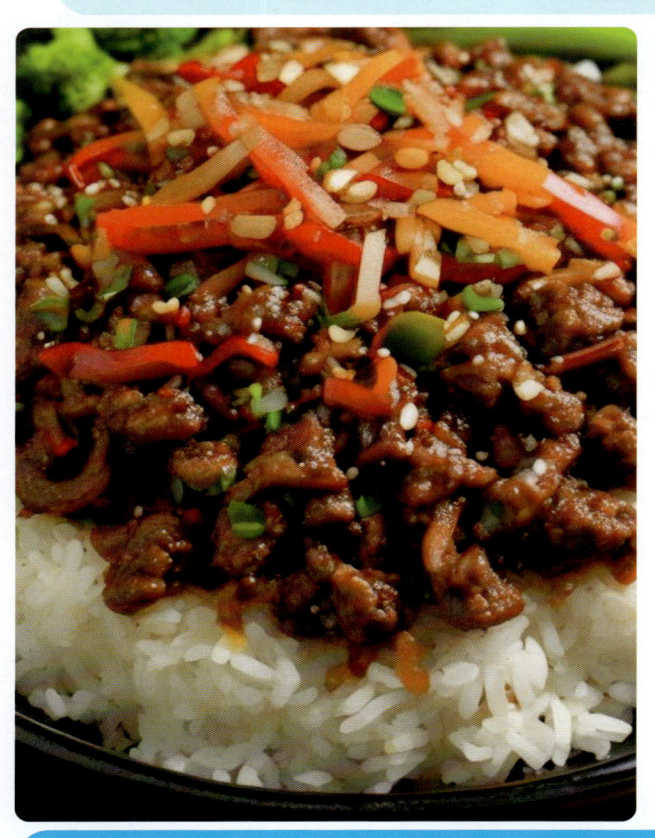

Ingredients   **Servings: 1**

Chicken and Rice:
- 6 oz. or 3/4 cup lean ground beef
- 1/2 cup cooked rice
- 2 cups frozen bell peppers and onions
- 1/2 tbsp gochujang (Korean chili paste)
- 1 tbsp soy sauce
- 1 tbsp sesame oil
- 1 tsp garlic powder
- ½ tsp black pepper
- ¼ tsp salt
- 1 tbsp sesame seeds

Optional Sides
- Salad (2 cups greens, 1 tbsp extra virgin olive oil, 2 tbsp balsamic - 307c, 4P, 11C, 27F)
- Protein shake (2 cups almond milk, 1 scoop Dummy Supps - 190c, 26P, 9C, 6F)

Instructions
1. Heat a pan over medium heat with cooking spray.
2. Add frozen bell peppers and onions to the pan and sauté for 4-5 minutes, stirring occasionally, until softened and excess moisture evaporates. Remove from the pan and set aside.
3. In the same pan, add sesame oil and ground beef. Season with garlic powder, black pepper, and salt, then cook for 5-7 minutes, breaking it up as it browns.
4. Stir in gochujang and soy sauce, mixing well to coat the beef evenly. Simmer for 1-2 minutes.
5. Add ½ cup water and ¼ cup rice to a pot, bring to a boil on high heat, then reduce to low, cover, and cook for 5-7 minutes or microwave rice.
6. Add cooked rice and sautéed vegetables back into the pan, stirring until everything is combined and heated through.
7. Sprinkle sesame seeds over the mixture before serving.

INDIVIDUAL MEAL PREP

BEEF GYRO

Calories: 650 **Protein: 54** **Carbs: 43** **Fat: 16**

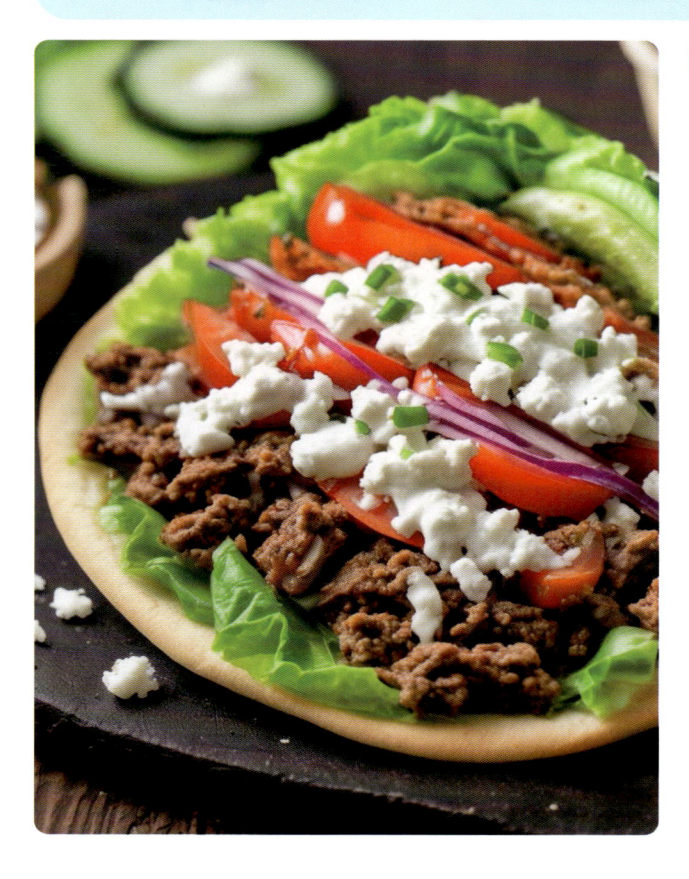

Ingredients Servings: 1

Gyro:

- 6 oz. or 3/4 cup lean ground beef
- 1 (8 oz. Joseph's Low Carb) pita
- 2 tbsp cucumbers
- 2 tbsp diced tomatoes
- 1/2 cup lettuce
- 2 tbsp red onion
- 2 tbsp banana peppers
- 2 tbsp low-fat feta
- 1 tsp garlic powder
- 1 tsp onion powder
- 1/2 tsp black pepper
- 1/4 tsp salt

Tzatziki:

- 1/2 cup nonfat plain greek yogurt
- 2 tbsp cucumber
- 2 tsp lemon juice
- 1 tsp dill
- 1/2 tsp black pepper
- 1/4 tsp salt

Optional Sides

- Salad (2 cups greens, 1 tbsp extra virgin olive oil, 2 tbsp balsamic - 307c, 4P, 11C, 27F)
- Protein shake (2 cups almond milk, 1 scoop Dummy Supps - 190c, 26P, 9C, 6F)
- Avocado (1/2 whole - 120c, 2P, 6C, 11F)

Instructions

1. Dice cucumber, tomatoes, and onions.
2. Cook ground beef in a pan with garlic powder, onion powder, salt, and black pepper over medium-high heat for 8-10 minutes until fully cooked.
3. To bowl, add tzatziki ingredients and mix well.
4. Warm pita in a pan or microwave.
5. Layer pita with lettuce, tomatoes, cucumbers, red onion, banana peppers, feta cheese, and cooked beef.
6. Drizzle with tzatziki sauce and fold or wrap the pita.

INDIVIDUAL MEAL PREP

STEAK FAJITA BOWL

Calories: 630 **Protein: 49** **Carbs: 31** **Fat: 27**

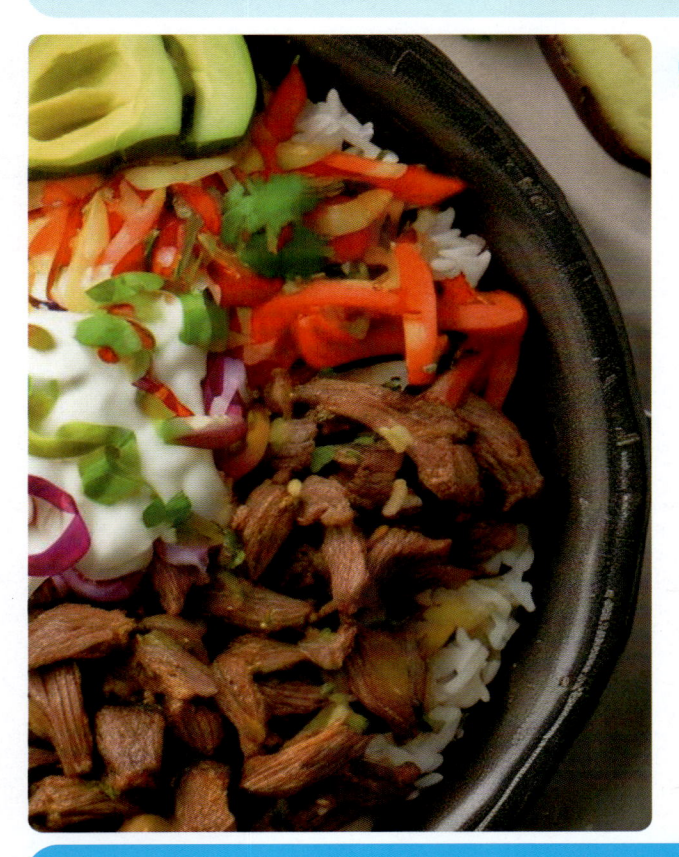

Ingredients **Servings: 1**

Bowl:
- 1 cup (8 oz.) carne asada/shaved beef
- 1/2 cup cooked rice
- 2 tbsp green chilies
- 1/4 red onion
- 1/2 bell pepper
- 2 tbsp mexican cheese
- 2 tsp lime juice
- 2 tbsp taco seasoning

Optional Sides

- Salad (2 cups greens, 1 tbsp extra virgin olive oil, 2 tbsp balsamic - 307c, 4P, 11C, 27F)
- Protein shake (2 cups almond milk, 1 scoop Dummy Supps - 190c, 26P, 9C, 6F)
- Hot sauce (1 tsp - 1c, 0P, 0C, 0F)
- Avocado (1/2 whole - 120c, 2P, 6C, 11F)

Instructions

1. Slice peppers and onions.
2. Heat a pan with cooking spray on medium-high. Add beef, taco seasoning, and green chilies. Cook for 6-8 minutes until fully cooked.
3. Add sliced onions and bell peppers to the pan and sauté for 5 minutes until softened.
4. Add 1/2 cup water and 1/4 cup rice in pot, bring to boil on high heat, turn to low, cover, and cook for 5-7 minutes or microwave rice.
5. Assemble the bowl: layer rice, beef, onions, and peppers.
6. Top with Mexican cheese and lime juice.

INDIVIDUAL MEAL PREP

CHIPOTLE CHICKEN WRAP

Calories: 414 **Protein: 51** **Carbs: 16** **Fat: 14**

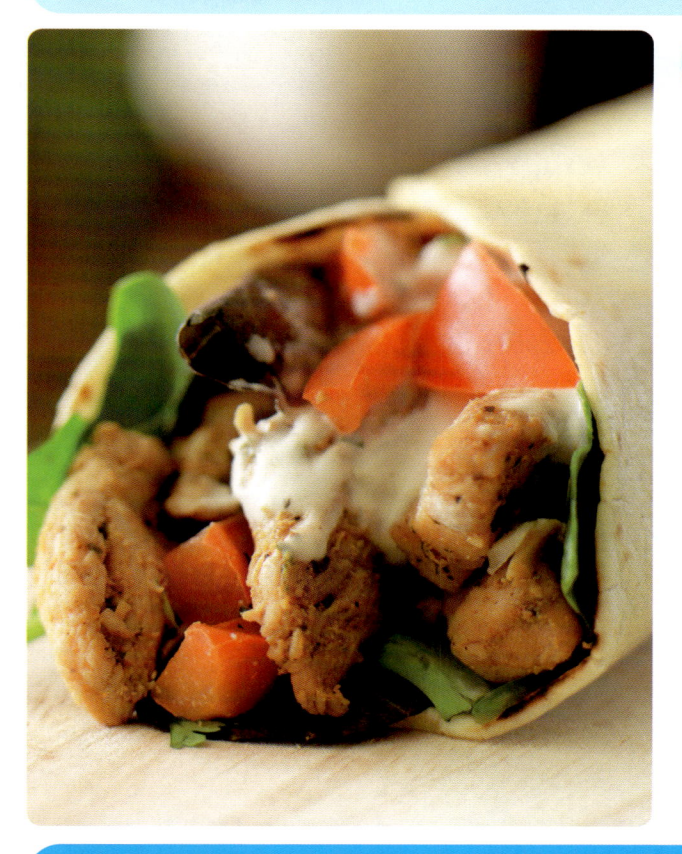

Ingredients — Servings: 1

Wrap:
- 1 (6 oz.) chicken breast
- 1 (12 oz.) Mission low carb tortilla
- 1/4 cup lettuce
- 2 tbsp diced tomatoes
- 2 tbsp red onion
- 1 slice cheddar cheese
- 1 tsp garlic powder
- 1 tsp onion powder
- 1/2 tsp black pepper

Chipotle Ranch:
- 1/4 cup nonfat plain greek yogurt
- 2 tsp taco seasoning
- 2 tsp lime juice

Optional Sides
- Salad (2 cups greens, 1 tbsp extra virgin olive oil, 2 tbsp balsamic - 307c, 4P, 11C, 27F)
- Protein shake (2 cups almond milk, 1 scoop Dummy Supps - 190c, 26P, 9C, 6F)
- Avocado (1/2 whole - 120c, 2P, 6C, 11F)

Instructions
1. Dice lettuce, tomatoes, onion. Dice chicken into bite-sized pieces.
2. Heat a pan with cooking spray on medium-high. Add chicken and listed seasonings.
3. Cook for 8-10 minutes until fully cooked.
4. In a small mixing bowl add the listed ingredients for chipotle ranch. Mix well.
5. Warm low-carb tortilla in a pan or microwave.
6. To tortilla combine chicken, chipotle ranch, slice of cheese, and diced vegetables.
7. Wrap tightly and serve.

INDIVIDUAL MEAL PREP

BUFFALO CHICKEN WRAP

Calories: 420   **Protein: 51**   **Carbs: 16**   **Fat: 14**

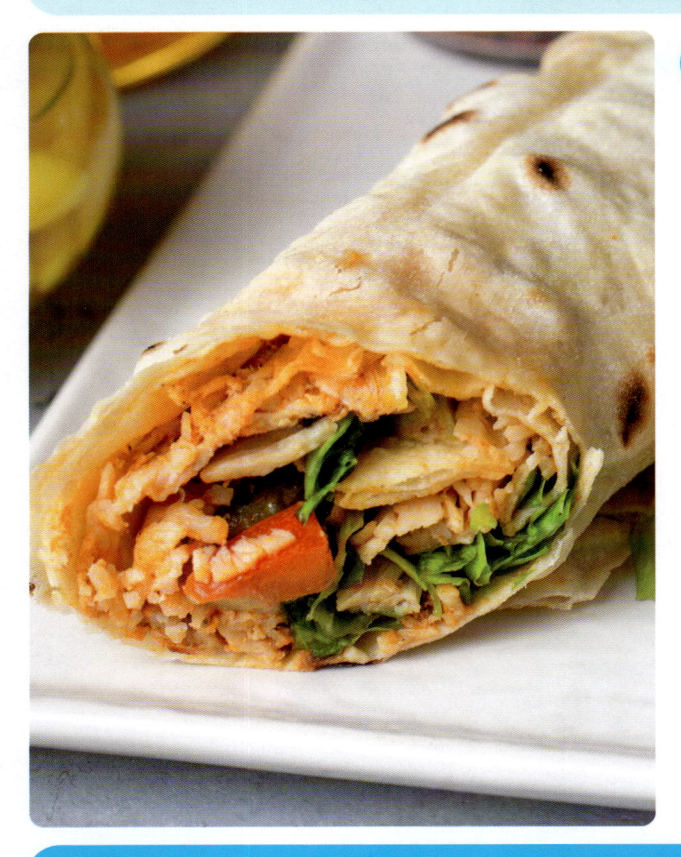

Ingredients   Servings: 1

Wrap:
- 1 (6 oz.) chicken breast
- 1 (12 oz.) Mission low carb tortilla
- 1/4 cup lettuce
- 2 tbsp tomatoes
- 2 tbsp red onion
- 1 slice cheddar cheese
- 1 tsp garlic powder
- 1 tsp onion powder
- 1/2 tsp black pepper

Buffalo Sauce:
- 1/4 cup nonfat plain greek yogurt
- 2 tbsp buffalo sauce
- 2 tsp lime juice

Optional Sides
- Salad (2 cups greens, 1 tbsp extra virgin olive oil, 2 tbsp balsamic - 307c, 4P, 11C, 27F)
- Protein shake (2 cups almond milk, 1 scoop Dummy Supps - 190c, 26P, 9C, 6F)
- Avocado (1/2 whole - 120c, 2P, 6C, 11F)

Instructions
1. Dice lettuce, tomatoes, onion. Dice chicken into bite-sized pieces.
2. Heat a pan with cooking spray on medium-high. Add chicken and listed seasonings.
3. Cook for 8-10 minutes until fully cooked.
4. In a small mixing bowl add the listed ingredients for buffalo sauce. Mix well.
5. Warm low-carb tortilla in a pan or microwave.
6. To tortilla combine chicken, buffalo sauce, slice of cheese, diced vegetables.
7. Wrap tightly and serve.

INDIVIDUAL MEAL PREP

CHICKEN CAESAR WRAP

Calories: 501 **Protein: 62** **Carbs: 30** **Fat: 12**

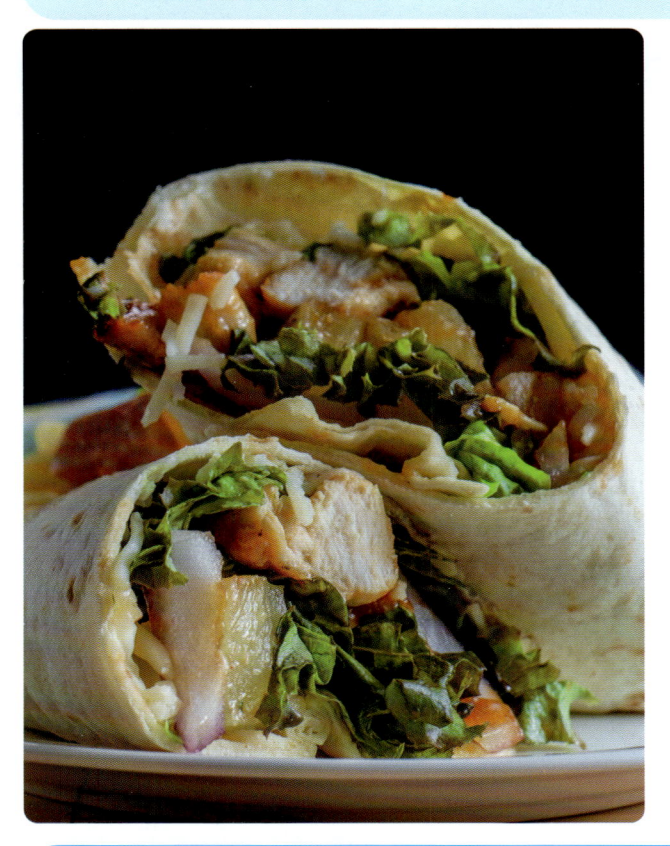

Ingredients **Servings: 1**

Wrap:
- 1 (6 oz.) chicken breast
- 1 (12 oz.) Mission low carb tortilla
- 1/4 cup romaine
- 2 tbsp parmesan cheese
- 2 tbsp (Primal Kitchen) caesar salad dressing
- 2 tbsp croutons
- 1/4 tsp salt
- 1/2 tsp black pepper

Optional Sides
- Salad (2 cups greens, 1 tbsp extra virgin olive oil, 2 tbsp balsamic - 307c, 4P, 11C, 27F)
- Protein shake (2 cups almond milk, 1 scoop Dummy Supps - 190c, 26P, 9C, 6F)
- Avocado (1/2 whole - 120c, 2P, 6C, 11F)

Instructions
1. Dice romaine lettuce. Dice chicken into bite-sized pieces.
2. Heat a pan with cooking spray on medium-high. Add chicken and listed seasonings.
3. Cook for 8-10 minutes until fully cooked.
4. Combine chicken, lettuce, parmesan cheese, croutons, and caesar salad dressing into bowl and mix well.
5. Warm low-carb tortilla in a pan or microwave.
6. To tortilla combine salad.
7. Wrap tightly and serve.

INDIVIDUAL MEAL PREP

CHICKEN BACON RANCH WRAP

Calories: 495 **Protein: 48** **Carbs: 12** **Fat: 26**

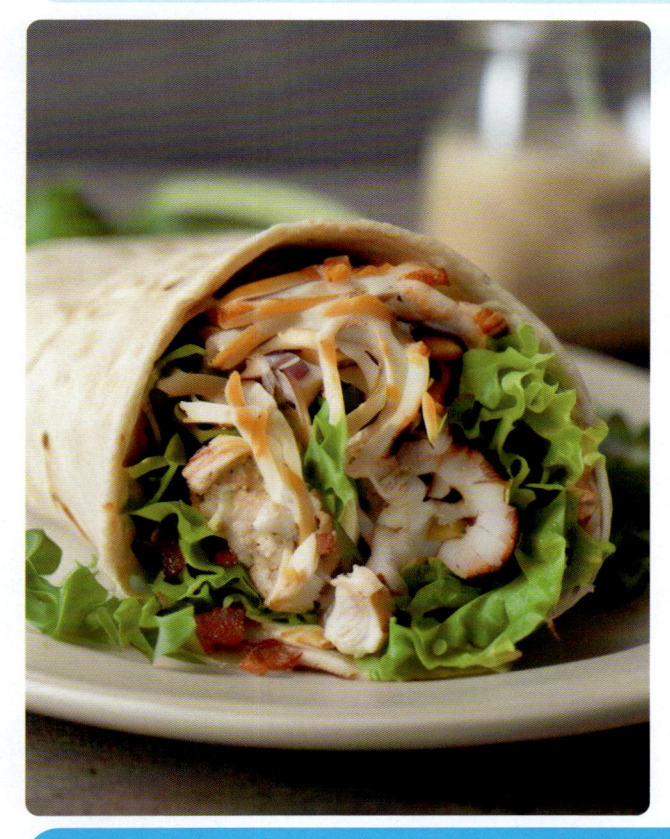

Ingredients **Servings: 1**

Wrap:
- 1 (6 oz.) chicken breast
- 1 (12 oz.) Mission low carb tortilla
- 1 tbsp minced garlic
- 2 slices turkey bacon
- 2 tbsp parmesan cheese
- 1 tsp garlic powder
- 1 tsp onion powder
- 1/2 tsp black pepper

Protein Ranch:
- 1/4 cup nonfat plain greek yogurt
- 2 tsp ranch seasoning
- 2 tsp lime juice

Optional Sides
- Salad (2 cups greens, 1 tbsp extra virgin olive oil, 2 tbsp balsamic - 307c, 4P, 11C, 27F)
- Protein shake (2 cups almond milk, 1 scoop Dummy Supps - 190c, 26P, 9C, 6F)
- Avocado (1/2 whole - 120c, 2P, 6C, 11F)

Instructions
1. Dice chicken breast into bite-sized pieces.
2. Season with garlic powder, onion powder, and black pepper.
3. Heat a pan with cooking spray on medium-high. Add minced garlic and chicken.
4. Cook for 8-10 minutes until fully cooked.
5. Cook turkey bacon in the same pan until crispy, then chop into small pieces.
6. In bowl, mix ingredients for protein ranch.
7. Warm low-carb tortilla in a pan or microwave.
8. Fill the tortilla with chicken, turkey bacon, parmesan cheese, and a drizzle of protein ranch.
9. Wrap tightly and serve.

INDIVIDUAL MEAL PREP

CHICKEN GYRO

Calories: 510 **Protein: 60** **Carbs: 44** **Fat: 12**

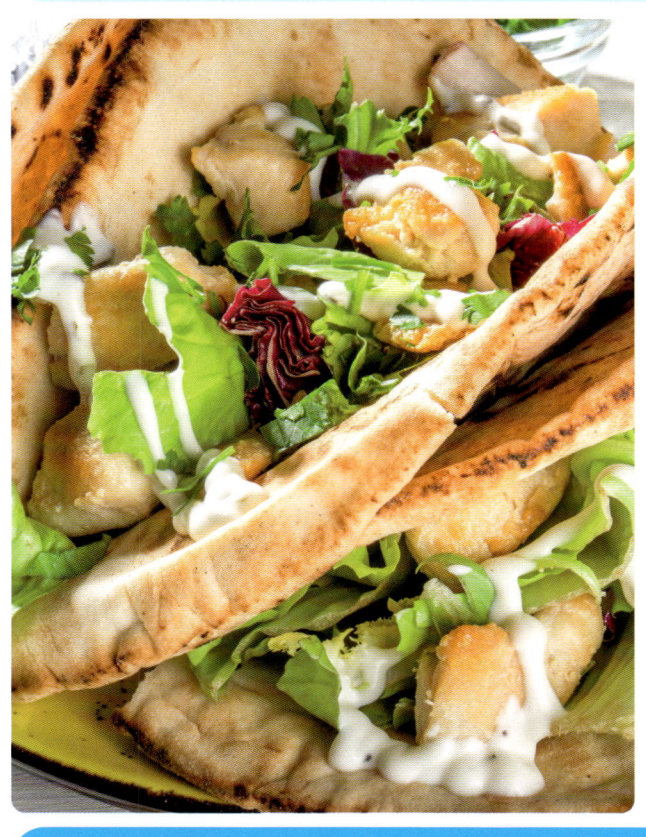

Ingredients **Servings: 1**

Gyro:
- 1 (6 oz.) chicken breast
- 1 (8 oz.) pita
- 1/2 cup cucumbers
- 1/2 cup tomatoes
- 1/2 cup lettuce
- 1/4 cup red onion
- 2 tbsp banana peppers
- 2 tbsp low-fat feta
- 1 tsp garlic powder
- 1 tsp onion powder
- 1/4 tsp salt
- 1/2 tsp black pepper

Tzatziki:
- 1/2 cup nonfat plain greek yogurt
- 2 tbsp cucumber
- 2 tsp lemon juice
- 1/4 tsp salt
- 1/2 tsp black pepper
- 1 tsp dill

Optional Sides
- Salad (2 cups greens, 1 tbsp extra virgin olive oil, 2 tbsp balsamic - 307c, 4P, 11C, 27F)
- Protein shake (2 cups almond milk, 1 scoop Dummy Supps - 190c, 26P, 9C, 6F)
- Avocado (1/2 whole - 120c, 2P, 6C, 11F)

Instructions
1. Dice cucumber, tomatoes, and onions.
2. Dice chicken into bite-sized pieces. Heat a pan with cooking spray on medium-high.
3. Add chicken and listed seasonings. Cook for 8-10 minutes until fully cooked.
4. To bowl, add tzatziki ingredients and mix well.
5. Warm pita in a pan or microwave.
6. Layer pita with lettuce, tomatoes, cucumbers, red onion, banana peppers, feta cheese, and cooked chicken.
7. Drizzle with tzatziki sauce and fold or wrap the pita.

INDIVIDUAL MEAL PREP

TURKEY CLUB WRAP

Calories: 456 **Protein: 43** **Carbs: 25** **Fat: 13**

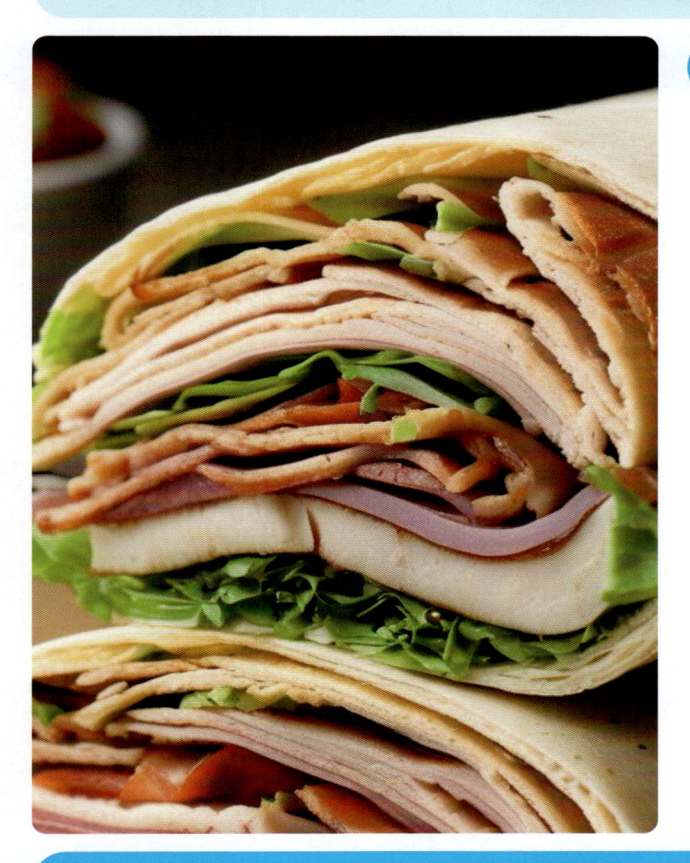

Ingredients Servings: 1

Wrap:
- 5 slices turkey breast
- 1 (12 oz.) Mission low carb tortilla
- 1/4 cup lettuce
- 2 tbsp tomatoes
- 2 tbsp sweet onion
- 1 slice cheddar cheese
- 2 slices turkey bacon
- 2 tbsp lite mayonnaise

Optional Sides
- Salad (2 cups greens, 1 tbsp extra virgin olive oil, 2 tbsp balsamic - 307c, 4P, 11C, 27F)
- Protein shake (2 cups almond milk, 1 scoop Dummy Supps - 190c, 26P, 9C, 6F)
- Avocado (1/2 whole - 120c, 2P, 6C, 11F)

Instructions

1. Dice lettuce, tomatoes, and onion.
2. Add turkey bacon in microwave for 2 minutes or air fry/bake at 400°F for 8-10 minutes.
3. Warm low-carb tortilla in a pan or microwave.
4. To tortilla combine turkey breast, lettuce, tomato, onion, sliced cheese, turkey bacon, and mayo.
5. Wrap tightly and serve.

INDIVIDUAL MEAL PREP

CHICKEN QUESADILLA

Calories: 390 **Protein: 49** **Carbs: 20** **Fat: 16**

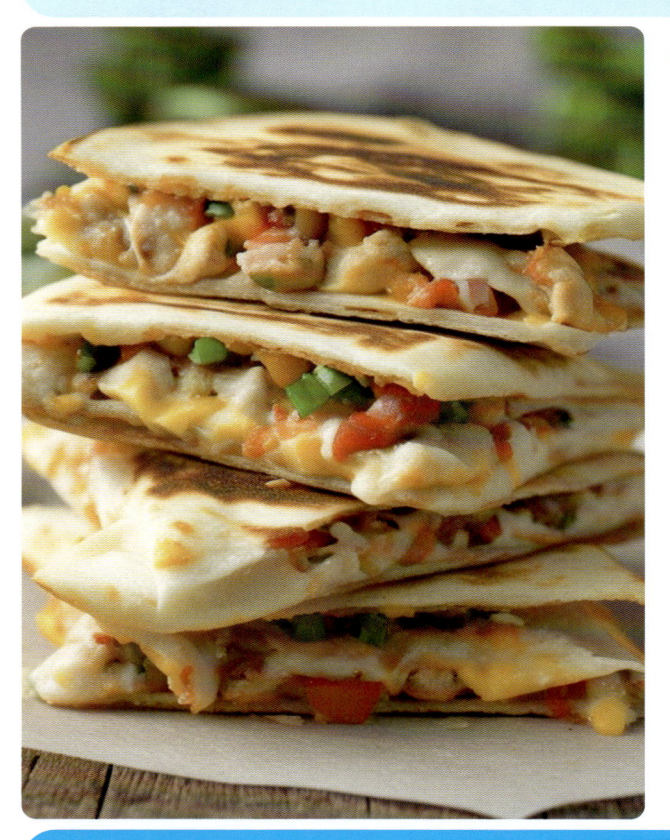

Ingredients **Servings: 1**

Quesadilla:
- 1 (6 oz.) chicken breast
- 1 (12 oz.) low-carb tortilla
- 2 tbsp green chilis
- 1/4 cup onion
- 1/4 cup bell pepper
- 1/2 cup shredded cheese
- 2 tsp taco seasoning

Optional Sides
- Salad (2 cups greens, 1 tbsp olive oil, 2 tbsp balsamic - 307c, 4P, 11C, 27F)
- Protein shake (2 cups almond milk, 1 scoop Dummy Supps - 200c, 28P, 5C, 7F)
- Salsa (2 tbsp - 10c, 0P, 2C, 0F)
- Hot sauce (1 tsp - 1c, 0P, 0C, 0F)
- Avocado (1/2 whole - 120c, 2P, 6C, 11F)

Instructions
1. Slice peppers and onions.
2. Dice chicken into bite-sized pieces and mix with taco seasoning and green chilis.
3. Cook chicken in a pan with cooking spray on medium-high heat for 8-10 minutes until fully cooked. Remove.
4. In the same pan, cook diced onions and bell peppers with cooking spray for 5 minutes until softened. Remove.
5. Add a tortilla to the pan with cooking spray on medium-low heat.
6. Add shredded cheese, chicken, onions, and peppers to one half of the tortilla.
7. Fold the tortilla in half and cook for 2-3 minutes on each side until the cheese is melted and the tortilla is golden and crispy.

INDIVIDUAL MEAL PREP

LOADED BLT SANDWICH

Calories: 588 **Protein: 45** **Carbs: 41** **Fat: 34**

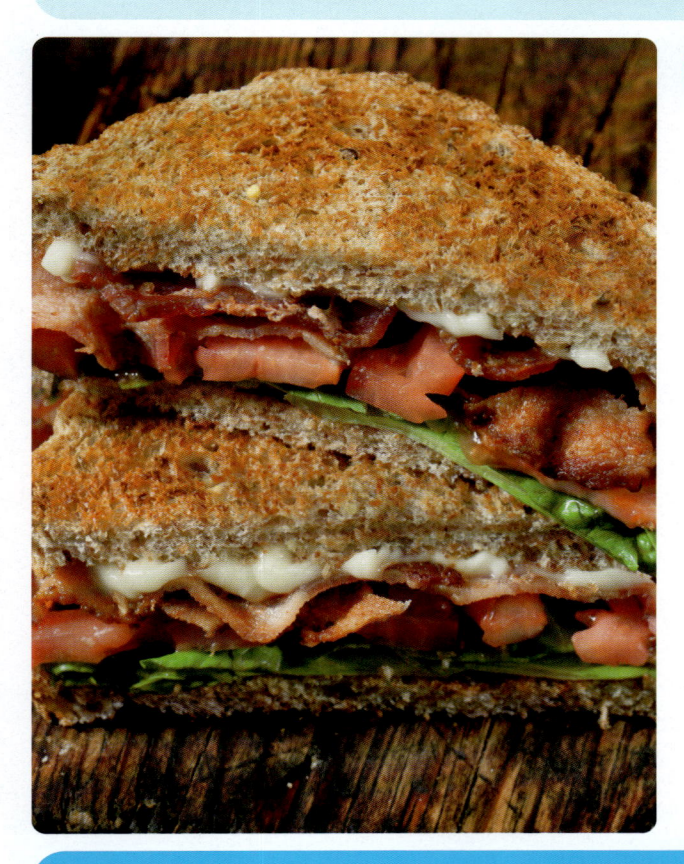

Ingredients **Servings: 1**

Sandwich:
- 5 slices turkey breast
- 2 slices 647 low carb bread
- 1/4 cup lettuce
- 2 slices tomato
- 1 slice cheddar cheese
- 2 slices turkey bacon
- 1/2 avocado
- 2 tbsp lite mayonnaise

Optional Sides
- Salad (2 cups greens, 1 tbsp extra virgin olive oil, 2 tbsp balsamic - 307c, 4P, 11C, 27F)
- Protein shake (2 cups almond milk, 1 scoop Dummy Supps - 190c, 26P, 9C, 6F)

Instructions
1. Dice lettuce, tomatoes, and onion.
2. Slice avocado.
3. Cook turkey bacon in microwave for 2 minutes or air fry/bake at 400°F for 8 minutes.
4. Toast bread.
5. To bread combine turkey breast, lettuce, tomato, sliced cheese, turkey bacon, sliced avocado and mayo.
6. Form sandwich.

INDIVIDUAL MEAL PREP

LOADED CHICKEN SANDWICH

Calories: 576 **Protein: 48** **Carbs: 33** **Fat: 33**

Ingredients **Servings: 1**

Sandwich:
- 1 (6 oz.) chicken breast
- 2 647 low carb bread
- 2 slices tomato
- 2 slice cheddar cheese
- 4 slices turkey bacon
- 1/2 whole avocado
- 4 tbsp lite mayonnaise
- 1 tsp garlic powder
- 1 tsp onion powder
- 1/4 tsp salt
- 1/2 tsp black pepper

Optional Sides

- Salad (2 cups greens, 1 tbsp extra virgin olive oil, 2 tbsp balsamic - 307c, 4P, 11C, 27F)
- Protein shake (2 cups almond milk, 1 scoop Dummy Supps - 190c, 26P, 9C, 6F)

Instructions

1. Slice tomatoes. Butterfly chicken breast and season with listed seasonings.
2. Cook chicken in a pan with cooking spray over medium heat for 4-5 minutes per side until fully cooked.
3. Cook turkey bacon in the same pan until crispy.
4. Toast bread slices in a toaster or pan.
5. Spread 2 tbsp of lite mayonnaise on each slice of bread. Layer each sandwich with one piece of chicken, cheddar cheese, turkey bacon, sliced avocado, and tomato.

INDIVIDUAL MEAL PREP

CHICKEN SALAD SANDWICH

Calories: 519 **Protein: 56** **Carbs: 29** **Fat: 23**

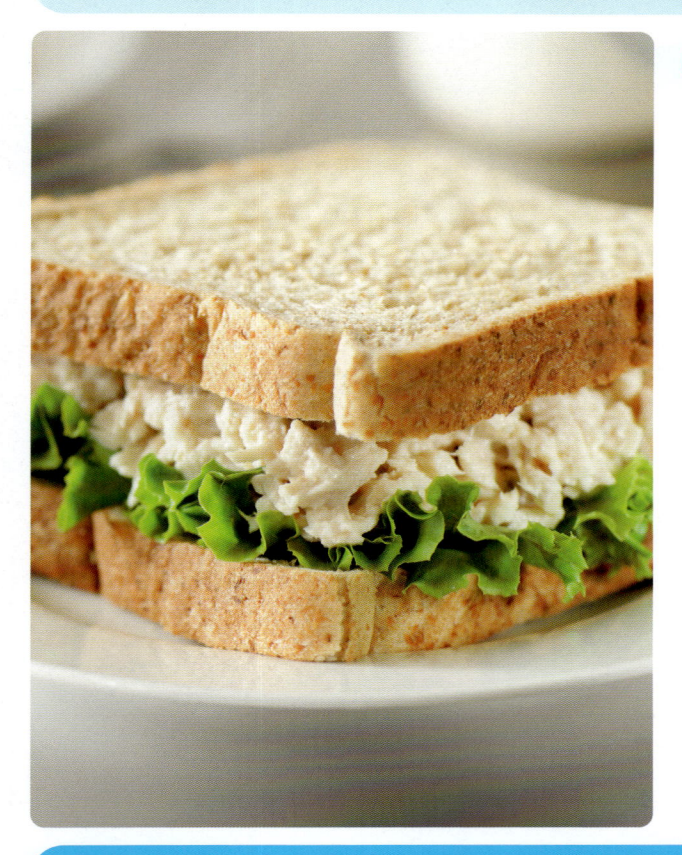

Ingredients   Servings: 1

Sandwich:
- 1 cup canned chicken breast
- 2 slices 647 low carb bread
- 1/4 cup lite mayonnaise
- 1/2 cup lettuce
- 1/4 cup dill pickles
- 1 tsp garlic powder
- 1 tsp onion powder
- 1/4 tsp salt
- 1/2 tsp black pepper

Optional Sides

- Salad (2 cups greens, 1 tbsp extra virgin olive oil, 2 tbsp balsamic - 307c, 4P, 11C, 27F)
- Protein shake (2 cups almond milk, 1 scoop Dummy Supps - 190c, 26P, 9C, 6F)
- Avocado (1/2 whole - 120c, 2P, 6C, 11F)

Instructions

1. Slice celery and dill pickles.
2. Drain canned chicken breast and add to a mixing bowl.
3. Combine chicken with celery, pickles, mayonnaise, salt, black pepper, garlic powder, and onion powder. Mix well.
4. Toast bread slices in a toaster or pan.
5. Spread chicken salad mixture onto each slice of bread.

INDIVIDUAL MEAL PREP

BUFFALO CHICKEN GRILLED CHEESE

Calories: 568 **Protein: 62** **Carbs: 29** **Fat: 27**

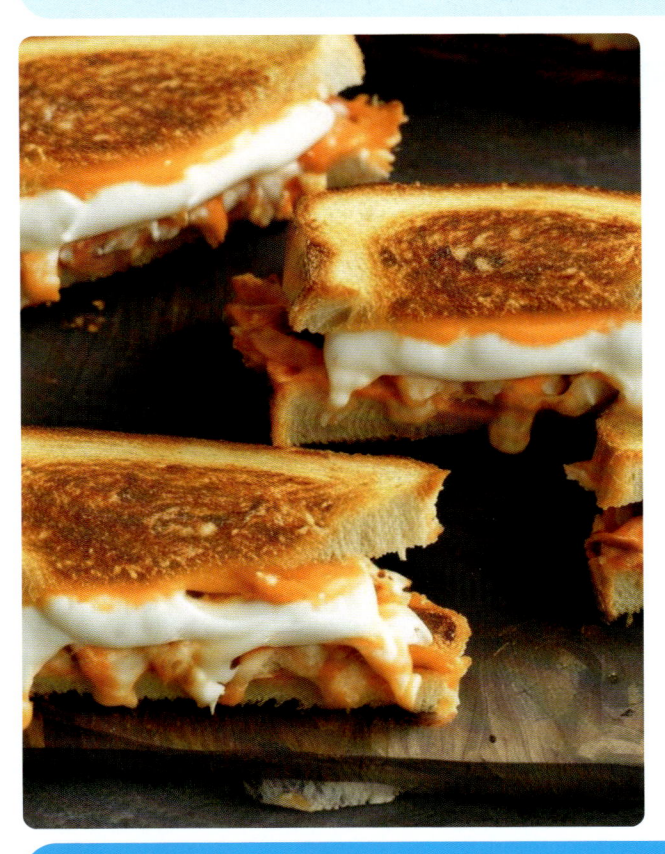

Ingredients Servings: 1

Sandwich:
- 1 cup canned chicken breast
- 2 slices 647 low carb bread
- 2 tbsp Buffalo wing sauce
- 2 tbsp whipped cream cheese
- 1 slice pepper jack cheese
- 1 tbsp butter
- 1/2 tsp cayenne pepper
- 1/2 tsp onion powder
- 1/4 tsp salt
- 1/2 tsp black pepper

Optional Sides
- Salad (2 cups greens, 1 tbsp extra virgin olive oil, 2 tbsp balsamic - 307c, 4P, 11C, 27F)
- Protein shake (2 cups almond milk, 1 scoop Dummy Supps - 190c, 26P, 9C, 6F)
- Avocado (1/2 whole - 120c, 2P, 6C, 11F)

Instructions
1. Drain canned chicken breast and add to a mixing bowl.
2. Mix chicken with Buffalo wing sauce, whipped cream cheese, and listed ingredients until well combined.
3. Spread the buffalo chicken mixture onto one slice of bread.
4. Place the pepper jack cheese on top of the chicken mixture, then cover with the second slice of bread.
5. Heat a skillet over medium heat and spread 1/2 tbsp butter on each side of bread.
6. Grill the sandwich in the skillet for 2-3 minutes per side until the bread is golden brown and the cheese is melted.

INDIVIDUAL MEAL PREP

CHIPOTLE CHICKEN GRILLED CHEESE

Calories: 568 **Protein: 62** **Carbs: 29** **Fat: 27**

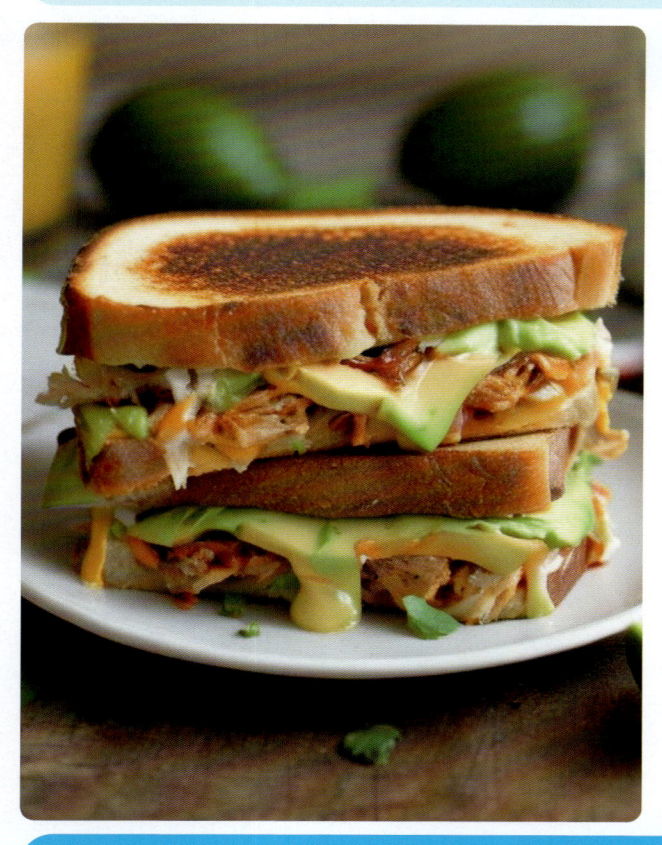

Ingredients **Servings: 1**

Sandwich:
- 1 cup canned chicken breast
- 2 slices 647 low carb bread
- 2 tbsp green chilies
- 1 slice pepper jack cheese
- 1/2 avocado
- 1/4 cup lite mayo
- 1 tbsp butter
- 2 tsp taco seasoning

Optional Sides
- Salad (2 cups greens, 1 tbsp extra virgin olive oil, 2 tbsp balsamic - 307c, 4P, 11C, 27F)
- Protein shake (2 cups almond milk, 1 scoop Dummy Supps - 190c, 26P, 9C, 6F)

Instructions
1. Drain canned chicken breast and add to a mixing bowl.
2. Mix chicken with green chilies, lite mayo, and taco seasoning until well combined.
3. Spread the chicken mixture onto one slice of bread.
4. Place pepper jack cheese on top of the chicken mixture, then spread mashed avocado on the second slice of bread and place it on top to form a sandwich.
5. Heat a skillet over medium heat and spread 1/2 tbsp butter on each side of the sandwich.
6. Grill the sandwich in the skillet for 2-3 minutes per side until the bread is golden brown and the cheese is melted.

INDIVIDUAL MEAL PREP

LOADED TURKEY SANDWICH

Calories: 520 **Protein: 51** **Carbs: 34** **Fat: 27**

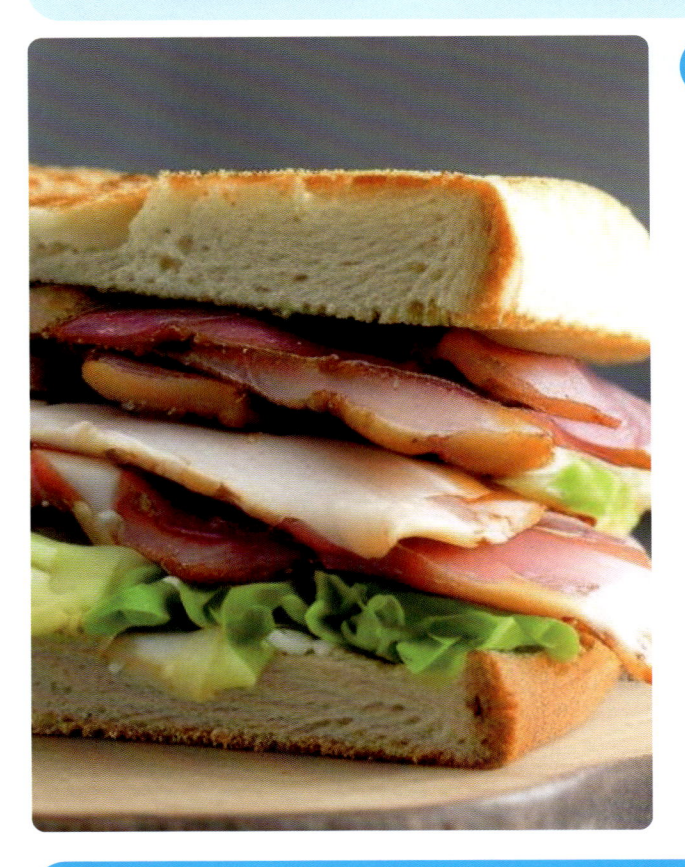

Ingredients **Servings: 1**

Sandwich:
- 4 slices turkey breast
- 2 slices low-calorie bread
- 1 slice cheese
- 2 slices of turkey bacon
- 1/2 whole avocado
- 2 slices lettuce
- 2 slices tomato
- 1 tbsp lite mayonnaise
- 1 tbsp everything but the bagel seasoning

Optional Sides

- Salad (2 cups greens, 1 tbsp extra virgin olive oil, 2 tbsp balsamic - 307c, 4P, 11C, 27F)
- Protein shake (2 cups almond milk, 1 scoop Dummy Supps - 190c, 26P, 9C, 6F)

Instructions

1. Toast bread if desired.
2. Cook turkey bacon in a pan over medium heat until crispy.
3. Mash avocado and spread onto one slice of bread. Top with bagel seasoning.
4. Spread lite mayonnaise onto the other slice of bread.
5. Layer turkey breast, cheese, turkey bacon, lettuce, and tomato.
6. Top with the second slice of bread.

INDIVIDUAL MEAL PREP

SALMON RICE & BROCCOLI

Calories: 559   **Protein: 40**   **Carbs: 25**   **Fat: 28**

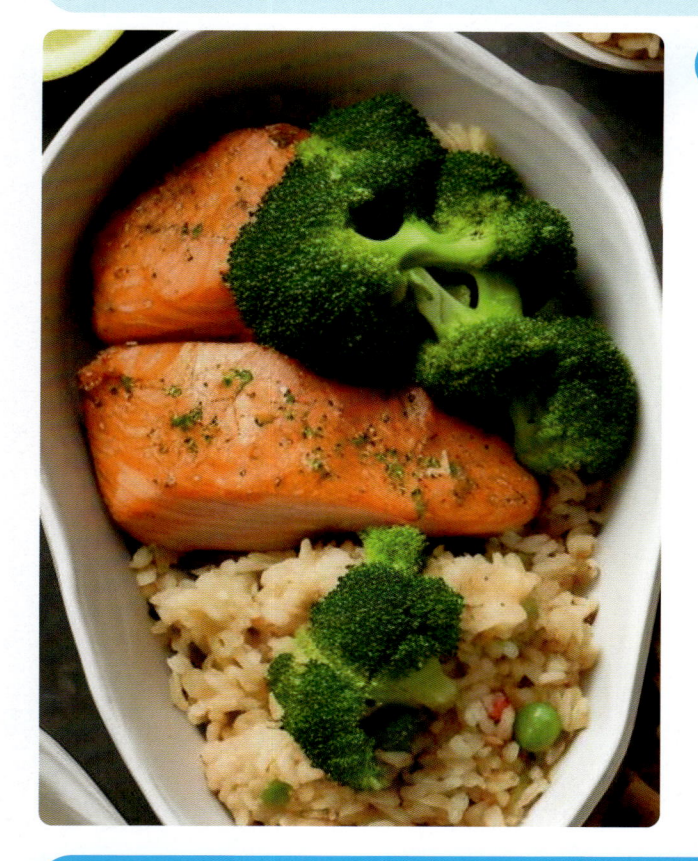

Ingredients   **Servings: 1**

Salmon:
- 1 (6 oz.) salmon fillet
- 1/2 cup cooked rice
- 1 cup broccoli florets
- 1 tbsp extra virgin olive oil
- 1/2 tsp garlic powder
- 1/2 tsp onion powder
- 1/4 tsp salt
- 1/2 tsp black pepper
- 2 tsp lemon juice

Optional Sides

- Salad (2 cups greens, 1 tbsp extra virgin olive oil, 2 tbsp balsamic - 307c, 4P, 11C, 27F)
- Protein shake (2 cups almond milk, 1 scoop Dummy Supps - 190c, 26P, 9C, 6F)
- Avocado (1/2 whole - 120c, 2P, 6C, 11F)

Instructions

1. Preheat a pan with olive oil on medium heat.
2. Season salmon with garlic powder, onion powder, paprika, salt, and pepper.
3. Cook salmon for 3-4 minutes per side until fully cooked. Remove from pan.
4. In the same pan, sauté broccoli with a pinch of salt and pepper for 5-7 minutes until tender.
5. Add 1/2 cup water and 1/4 cup rice in pot, bring to boil on high heat, turn to low, cover, and cook for 5-7 minutes or microwave rice.
6. Drizzle lemon juice over the salmon, add rice and broccoli and serve.

INDIVIDUAL MEAL PREP

SWEET & SPICY SALMON

Calories: 500 **Protein: 40** **Carbs: 25** **Fat: 28**

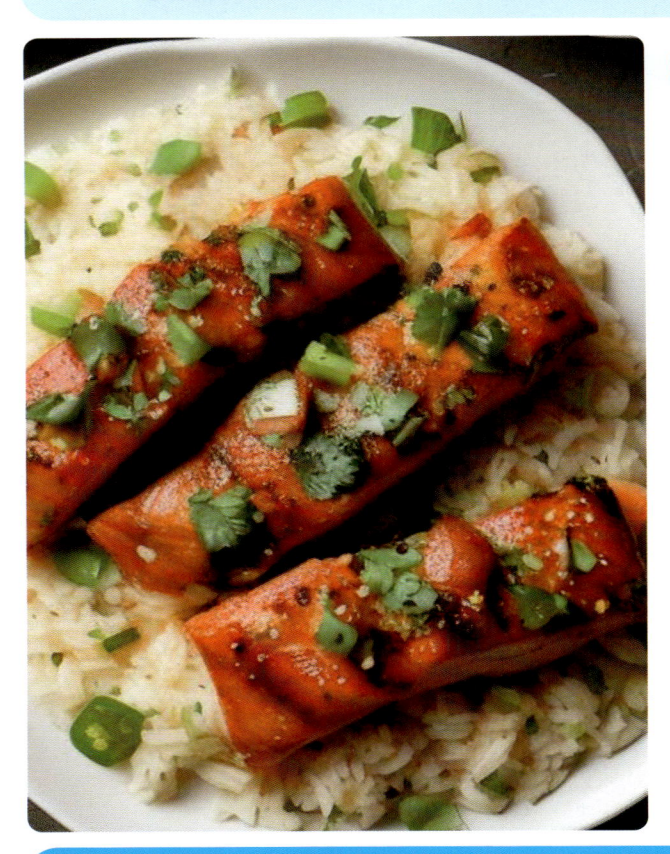

Ingredients Servings: 1

Salmon:
- 1 (6 oz.) salmon fillet
- 1/2 cup cooked rice
- 1 cup broccoli florets
- 1 tbsp extra virgin olive oil
- 1/2 tsp garlic powder
- 1/2 tsp onion powder
- 1/4 tsp salt
- 1/2 tsp black pepper
- 1 tbsp sesame seeds

Sweet & Spicy Sauce:
- 2 tbsp honey
- 2 tbsp soy sauce
- 1 tbsp sriracha
- 1 tsp minced garlic
- 1 tsp minced ginger

Optional Sides

- Salad (2 cups greens, 1 tbsp extra virgin olive oil, 2 tbsp balsamic - 307c, 4P, 11C, 27F)
- Protein shake (2 cups almond milk, 1 scoop Dummy Supps - 190c, 26P, 9C, 6F)
- Avocado (1/2 whole - 120c, 2P, 6C, 11F)

Instructions

1. Preheat a pan with olive oil on medium heat.
2. Season salmon with garlic powder, onion powder, paprika, salt, and pepper.
3. Cook salmon for 3-4 minutes per side until nearly cooked through. Remove and set aside.
4. In the same pan, add ingredients to sweet and spicy sauce. Stir and cook for 1-2 minutes until sauce thickens slightly.
5. Return salmon to the pan for 2 minutes to coat the salmon.
6. In another pan, sauté broccoli with a pinch of salt and pepper for 5-7 minutes until tender.
7. Add 1/2 cup water and 1/4 cup rice in pot, bring to boil on high heat, turn to low, cover, and cook for 5-7 minutes or microwave rice.
8. Add sesame seeds over the salmon, add rice and broccoli and serve.

INDIVIDUAL MEAL PREP

GARLIC PARMESAN SALMON BITES

Calories: 550 **Protein: 43** **Carbs: 40** **Fat: 18**

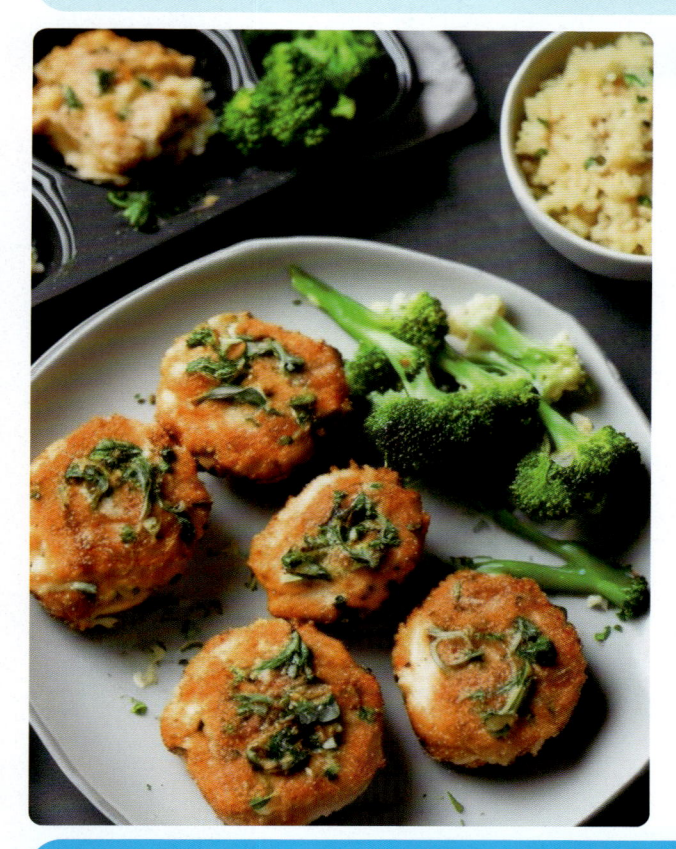

Ingredients   Servings: 1

Salmon:
- 1 (6 oz.) salmon fillet
- 1/2 cup cooked rice
- 1 cup broccoli florets
- 1/4 cup panko bread crumbs
- 2 tbsp parmesan cheese
- 1 tsp olive oil
- 1/2 tsp garlic powder
- 1/2 tsp onion powder
- 1/2 tsp paprika
- 1/4 tsp salt
- 1/4 tsp black pepper
- 1 tbsp Dijon mustard
- 2 tsp lemon juice

Optional Sides

- Salad (2 cups greens, 1 tbsp extra virgin olive oil, 2 tbsp balsamic - 307c, 4P, 11C, 27F)
- Protein shake (2 cups almond milk, 1 scoop Dummy Supps - 190c, 26P, 9C, 6F)
- Avocado (1/2 whole - 120c, 2P, 6C, 11F)

Instructions

1. Preheat oven to 400°F.
2. In a bowl, mix panko, parmesan, garlic powder, onion powder, paprika, salt, and black pepper.
3. Add Dijon mustard and olive oil to a bowl and whisk.
4. Brush salmon fillet with Dijon mustard dressing, then add panko mixture into the bowl to cover salmon.
5. Place salmon on a baking sheet.
6. Bake for 12-15 minutes until golden and cooked through.
7. While salmon bakes, steam broccoli for 4-5 minutes until tender.
8. Add 1/2 cup water and 1/4 cup rice in pot, bring to boil on high heat, turn to low, cover, and cook for 5-7 minutes or microwave rice.
9. Divide rice and broccoli into meal prep containers.
10. Place salmon on top and squeeze fresh lemon juice before serving.

INDIVIDUAL MEAL PREP

BLACKENED SALMON, POTATOES & SPINACH

Calories: 460 **Protein: 44** **Carbs: 29** **Fat: 18**

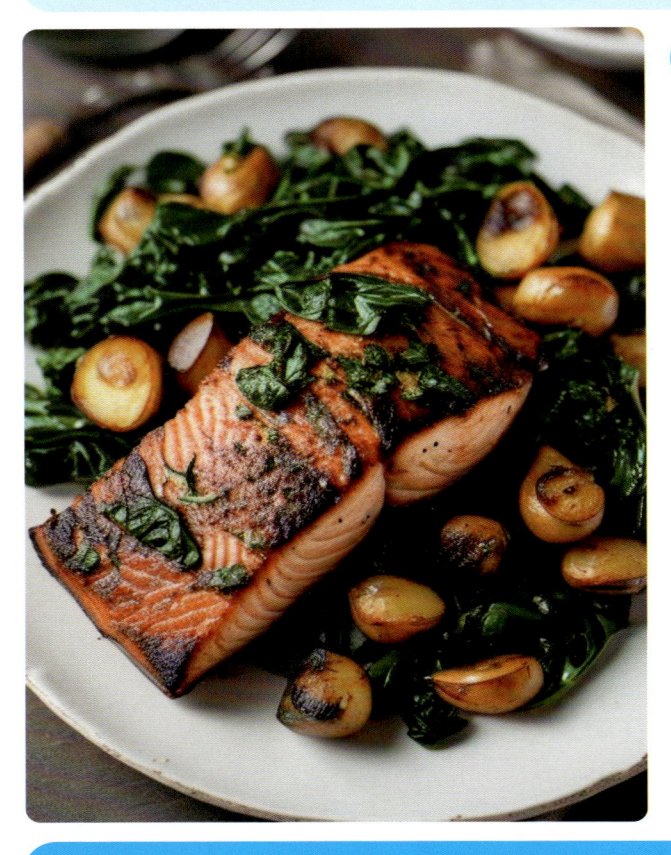

Ingredients Servings: 1

Salmon:
- 1 (6 oz.) salmon fillet
- 1 (6 oz.) russet potato
- 1 cup baby spinach
- 1 tbsp minced garlic
- 2 tsp olive oil
- 1 tbsp cajun seasoning
- 1 tsp garlic powder
- 1 tsp onion powder
- 1 tsp paprika
- 1/2 tsp black pepper
- 1/2 tsp salt
- 2 tsp lemon juice

Optional Sides
- Salad (2 cups greens, 1 tbsp extra virgin olive oil, 2 tbsp balsamic - 307c, 4P, 11C, 27F)
- Protein shake (2 cups almond milk, 1 scoop Dummy Supps - 190c, 26P, 9C, 6F)
- Avocado (1/2 whole - 120c, 2P, 6C, 11F)

Instructions
1. Preheat oven to 425°F.
2. Dice potato and toss with 1 tsp olive oil, ½ tsp salt, ½ tsp black pepper, ½ tsp garlic powder, and ½ tsp paprika.
3. Spread potatoes on a baking sheet and roast for 30-35 minutes, flipping halfway.
4. Pat salmon dry and coat with ½ tsp olive oil.
5. Mix Cajun seasoning, garlic powder, onion powder, paprika, black pepper, and salt. Rub onto salmon.
6. Heat a pan over medium-high heat. Cook salmon for 3-4 minutes per side until blackened and flaky.
7. Heat a pan over medium heat with ½ tsp olive oil. Add minced garlic and cook for 30 seconds.
8. Add spinach, salt, and black pepper. Sauté for 1-2 minutes until wilted.
9. Plate rice, roasted potatoes, and sautéed spinach.
10. Place salmon on top and squeeze fresh lemon juice before serving.

INDIVIDUAL MEAL PREP

SAUSAGE PEPPERS ONIONS

Calories: 448 **Protein: 30** **Carbs: 30** **Fat: 16**

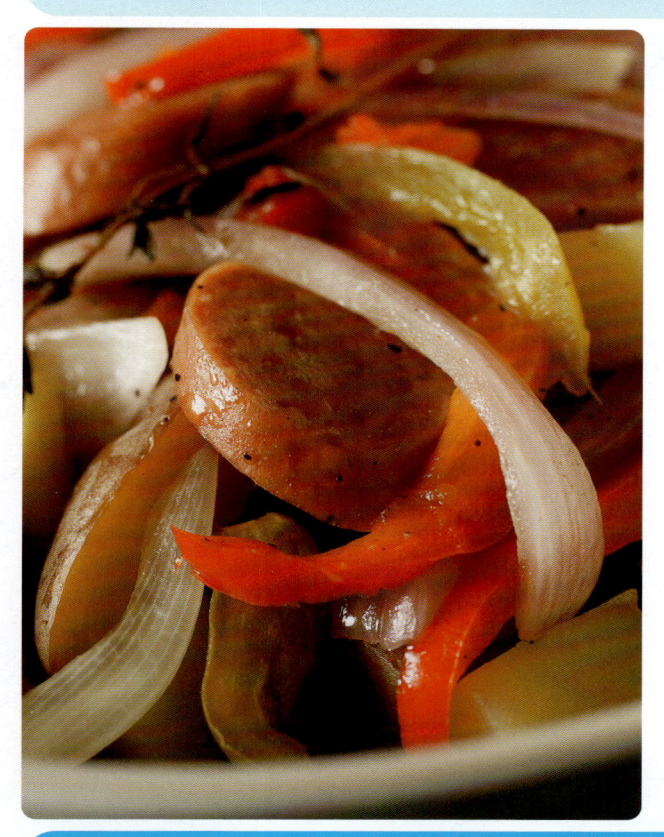

Ingredients **Servings: 1**

Sausage
- 2 (4 oz.) chicken sausages
- 1/2 cup cooked rice
- 1 cup mixed frozen peppers and onions
- 1 tsp garlic powder
- 1 tsp onion powder
- 1/4 tsp salt
- 1/2 tsp black pepper

Optional Sides
- Salad (2 cups greens, 1 tbsp extra virgin olive oil, 2 tbsp balsamic - 307c, 4P, 11C, 27F)
- Protein shake (2 cups almond milk, 1 scoop Dummy Supps - 190c, 26P, 9C, 6F)
- Avocado (1/2 whole - 120c, 2P, 6C, 11F)

Instructions
1. Slice chicken sausage into bite sized pieces.
2. Heat a pan with cooking spray on medium-high. Add chicken sausage and listed seasonings.
3. Cook for 4-5 minutes until re-warmed.
4. Add 1/2 cup water and 1/4 cup rice in pot, bring to boil on high heat, turn to low, cover, and cook for 5-7 minutes or microwave rice.
5. Add frozen peppers and onions to microwave for 4-5 minutes.
6. Combine ingredients.

INDIVIDUAL MEAL PREP

OPTIONAL ADD ON'S

ADD ON'S

- **Protein Shake:** 1 scoop Dummy Supps Whey, 2 cups almond milk (190c, 26P, 9C, 6F)
- **Chocolate PB Shake:** 1 scoop Dummy Supps Chocolate Whey, 2 cups almond milk (190c, 26P, 9C, 6F)
- **Side Salad:** 2 cups greens, 2 tbsp olive oil, 2 tbsp balsamic: (307c, 4P, 11C, 27F)
- **PB&J Sandwich:** 2 slices 647 bread, 2 tbsp PB2, 1 tbsp water, 2 tbsp SF jam (160c, 9P, 31C, 3F)
- **PB & Banana Sandwich:** 2 slices 647 bread, 2 tbsp PB2, 1 tbsp water, 1 banana, 1 tsp cinnamon (235c, 10P, 50C, 3F)
- **Hard Boiled Eggs:** 2 eggs (144c, 12P, 0C, 10F)
- **Turkey Rice Cake:** 2 salted rice cakes, 2 slices turkey breast, 1 slice cheese, 1 tbsp lite mayo (220c, 16P, 25C, 8F)
- **Turkey Roll Ups:** 4 slices turkey breast (119c, 17P, 2C, 4F)
- **Mixed nuts:** 1/4 cup (217c, 7P, 21C, 21F)

- **Raspberries:** 1 cup (80c, 1P, 18C, 1F)
- **Blackberries:** 1 cup (80c, 1P, 18C, 1F)
- **Apple:** 1 whole (100c, 1P, 28C, 0F)
- **Strawberries:** 2 cups diced (100c, 1P, 23C, 1F)
- **Grapes:** 2 cups (200c, 1P, 54C, 0F)
- **Apple & PB:** 1 whole apple, 2 tbsp PB2, 1 tbsp water (154c, 6P, 33C, 2F)
- **Blueberries:** 1 cup (80c, 1P, 22C, 0F)
- **Clementines:** 2 whole (70c, 1P, 18C, 0F)
- **Veggies & Ranch:** 1 cup nonfat plain greek yogurt, 2 tsp ranch seasoning, 5 stalks celery/10 baby carrots (250c, 22P, 9C, 0F)
- **Veggies & Taco Dip:** 1 cup nonfat plain greek yogurt, 2 tsp taco seasoning, 5 stalks celery/10 baby carrots (250c, 22P, 9C, 0F)
- **Lite Popcorn:** 2 cups (150c, 2P, 15C, 10F)
- **Greek Yogurt:** 3/4 cup non fat plain, 1/2 cup berries (150c, 25P, 30C, 1F)

INDIVIDUAL MEAL PREP

OPTIONAL ADD ON'S

SAUCES

- **Tzatziki Sauce:** 1/2 cup nonfat plain greek yogurt, 1/4 cup grated cucumber, 1 tbsp dill, 2 tsp lemon juice, 1/2 tsp olive oil. 1/4 tsp salt (100c, 11P, 11C, 2F)
- **Protein Ranch:** 1/2 cup nonfat plain greek yogurt, 2 tsp ranch dressing seasoning (80c, 11P, 4C, 2F)
- **Protein Taco Dip:** 1/2 cup nonfat plain greek yogurt, 2 tsp taco dressing seasoning (80c, 11P, 4C, 2F)
- **Hot Sauce:** 2 tbsp (0c, 0P, 0C, 0F)
- **Salsa:** 2 tbsp (10c, 0P, 3C, 0F)
- **Lite Sour Cream:** 2 tbsp (35c, 2P, 2C, 3F)
- **Marinara:** 1/2 cup (50c, 2P, 11C, 1F)
- **Yellow Mustard:** 2 tbsp (1P, 0C, 0F)
- **Low Sodium Soy Sauce:** 1 tbsp (10c, 1P, 1C, 0F)
- **Hummus:** 1 tbsp (36c, 1P, 2C, 3F)
- **Balsamic Glaze:** 1 tbsp (25c, 0P, 6C, 0F)
- **Olive Oil:** 1 tbsp (120c, 0P, 0C, 14F)
- **Balsamic Vinegar:** 1 tbsp (14c, 0P, 3C, 0F)
- **G Hughes Teriyaki:** 2 tbsp (10c, 0P, 2C, 0F)
- **G Hughes Thai Chili:** 2 tbsp (10c, 0P, 2C, 0F)
- **G Hughes Burger Sauce:** 2 tbsp (100c, 0P, 2C, 10F)
- **G Hughes Stir Fry:** 2 tbsp (10c, 0P, 2C, 0F)
- **G Hughes BBQ:** 2 tbsp (10c, 0P, 2C, 0F)
- **G Hughes Sweet & Spicy:** 2 tbsp (10c, 0P, 2C, 0F)
- **G Hughes Ketchup:** 2 tbsp (5c, 0P, 2C, 0F)
- **G Hughes Sweet Chili Sauce:** 2 tbsp (100c, 0P, 2C, 10F)

BULK MEAL PREP

CROCKPOT MEAL PREPS

BULK RECIPES TO LAST YOU ALL WEEK

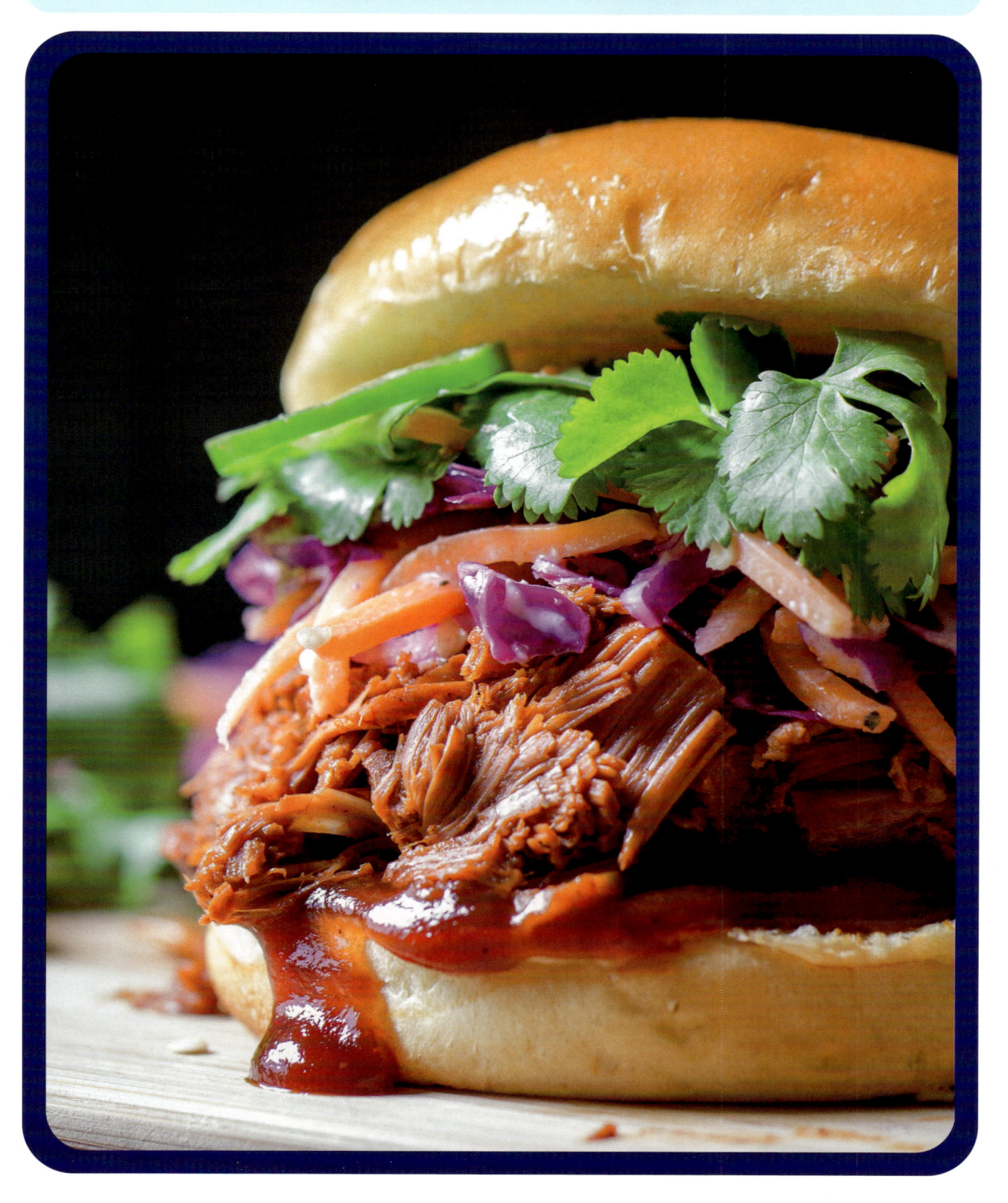

CROCKPOT MEAL PREPS

BUFFALO DIP BOWLS

Calories: 500   **Protein: 57**   **Carbs: 23**   **Fat: 15**

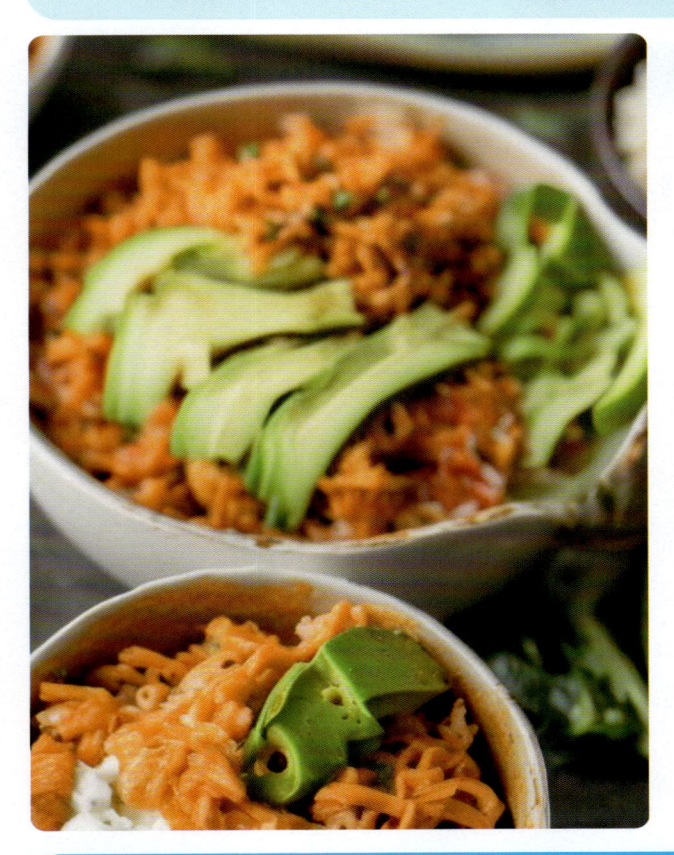

Ingredients   Servings: 8 (1 1/2 CUP)

Buffalo Dip:
- 3 lb chicken breast
- 1 cup dry rice
- 1/2 cup buffalo wing sauce
- 2 tbsp minced garlic
- 1/2 cup whipped cream cheese
- 1 cup shredded cheddar cheese
- 2 (1 oz.) packets ranch seasoning
- 1 bunch chives

Optional Sides
- Salad (2 cups greens, 1 tbsp extra virgin olive oil, 2 tbsp balsamic - 307c, 4P, 11C, 27F)
- Protein shake (2 cups almond milk, 1 scoop Dummy Supps - 190c, 26P, 9C, 6F)
- Avocado (1/2 whole - 120c, 2P, 6C, 11F)

Instructions
1. Add chicken breasts, ranch seasoning, buffalo wing sauce, minced garlic, and ranch seasoning to the crockpot.
2. Cook on high for 3-4 hours or low for 5-6 hours.
3. Shred the cooked chicken directly in the crockpot.
4. Add 2 cups water and rice in pot, bring to boil on high heat, turn to low, cover, and cook for 10 minutes.
5. Stir in whipped cream cheese and shredded cheddar cheese until melted and combined.
6. Garnish with chopped chives before serving.

CROCKPOT MEAL PREPS

BUFFALO CHICKEN PASTA

Calories: 450 **Protein: 52** **Carbs: 34** **Fat: 12**

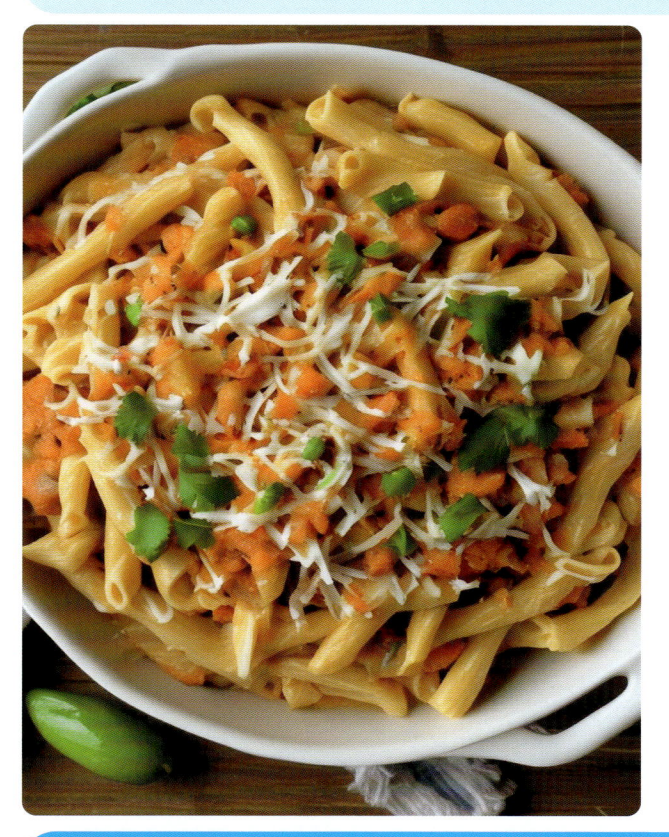

Ingredients   Servings: 8 (1 1/2 CUP)

Buffalo Pasta:
- 3 lb chicken breast
- c1 (14.5 oz.) box protein/chickpea pasta
- 2 bell peppers
- 1 sweet onion
- 2 jalapeno peppers
- 1/2 cup buffalo wing sauce
- 2 tbsp minced garlic
- 1/2 cup whipped cream cheese
- 1 cup shredded cheddar cheese
- 2 (1 oz.) packets ranch seasoning
- 1 bunch chives

Optional Sides
- Salad (2 cups greens, 1 tbsp extra virgin olive oil, 2 tbsp balsamic - 307c, 4P, 11C, 27F)
- Protein shake (2 cups almond milk, 1 scoop Dummy Supps - 190c, 26P, 9C, 6F)
- Avocado (1/2 whole - 120c, 2P, 6C, 11F)

Instructions
1. Dice bell peppers, onion, and jalapeños.
2. Add chicken, diced veggies, ranch seasoning, buffalo wing sauce, minced garlic, and low-sodium bone broth to the crockpot.
3. Cook on high for 3-4 hours or low for 4-5 hours.
4. Shred chicken in the crockpot. Stir in whipped cream cheese and cheddar cheese until melted.
5. Boil pasta for 9-11 minutes. Drain.
6. Mix pasta into the crockpot and stir well.
7. Garnish with chopped chives before serving.

CROCKPOT MEAL PREPS

CHICKEN ALFREDO PASTA

Calories: 500   **Protein: 60**   **Carbs: 34**   **Fat: 13**

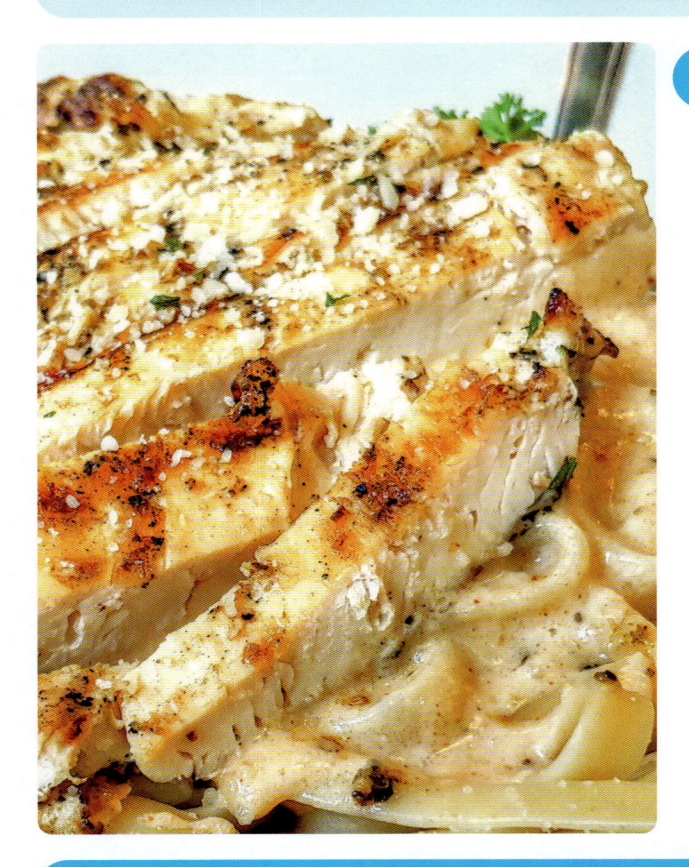

Ingredients   Servings: 10 (1 1/2 CUP)

Chicken Alfredo:
- 3 lb chicken breast
- 1 (14.5 oz.) box protein pasta/chickpea pasta
- 1 bunch parsley
- 2 tbsp Italian seasoning
- 2 tbsp garlic powder
- 1 tbsp onion powder
- 1 tsp black pepper

Alfredo Sauce:
- 3 cups low-fat cottage cheese
- 1 cup low fat mozzarella cheese
- 1/2 cup parmesan cheese
- 2 tbsp minced garlic
- 1/4 cup 1% milk

Optional Sides
- Salad (2 cups greens, 1 tbsp extra virgin olive oil, 2 tbsp balsamic - 307c, 4P, 11C, 27F)
- Protein shake (2 cups almond milk, 1 scoop Dummy Supps - 190c, 26P, 9C, 6F)

Instructions
1. Add chicken and listed seasonings to the crockpot.
2. Cook on high for 3-4 hours or low for 5-6 hours.
3. Shred chicken in the crockpot.
4. Blend cottage cheese, parmesan, mozzarella, minced garlic, and milk until smooth.
5. Boil pasta for 9-11 minutes. Drain.
6. Stir cheese sauce and pasta into the crockpot until well combined.
7. Garnish with chopped parsley before serving.

CROCKPOT MEAL PREPS

CHICKEN PARM PASTA

Calories: 540 **Protein: 57** **Carbs: 40** **Fat: 16**

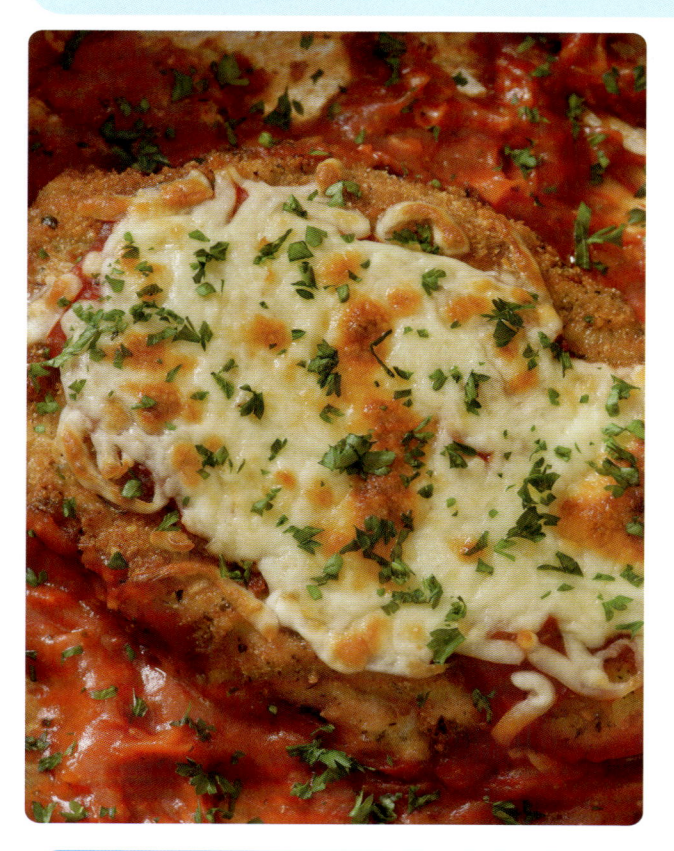

Ingredients **Servings: 10 (1 1/2 CUP)**

Chicken Parm:
- 3 lb chicken breast
- 1 (14.5 oz.) box protein pasta/chickpea pasta
- 2 tbsp minced garlic
- 1 cup low fat mozzarella cheese
- 1/2 cup parmesan cheese
- 1 (15 oz.) container low fat ricotta cheese
- 1 (24 oz.) container marinara sauce
- 1 bunch parsley
- 2 tbsp Italian seasoning
- 2 tbsp garlic powder
- 1 tbsp onion powder
- 1 tsp black pepper

Optional Sides

- Salad (2 cups greens, 1 tbsp extra virgin olive oil, 2 tbsp balsamic - 307c, 4P, 11C, 27F)
- Protein shake (2 cups almond milk, 1 scoop Dummy Supps - 190c, 26P, 9C, 6F)

Instructions

1. Add chicken, marinara sauce, minced garlic, and listed seasonings to the crockpot.
2. Cook on high for 3-4 hours or low for 5-6 hours.
3. Shred chicken in the crockpot. Stir in mozzarella, parmesan, and ricotta cheese until melted.
4. Boil pasta for 9-11 minutes. Drain.
5. Add pasta to the crockpot and mix well.
6. Garnish with chopped parsley before serving.

CROCKPOT MEAL PREPS

SPICY GARLIC PASTA

Calories: 500 **Protein: 53** **Carbs: 33** **Fat: 15**

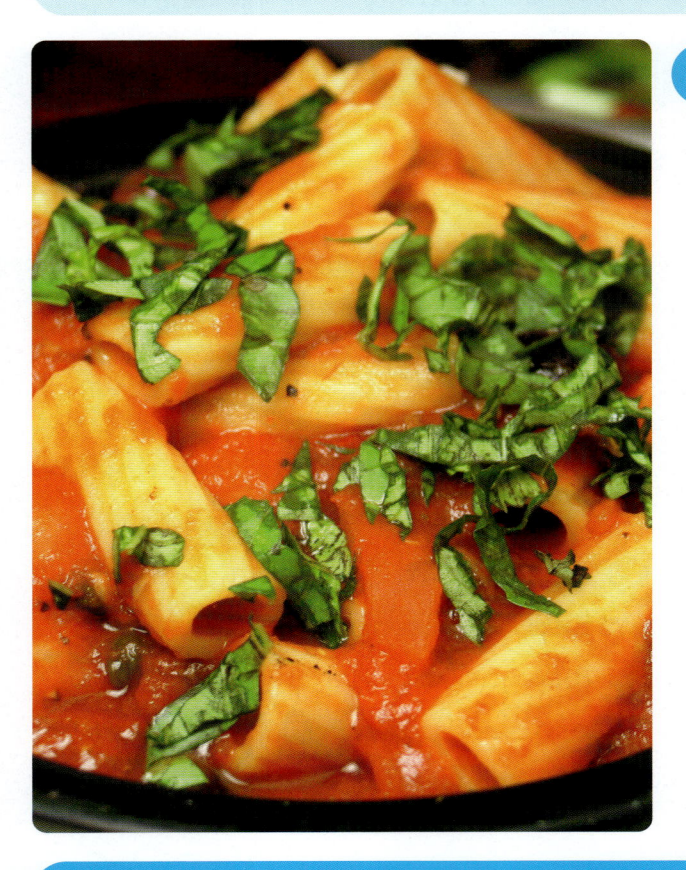

Ingredients — Servings: 10 (1 1/2 CUP)

Pasta:
- 3 lb chicken breast
- 1 (14.5 oz.) box protein/chickpea pasta
- 2 tbsp minced garlic
- 1 (24 oz.) bottle fra diavolo sauce
- 1 (15 oz.) container part skim ricotta cheese
- 1/4 cup parmesan cheese
- 1 bunch parsley
- 2 tbsp Italian seasoning
- 2 tbsp garlic powder
- 1 tbsp onion powder
- 1 tsp black pepper
- 1 tsp crushed red pepper

Optional Sides

- Salad (2 cups greens, 1 tbsp extra virgin olive oil, 2 tbsp balsamic - 307c, 4P, 11C, 27F)
- Protein shake (2 cups almond milk, 1 scoop Dummy Supps - 190c, 26P, 9C, 6F)

Instructions

1. Add chicken, fra diavolo sauce, minced garlic, and listed seasonings to the crockpot.
2. Cook on high for 3-4 hours or low for 5-6 hours.
3. Shred chicken in the crockpot. Stir in ricotta and parmesan cheese until well combined.
4. Boil pasta for 9-11 minutes. Drain.
5. Add cooked pasta to the crockpot and mix thoroughly.
6. Garnish with chopped parsley before serving.

CROCKPOT MEAL PREPS

CHIPOTLE CHICKEN PASTA

Calories: 530   **Protein: 63**   **Carbs: 39**   **Fat: 14**

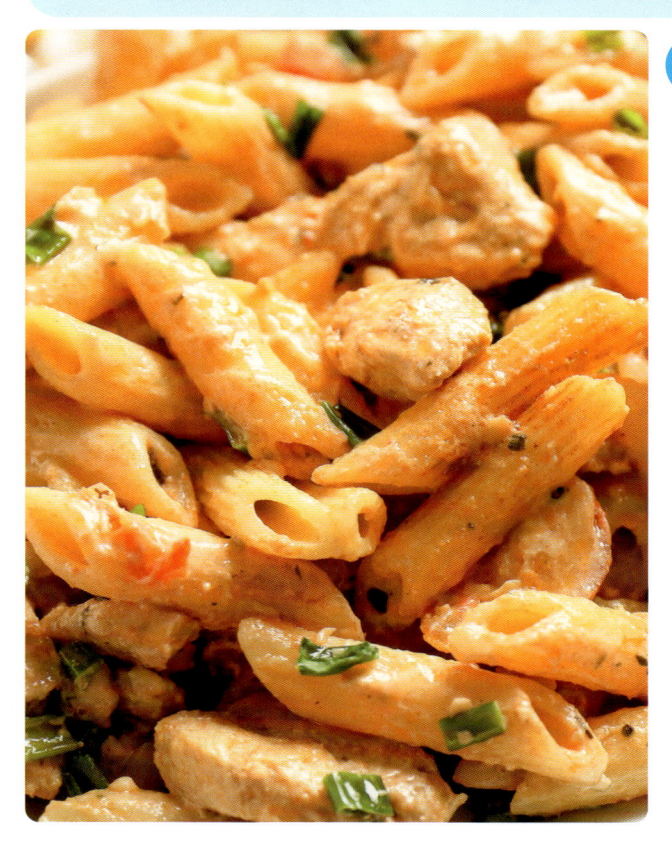

Ingredients   Servings: 10 (1 1/2 CUP)

Pasta:
- 3 lb chicken breast
- 1 (14.5 oz.) box protein/chickpea pasta
- 2 tbsp minced garlic
- 1 sweet onion
- 2 bell peppers
- 2 jalapeno peppers
- 4 cups spinach

Cajun Sauce:
- 3 cups low fat cottage cheese
- 2 cups shredded cheddar cheese
- 1 (7 oz.) can chipotle peppers in adobo sauce
- 1 lime
- 1/4 cup 1% milk

Optional Sides
- Salad (2 cups greens, 1 tbsp extra virgin olive oil, 2 tbsp balsamic - 307c, 4P, 11C, 27F)
- Protein shake (2 cups almond milk, 1 scoop Dummy Supps - 190c, 26P, 9C, 6F)

Instructions
1. Dice onion, bell peppers, and jalapeños.
2. Add chicken, minced garlic, onion, bell peppers, and jalapeños to the crockpot.
3. Cook on high for 3-4 hours or low for 5-6 hours.
4. Blend cottage cheese, cheddar cheese, chipotle peppers, lime juice, and milk until smooth.
5. Cook pasta for 9-11 minutes. Drain.
6. Add spinach, pasta, and blended sauce to the crockpot. Stir until combined.
7. Cook on low for 10-15 minutes until warmed through.

CROCKPOT MEAL PREPS

CHEESY CHICKEN MAC & CHEESE

Calories: 560 **Protein: 64** **Carbs: 41** **Fat: 16**

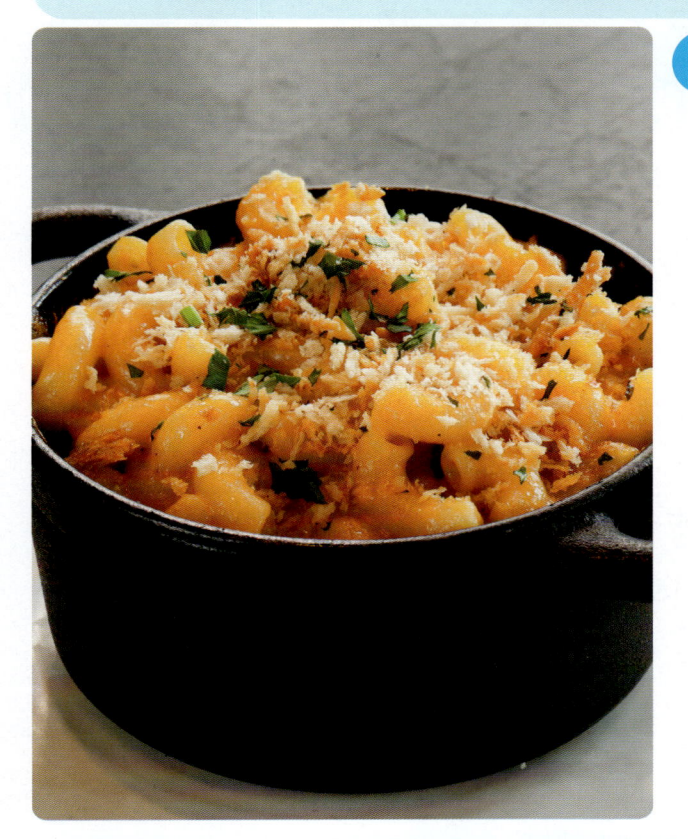

Ingredients   Servings: 10 (1 1/2 CUP)

Pasta:
- 3 lb chicken breast
- 1 (14.5 oz.) box protein/chickpea pasta
- 2 tbsp minced garlic
- 1 sweet onion
- 2 bell peppers
- 1 (10 oz.) can green chilies
- 1 (15 oz.) can fire roasted tomatoes
- 1 (10 oz.) can red enchilada sauce

Queso Sauce:
- 3 cups low fat cottage cheese
- 1/2 cup whipped cream cheese
- 2 cups shredded cheddar cheese
- 1/4 cup 1% milk

Optional Sides
- Salad (2 cups greens, 1 tbsp extra virgin olive oil, 2 tbsp balsamic - 307c, 4P, 11C, 27F)
- Protein shake (2 cups almond milk, 1 scoop Dummy Supps - 190c, 26P, 9C, 6F)

Instructions
1. Dice onion and bell peppers.
2. Add chicken, minced garlic, onion, bell peppers, green chilies, fire-roasted tomatoes, and enchilada sauce to the crockpot.
3. Cook on high for 3-4 hours or low for 5-6 hours.
4. Blend cottage cheese, whipped cream cheese, cheddar cheese, and milk until smooth to make the queso.
5. Cook pasta for 9-11 minutes. Drain.
6. Shred chicken in the crockpot, then stir in the blended queso and cooked pasta.
7. Mix well and cook on low for 10-15 minutes until warmed through.

CROCKPOT MEAL PREPS

HOT HONEY CHICKEN BOWLS

Calories: 460 **Protein: 54** **Carbs: 34** **Fat: 10**

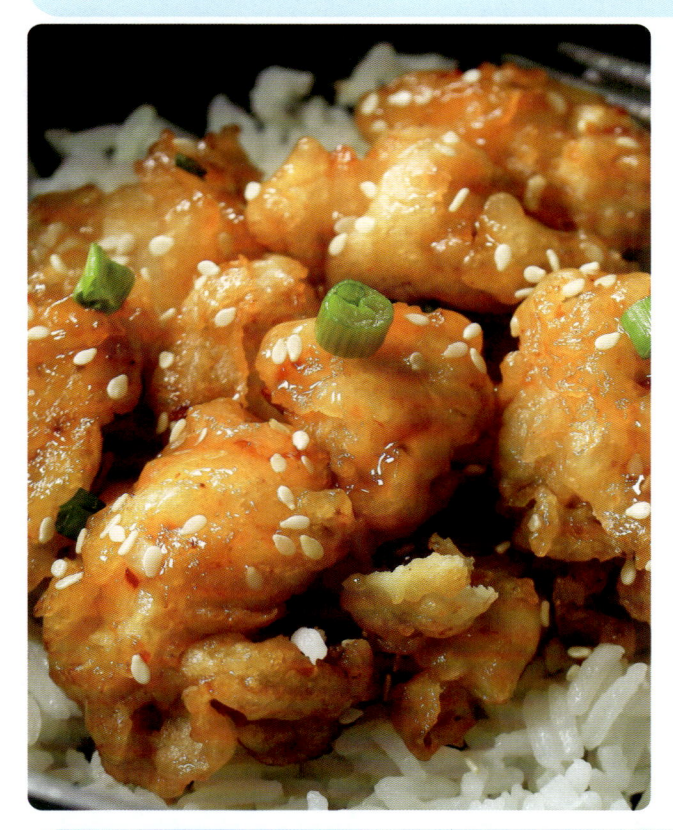

Ingredients   Servings: 8 (1 1/2 CUP)

Hot Honey Bowls:
- 3 lb chicken breast
- 1/2 bone broth
- 1 cup dry rice
- 2 tbsp minced garlic
- 3 tbsp low sodium soy sauce
- 4 tbsp honey
- 2 tbsp sriracha
- 1 tbsp gochujang (Korean chili paste)
- 1 (10 oz.) can chipotle peppers in adobo sauce
- 1 lime
- 1 tbsp onion powder
- 1 tbsp black pepper
- 1/4 tsp salt
- 1 tbsp sesame seeds

Optional Sides

- Salad (2 cups greens, 1 tbsp extra virgin olive oil, 2 tbsp balsamic - 307c, 4P, 11C, 27F)
- Protein shake (2 cups almond milk, 1 scoop Dummy Supps - 190c, 26P, 9C, 6F)

Instructions

1. Blend chipotle peppers, minced garlic, soy sauce, honey, and sriracha until smooth.
2. Add chicken, blendeded sauce, bone broth, lime juice, and listed seasoinings to the crockpot.
3. Cook on high for 3-4 hours or low for 5-6 hours.
4. Add 2 cups water and rice in pot, bring to boil on high heat, turn to low, cover, and cook for 10 minutes.
5. Shred chicken in the crockpot and stir well.
6. Serve chicken over rice, and garnish with sesame seeds before serving.

CROCKPOT MEAL PREPS

SPICY JALAPENO MAC & CHEESE

Calories: 500   **Protein: 56**   **Carbs: 30**   **Fat: 17**

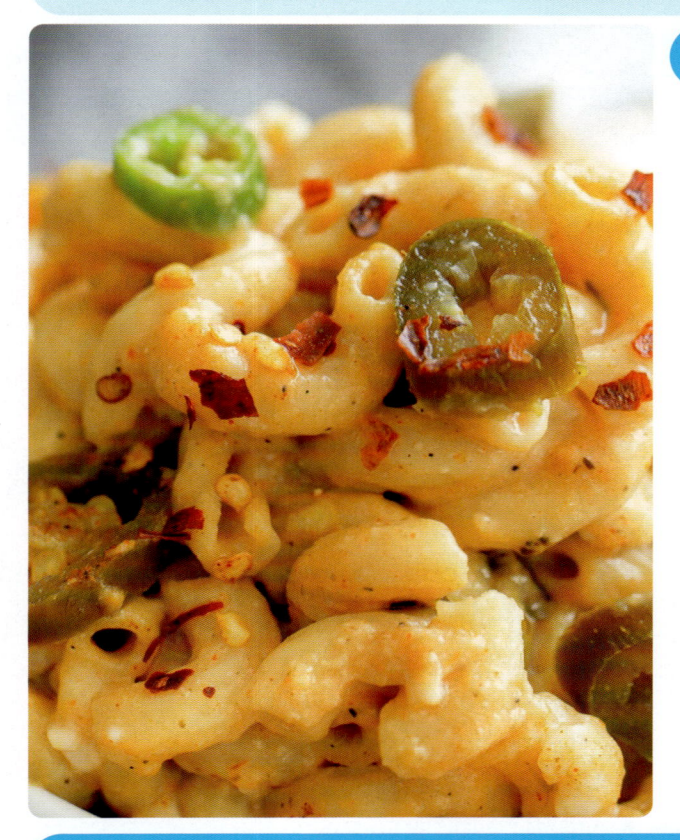

Ingredients   Servings: 12 (1 1/2 CUP)

Pasta:
- 3 lb chicken breast
- 1 (14.5 oz.) box protein/chickpea pasta
- 1 sweet onion
- 2 bell peppers
- 2 jalapeno peppers
- 1/4 cup jalapeno brine
- 12 slices turkey bacon
- 1 tbsp garlic powder
- 1 tbsp onion powder
- 1 tsp black pepper
- 1 tsp crushed red pepper flakes

Queso Sauce:
- 3 cups low fat cottage cheese
- 1/2 cup whipped cream cheese
- 2 cups shredded cheddar cheese
- 1/4 cup 1% milk

Optional Sides

- Salad (2 cups greens, 1 tbsp extra virgin olive oil, 2 tbsp balsamic - 307c, 4P, 11C, 27F)
- Protein shake (2 cups almond milk, 1 scoop Dummy Supps - 190c, 26P, 9C, 6F)

Instructions

1. Dice onion, bell peppers, and jalapeños.
2. Add chicken, diced vegetables, jalapeño brine, and listed seasonings to the crockpot.
3. Cook on high for 3-4 hours or low for 5-6 hours.
4. Cook turkey bacon in a pan until crispy. Chop into small pieces.
5. Blend cottage cheese, whipped cream cheese, cheddar cheese, and milk until smooth to make the queso sauce.
6. Cook pasta for 9-11 minutes. Drain.
7. Shred chicken in the crockpot, then stir in the queso sauce, cooked pasta, and chopped turkey bacon.
8. Mix well and cook on low for 10-15 minutes until warmed through.

CROCKPOT MEAL PREPS

SWEET AND SPICY CHICKEN

Calories: 470 **Protein: 53** **Carbs: 31** **Fat: 10**

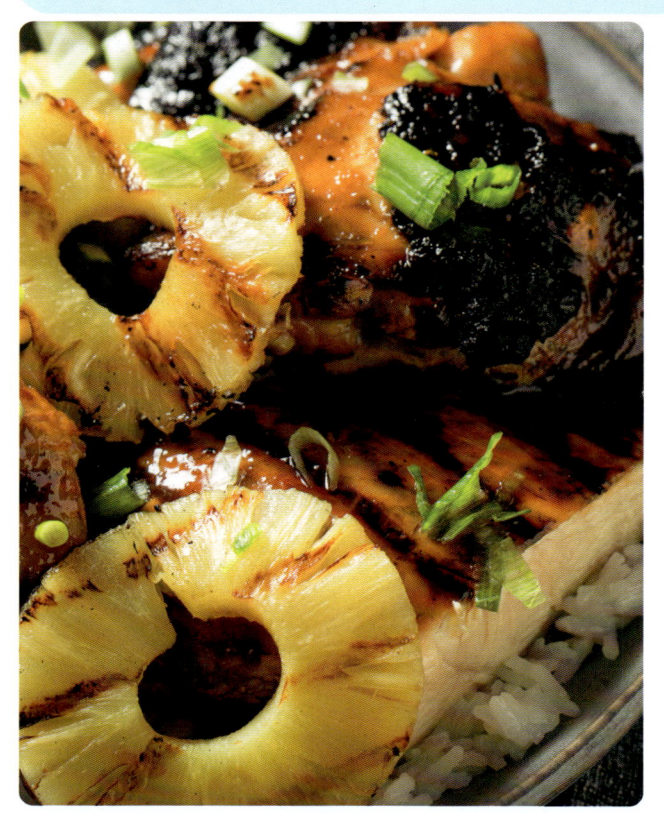

Ingredients   Servings: 8 (1 1/2 CUP)

Sweet & Spicy Chicken:
- 3 lb chicken breast
- 1 cup dry rice
- 1 red onion
- 2 jalapeño peppers
- 1 (15 oz.) can unsweetened diced pineapple
- 1 (12 oz.) container G Hughes sweet chili
- 1 bunch cilantro
- 2 tbsp garlic powder
- 2 tbsp onion powder
- 1 tsp black pepper
- 1/2 tsp cayenne pepper

Optional Sides
- Salad (2 cups greens, 1 tbsp extra virgin olive oil, 2 tbsp balsamic - 307c, 4P, 11C, 27F)
- Protein shake (2 cups almond milk, 1 scoop Dummy Supps - 190c, 26P, 9C, 6F)
- Avocado (1/2 whole - 120c, 2P, 6C, 11F)

Instructions
1. Dice red onion and jalapeño peppers.
2. Add chicken, sweet chili sauce, and listed seasonings to the crockpot.
3. Cook on high for 3-4 hours or low for 5-6 hours.
4. Shred chicken in the crockpot and stir to mix flavors.
5. Add diced vegetables and drained pineapple and cook on low for 30 minutes.
6. Add 2 cups water and rice in pot, bring to boil on high heat, turn to low, cover, and cook for 10 minutes.
7. Serve chicken and sauce over rice.
8. Garnish with chopped cilantro before serving.

CROCKPOT MEAL PREPS

TINGA TACO BOWLS

Calories: 440 **Protein: 53** **Carbs: 29** **Fat: 11**

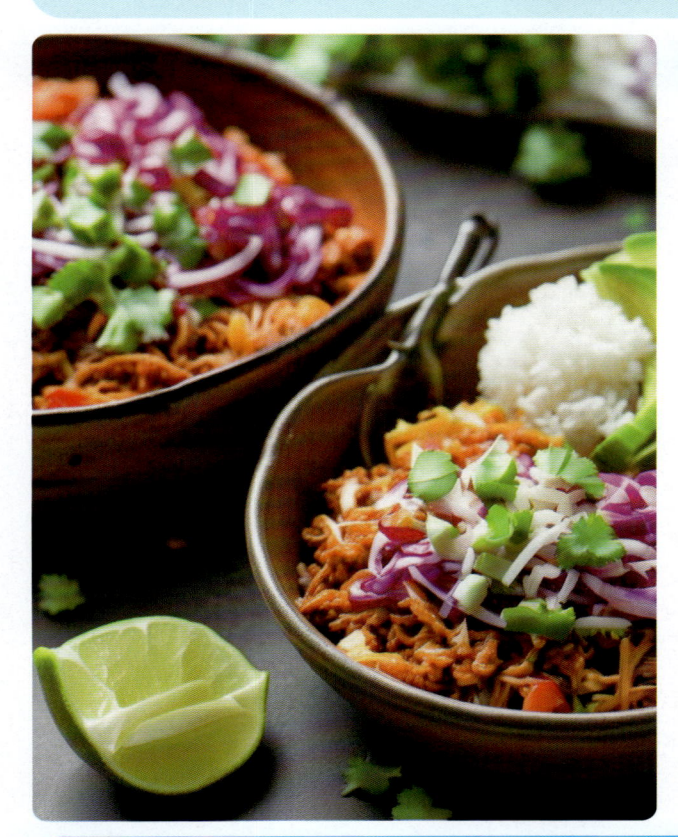

Ingredients **Servings: 8 (1 1/2 CUP)**

Tinga Tacos:
- 3 lb chicken breast
- 1 cup dry rice
- 1 red onion
- 2 jalapeno peppers
- 5 roma tomatoes
- 1 (10 oz.) can green chilies
- 1 (7 oz.) can chipotle peppers in adobo sauce
- 1 (10 oz.) can red enchilada sauce
- 1 lime
- 1 (1 oz.) packet taco seasoning

Optional Sides

- Salad (2 cups greens, 1 tbsp extra virgin olive oil, 2 tbsp balsamic - 307c, 4P, 11C, 27F)
- Protein shake (2 cups almond milk, 1 scoop Dummy Supps - 190c, 26P, 9C, 6F)
- Avocado (1/2 whole - 120c, 2P, 6C, 11F)

Instructions

1. Dice red onion, jalapeños, and tomatoes.
2. Blend green chilies and chipotle peppers until smooth.
3. Add chicken, diced vegetables, blended peppers, enchilada sauce, taco seasoning, and juice from the lime to the crockpot.
4. Cook on high for 3-4 hours or low for 5-6 hours.
5. Shred chicken in the crockpot and mix well.
6. Add 2 cups water and rice in pot, bring to boil on high heat, turn to low, cover, and cook for 10 minutes.
7. Serve tinga chicken over rice.

CROCKPOT MEAL PREPS

TACO PASTA SALAD

Calories: 490   **Protein: 52**   **Carbs: 39**   **Fat: 14**

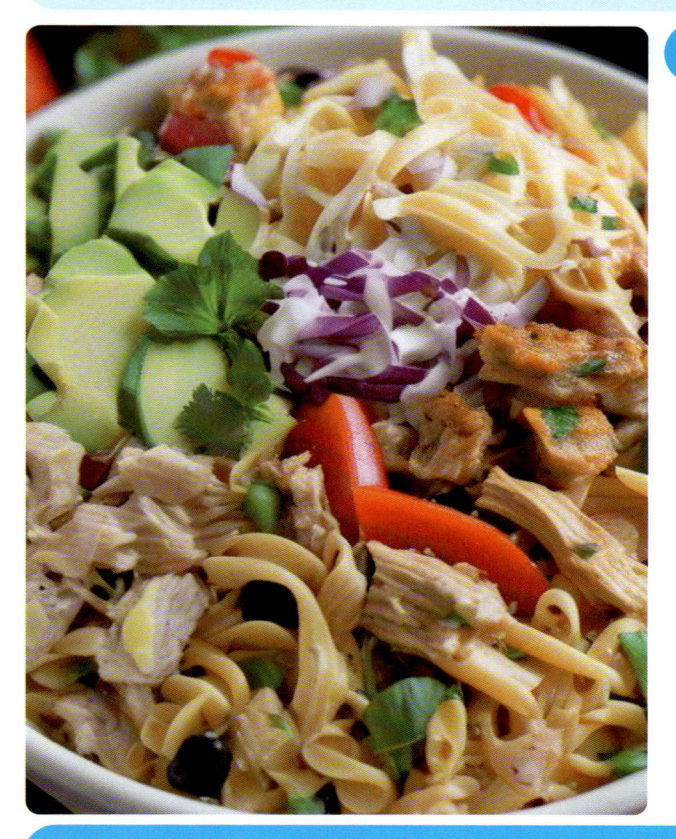

Ingredients — Servings: 10 (1 1/2 CUP)

Pasta:
- 3 lb chicken breast
- 1 (14 oz.) box protein pasta
- 2 bell peppers
- 1 red onion
- 2 jalapeno's
- 1 (15 oz.) can diced tomatoes
- 1 (15 oz.) can black beans
- 1 tbsp tomato paste
- 1/2 cup red enchilada sauce
- 1/2 cup red wine vinegar
- 1/2 cup olive oil
- 1 tbsp Worcestershire sauce
- 1 (1 oz.) packet taco seasoning

Optional Sides
- Salad (2 cups greens, 1 tbsp extra virgin olive oil, 2 tbsp balsamic - 307c, 4P, 11C, 27F)
- Protein shake (2 cups almond milk, 1 scoop Dummy Supps - 190c, 26P, 9C, 6F)
- Avocado (1/2 whole - 120c, 2P, 6C, 11F)

Instructions
1. Place chicken breast and taco seasoning into the crockpot.
2. Cook on high for 4 hours or low for 6 hours until tender.
3. Chop bell peppers, red onion, and jalapeños while the chicken cooks.
4. In a bowl, combine enchilada sauce, red wine vinegar, olive oil, Worcestershire sauce, diced tomatoes, and tomato paste in order, then mix well.
5. Once the chicken is done, shred it and add the chopped vegetables.
6. Cook pasta according to package instructions, then drain.
7. Combine pasta, chicken, and dressing, then toss to coat.
8. Serve warm or chilled.

CROCKPOT MEAL PREPS

SOUTHWEST CHICKEN BOWLS

Calories: 460   **Protein: 56**   **Carbs: 32**   **Fat: 11**

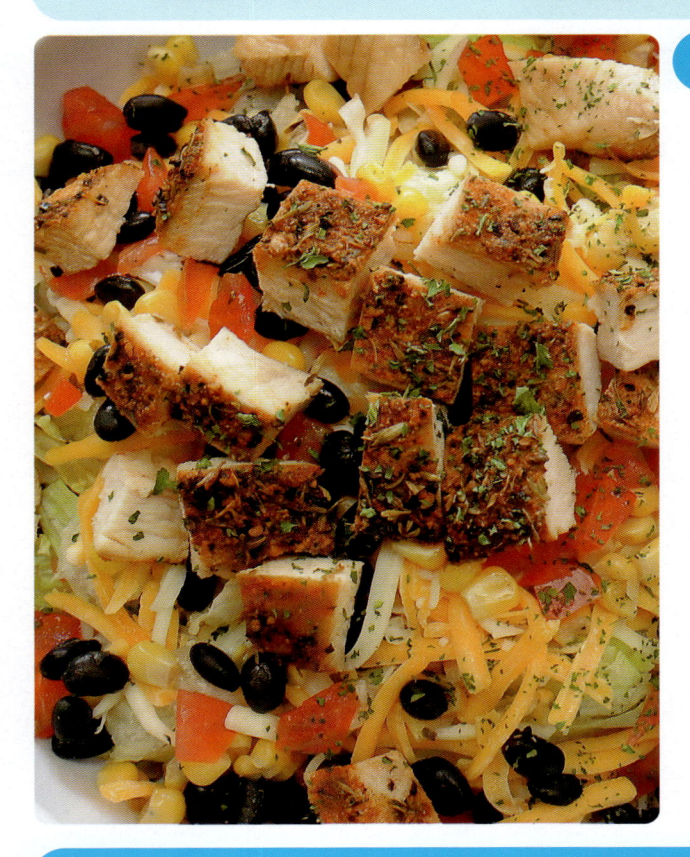

Ingredients   Servings: 10 (1 1/2 CUP)

Southwest Bowls:
- 3 lb chicken breast
- 1 cup dry rice
- 1 sweet onion
- 2 bell peppers
- 2 jalapeno peppers
- 5 roma tomatoes
- 1 (10 oz.) can green chilies
- 1 (15 oz.) can black beans
- 1 bunch cilantro
- 2 cups low fat cottage cheese
- 1 cup shredded cheese
- 1 lime
- 2 (1 oz.) packets taco seasoning

Optional Sides
- Salad (2 cups greens, 1 tbsp extra virgin olive oil, 2 tbsp balsamic - 307c, 4P, 11C, 27F)
- Protein shake (2 cups almond milk, 1 scoop Dummy Supps - 190c, 26P, 9C, 6F)
- Avocado (1/2 whole - 120c, 2P, 6C, 11F)

Instructions

1. Dice onion, bell peppers, jalapeños, and tomatoes.
2. Add chicken, green chilies, black beans, and taco seasoning to the crockpot.
3. Cook on high for 3-4 hours or low for 5-6 hours.
4. Blend cottage cheese, shredded cheese, and juice from one lime until smooth.
5. Shred chicken in the crockpot, stir in the blended cheese sauce, and mix well.
6. Add diced vegetables and cook for 30 minutes on low.
7. Add 2 cups water and rice in pot, bring to boil on high heat, turn to low, cover, and cook for 10 minutes.
8. Serve over rice and garnish with chopped cilantro.

CROCKPOT MEAL PREPS

CILANTRO LIME CHICKEN BOWLS

Calories: 470 **Protein: 62** **Carbs: 27** **Fat: 11**

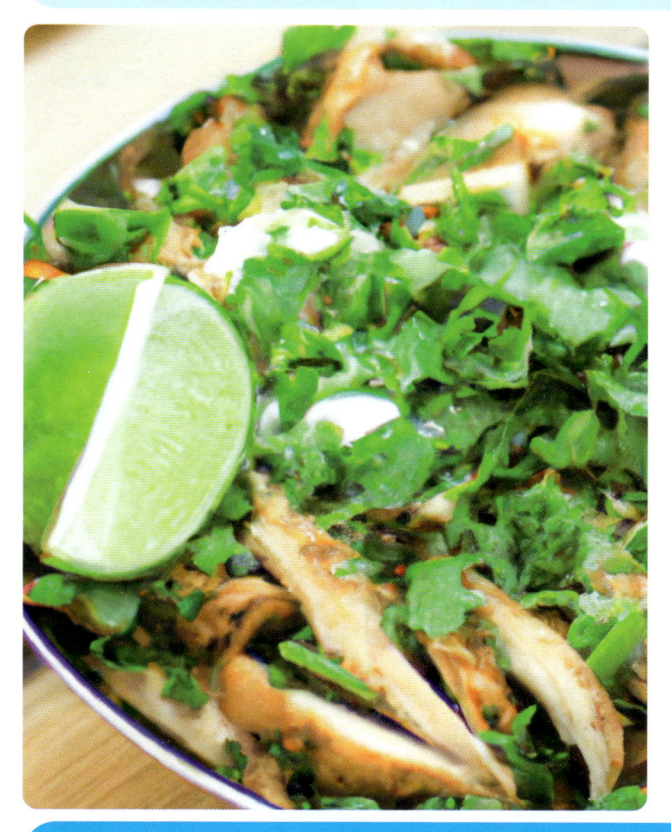

Ingredients **Servings: 8 (1 1/2 CUP)**

Cilantro Lime Bowls:
- 3 lb chicken breast
- 1 cup dry rice
- 1 red onion
- 2 bell peppers
- 2 cups cottage cheese
- 1 (10 oz.) can green chilies
- 1 bunch cilantro
- 1 lime
- 2 (1 oz.) packets taco seasoning

Optional Sides

- Salad (2 cups greens, 1 tbsp extra virgin olive oil, 2 tbsp balsamic - 307c, 4P, 11C, 27F)
- Protein shake (2 cups almond milk, 1 scoop Dummy Supps - 190c, 26P, 9C, 6F)
- Avocado (1/2 whole - 120c, 2P, 6C, 11F)

Instructions

1. Dice red onion, bell peppers, and jalapeños.
2. Add chicken, diced vegetables, and taco seasoning to the crockpot.
3. Cook on high for 3-4 hours or low for 5-6 hours.
4. Blend cottage cheese, cilantro, and lime juice until smooth.
5. Shred chicken in the crockpot and stir well.
6. Add blended cottage cheese mixture to crockpot and stir until well combined.
7. Add 2 cups water and rice in pot, bring to boil on high heat, turn to low, cover, and cook for 10 minutes.
8. Serve over rice and garnish with chopped cilantro.

CROCKPOT MEAL PREPS

BUFFALO CHICKEN BOWLS

Calories: 450   **Protein: 49**   **Carbs: 24**   **Fat: 20**

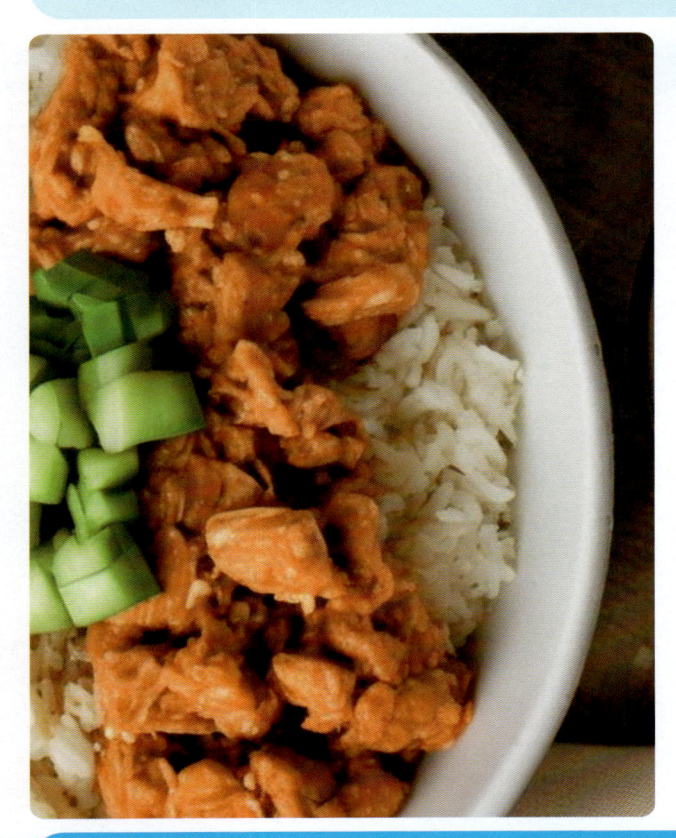

Ingredients   Servings: 8 (1 1/2 CUP)

Buffalo Chicken Bowls:
- 3 lb chicken breast
- 1 cup dry rice
- 1 red onion
- 2 jalapeno peppers
- 2 cups cottage cheese
- 1/2 cup buffalo sauce
- 1 cup shredded cheese
- 2 (1 oz.) packets ranch dressing seasoning

Optional Sides
- Salad (2 cups greens, 1 tbsp extra virgin olive oil, 2 tbsp balsamic - 307c, 4P, 11C, 27F)
- Protein shake (2 cups almond milk, 1 scoop Dummy Supps - 190c, 26P, 9C, 6F)
- Avocado (1/2 whole - 120c, 2P, 6C, 11F)

Instructions
1. Dice red onion and jalapeños.
2. Add chicken, diced vegetables, and ranch dressing seasoning to the crockpot.
3. Cook on high for 3-4 hours or low for 5-6 hours.
4. Add 2 cups water and rice in pot, bring to boil on high heat, turn to low, cover, and cook for 10 minutes.
5. Shred chicken in the crockpot.
6. Blend cottage cheese, buffalo sauce, and shredded cheese until smooth. Add to the crockpot and stir well.
7. Serve buffalo chicken over rice.

CROCKPOT MEAL PREPS

SWEET & SPICY CHICKEN BOWLS

Calories: 450   **Protein: 53**   **Carbs: 28**   **Fat: 10**

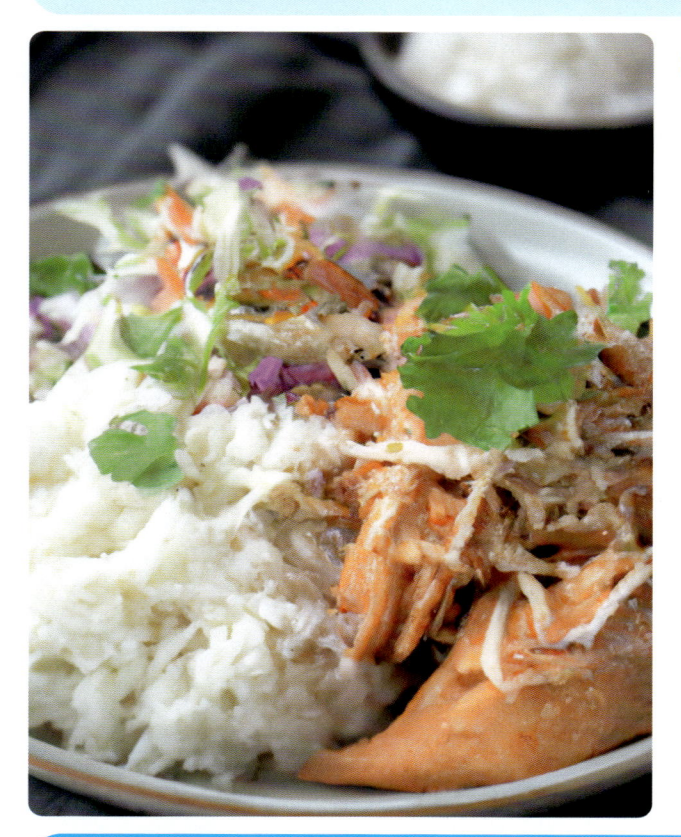

Ingredients — Servings: 8 (1 1/2 CUP)

Sweet & Spicy Bowls:
- 3 lb chicken breast
- 1 cup dry rice
- 1 red onion
- 2 bell peppers
- 2 jalapeno peppers
- 1 (18 oz.) container G Hughes sweet chili sauce
- 1 tbsp garlic powder
- 1 tbsp onion powder

Asian Slaw:
- 1 (14 oz.) bag coleslaw mix
- 1 bunch cilantro
- 4 tbsp red wine vinegar
- 2 tbsp low sodium soy sauce
- 2 tsp monk fruit sweetener

Optional Sides

- Salad (2 cups greens, 1 tbsp extra virgin olive oil, 2 tbsp balsamic - 307c, 4P, 11C, 27F)
- Protein shake (2 cups almond milk, 1 scoop Dummy Supps - 190c, 26P, 9C, 6F)

Instructions

1. Dice red onion, bell peppers, and jalapeños.
2. Add chicken, diced vegetables, sweet chili sauce, and listed seasonings to the crockpot.
3. Cook on high for 3-4 hours or low for 5-6 hours.
4. Shred chicken in the crockpot and stir well.
5. Add 2 cups water and rice in pot, bring to boil on high heat, turn to low, cover, and cook for 10 minutes.
6. Combine coleslaw mix, chopped cilantro, red wine vinegar, soy sauce, and monk fruit sweetener in a bowl. Mix well.
7. Serve chicken over rice with a side of Asian slaw.

CROCKPOT MEAL PREPS

CILANTRO LIME BURRITOS

Calories: 350 **Protein: 45** **Carbs: 10** **Fat: 10**

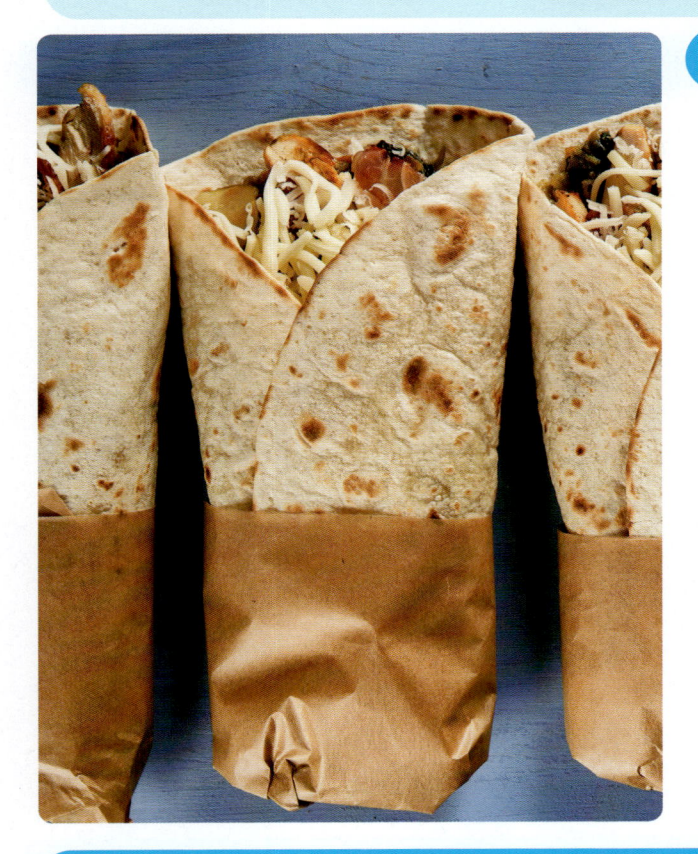

Ingredients — Servings: 12 (1 1/2 CUP)

Burritos:
- 3 lb chicken breast
- 12 (12 oz.) Mission low carb tortillas
- 1 sweet onion
- 2 bell peppers
- 2 jalapeno peppers
- 2 cups cottage cheese
- 1 (10 oz.) can green chilies
- 1 bunch cilantro
- 1 lime
- 2 (1 oz.) packets taco seasoning

Optional Sides
- Salad (2 cups greens, 1 tbsp extra virgin olive oil, 2 tbsp balsamic - 307c, 4P, 11C, 27F)
- Protein shake (2 cups almond milk, 1 scoop Dummy Supps - 190c, 26P, 9C, 6F)
- Avocado (1/2 whole - 120c, 2P, 6C, 11F)

Instructions
1. Dice red onion, bell peppers, and jalapeños.
2. Add chicken, diced vegetables, and taco seasoning to the crockpot.
3. Cook on high for 3-4 hours or low for 5-6 hours.
4. Blend cottage cheese, cilantro, and lime juice until smooth.
5. Shred chicken in the crockpot and stir well.
6. Add blended cottage cheese mixture to crockpot and stir until well combined.
7. Fill tortillas with chicken mixture and roll into burritos.
8. Serve warm or freeze for meal prep.

CROCKPOT MEAL PREPS

SMOTHERED CHIPOTLE CHICKEN BURRITOS

Calories: 350   **Protein: 45**   **Carbs: 28**   **Fat: 10**

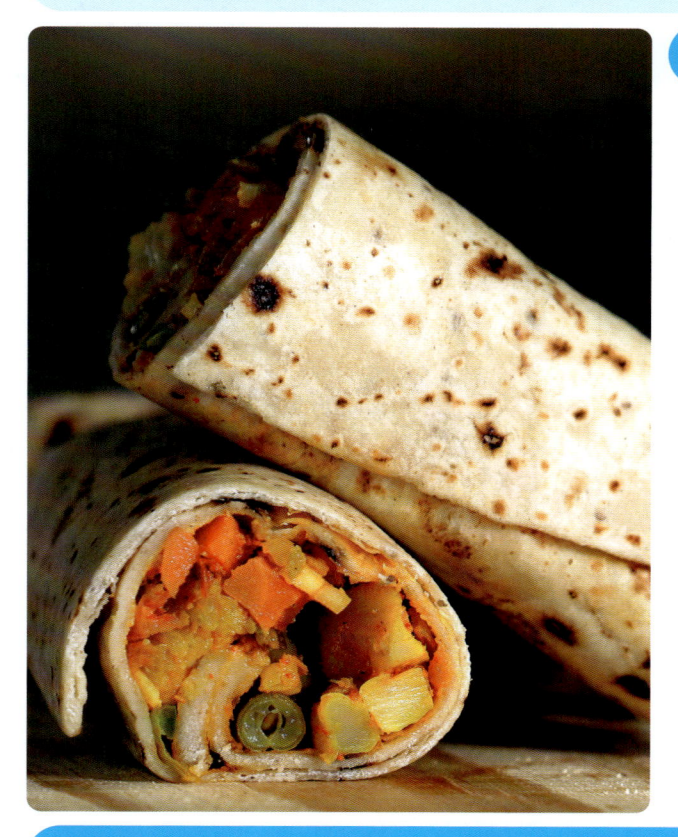

Ingredients   Servings: 12 (1 1/2 CUP)

Burritos:
- 3 lb chicken breast
- 12 (12 oz.) Mission low carb tortillas
- 2 white onions
- 2 bell peppers
- 2 jalapeno peppers
- 2 tbsp minced garlic
- 1 (10 oz.) can diced tomatoes
- 1 cup shredded cheese
- 1 (10 oz.) can chipotle peppers in adobo
- 1 1/2 cups enchilada sauce
- 1 bunch cilantro
- 1 lime
- 2 (1 oz.) packets taco seasoning

Optional Sides
- Salad (2 cups greens, 1 tbsp extra virgin olive oil, 2 tbsp balsamic - 307c, 4P, 11C, 27F)
- Protein shake (2 cups almond milk, 1 scoop Dummy Supps - 190c, 26P, 9C, 6F)
- Avocado (1/2 whole - 120c, 2P, 6C, 11F)

Instructions
1. Blend chipotle peppers until smooth.
2. Dice white onions, bell peppers, and jalapeños.
3. Add chicken, blended chipotle peppers, diced vegetables, minced garlic, diced tomatoes, taco seasoning, and juice from the lime to the crockpot.
4. Cook on high for 3-4 hours or low for 5-6 hours.
5. Shred chicken in the crockpot and stir well.
6. Fill tortillas with the chipotle chicken mixture.
7. Top with enchilada sauce, diced white onion, and chopped cilantro before serving.

CROCKPOT MEAL PREPS

BUFFALO CHICKEN BURRITOS

Calories: 330   **Protein: 46**   **Carbs: 22**   **Fat: 10**

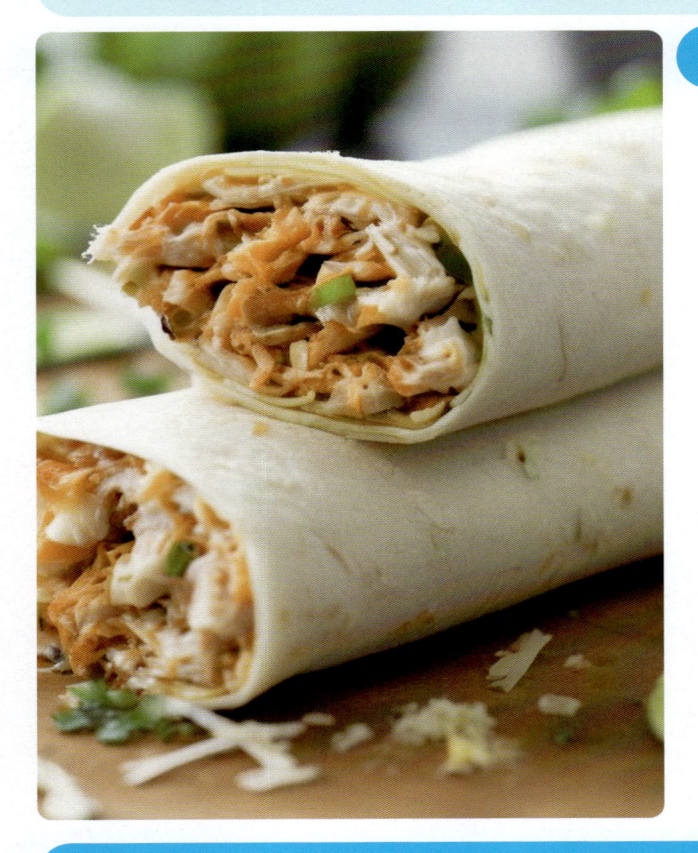

Ingredients   **Servings: 12 (1 1/2 CUP)**

Burritos:
- 3 lb chicken breast
- 12 (12 oz.) Mission low carb tortillas
- 1 red onion
- 2 jalapeno peppers
- 2 cups cottage cheese
- 1/2 cup buffalo sauce
- 1 cup shredded cheese
- 2 (1 oz.) packets ranch dressing seasonings

Optional Sides

- Salad (2 cups greens, 1 tbsp extra virgin olive oil, 2 tbsp balsamic - 307c, 4P, 11C, 27F)
- Protein shake (2 cups almond milk, 1 scoop Dummy Supps - 190c, 26P, 9C, 6F)
- Avocado (1/2 whole - 120c, 2P, 6C, 11F)

Instructions

1. Dice red onion, bell peppers, and jalapeños.
2. Add chicken, diced vegetables and ranch dressing seasoning to the crockpot.
3. Cook on high for 3-4 hours or low for 4-5 hours.
4. Shred chicken in the crockpot.
5. Blend cottage cheese, shredded cheese, and buffalo sauce until smooth. Add to the crockpot and stir well.
6. Fill tortillas with the buffalo chicken mixture and roll tightly into burritos.
7. Serve warm or freeze for meal prep.

CROCKPOT MEAL PREPS

CHEESY CHICKEN AND RICE BURRITOS

Calories: 450 **Protein: 53** **Carbs: 37** **Fat: 15**

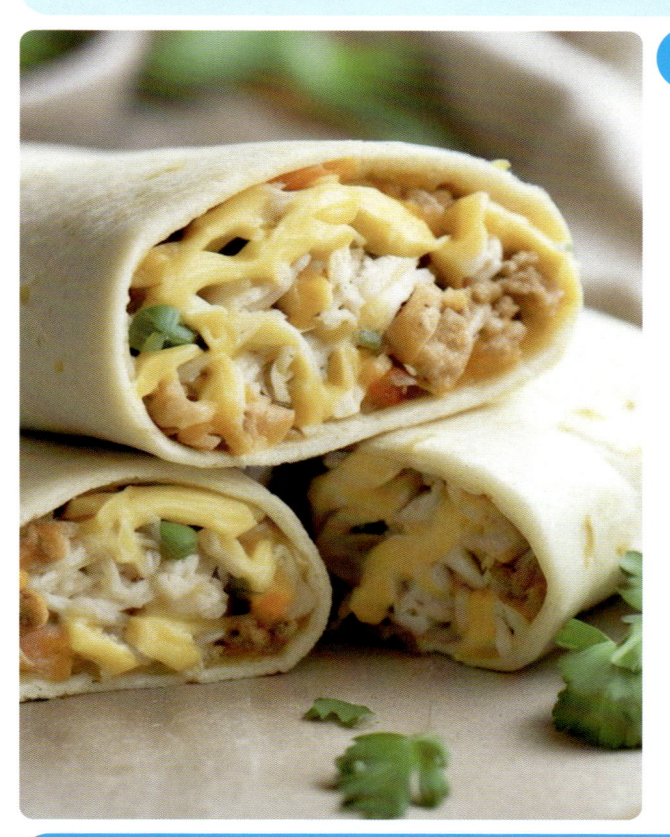

Ingredients **Servings: 12 (1 1/2 CUP)**

Burritos:
- 3 lb chicken breast
- 12 (12 oz.) Mission low carb tortillas
- 1 cup dry rice
- 1 sweet onion
- 2 bell peppers
- 2 (1 oz.) packets taco seasoning

Queso Sauce:
- 3 cups low fat cottage cheese
- 2 cups shredded cheddar cheese
- 1 (7 oz.) can green chiles

Optional Sides
- Salad (2 cups greens, 1 tbsp extra virgin olive oil, 2 tbsp balsamic - 307c, 4P, 11C, 27F)
- Protein shake (2 cups almond milk, 1 scoop Dummy Supps - 190c, 26P, 9C, 6F)
- Avocado (1/2 whole - 120c, 2P, 6C, 11F)

Instructions
1. Dice onion and bell peppers.
2. Add chicken, diced vegetables, and taco seasoning to the crockpot.
3. Cook on high for 3-4 hours or low for 5-6 hours.
4. Shred chicken in the crockpot and stir well.
5. Add 2 cups water and rice in pot, bring to boil on high heat, turn to low, cover, and cook for 10 minutes.
6. Blend cottage cheese, cheddar cheese, and chipotle peppers until smooth to make the queso sauce.
7. Add blended queso sauce to crockpot.
8. Fill tortillas with the cheesy chicken and rice mixture. Roll into burritos and serve.

CROCKPOT MEAL PREPS

SWEET & SPICY SANDWICHES

Calories: 400 **Protein: 40** **Carbs: 35** **Fat: 8**

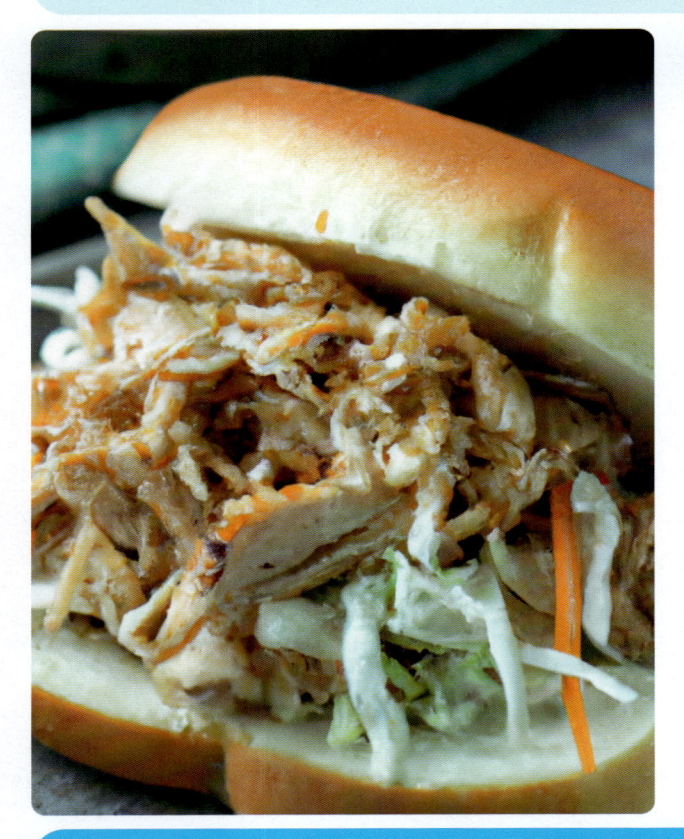

Ingredients   Servings: 8 (1 1/2 CUP)

Sweet & Spicy Chicken:
- 2 lb chicken breast
- 1 (18 oz.) container G Hughes BBQ
- 8 (647 low carb) buns
- 1 tbsp garlic powder
- 1 tbsp onion powder
- 1 tsp black pepper

Coleslaw:
- 1 (14 oz.) bag coleslaw mix
- 1 bunch cilantro
- 4 tbsp red wine vinegar
- 2 tbsp low sodium soy sauce
- 2 tsp monk fruit sweetener

Optional Sides
- Salad (2 cups greens, 1 tbsp extra virgin olive oil, 2 tbsp balsamic - 307c, 4P, 11C, 27F)
- Protein shake (2 cups almond milk, 1 scoop Dummy Supps - 190c, 26P, 9C, 6F)
- Avocado (1/2 whole - 120c, 2P, 6C, 11F)

Instructions
1. Add chicken, BBQ sauce, minced garlic, garlic powder, onion powder, and black pepper to the crockpot.
2. Cook on high for 3-4 hours or low for 5-6 hours.
3. Shred chicken in the crockpot and mix well.
4. Combine coleslaw mix, mayonnaise, vinegar, and sweetener in a bowl. Mix thoroughly.
5. Serve pulled BBQ chicken on low-carb buns topped with coleslaw.

CROCKPOT MEAL PREPS

BBQ CHICKEN SANDWICHES

Calories: 400 **Protein: 55** **Carbs: 15** **Fat: 23**

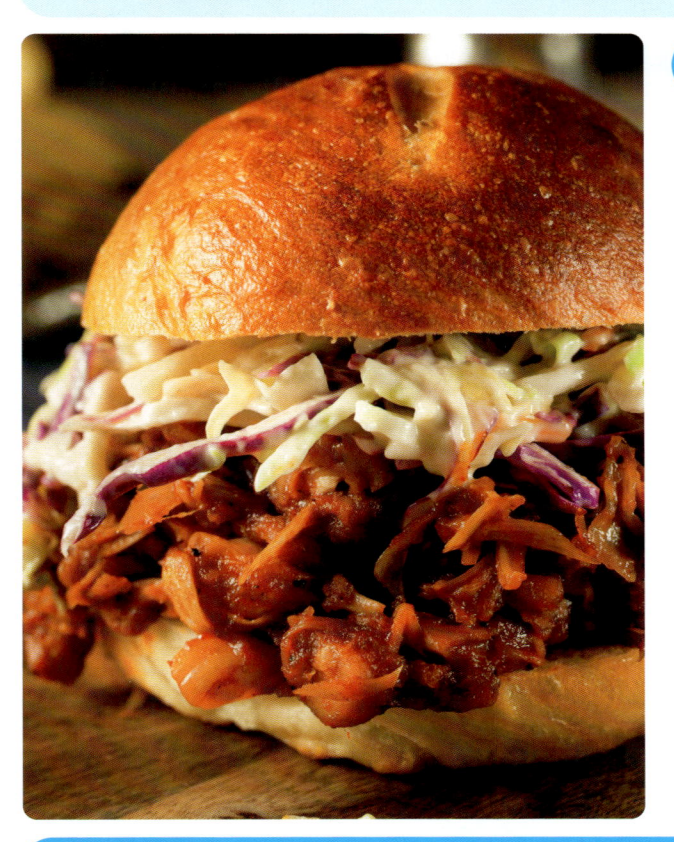

Ingredients   Servings: 8 (1 1/2 CUP)

BBQ Chicken:
- 2 lb chicken breast
- 1 (18 oz.) container G Hughes BBQ
- 8 (647 low carb) buns
- 2 tbsp minced garlic
- 1 tbsp garlic powder
- 1 tbsp onion powder
- 1 tsp black pepper

Coleslaw:
- 1 (14 oz.) bag coleslaw mix
- 1 cup lite mayonnaise
- 2 tbsp red wine vinegar
- 2 tsp monk fruit sweetener

Optional Sides
- Salad (2 cups greens, 1 tbsp extra virgin olive oil, 2 tbsp balsamic - 307c, 4P, 11C, 27F)
- Protein shake (2 cups almond milk, 1 scoop Dummy Supps - 190c, 26P, 9C, 6F)
- Avocado (1/2 whole - 120c, 2P, 6C, 11F)

Instructions
1. Add chicken, BBQ sauce, minced garlic, garlic powder, onion powder, and black pepper to the crockpot.
2. Cook on high for 3-4 hours or low for 5-6 hours.
3. Shred chicken in the crockpot and mix well.
4. Combine coleslaw mix, mayonnaise, vinegar, and sweetener in a bowl. Mix thoroughly.
5. Serve pulled BBQ chicken on low-carb buns topped with coleslaw.

CROCKPOT MEAL PREPS

BUFFALO CHICKEN SANDWICHES

Calories: 410   **Protein: 57**   **Carbs: 15**   **Fat: 24**

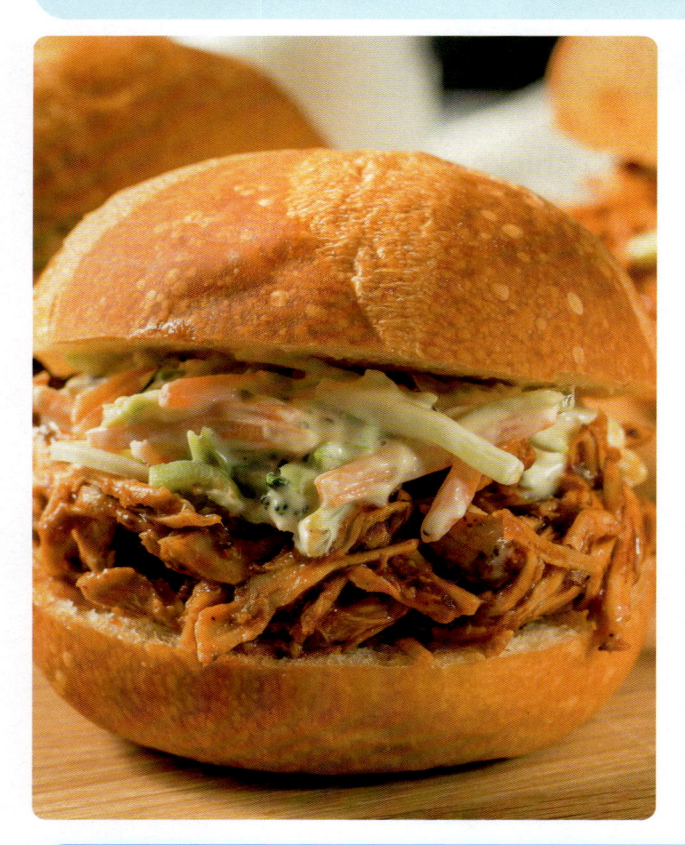

Ingredients   Servings: 8 (1 1/2 CUP)

Buffalo Chicken:
- 2 lb chicken breast
- 1/2 cup red hot
- 1/2 cup nonfat plain greek yogurt
- 8 low carb buns
- 2 cups shredded lettuce
- 1 packet ranch dressing seasoning
- 1 tsp black pepper

Coleslaw:
- 1 (14 oz.) bag coleslaw mix
- 1 cup lite mayonnaise
- 2 tbsp red wine vinegar
- 2 tsp monk fruit sweetener

Optional Sides

- Salad (2 cups greens, 1 tbsp extra virgin olive oil, 2 tbsp balsamic - 307c, 4P, 11C, 27F)
- Protein shake (2 cups almond milk, 1 scoop Dummy Supps - 190c, 26P, 9C, 6F)
- Cheese (1 slice - 80c, 5P, 0C, 7F)
- Dill Pickles (4 slices - 5c, 0P, 1C, 0F)

Instructions

1. Add chicken, hot sauce, ranch seasoning, and black pepper to the crockpot.
2. Cook on high for 3-4 hours or low for 5-6 hours.
3. Shred chicken in the crockpot and stir in Greek yogurt.
4. Combine coleslaw mix, mayonnaise, vinegar, and sweetener in a bowl. Mix well.
5. Serve buffalo chicken on low-carb buns with shredded lettuce and coleslaw.

CROCKPOT MEAL PREPS

MOMMA'S LASAGNA

Calories: 550 **Protein: 53** **Carbs: 35** **Fat: 23**

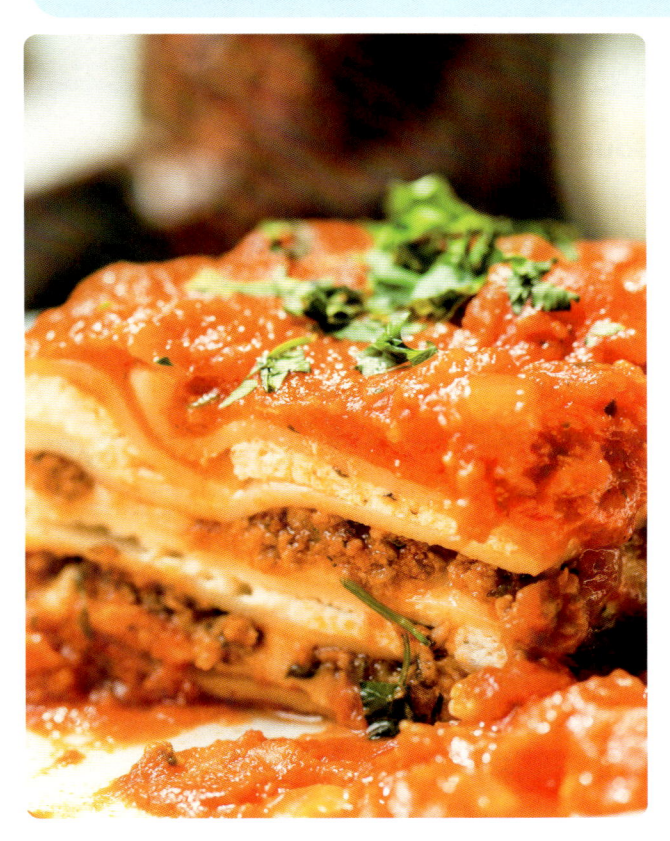

Ingredients   Servings: 8 (1 1/2 CUP)

Lasagna:
- 3 lb lean ground turkey/beef
- 4 tablespoons minced garlic
- 1 (30 oz.) can tomato sauce
- 1/2 box oven-ready lasagna noodles
- 1 (15 oz.) container skim ricotta cheese
- 2 cups low-fat mozzarella cheese
- 1 bunch parsley
- 2 tbsp Italian seasoning
- 2 tbsp minced garlic
- 1 tbsp onion powder
- 1 tsp black pepper
- 2 tsp crushed red pepper flakes

Optional Sides
- Salad (2 cups greens, 1 tbsp extra virgin olive oil, 2 tbsp balsamic - 307c, 4P, 11C, 27F)
- Protein shake (2 cups almond milk, 1 scoop Dummy Supps - 190c, 26P, 9C, 6F)

Instructions
1. Cook ground beef/turkey and listed seasonings in a pan for 8-10 minutes.
2. Add 3/4 of the tomato sauce to the cooked meat and stir.
3. Spread 1/4 of the tomato sauce on the bottom of the crockpot.
4. Layer oven-ready lasagna noodles over the sauce.
5. Spoon ricotta and mozzarella cheese over the noodles.
6. Add a layer of the meat and tomato sauce mixture.
7. Repeat layers of noodles, cheese, and meat until all ingredients are used.
8. Cover and cook on high for 50-60 minutes.
9. Dice parsley, sprinkle on top, and serve.

CROCKPOT MEAL PREPS

CHICKEN TORTILLA SOUP

Calories: 430 **Protein: 65** **Carbs: 37** **Fat: 11**

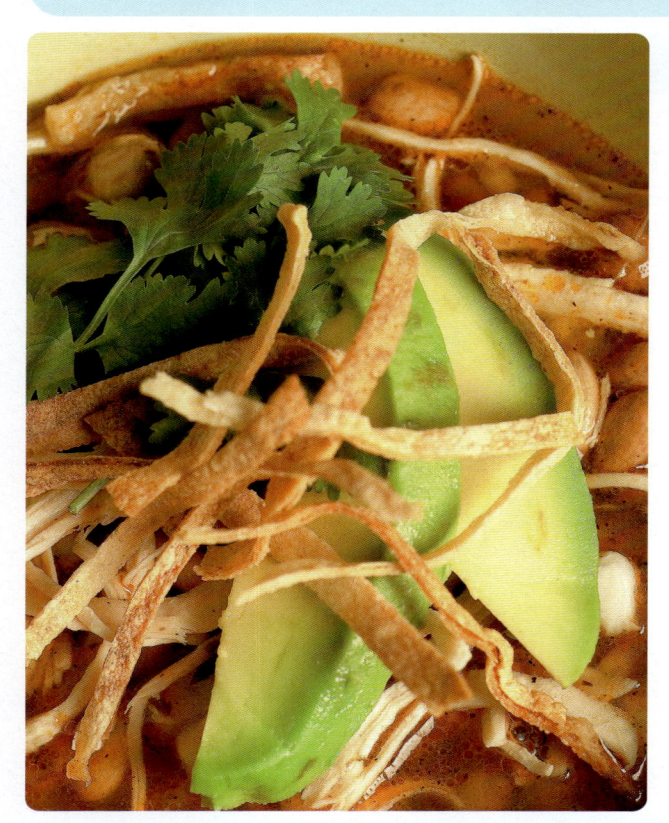

Ingredients — Servings: 8 (1 1/2 CUP)

Soup:
- 3 lb chicken breast
- 2 (30 oz.) containers bone broth
- 3 (15 oz.) cans diced tomatoes
- 1 cup tomato sauce
- 1 (7 oz.) container diced green chilies
- 2 teaspoons olive oil
- 4 tablespoons minced garlic
- 1 sweet onion
- 2 bell peppers
- 2 jalapeno peppers
- 1 cup shredded mexican blend cheese
- 2 (1 oz.) packets taco seasoning
- 1/2 teaspoon cayenne pepper

Optional Sides
- Avocado (1/2 whole - 20c, 2P, 6C, 11F)
- Tortilla strips (1/4 cup - 30c, 0P, 4C, 2F)
- Lite sour cream (2 tbsp - 35c, 1P, 2C, 3F)

Instructions
1. Dice onion, jalapeño, and green pepper.
2. Heat olive oil in a pan over medium heat. Sauté onion, jalapeño, green pepper, and garlic for 5 minutes.
3. Add chicken, onion, sauteed vegetables, bone broth, diced tomatoes, tomato sauce, green chilies, taco seasoning, and cayenne pepper to the crockpot.
4. Cook on high for 3-4 hours or low for 4-5 hours.
5. Shred chicken in the crockpot and stir well.
6. Serve soup topped with shredded Mexican blend cheese.

CROCKPOT MEAL PREPS

CLASSIC BEEF STEW

Calories: 450   **Protein: 47**   **Carbs: 23**   **Fat: 16**

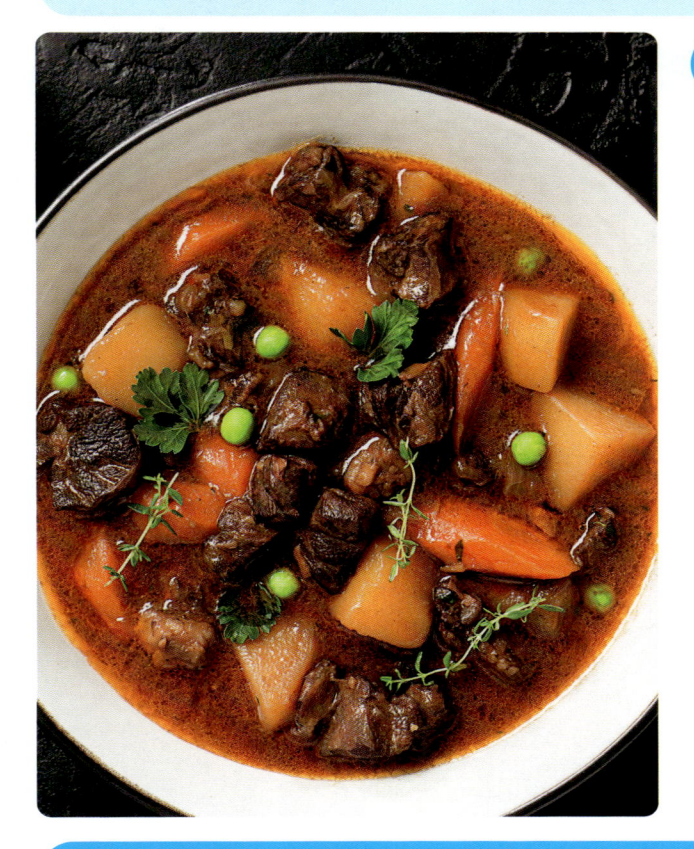

Ingredients   Servings: 8 (1 1/2 CUP)

Soup:
- 3 lb beef stew tips
- 2 (30 oz.) containers bone broth
- 4 tbsp minced garlic
- 1 lb carrots
- 1 lb celery
- 1 yellow onion
- 1 lb bag yellow potatoes
- 1/2 cup red wine vinegar
- 2 (1 oz.) packets beef onion soup mix

Optional Sides

- Salad (2 cups greens, 1 tbsp extra virgin olive oil, 2 tbsp balsamic - 307c, 4P, 11C, 27F)
- Protein shake (2 cups almond milk, 1 scoop Dummy Supps - 190c, 26P, 9C, 6F)

Instructions

1. Dice carrots, celery, onions, and potatoes into bite-sized pieces.
2. Add beef stew tips, minced garlic, diced vegetables, bone broth, red wine vinegar, and beef onion soup mix to the crockpot.
3. Cook on high for 4-5 hours or low for 4-5 hours, until beef is tender and vegetables are cooked through.
4. Stir before serving.

CROCKPOT MEAL PREPS

CHICKEN NOODLE SOUP

Calories: 460   **Protein: 48**   **Carbs: 37**   **Fat: 14**

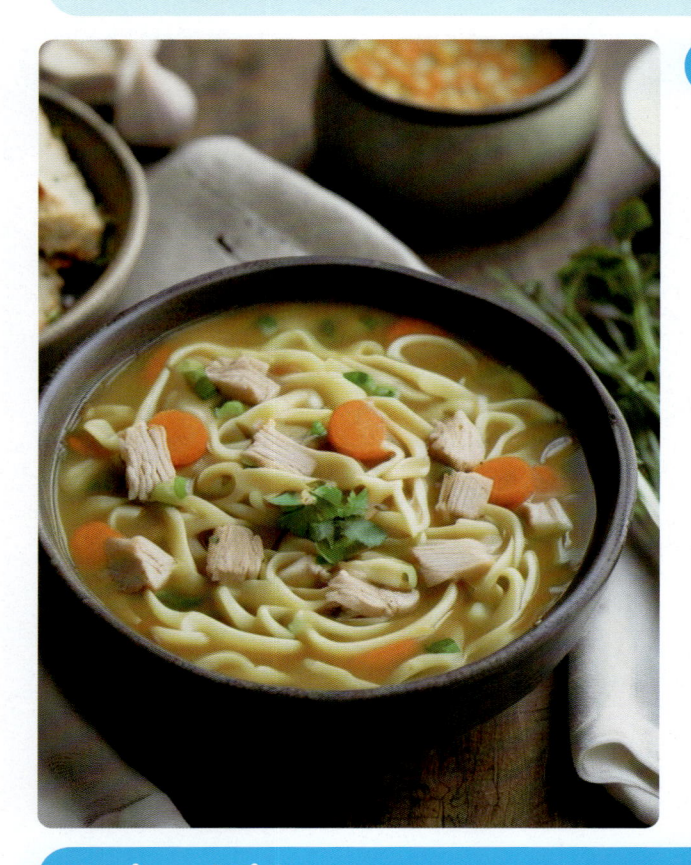

Ingredients   Servings: 10 (1 1/2 CUP)

Soup:
- 3 lb chicken breast
- 1 (15 oz.) box protein pasta
- 2 (30 oz.) containers bone broth
- 4 tbsp minced garlic
- 1 yellow onion
- 1 lb celery
- 1 lb carrots
- 1 tsp thyme
- 1 tsp rosemary
- 1/2 tsp salt
- 1 tsp black pepper
- 4 tsp chicken bouillon

Optional Sides

- Salad (2 cups greens, 1 tbsp extra virgin olive oil, 2 tbsp balsamic - 307c, 4P, 11C, 27F)
- Protein shake (2 cups almond milk, 1 scoop Dummy Supps - 190c, 26P, 9C, 6F)

Instructions

1. Dice onion and celery.
2. Add chicken, onion, celery, minced garlic, thyme, rosemary, salt, black pepper, chicken bouillon, and bone broth to the crockpot.
3. Cook on high for 3-4 hours or low for 5-6 hours.
4. Shred chicken in the crockpot.
5. Add protein pasta and cook on high for 20-30 minutes until tender.
6. Stir well and serve warm.

CROCKPOT MEAL PREPS

CRACK CHICKEN SOUP

Calories: 620 **Protein: 56** **Carbs: 38** **Fat: 29**

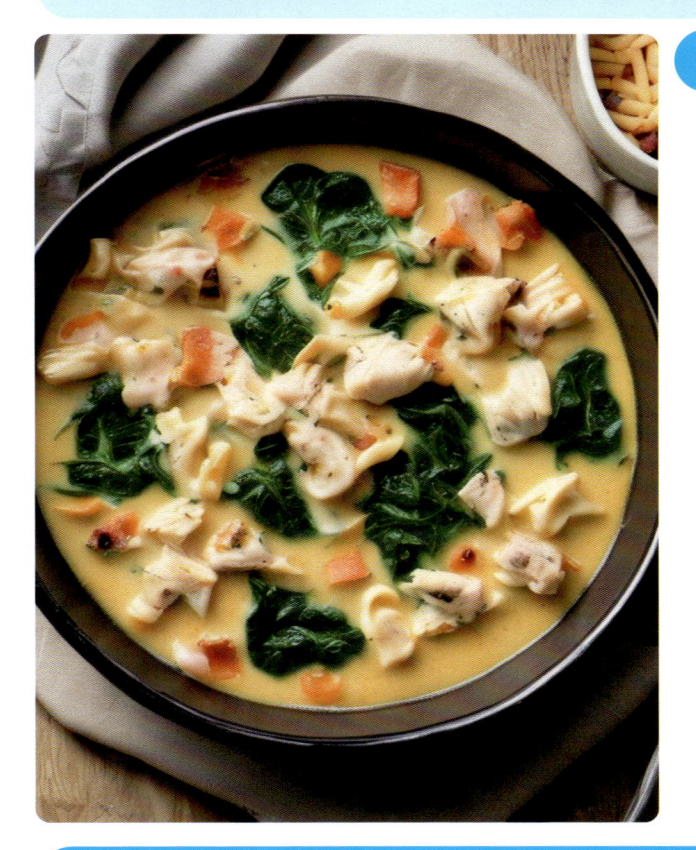

Ingredients   Servings: 10 (1 1/2 CUP)

Soup:
- 3 lb chicken breast
- 1 (15 oz.) box protein pasta
- 10 slices turkey bacon
- 2 (30 oz.) containers bone broth
- 4 tbsp minced garlic
- 2 (16 oz.) containers baby spinach
- 2 (8 oz.) container whipped cream cheese
- 2 cups shredded cheddar cheese
- 1 bunch green onions
- 2 (1 oz.) packets ranch dressing seasoning

Optional Sides
- Salad (2 cups greens, 1 tbsp extra virgin olive oil, 2 tbsp balsamic - 307c, 4P, 11C, 27F)
- Protein shake (2 cups almond milk, 1 scoop Dummy Supps - 190c, 26P, 9C, 6F)

Instructions
1. Dice turkey bacon and green onions.
2. Add chicken, turkey bacon, minced garlic, ranch dressing seasoning, bone broth, and whipped cream cheese to the crockpot.
3. Cook on high for 3-4 hours or low for 5-6 hours.
4. Shred chicken in the crockpot.
5. Stir in shredded cheddar cheese and baby spinach. Cook on high for 20-25 minutes until spinach is wilted and cheese is melted.
6. Add protein pasta and cook on high for 20-30 minutes until pasta is tender.
7. Stir well and top with green onions before serving.

CROCKPOT MEAL PREPS

NACHO SOUP

Calories: 430 **Protein: 60** **Carbs: 8** **Fat: 12**

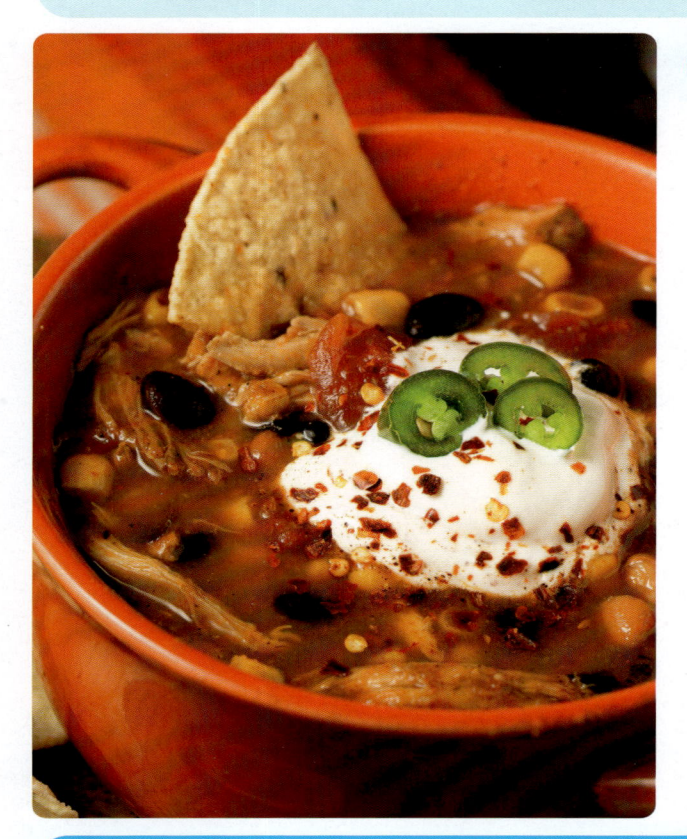

Ingredients   Servings: 8 (1 1/2 CUP)

Soup:
- 3 lb chicken breast
- 1 white onion
- 2 jalapeno peppers
- 3 tablespoons minced garlic
- 1 (15 oz.) can fire-roasted diced tomatoes
- 1 (15 oz.) can black beans
- 1 (15 oz.) can corn
- 6 cups bone broth
- 1 cup 1% milk
- 1 1/2 cups shredded cheese
- 1 bunch cilantro
- 2 (1 oz.) taco seasoning packets

Optional Sides
- Lite sour cream (2 tbsp - 35c, 1P, 2C, 3F)
- Avocado (1/2 whole - 120c, 2P, 6C, 11F)
- Tortilla strips (1/4 cup - 30c, 0P, 4C, 2F)

Instructions
1. Dice white onion and jalapeños. Chop cilantro and set aside.
2. Add chicken breast, onion, jalapeños, minced garlic, fire-roasted diced tomatoes, black beans, corn, bone broth, taco seasoning, and half of the chopped cilantro to the crockpot.
3. Cook on high for 3-4 hours or low for 5-6 hours until chicken is tender.
4. Shred chicken in the crockpot and stir well.
5. Stir in milk and shredded cheese, cooking for 10-15 minutes until melted and creamy.
6. Garnish with remaining cilantro before serving.

INDIVIDUAL MEAL PREP

OPTIONAL ADD ON'S

ADD ON'S

- **Protein Shake:** 1 scoop Dummy Supps Whey, 2 cups almond milk (190c, 26P, 9C, 6F)
- **Chocolate PB Shake:** 1 scoop Dummy Supps Chocolate Whey, 2 cups almond milk (190c, 26P, 9C, 6F)
- **Side Salad:** 2 cups greens, 2 tbsp olive oil, 2 tbsp balsamic: (307c, 4P, 11C, 27F)
- **PB&J Sandwich:** 2 slices 647 bread, 2 tbsp PB2, 1 tbsp water, 2 tbsp SF jam (160c, 9P, 31C, 3F)
- **PB & Banana Sandwich:** 2 slices 647 bread, 2 tbsp PB2, 1 tbsp water, 1 banana, 1 tsp cinnamon (235c, 10P, 50C, 3F)
- **Hard Boiled Eggs:** 2 eggs (144c, 12P, 0C, 10F)
- **Turkey Rice Cake:** 2 salted rice cakes, 2 slices turkey breast, 1 slice cheese, 1 tbsp lite mayo (220c, 16P, 25C, 8F)
- **Turkey Roll Ups:** 4 slices turkey breast (119c, 17P, 2C, 4F)
- **Mixed nuts:** 1/4 cup (217c, 7P, 21C, 21F)

- **Raspberries:** 1 cup (80c, 1P, 18C, 1F)
- **Blackberries:** 1 cup (80c, 1P, 18C, 1F)
- **Apple:** 1 whole (100c, 1P, 28C, 0F)
- **Strawberries:** 2 cups diced (100c, 1P, 23C, 1F)
- **Grapes:** 2 cups (200c, 1P, 54C, 0F)
- **Apple & PB:** 1 whole apple, 2 tbsp PB2, 1 tbsp water (154c, 6P, 33C, 2F)
- **Blueberries:** 1 cup (80c, 1P, 22C, 0F)
- **Clementines:** 2 whole (70c, 1P, 18C, 0F)
- **Veggies & Ranch:** 1 cup nonfat plain greek yogurt, 2 tsp ranch seasoning, 5 stalks celery/10 baby carrots (250c, 22P, 9C, 0F)
- **Veggies & Taco Dip:** 1 cup nonfat plain greek yogurt, 2 tsp taco seasoning, 5 stalks celery/10 baby carrots (250c, 22P, 9C, 0F)
- **Lite Popcorn:** 2 cups (150c, 2P, 15C, 10F)
- **Greek Yogurt:** 3/4 cup non fat plain, 1/2 cup berries (150c, 25P, 30C, 1F)

INDIVIDUAL MEAL PREP

OPTIONAL ADD ON'S

SAUCES

- **Tzatziki Sauce:** 1/2 cup nonfat plain greek yogurt, 1/4 cup grated cucumber, 1 tbsp dill, 2 tsp lemon juice, 1/2 tsp olive oil. 1/4 tsp salt (100c, 11P, 11C, 2F)
- **Protein Ranch:** 1/2 cup nonfat plain greek yogurt, 2 tsp ranch dressing seasoning (80c, 11P, 4C, 2F)
- **Protein Taco Dip:** 1/2 cup nonfat plain greek yogurt, 2 tsp taco dressing seasoning (80c, 11P, 4C, 2F)
- **Hot Sauce:** 2 tbsp (0c, 0P, 0C, 0F)
- **Salsa:** 2 tbsp (10c, 0P, 3C, 0F)
- **Lite Sour Cream:** 2 tbsp (35c, 2P, 2C, 3F)
- **Marinara:** 1/2 cup (50c, 2P, 11C, 1F)
- **Yellow Mustard:** 2 tbsp (1P, 0C, 0F)
- **Low Sodium Soy Sauce:** 1 tbsp (10c, 1P, 1C, 0F)
- **Hummus:** 1 tbsp (36c, 1P, 2C, 3F)
- **Balsamic Glaze:** 1 tbsp (25c, 0P, 6C, 0F)
- **Olive Oil:** 1 tbsp (120c, 0P, 0C, 14F)
- **Balsamic Vinegar:** 1 tbsp (14c, 0P, 3C, 0F)
- G Hughes Teriyaki: 2 tbsp (10c, 0P, 2C, 0F)
- G Hughes Thai Chili: 2 tbsp (10c, 0P, 2C, 0F)
- G Hughes Burger Sauce: 2 tbsp (100c, 0P, 2C, 10F)
- G Hughes Stir Fry: 2 tbsp (10c, 0P, 2C, 0F)
- G Hughes BBQ: 2 tbsp (10c, 0P, 2C, 0F)
- G Hughes Sweet & Spicy: 2 tbsp (10c, 0P, 2C, 0F)
- G Hughes Ketchup: 2 tbsp (5c, 0P, 2C, 0F)
- G Hughes Sweet Chili Sauce: 2 tbsp (100c, 0P, 2C, 10F)

BULK MEAL PREP

MULTIPLE MEAL PREPS

BULK RECIPES TO LAST YOU ALL WEEK

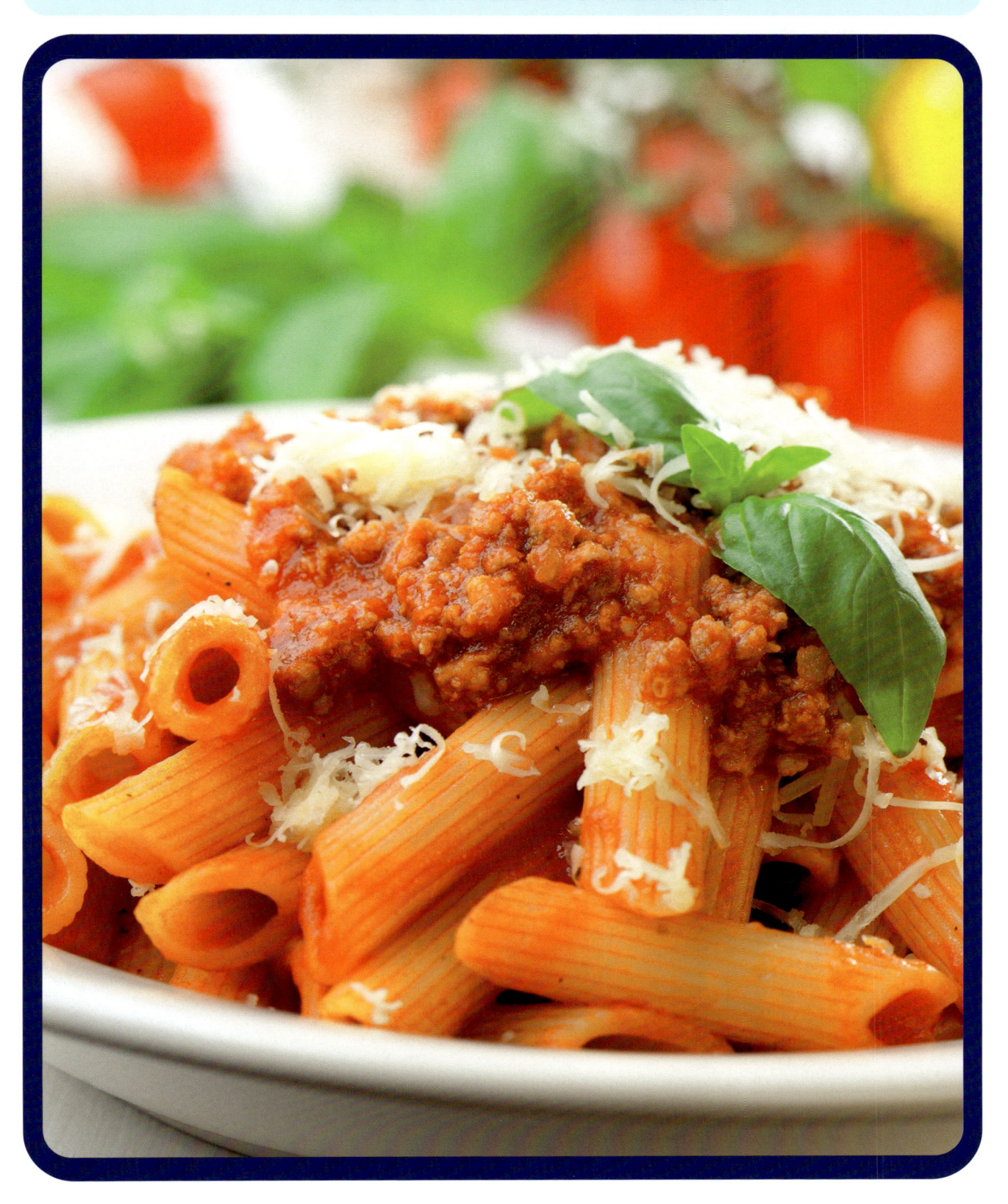

MULTIPLE MEAL PREPS

HAMBURGER HELPER

Calories: 550   **Protein: 54**   **Carbs: 31**   **Fat: 26**

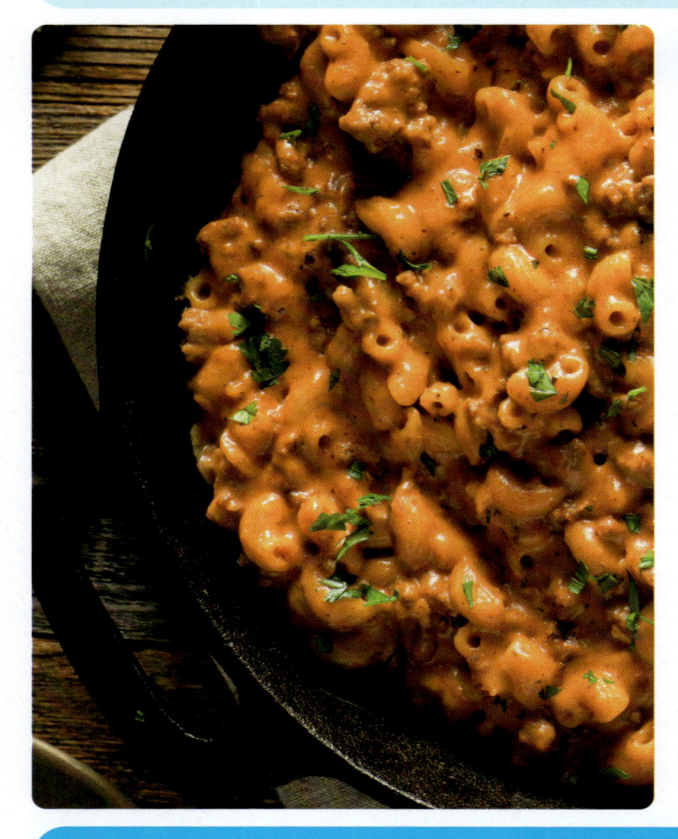

Ingredients   Servings: 8 (1 1/2 CUP)

Hamburger Helper:
- 3 lb lean ground beef/turkey
- 1 yellow onion
- 3 tbsp tomato paste
- 4 cups bone broth
- 1 (14.5 oz.) box protein pasta
- 2 cups shredded cheddar cheese
- 2 tbsp minced garlic
- 2 tbsp garlic powder
- 1 tbsp chili powder
- 1 tsp paprika
- 1 tsp black pepper

Optional Sides
- Salad (2 cups greens, 1 tbsp extra virgin olive oil, 2 tbsp balsamic - 307c, 4P, 11C, 27F)
- Protein shake (2 cups almond milk, 1 scoop Dummy Supps - 190c, 26P, 9C, 6F)

Instructions
1. Dice yellow onion.
2. Heat a pan over medium heat. Add diced onion and minced garlic. Cook for 2-3 minutes until softened.
3. Add ground beef/turkey and cook for 8-10 minutes until browned.
4. Stir in tomato paste, garlic powder, chili powder, paprika, and black pepper. Cook for 1 minute.
5. Pour in bone broth and bring to a boil.
6. Add protein pasta, reduce heat, and simmer for 9-11 minutes, stirring occasionally until pasta is tender.
7. Stir in shredded cheddar cheese until melted and creamy.
8. Serve warm.

MULTIPLE MEAL PREPS

CHEESEBURGER BOWLS

Calories: 540 **Protein: 50** **Carbs: 33** **Fat: 25**

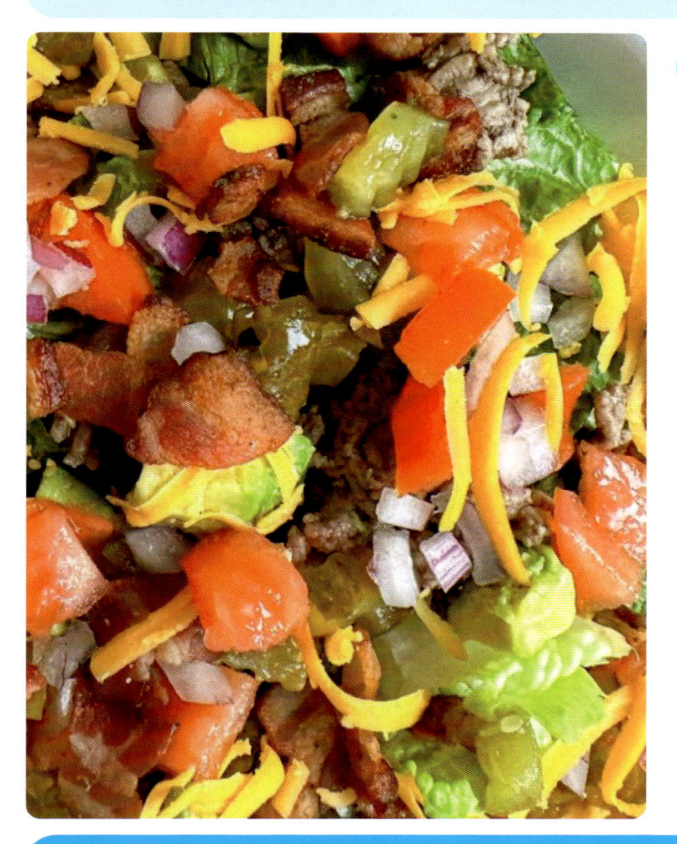

Ingredients   Servings: 8 (1 1/2 CUP)

Bowls:
- 3 lb lean ground beef
- 1 1/2 cup dry rice
- 6 cups shredded lettuce
- 3 cups shredded cheese
- 2 tablespoons garlic powder
- 1 tablespoon onion powder
- 1/2 teaspoon salt
- 1 teaspoon black pepper

Optional Sides

- 2 tbsp simply ketchup (40c, 0P, 8C, 0F)
- 2 tbsp lite mayonnaise (70c, 0P, 2C, 7F)
- 2 tbsp dill relish (10c, 0P, 0C, 0F)
- 2 tbsp yellow mustard (5c, 0P, 0C, 0F)
- 2 tbsp white onion (8c, 0P, 2C, 0F)
- 2 tbsp diced tomatoes (6c, 0P, 1C, 0F)
- 2 slices turkey bacon (80c, 12P, 1C, 6P)

Instructions

1. Heat a pan over medium heat. Cook ground beef with listed seasonings for 7-8 minutes until browned.
2. Add 3 cups water and rice in pot, bring to boil on high heat, turn to low, cover, and cook for 10 minutes.
3. Assemble bowls with a base of shredded lettuce and scoop of rice. Add cooked ground beef.
4. Top each bowl with shredded cheese.
5. Add any additional sides.

MULTIPLE MEAL PREPS

BURGER & FRIES BOWL

Calories: 480 **Protein: 42** **Carbs: 25** **Fat: 20**

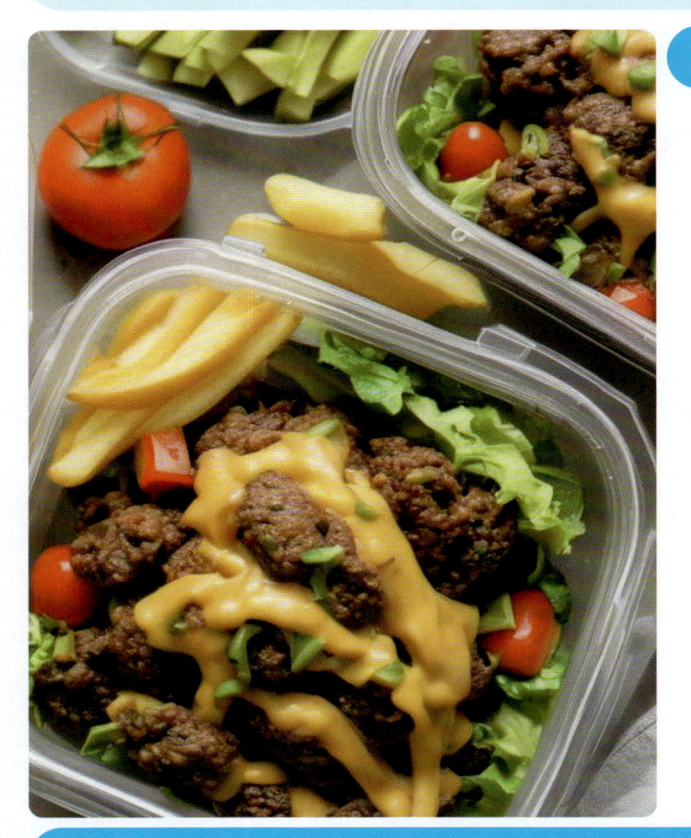

Ingredients   Servings: 10 (1 1/2 CUP)

Bowls:
- 3 lb ground beef/turkey
- 6 (6 oz.) russet potatoes
- 2 tbsp olive oil
- 1 1/2 cups shredded cheese
- 4 tbsp garlic powder
- 2 tbsp onion powder
- 4 tsp paprika
- 1 tsp salt
- 2 tsp black pepper

Optional Sides

- 2 tbsp simply ketchup (40c, 0P, 8C, 0F)
- 2 tbsp lite mayonnaise (70c, 0P, 2C, 7F)
- 2 tbsp dill relish (10c, 0P, 0C, 0F)
- 2 tbsp yellow mustard (5c, 0P, 0C, 0F)
- 2 tbsp white onion (8c, 0P, 2C, 0F)
- 2 tbsp diced tomatoes (6c, 0P, 1C, 0F)
- 2 slices turkey bacon (80c, 12P, 1C, 6P)

Instructions

1. Preheat oven to 400°F.
2. Dice potatoes into bite-sized pieces and toss with olive oil, and one half the listed seasonings.
3. Spread potatoes on a baking sheet and bake for 25-30 minutes until crispy, flipping halfway.
4. Heat a pan over medium heat with cooking spray. Add ground beef and other half of listed seasonings and cook for 10-12 minutes until fully cooked.
5. Divide roasted potatoes into bowls. Top with cooked beef and shredded cheese.
6. Add any additional toppings.

MULTIPLE MEAL PREPS

BUFFALO CHICKEN AND FRIES

Calories: 470 **Protein: 52** **Carbs: 20** **Fat: 16**

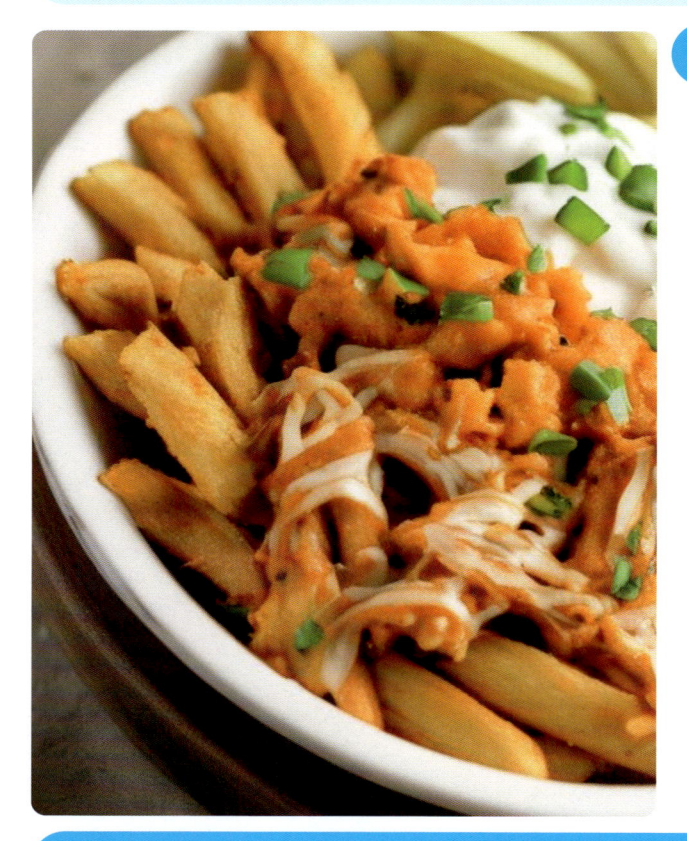

Ingredients — Servings: 10 (1 1/2 CUP)

Bowls:
- 3 lb chicken breast
- 6 (6 oz.) russet potatoes
- 2 tbsp olive oil
- 2 cups low fat cottage cheese
- 1/2 cup buffalo wing sauce
- 1 1/2 cups shredded cheese
- 4 tbsp garlic powder
- 2 tbsp onion powder
- 4 tsp paprika
- 1 tsp salt
- 2 tsp black pepper
- 1 bunch parsley

Optional Sides
- Salad (2 cups greens, 1 tbsp extra virgin olive oil, 2 tbsp balsamic - 307c, 4P, 11C, 27F)
- Protein shake (2 cups almond milk, 1 scoop Dummy Supps - 190c, 26P, 9C, 6F)

Instructions

1. Preheat oven to 400°F.
2. Dice potatoes into bite-sized pieces and toss with olive oil, and one half the listed seasonings.
3. Spread potatoes on a baking sheet and bake for 25-30 minutes until crispy, flipping halfway.
4. Dice chicken into bite-sized pieces.
5. Heat a pan over medium heat with cooking spray. Add chicken and season with the remaining half of the listed seasonings. Cook for 10-12 minutes until fully cooked.
6. Blend cottage cheese, shredded cheese, and buffalo wing sauce until smooth to make the buffalo cheese sauce. Heat in a pan over low heat until warm.
7. Divide fries into bowls. Top with cooked chicken and buffalo cheese sauce
8. Garnish with chopped parsley.

MULTIPLE MEAL PREPS

CHIPOTLE STEAK & FRIES

Calories: 500 **Protein:** 42 **Carbs:** 26 **Fat:** 25

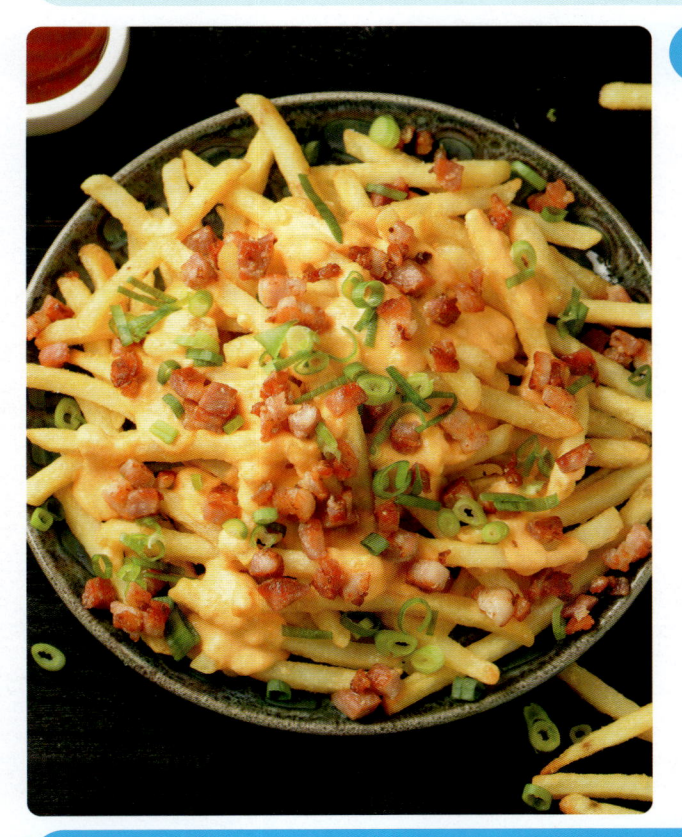

Ingredients — Servings: 10 (1 1/2 CUP)

Bowls:
- 3 lb steak (shaved, ribeye, sirloin, filet)
- 6 (6 ounce) russet potatoes
- 1 tablespoon olive oil
- 2 tablespoons garlic powder
- 2 tablespoons onion powder
- 2 teaspoons paprika
- 2 teaspoons salt
- 2 teaspoons black pepper

Chipotle Queso:
- 3 cups low fat cottage cheese
- 1 (10 oz.) can chipotle peppers in adobo
- 1 1/2 cups shredded cheese

Optional Sides
- Salad (2 cups greens, 1 tbsp extra virgin olive oil, 2 tbsp balsamic - 307c, 4P, 11C, 27F)
- Protein shake (2 cups almond milk, 1 scoop Dummy Supps - 190c, 26P, 9C, 6F)

Instructions
1. Preheat oven to 400°F.
2. Cut potatoes into fries and toss with olive oil and half the listed seasonings.
3. Spread on a baking sheet and bake for 25-30 minutes, flipping halfway.
4. Slice steak into thin strips.
5. Heat a pan over medium-high heat. Add steak and season with remaining half of the seasonings. Cook for 4-6 minutes, stirring occasionally.
6. Blend cottage cheese and chipotle peppers until smooth to make the chipotle queso. Heat in a pan over low heat until warm.
7. Divide fries into bowls and top with cooked steak and shredded cheese.
8. Drizzle with chipotle queso before serving.

MULTIPLE MEAL PREPS

SOUTHWEST MAC & CHEESE

Calories: 480 **Protein: 49** **Carbs: 27** **Fat: 21**

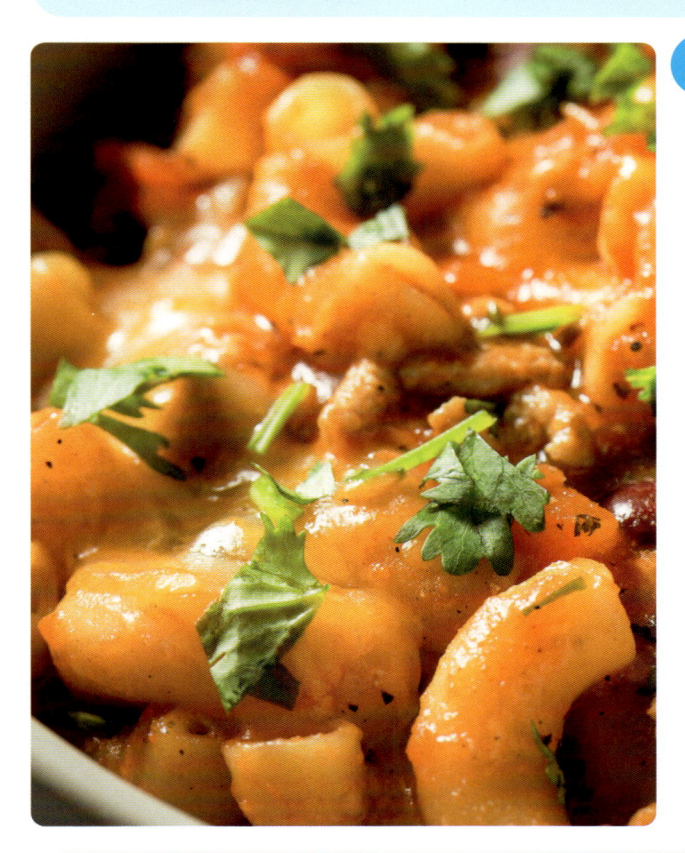

Ingredients — Servings: 10 (1 1/2 CUP)

Pasta:
- 3 lb lean ground beef/turkey
- 1 (14.5 oz.) box protein pasta
- 1 yellow onion
- 2 bell peppers
- 2 jalapeno peppers
- 1 (15 oz.) can diced tomatoes
- 4 cups low fat cottage cheese
- 1 (10 oz.) can green chilies
- 2 cups shredded sharp cheddar cheese
- 1 (1 oz.) packet taco seasoning
- 2 tbsp garlic powder
- 1 tbsp onion powder
- 1 tsp black pepper

Optional Sides

- Salad (2 cups greens, 1 tbsp extra virgin olive oil, 2 tbsp balsamic - 307c, 4P, 11C, 27F)
- Protein shake (2 cups almond milk, 1 scoop Dummy Supps - 190c, 26P, 9C, 6F)

Instructions

1. Dice onion and bell peppers.
2. Heat a pan over medium heat. Add onion and bell peppers, cooking for 5-7 minutes until softened.
3. Add ground beef/turkey to the pan. Stir in taco seasoning, garlic powder, onion powder, and black pepper. Cook for 10-12 minutes until browned.
4. Stir in diced tomatoes and green chilies. Simmer for 5 minutes.
5. Cook pasta for 9-11 minutes. Drain.
6. Blend cottage cheese until smooth, then mix in shredded cheddar cheese.
7. Add pasta to the pan and stir in the cheese sauce until evenly coated.

MULTIPLE MEAL PREPS

PASTA SALAD

Calories: 530 **Protein: 53** **Carbs: 29** **Fat: 20**

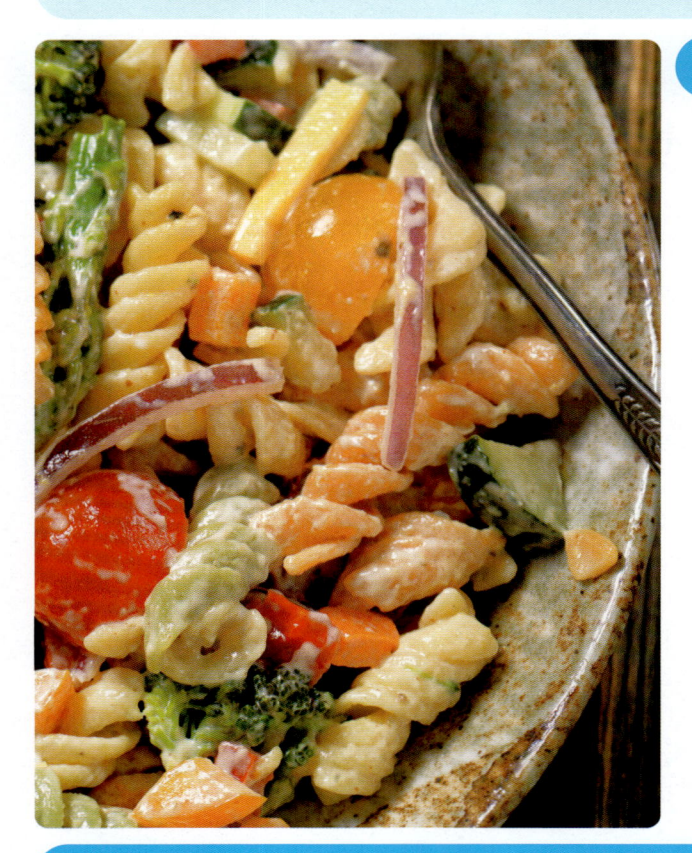

Ingredients **Servings: 10 (1 1/2 CUP)**

Pasta:
- 3 lb chicken breast
- 1 (14 oz.) box protein pasta
- 1 (10 oz.) container cherry tomatoes
- 1 large cucumber
- 1 red onion
- 1 (8 oz.) block reduced fat cheddar cheese
- 1 (12 oz.) G Hughes Italian dressing
- 1 tbsp garlic powder
- 1 tbsp onion powder
- 1/4 tsp salt
- 1 tsp pepper
- 1 bunch parsley

Optional Sides

- Salad (2 cups greens, 1 tbsp extra virgin olive oil, 2 tbsp balsamic - 307c, 4P, 11C, 27F)
- Protein shake (2 cups almond milk, 1 scoop Dummy Supps - 190c, 26P, 9C, 6F)

Instructions

1. Dice chicken into bite-sized pieces.
2. Heat a pan over medium heat with cooking spray. Add chicken, garlic powder, onion powder, salt, and pepper. Cook for 10-12 minutes until fully cooked.
3. Dice cherry tomatoes, cucumber, red onion, and cheddar cheese into small cubes.
4. In a large bowl, combine pasta, chicken, tomatoes, cucumber, red onion, cheddar cheese, and chopped parsley.
5. Cook pasta for 9-11 minutes. Drain.
6. Pour Italian dressing over the mixture and toss until evenly coated.

MULTIPLE MEAL PREPS

GREEK PASTA SALAD

Calories: 500 **Protein: 51** **Carbs: 30** **Fat: 17**

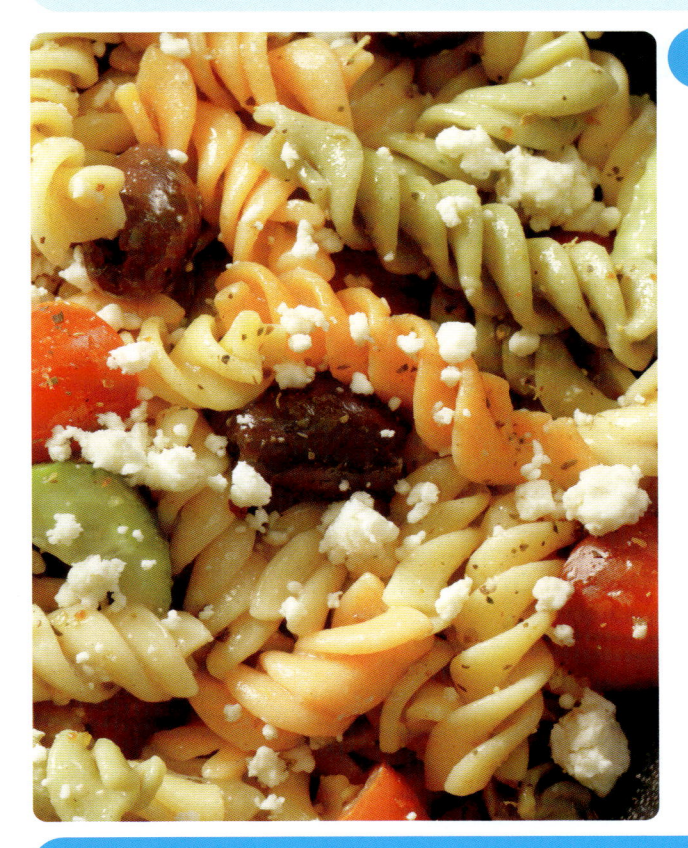

Ingredients — Servings: 10 (1 1/2 CUP)

Pasta:
- 3 lb chicken breast
- 1 (14 oz.) box protein pasta
- 1 (5 oz.) turkey pepperoni package
- 1 (10 oz.) container cherry tomatoes
- 1 large cucumber
- 1 red onion
- 1/2 cup black olives
- 1 (6 oz.) container feta cheese
- 1 (12 oz.) G Hughes Italian dressing
- 1 lemon
- 1 tbsp garlic powder
- 1 tbsp onion powder
- 1/4 tsp salt
- 1 tsp pepper
- 1 bunch parsley

Optional Sides

- Salad (2 cups greens, 1 tbsp extra virgin olive oil, 2 tbsp balsamic - 307c, 4P, 11C, 27F)
- Protein shake (2 cups almond milk, 1 scoop Dummy Supps - 190c, 26P, 9C, 6F)

Instructions

1. Dice chicken into bite-sized pieces.
2. Heat a pan over medium heat with cooking spray. Add chicken, garlic powder, onion powder, salt, and pepper. Cook for 10-12 minutes until fully cooked.
3. Dice cherry tomatoes, cucumber, red onion, and cheddar cheese into small cubes.
4. In a large bowl, combine pasta, chicken, tomatoes, cucumber, red onion, cheddar cheese, and chopped parsley.
5. Cook pasta for 9-11 minutes. Drain.
6. Pour Italian dressing over the mixture and toss until evenly coated.

MULTIPLE MEAL PREPS

THAI PEANUT CHICKEN PASTA SALAD

Calories: 600   **Protein: 56**   **Carbs: 38**   **Fat: 25**

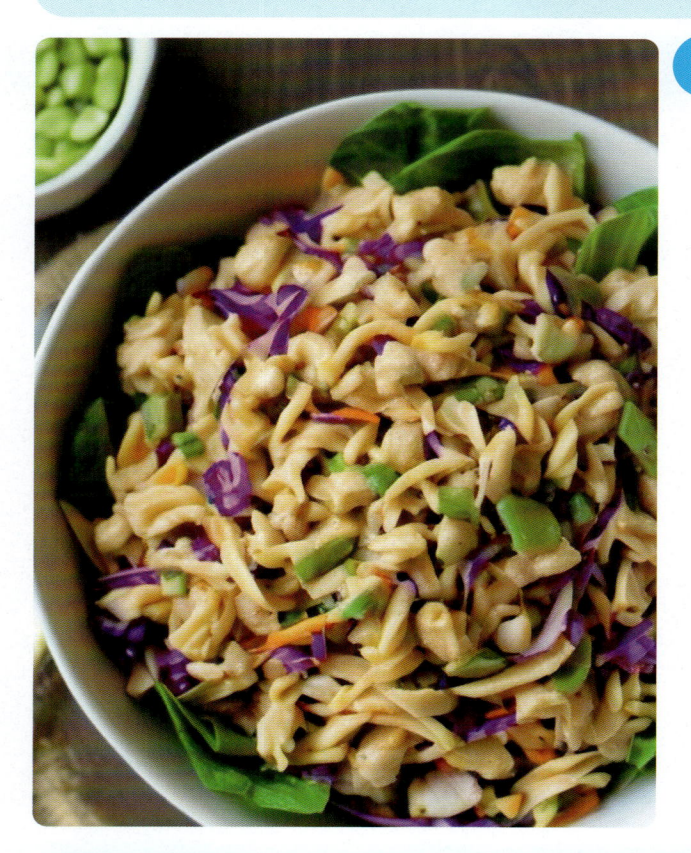

Ingredients   Servings: 10 (1 1/2 CUP)

Salad:
- 3 lb chicken breast
- 1 (14.5 oz.) box protein pasta
- 2 (16 oz.) bags asian slaw mix
- 2 tbsp minced garlic
- 1 tbsp minced ginger
- 1 tbsp sesame oil
- 4 tbsp low-sodium soy sauce
- 2 tbsp zero calorie brown sugar
- 1 large cucumber
- 1 red bell pepper
- 1 bunch cilantro
- 1/4 cup peanuts

Peanut Dressing:
- 1 cup smooth peanut butter
- 2 tbsp minced garlic
- 1 lime
- 2 tbsp low-sodium soy sauce
- 1 tbsp rice wine vinegar
- 2 tsp sriracha
- 6 tbsp warm water

Optional Sides
- Salad (2 cups greens, 1 tbsp extra virgin olive oil, 2 tbsp balsamic - 307c, 4P, 11C, 27F)
- Protein shake (2 cups almond milk, 1 scoop Dummy Supps - 190c, 26P, 9C, 6F)

Instructions
1. Dice cucumber and red bell pepper. Chop cilantro.
2. Heat a pan over medium heat with sesame oil. Add chicken, minced garlic, minced ginger, soy sauce, and brown sugar. Cook for 10-12 minutes until fully cooked.
3. Blend peanut butter, minced garlic, lime juice, soy sauce, rice wine vinegar, sriracha, and warm water until smooth to make the peanut sauce.
4. Cook pasta for 9-11 minutes. Drain.
5. In a large bowl, combine pasta, Asian slaw mix, cucumber, red bell pepper, and chopped cilantro.
6. Add cooked chicken and toss with peanut sauce until evenly coated.
7. Top with peanuts before serving.

MULTIPLE MEAL PREPS

CILANTRO LIME CHICKEN

Calories: 450 **Protein: 48** **Carbs: 26** **Fat: 13**

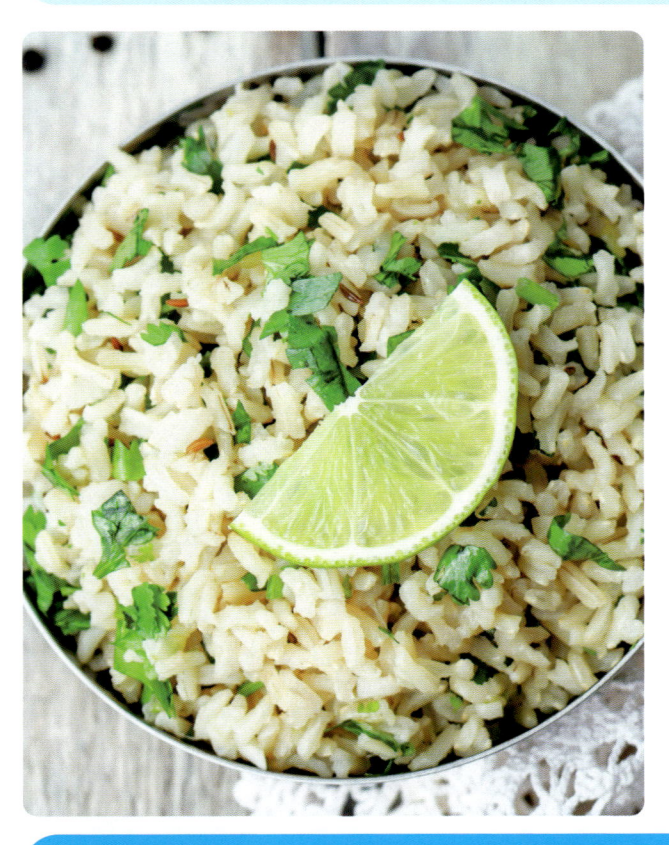

Ingredients   Servings: 6 (1 1/2 CUP)

Bowls:
- 2 lb chicken breast
- 1 1/2 cup dry rice
- 2 tablespoons olive oil
- 2 limes
- 1 bunch cilantro
- 2 tbsp minced garlic
- 2 tbsp garlic powder
- 1 tablespoon onion powder
- 1 teaspoon paprika
- 1 teaspoon chili powder

Optional Sides

- Salad (2 cups greens, 1 tbsp extra virgin olive oil, 2 tbsp balsamic - 307c, 4P, 11C, 27F)
- Protein shake (2 cups almond milk, 1 scoop Dummy Supps - 190c, 26P, 9C, 6F)
- Avocado (1/2 whole - 120c, 2P, 6C, 11F)

Instructions

1. Dice chicken into bite-sized pieces.
2. In a bowl, mix olive oil, juice from both limes, minced garlic, and listed seasonings.
3. Toss chicken in the marinade and let sit for 10 minutes.
4. Heat a pan over medium heat and cook chicken for 6-8 minutes, stirring occasionally, until fully cooked.
5. Add 3 cups water and rice in pot, bring to boil on high heat, turn to low, cover, and cook for 10 minutes.
6. Chop cilantro and mix half into the rice.
7. Serve chicken over rice and top with remaining cilantro.

MULTIPLE MEAL PREPS

TERIYAKI CHICKEN

Calories: 550 **Protein: 54** **Carbs: 34** **Fat: 5**

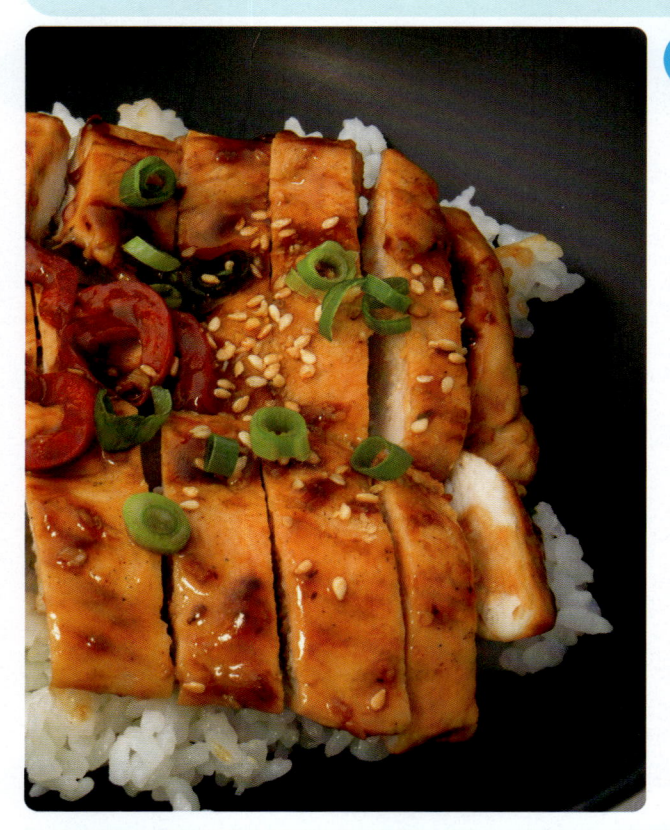

Ingredients **Servings: 6 (1 1/2 CUP)**

Bowls:
- 2 lb chicken breast
- 1 cup dry rice
- 1 red onion
- 2 bell peppers
- 1 jalapeno pepper
- 4 tablespoons minced garlic
- 1/2 (12 oz.) container G Hughes teriyaki
- 1 tablespoon garlic powder
- 1 teaspoon black pepper
- 1/2 teaspoon red pepper flakes
- 1 tablespoon sesame seeds

Optional Sides

- Salad (2 cups greens, 1 tbsp extra virgin olive oil, 2 tbsp balsamic - 307c, 4P, 11C, 27F)
- Protein shake (2 cups almond milk, 1 scoop Dummy Supps - 190c, 26P, 9C, 6F)
- Avocado (1/2 whole - 120c, 2P, 6C, 11F)

Instructions

1. Dice red onion, bell peppers, and jalapeño.
2. Dice chicken into bite-sized pieces.
3. Heat a pan over medium heat with cooking spray. Add onion, bell peppers, and jalapeño. Cook for 4-5 minutes until softened.
4. Add chicken, minced garlic, garlic powder, black pepper, and red pepper flakes. Cook for 10-12 minutes until fully cooked.
5. Add 2 cups water and rice to a pot. Bring to a boil on high heat, then turn to low, cover, and cook for 10 minutes.
6. Divide rice into bowls and top with teriyaki chicken.
7. Add teriyaki sauce on top of each of the bowls with sesame seeds.

MULTIPLE MEAL PREPS

PHILLY CHEESESTEAK BOWLS

Calories: 580 **Protein: 54** **Carbs: 31** **Fat: 20**

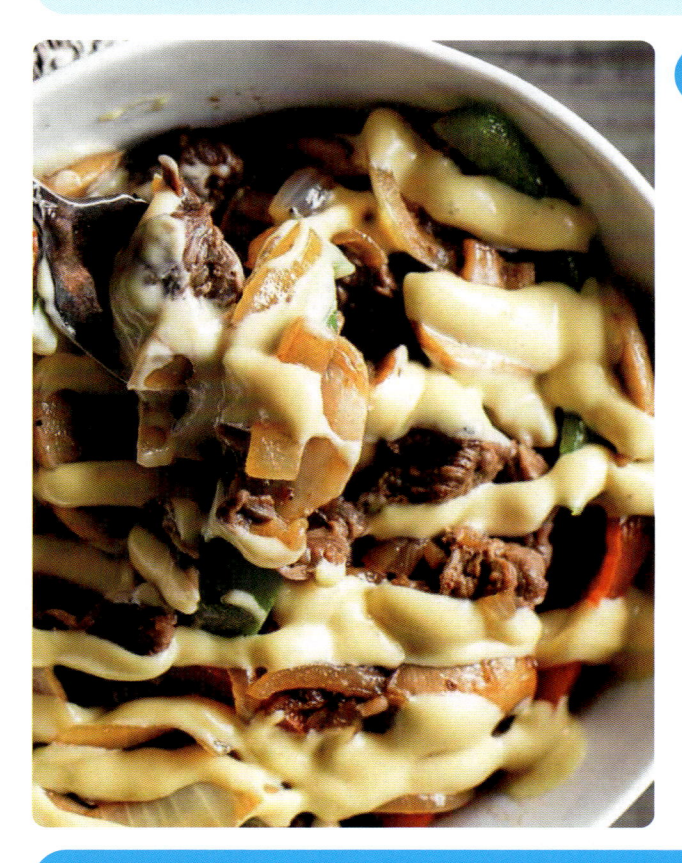

Ingredients Servings: 6 (1 1/2 CUP)

Bowls:
- 3 lb lean ground beef/turkey
- 1 cup dry rice
- 1 sweet onion
- 2 bell peppers
- 2 tbsp minced garlic
- 6 slices provolone cheese
- 2 tablespoons garlic powder
- 1 tablespoon chili powder
- 1 teaspoon salt
- 1 teaspoon black pepper

Optional Sides
- Salad (2 cups greens, 1 tbsp extra virgin olive oil, 2 tbsp balsamic - 307c, 4P, 11C, 27F)
- Protein shake (2 cups almond milk, 1 scoop Dummy Supps - 190c, 26P, 9C, 6F)
- Avocado (1/2 whole - 120c, 2P, 6C, 11F)

Instructions
1. Dice sweet onion and bell peppers.
2. Heat a pan over medium heat. Add onion and bell peppers. Cook for 4-5 minutes until softened. Remove from pan and set aside.
3. Add ground beef/turkey to the pan with minced garlic, garlic powder, chili powder, salt, and black pepper. Cook for 10-12 minutes until browned.
4. Return cooked onions and bell peppers to the pan and stir to combine.
5. Add 2 cups water and rice to a pot. Bring to a boil on high heat, then turn to low, cover, and cook for 10 minutes.
6. Divide cooked rice into bowls and top with the beef mixture.
7. Place a slice of provolone cheese over each bowl and let melt before serving.

MULTIPLE MEAL PREPS

LEMON CHICKEN AND RICE

Calories: 590 **Protein: 52** **Carbs: 40** **Fat: 13**

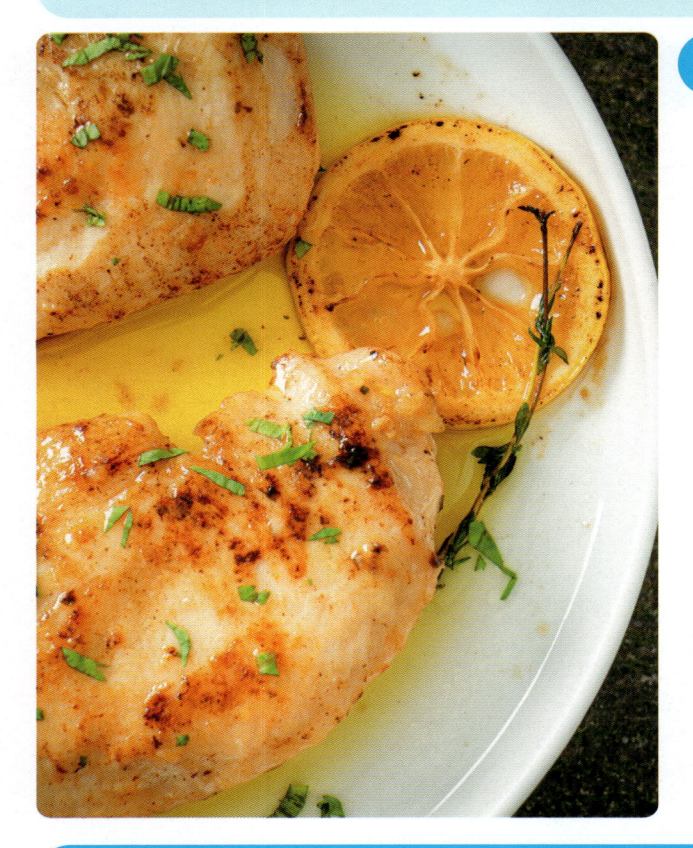

Ingredients **Servings: 6 (1 1/2 CUP)**

Bowls:
- 2 lb chicken breast
- 1 cup dry rice
- 2 tbsp minced garlic
- 2 lemons
- 2 tbsp capers
- 1/4 cup Italian blended cheese
- 3 cups arugula
- 2 tbsp balsamic vinegar
- 2 tbsp garlic powder
- 1 tbsp onion powder
- 1/4 tsp salt
- 1/2 tsp black pepper

Optional Sides
- Salad (2 cups greens, 1 tbsp extra virgin olive oil, 2 tbsp balsamic - 307c, 4P, 11C, 27F)
- Protein shake (2 cups almond milk, 1 scoop Dummy Supps - 190c, 26P, 9C, 6F)

Instructions
1. Dice chicken into bite-sized pieces.
2. Heat a pan over medium heat with cooking spray. Add chicken, minced garlic, garlic powder, onion powder, salt, and black pepper. Cook for 6-8 minutes until fully cooked.
3. Squeeze juice from both lemons over the chicken. Stir in capers and cook for 1-2 minutes.
4. Toss arugula with balsamic vinegar in a bowl.
5. Add 3 cups water and rice to a pot. Bring to a boil on high heat, then turn to low, cover, and cook for 10 minutes.
6. Divide rice, chicken, and arugula into meal prep containers.
7. Top with Italian blended cheese before serving.

MULTIPLE MEAL PREPS

BEEF NACHO BOWLS & PROTEIN QUESO

Calories: 500 **Protein: 41** **Carbs: 31** **Fat: 18**

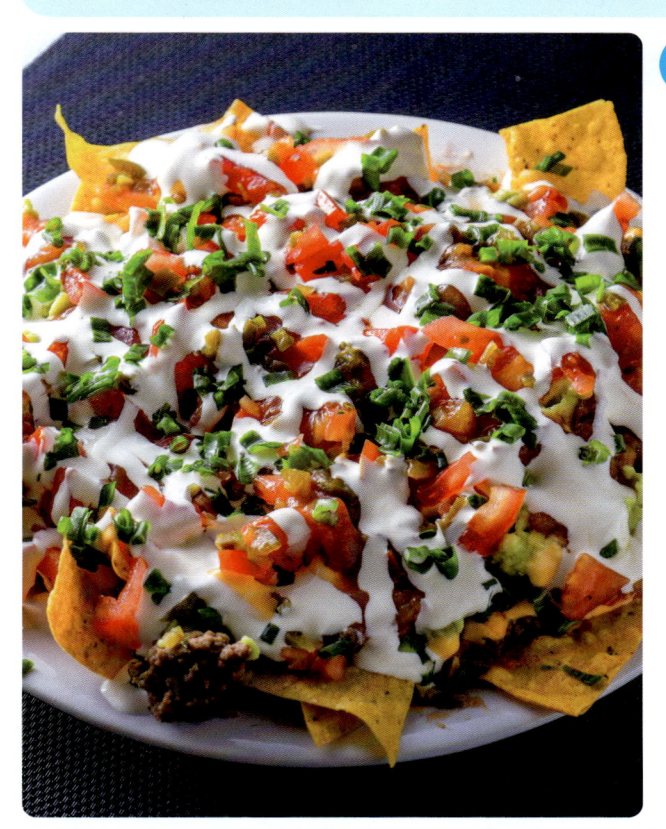

Ingredients — Servings: 8 (1 1/2 CUP)

Bowl:
- 3 lb ground turkey/beef
- 1 cup dry rice
- 1/2 red onion
- 1 (15 oz.) can diced tomatoes
- 1 (10 oz.) can green chilies
- 1 (15 oz.) can black beans
- 2 jalapeno peppers
- 2 avocados
- 1 bunch cilantro
- 2 limes
- 2 (1 oz.) packet taco seasoning

Protein Queso:
- 3 cups low fat cottage cheese
- 2 cups shredded cheddar cheese
- 1 (4 oz.) can green chilies
- 2 tbsp minced garlic

Optional Sides

- Salad (2 cups greens, 1 tbsp extra virgin olive oil, 2 tbsp balsamic - 307c, 4P, 11C, 27F)
- Protein shake (2 cups almond milk, 1 scoop Dummy Supps - 190c, 26P, 9C, 6F)

Instructions

1. Dice red onion and jalapeños. Dice avocados and chop cilantro.
2. Heat a pan over medium heat. Add ground turkey/beef, taco seasoning, and cook for 10-12 minutes until browned.
3. Blend cottage cheese, shredded cheddar cheese, green chilies, and minced garlic until smooth to make protein queso. Heat in a pan over low heat until warm.
4. Add 2 cups water and rice in pot, bring to boil on high heat, turn to low, cover, and cook for 10 minutes.
5. Heat black beans in a small bowl in the microwave for 1 minute.
6. Divide cooked rice into bowls. Top with beef, diced red onion, diced tomatoes, green chilies, black beans, diced jalapeños, avocado, and cilantro.
7. Drizzle with warm protein queso and serve with lime wedges.

MULTIPLE MEAL PREPS

BEEF AND RICE

Calories: 550   **Protein: 50**   **Carbs: 33**   **Fat: 25**

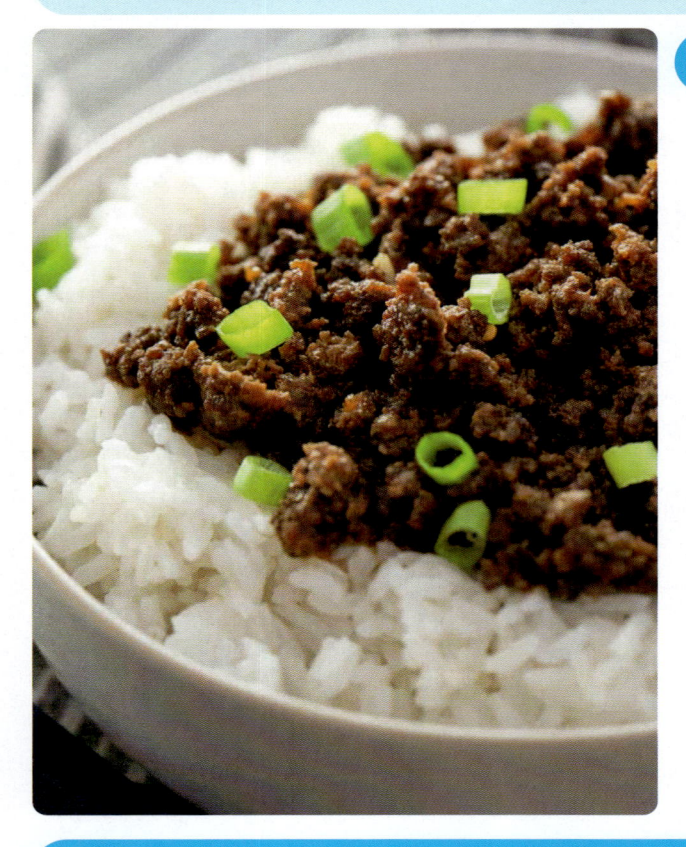

Ingredients   **Servings: 6 (1 1/2 CUP)**

Bowls:
- 3 lb lean ground beef/turkey
- 1 cup dry rice
- 2 tbsp olive oil
- 2 (12 oz.) bags frozen mixed vegetable
- 2 tbsp garlic powder
- 1 tbsp onion powder
- 1 tsp paprika
- 1 tsp chili powder

Optional Sides

- Salad (2 cups greens, 1 tbsp extra virgin olive oil, 2 tbsp balsamic - 307c, 4P, 11C, 27F)
- Protein shake (2 cups almond milk, 1 scoop Dummy Supps - 190c, 26P, 9C, 6F)
- Avocado (1/2 whole - 120c, 2P, 6C, 11F)

Instructions

1. Heat a pan over medium heat with olive oil. Add ground beef/turkey, garlic powder, onion powder, paprika, and chili powder. Cook for 6-8 minutes until browned.
2. In a separate pan, cook frozen mixed vegetables for 10-12 minutes until heated through.
3. Add 2 cups water and rice in pot, bring to boil on high heat, turn to low, cover, and cook for 10 minutes.
4. Divide cooked rice, beef, and vegetables evenly into meal prep containers.

MULTIPLE MEAL PREPS

ASIAN BEEF BOWLS

Calories: 490 **Protein: 45** **Carbs: 27** **Fat: 28**

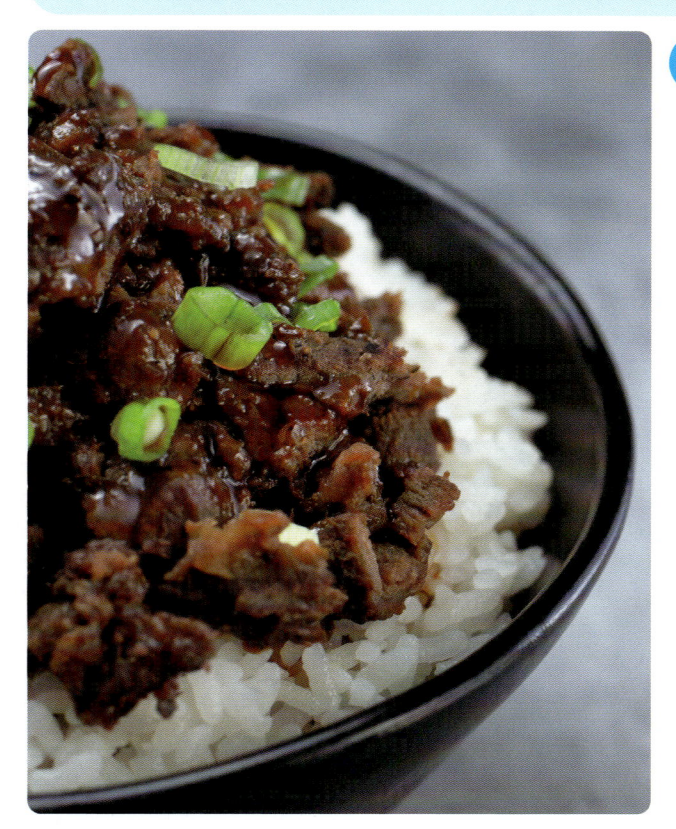

Ingredients — Servings: 6 (1 1/2 CUP)

Bowls:
- 3 lb lean ground beef/turkey
- 1 cup dry rice
- 2 tbsp minced garlic
- 2 tbsp minced ginger
- 1 white onion
- 2 bell peppers
- 2 jalapeno peppers
- 1/2 (12 oz.) container G Hughes sweet chili
- 2 tbsp garlic powder
- 1 tablespoon onion powder
- 1 teaspoon paprika
- 1 teaspoon chili powder
- 2 tbsp sesame seeds
- 1 bunch green onions

Optional Sides
- Salad (2 cups greens, 1 tbsp extra virgin olive oil, 2 tbsp balsamic - 307c, 4P, 11C, 27F)
- Protein shake (2 cups almond milk, 1 scoop Dummy Supps - 190c, 26P, 9C, 6F)
- Avocado (1/2 whole - 120c, 2P, 6C, 11F)

Instructions
1. Dice white onion, bell peppers, and jalapeños. Chop green onions.
2. Heat a pan over medium heat. Add onion, bell peppers, and jalapeños. Cook for 4-5 minutes until softened.
3. Add ground beef/turkey, minced garlic, minced ginger, garlic powder, onion powder, paprika, and chili powder. Cook for 6-8 minutes until browned.
4. Stir in sweet chili sauce and cook for 2-3 more minutes.
5. Add 2 cups water and rice to a pot. Bring to a boil on high heat, then turn to low, cover, and cook for 10 minutes.
6. Divide cooked rice into bowls. Top with beef mixture, sesame seeds, and chopped green onions.

MULTIPLE MEAL PREPS

ASIAN CHICKEN BOWLS

Calories: 440   **Protein: 54**   **Carbs: 27**   **Fat: 12**

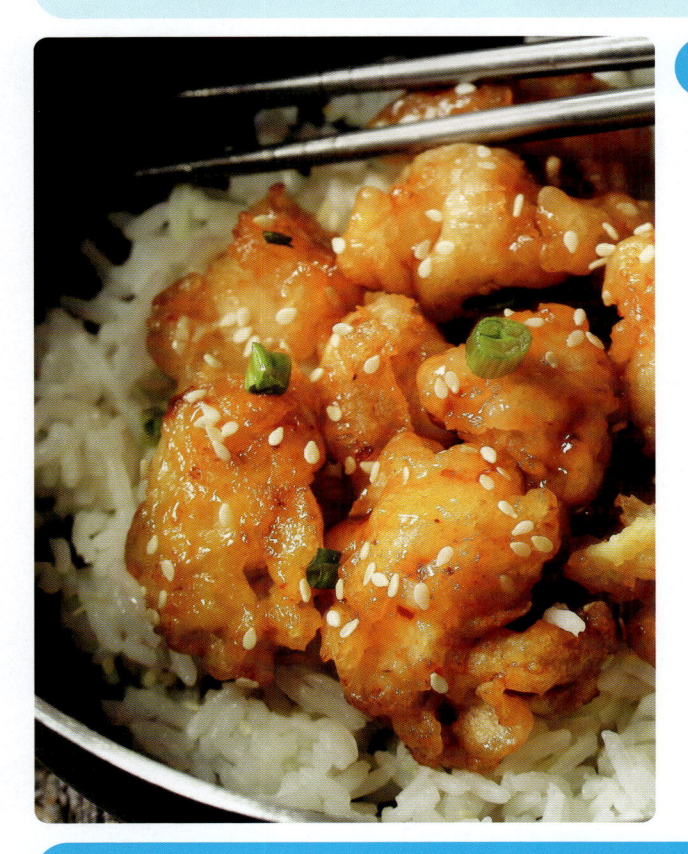

Ingredients — Servings: 6 (1 1/2 CUP)

Bowls:
- 3 lb chicken breast
- 1 cup dry rice
- 2 tbsp minced garlic
- 2 tbsp minced ginger
- 1 white onion
- 2 bell peppers
- 2 jalapeno peppers
- 1/2 (12 oz.) container G Hughes sweet chili
- 2 tbsp garlic powder
- 1 tablespoon onion powder
- 1 teaspoon paprika
- 1 teaspoon chili powder
- 2 tbsp sesame seeds
- 1 bunch green onions

Optional Sides
- Salad (2 cups greens, 1 tbsp extra virgin olive oil, 2 tbsp balsamic - 307c, 4P, 11C, 27F)
- Protein shake (2 cups almond milk, 1 scoop Dummy Supps - 190c, 26P, 9C, 6F)
- Avocado (1/2 whole - 120c, 2P, 6C, 11F)

Instructions
1. Dice white onion, bell peppers, and jalapeños. Chop green onions. Dice chicken into bite-sized pieces.
2. Heat a pan over medium heat. Add onion, bell peppers, and jalapeños. Cook for 4-5 minutes until softened.
3. Add chicken, minced garlic, minced ginger, garlic powder, onion powder, paprika, and chili powder. Cook for 6-8 minutes until fully cooked.
4. Stir in sweet chili sauce and cook for 2-3 more minutes.
5. Add 2 cups water and rice to a pot. Bring to a boil on high heat, then turn to low, cover, and cook for 10 minutes.
6. Divide cooked rice into bowls. Top with chicken mixture, sesame seeds, and chopped green onions.

MULTIPLE MEAL PREPS

CHICKEN AND RICE

Calories: 450 **Protein: 48** **Carbs: 25** **Fat: 17**

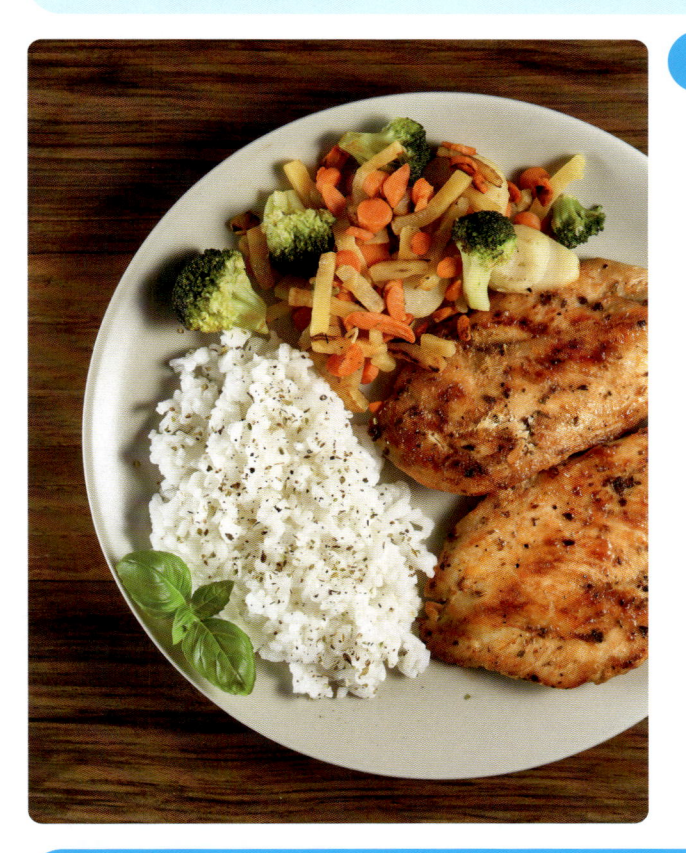

Ingredients   Servings: 8 (1 1/2 CUP)

Bowls:
- 3 lb chicken breast
- 1 cup dry rice
- 2 tablespoons olive oil
- 2 (12 oz.) bags frozen mixed vegetable
- 2 tbsp garlic powder
- 1 tablespoon onion powder
- 1 teaspoon paprika
- 1 teaspoon chili powder

Optional Sides
- Salad (2 cups greens, 1 tbsp extra virgin olive oil, 2 tbsp balsamic - 307c, 4P, 11C, 27F)
- Protein shake (2 cups almond milk, 1 scoop Dummy Supps - 190c, 26P, 9C, 6F)
- Avocado (1/2 whole - 120c, 2P, 6C, 11F)

Instructions
1. Dice chicken into bite-sized pieces.
2. Heat a pan over medium heat with olive oil. Add chicken, garlic powder, onion powder, paprika, and chili powder. Cook for 10-12 minutes until browned and fully cooked.
3. In a separate pan, cook frozen mixed vegetables for 5-7 minutes until heated through.
4. Add 2 cups water and rice in pot, bring to boil on high heat, turn to low, cover, and cook for 10 minutes.
5. Divide cooked rice, chicken, and vegetables evenly into meal prep containers.

MULTIPLE MEAL PREPS

CHEESY BACON RANCH CHICKEN BOWLS

Calories: 510 **Protein: 63** **Carbs: 26** **Fat: 16**

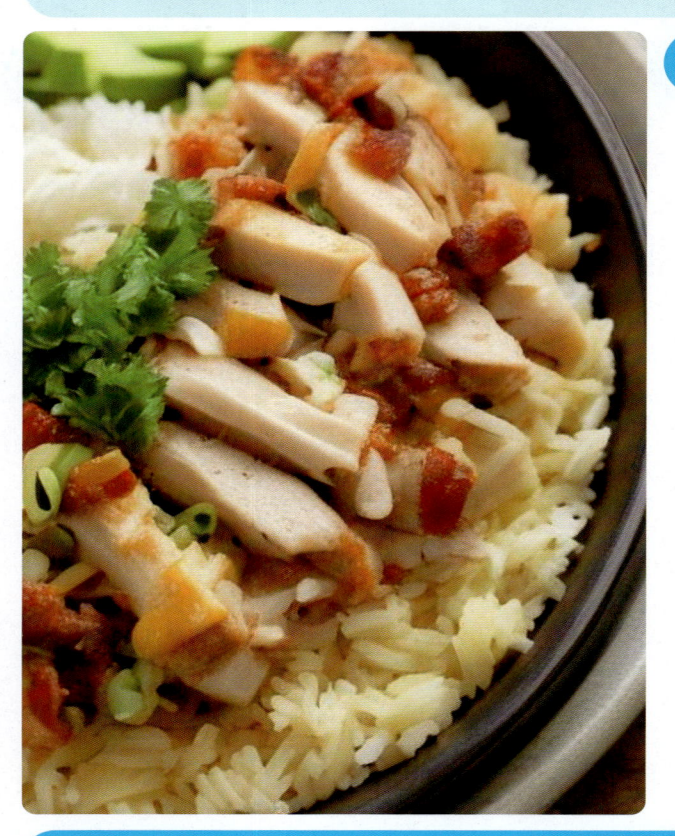

Ingredients   Servings: 6 (1 1/2 CUP)

Bowls:
- 2 lb chicken breast
- 1 cup dry rice
- 12 slices turkey bacon
- 1 cup part skim mozzarella cheese
- 1 (1 oz.) packet ranch dressing seasoning
- 1 tablespoon onion powder
- 1 teaspoon paprika
- 1 teaspoon chili powder
- 1 bunch cilantro

Optional Sides
- Salad (2 cups greens, 1 tbsp extra virgin olive oil, 2 tbsp balsamic - 307c, 4P, 11C, 27F)
- Protein shake (2 cups almond milk, 1 scoop Dummy Supps - 190c, 26P, 9C, 6F)
- Avocado (1/2 whole - 120c, 2P, 6C, 11F)

Instructions
1. Dice chicken into bite-sized pieces.
2. Heat a pan over medium heat. Add diced bacon and cook until crispy. Remove and set aside.
3. In the same pan, add chicken, ranch seasoning, onion powder, paprika, and chili powder. Cook for 8-10 minutes until fully cooked.
4. Stir in ½ of the cooked bacon and mozzarella cheese. Cook for 1-2 minutes until cheese is melted.
5. Add 2 cups water and rice in pot, bring to boil on high heat, turn to low, cover, and cook for 10 minutes.
6. Divide rice into bowls.
7. Top with cheesy bacon ranch chicken and remaining bacon.
8. Garnish with chopped cilantro before serving.

MULTIPLE MEAL PREPS

CHICKEN NACHO BOWLS & PROTEIN QUESO

Calories: 480   **Protein: 54**   **Carbs: 32**   **Fat: 14**

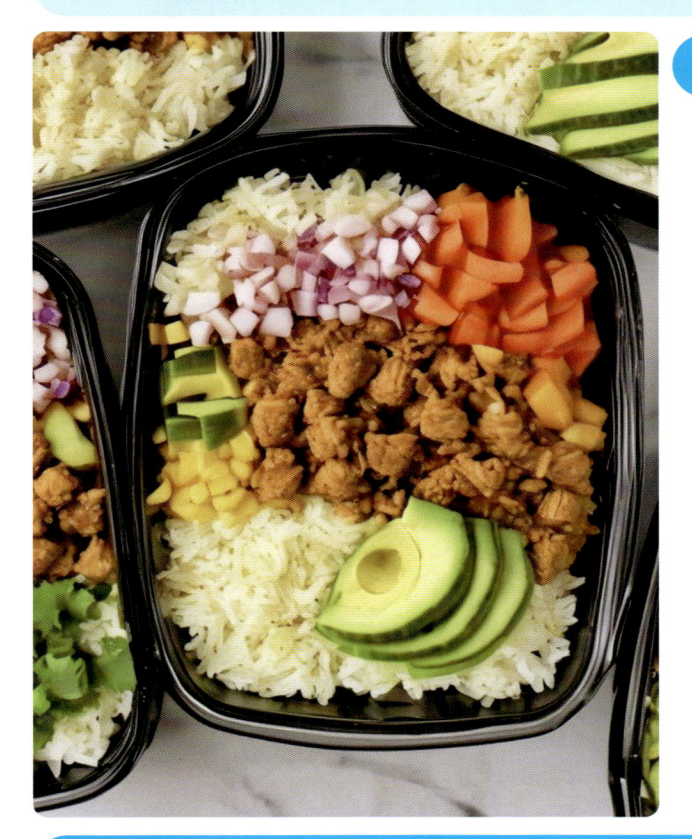

Ingredients   Servings: 8 (1 1/2 CUP)

Bowl:
- 3 lb chicken breast
- 1 cup dry rice
- 1/2 red onion
- 1 (15 oz.) can diced tomatoes
- 1 (10 oz.) can green chilies
- 1 (15 oz.) can black beans
- 2 jalapeno peppers
- 2 avocados
- 1 bunch cilantro
- 2 limes
- 2 (1 oz.) packet taco seasoning

Protein Queso:
- 3 cups low fat cottage cheese
- 2 cups shredded cheddar cheese
- 1 (4 oz.) can green chilies
- 2 tbsp minced garlic

Optional Sides

- Salad (2 cups greens, 1 tbsp extra virgin olive oil, 2 tbsp balsamic - 307c, 4P, 11C, 27F)
- Protein shake (2 cups almond milk, 1 scoop Dummy Supps - 190c, 26P, 9C, 6F)

Instructions

1. Dice red onion and jalapeños. Dice avocados and chop cilantro. Dice chicken into bite sized pieces.
2. Heat a pan over medium heat. Add diced chicken and taco seasoning. Cook for 10-12 minutes until fully cooked.
3. Blend cottage cheese, shredded cheddar cheese, green chilies, and minced garlic until smooth to make protein queso. Heat in a pan over low heat until warm.
4. Add 2 cups water and rice to a pot. Bring to a boil on high heat, then turn to low, cover, and cook for 10 minutes.
5. Heat black beans in a small bowl in the microwave for 1 minute.
6. Divide cooked rice into bowls. Top with chicken, diced red onion, diced tomatoes, green chilies, black beans, diced jalapeños, avocado, and cilantro.
7. Drizzle with warm protein queso and serve with lime wedges.

MULTIPLE MEAL PREPS

CLASSIC CHILI

Calories: 500 **Protein: 43** **Carbs: 30** **Fat: 16**

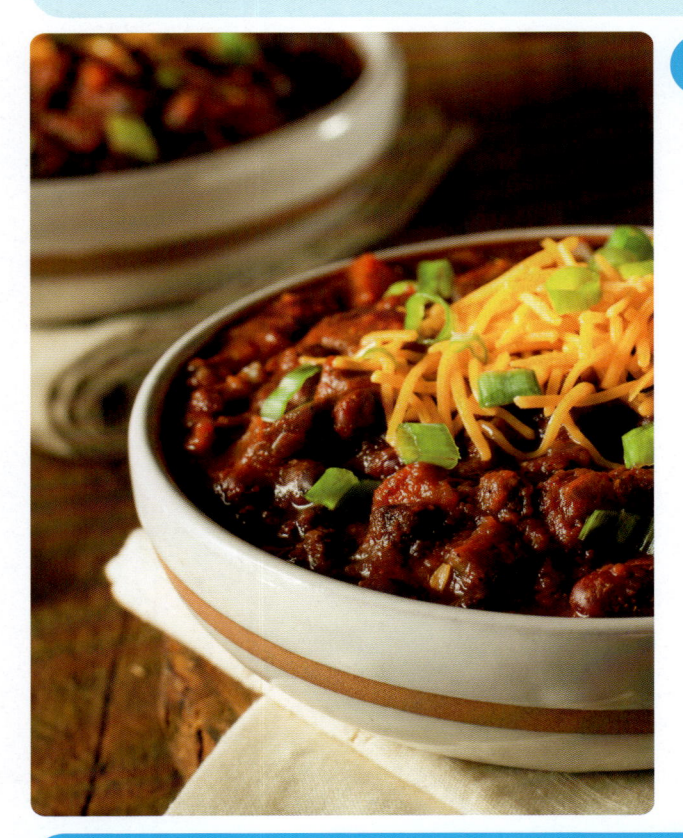

Ingredients   Servings: 8 (1 1/2 CUP)

Chili:
- 3 lb lean ground beef/turkey
- 4 tablespoons minced garlic
- 1 sweet onion
- 2 bell peppers
- 2 jalapeno peppers
- 1 (30 oz.) can diced tomatoes
- 1 (15 oz.) can kidney beans
- 1 (15 oz.) can low-sodium black beans
- 2 tbsp tomato paste
- 1 (1 oz.) packet chili seasoning
- 1 cup tomato sauce
- 1 bunch cilantro

Optional Sides
- Shredded cheese (1/4 cup - 110c, 7P, 9C, 1F)
- Lite sour cream (2 tbsp - 35c, 3P, 2C, 1F)
- White onion (2 tbsp - 0P, 2C, 0F)

Instructions
1. Dice onion, bell peppers, and jalapeños.
2. Heat a large pot over medium heat. Cook ground beef/turkey for 5-7 minutes until browned.
3. Add minced garlic, onion, bell peppers, and jalapeños. Cook for 5 minutes until softened.
4. Stir in diced tomatoes, kidney beans, black beans, tomato paste, chili seasoning, and tomato sauce.
5. Simmer on low heat for 20-25 minutes, stirring occasionally.
6. Chop cilantro and stir in before serving.

MULTIPLE MEAL PREPS

SPICY NACHO CHEESE TAQUITOS

Calories: 350 **Protein: 33** **Carbs: 10** **Fat: 15**

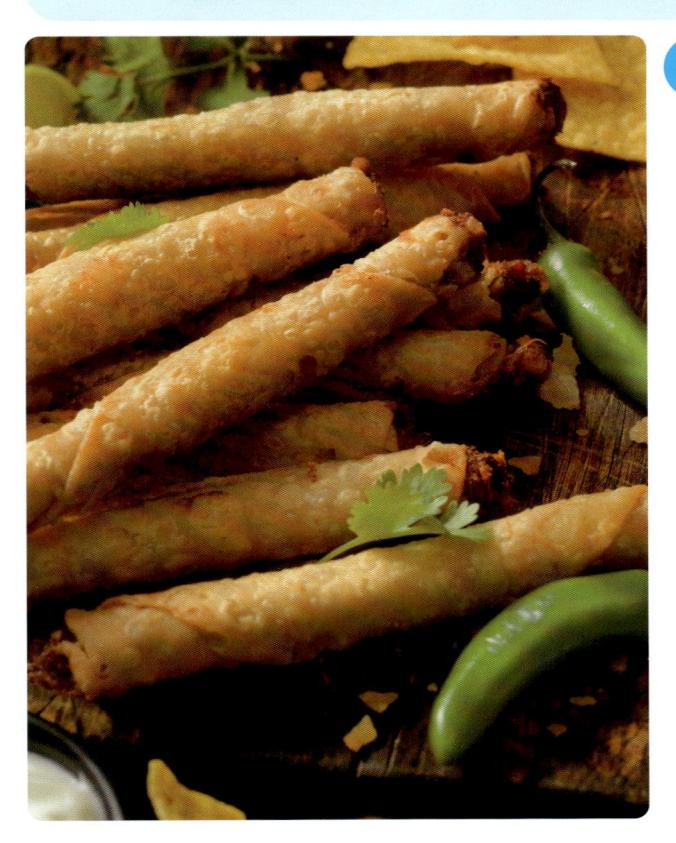

Ingredients **Servings: 10 (1 1/2 CUP)**

Taquitos:
- 2 lb ground beef/turkey
- 10 (12 oz.) Mission low carb tortillas
- 2 tbsp minced garlic
- 1 sweet onion
- 2 jalapeno peppers
- 1 tbsp tomato paste
- 1 (1 oz.) packet taco seasoning

Pico de Gallo:
- 2 cups low fat cottage cheese
- 1 cup shredded cheddar cheese
- 2 tbsp jalapeno brine
- 1/2 (7 oz.) can chipotle peppers in adobo sauce

Optional Sides
- Salad (2 cups greens, 1 tbsp extra virgin olive oil, 2 tbsp balsamic - 307c, 4P, 11C, 27F)
- Protein shake (2 cups almond milk, 1 scoop Dummy Supps - 190c, 26P, 9C, 6F)
- Avocado (1/2 whole - 120c, 2P, 6C, 11F)

Instructions
1. Dice onion and and jalapeños.
2. Heat a pan over medium heat and sauté onion and minced garlic for 3-4 minutes until softened.
3. Add ground beef/turkey to the pan. Cook with vegetables for 8-10 minutes until browned.
4. Stir in tomato paste and taco seasoning. Cook for 2-3 minutes.
5. Add cooked meat mixture on tortillas and roll tightly into taquitos.
6. Air fry at 400°F for 8-10 minutes or bake at 425°F for 12-15 minutes until crispy.
7. Blend cottage cheese, cheddar cheese, jalapeño brine, and chipotle peppers until smooth. Heat in a pan until warm and serve as a dipping sauce.

MULTIPLE MEAL PREPS

SOUTHERN DIRTY RICE

Calories: 490 **Protein: 46** **Carbs: 35** **Fat: 18**

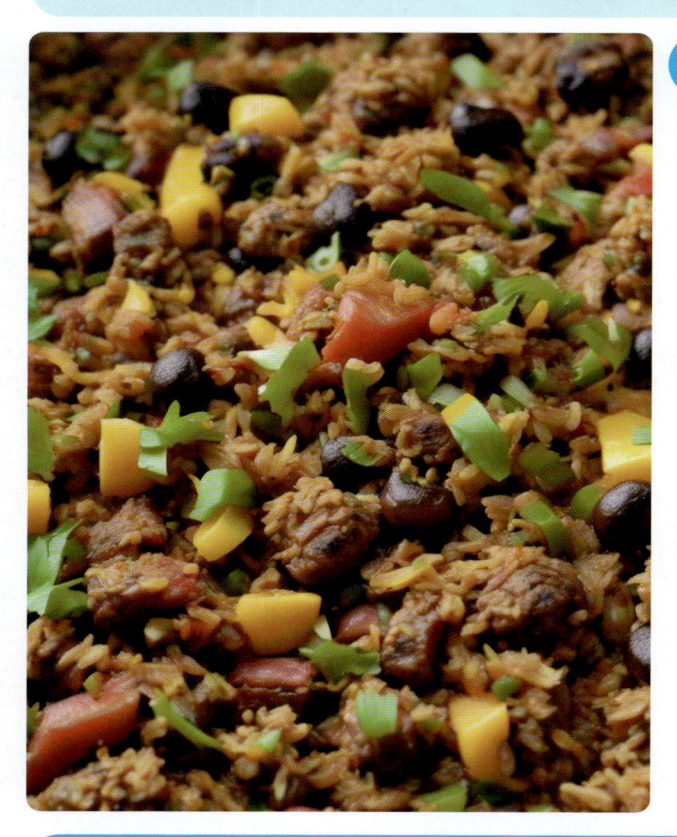

Ingredients — Servings: 12 (1 1/2 CUP)

Rice:
- 3 lb lean ground beef/turkey
- 4 (4 oz.) Andouille chicken sausages
- 1 cup dry rice
- 4 tbsp minced garlic
- 1 yellow onion
- 2 bell peppers
- 2 jalapeno peppers
- 1 (15 oz.) can crushed tomatoes
- 1 (15 oz.) can black beans
- 2 tbsp cajun seasoning
- 1 tbsp garlic powder
- 1 tsp red pepper flakes
- 1 tsp paprika
- 1/2 tsp black pepper
- 1 bunch parsley

Optional Sides

- Salad (2 cups greens, 1 tbsp extra virgin olive oil, 2 tbsp balsamic - 307c, 4P, 11C, 27F)
- Protein shake (2 cups almond milk, 1 scoop Dummy Supps - 190c, 26P, 9C, 6F)

Instructions

1. Dice onion, bell peppers, jalapeños, and Andouille sausages.
2. Heat a pan over medium heat. Add onion, bell peppers, and jalapeños. Cook for 3-5 minutes until softened.
3. Add ground beef/turkey and Andouille sausage to the pan. Stir in minced garlic, Cajun seasoning, and listed ingredients. Cook for 10-12 minutes until browned.
4. Stir in crushed tomatoes and black beans. Simmer for 5 minutes.
5. Add 2 cups water and rice to a pot. Bring to a boil on high heat, then turn to low, cover, and cook for 10 minutes.
6. Mix in cooked rice and stir until evenly combined.
7. Top with chopped parsley.

MULTIPLE MEAL PREPS

LOADED CLASSIC NACHOS

Calories: 400 **Protein: 40** **Carbs: 31** **Fat: 19**

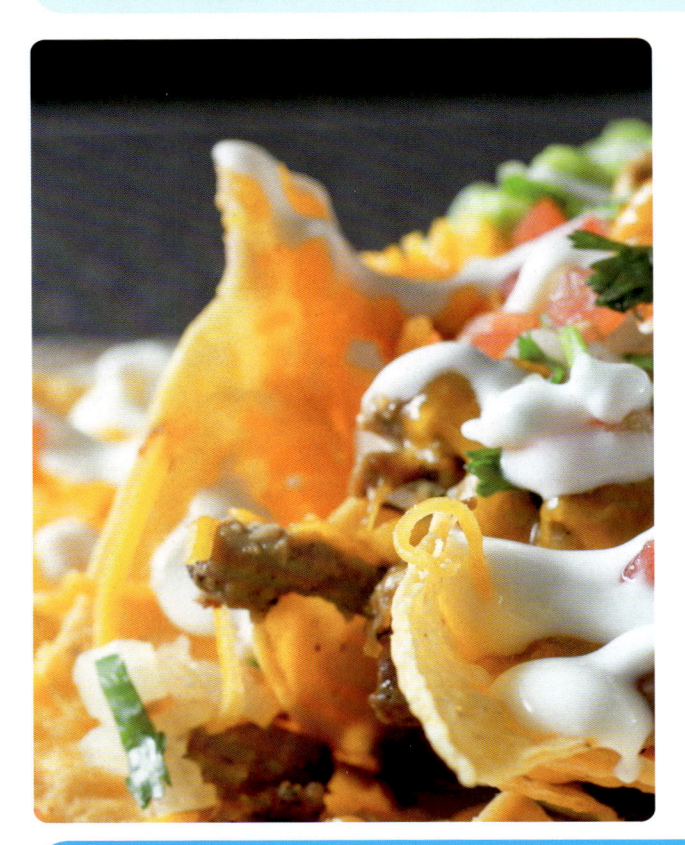

Ingredients — Servings: 4

Nachos:
- 1 (9 oz.) bag Mission low carb tortillas
- 1 lb lean ground turkey/beef
- 1 cup shredded lettuce
- 1/4 cup red onion
- 4 tbsp jalapeño peppers
- 1/4 cup black beans
- 1/2 cup diced tomatoes
- 1/2 (1 oz.) packet taco seasoning

Protein Queso:
- 1 cup low fat cottage cheese
- 1/2 cup shredded cheese
- 1 (10 oz.) container green chilies
- 1 tbsp packet taco seasonings
- 1 lime

Optional Sides

- Salad (2 cups greens, 1 tbsp extra virgin olive oil, 2 tbsp balsamic - 307c, 4P, 11C, 27F)
- Protein shake (2 cups almond milk, 1 scoop Dummy Supps - 190c, 26P, 9C, 6F)
- Avocado (1/2 whole - 120c, 2P, 6C, 11F)

Instructions

1. Cut tortillas into chips, toss with lime juice and salt.
2. Air fry at 350°F for 5 minutes, flip, and cook for 5-7 more minutes until crispy.
3. Dice red onion and jalapeños. Chop lettuce.
4. Heat a pan over medium heat. Add ground turkey/beef and taco seasoning. Cook for 6-8 minutes until browned.
5. Blend cottage cheese, shredded cheese, green chilies, taco seasoning, and lime juice until smooth to make protein queso. Heat in a pan over low heat until warm.
6. Spread chips on a plate. Top with cooked meat, black beans, diced tomatoes, red onion, jalapeños, and shredded lettuce.
7. Drizzle with warm protein queso and serve immediately.

MULTIPLE MEAL PREPS

CHEESY BEEF TAQUITOS

Calories: 320 **Protein: 29** **Carbs: 9** **Fat: 15**

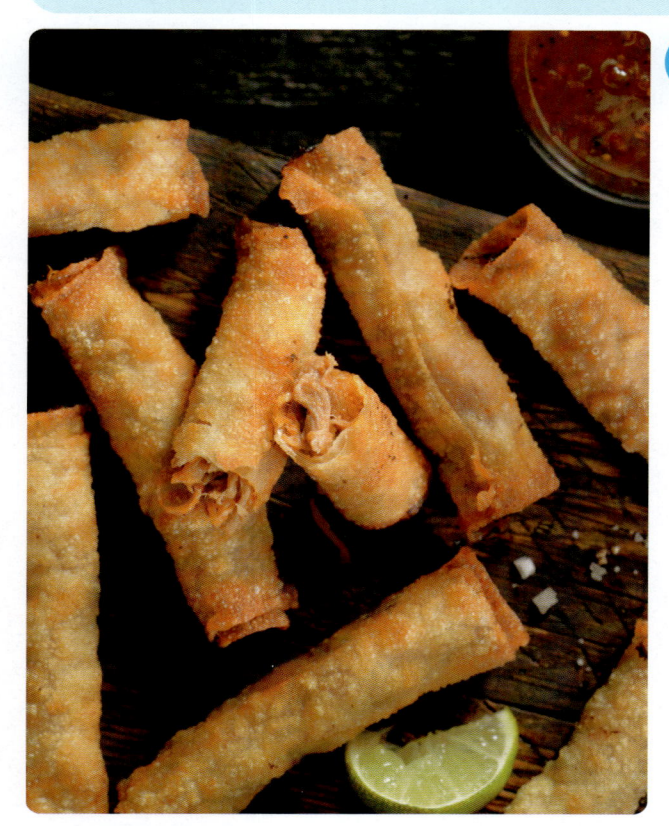

Ingredients Servings: 10 (1 1/2 CUP)

Taquitos:
- 2 lb ground beef/turkey
- 10 (12 oz.) Mission low carb tortillas
- 1 1/2 cups shredded mexican cheese
- 1 (7 oz.) can diced green chilies
- 1 (1 oz.) packet taco seasoning

Pico De Gallo:
- 5 roma tomatoes
- 1 red onion
- 2 jalapeno peppers
- 1 bunch cilantro
- 1 lime
- 1 tsp garlic powder
- 1/2 tsp salt

Optional Sides
- Salad (2 cups greens, 1 tbsp extra virgin olive oil, 2 tbsp balsamic - 307c, 4P, 11C, 27F)
- Protein shake (2 cups almond milk, 1 scoop Dummy Supps - 190c, 26P, 9C, 6F)
- Avocado (1/2 whole - 120c, 2P, 6C, 11F)

Instructions
1. Heat a pan over medium heat. Cook ground beef/turkey with for 5-7 minutes until browned.
2. Stir in taco seasoning and green chilies. Cook for 2-3 minutes. Remove from heat and mix in shredded cheese until melted.
3. Fill tortillas with the meat and cheese mixture. Roll tightly into taquitos.
4. Air fry at 400°F for 8-10 minutes or bake at 425°F for 12-15 minutes until crispy.
5. Dice tomatoes, red onion, and jalapeños. Mix with chopped cilantro, lime juice, garlic powder, and salt to make pico de gallo.
6. Serve taquitos with pico de gallo on the side.

MULTIPLE MEAL PREPS

BUFFALO MAC & CHEESE

Calories: 550 **Protein: 46** **Carbs: 36** **Fat: 27**

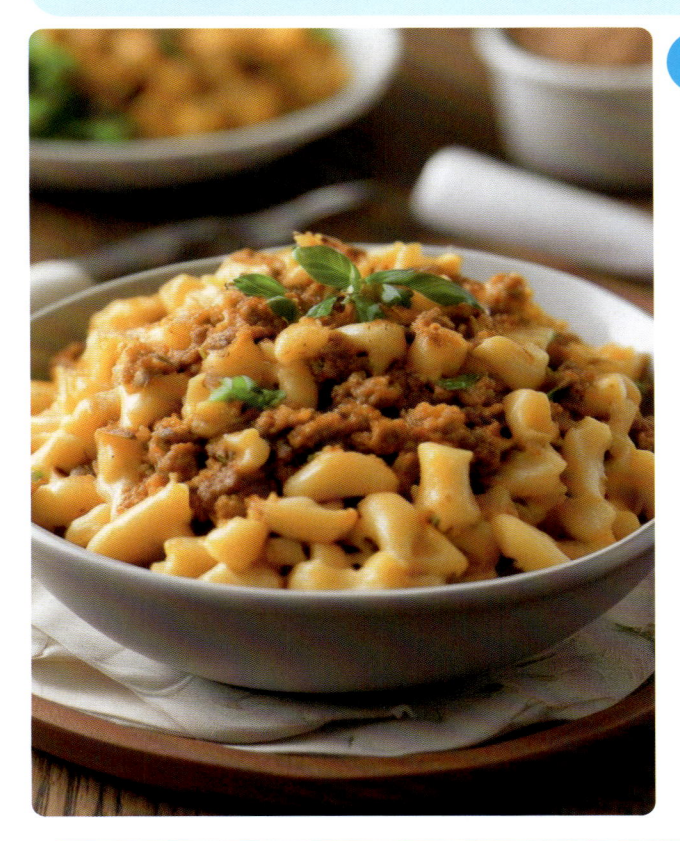

Ingredients — Servings: 10 (1 1/2 CUP)

Buffalo Mac & Cheese:
- 3 lb ground turkey/beef
- 1 (14.5 oz.) box protein/chickpea pasta
- 1 (1 oz.) package ranch seasoning
- 2 jalapeno peppers
- 2 tbsp minced garlic
- 1 bunch chives

Cheese Sauce:
- 3 cups low fat cottage cheese
- 2 cup shredded cheddar cheese
- 1/2 cup whipped cream cheese
- 1/2 cup buffalo wing sauce
- 1/4 cup 1% milk

Optional Sides
- Salad (2 cups greens, 1 tbsp extra virgin olive oil, 2 tbsp balsamic - 307c, 4P, 11C, 27F)
- Protein shake (2 cups almond milk, 1 scoop Dummy Supps - 190c, 26P, 9C, 6F)

Instructions
1. Dice jalapeños.
2. Spray a pan with cooking spray and heat to medium-high. Add jalapeños and sauté for 5 minutes.
3. Add ground turkey/beef, ranch seasoning, and minced garlic. Ccok for 10-12 minutes, until fully cooked.
4. Blend cheese sauce ingredients until smooth.
5. Boil pasta for 9-11 minutes. Drain.
6. Mix pasta into the pan with the meat mixture and stir well.
7. Garnish with chopped chives before serving.

MULTIPLE MEAL PREPS

BAKED ZITI

Calories: 650 **Protein: 48** **Carbs: 45** **Fat: 33**

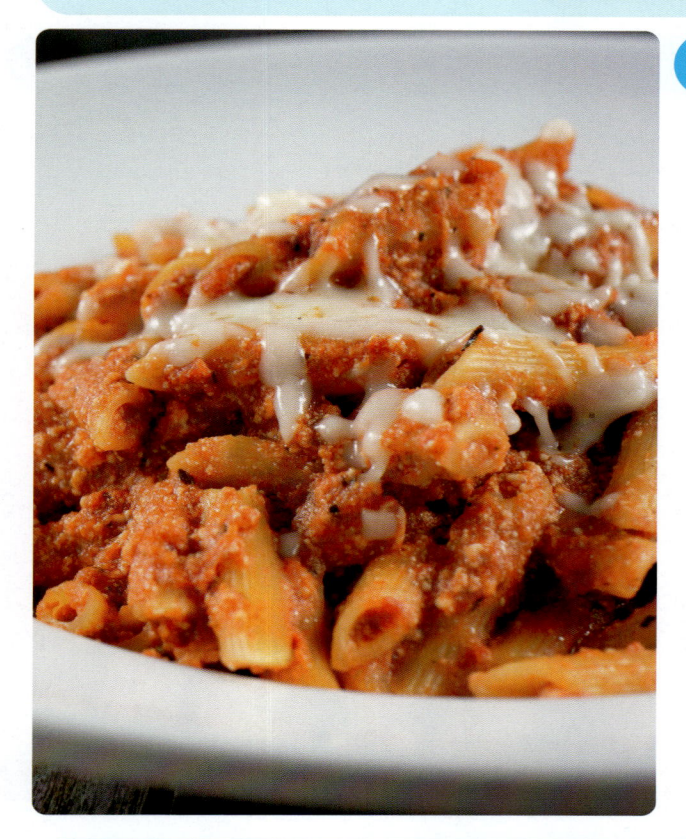

Ingredients Servings: 10 (1 1/2 CUP)

Pasta:
- 3 lb ground turkey/beef
- 1 (14.5 oz.) box protein/chickpea pasta
- 2 tbsp minced garlic
- 1 (24 oz.) bottle marinara sauce
- 1 (15 oz.) container part skim ricotta cheese
- 1 cup low-fat mozzarella cheese
- 1/4 cup parmesan cheese
- 1 bunch parsley
- 1 tbsp Italian seasoning
- 1 tbsp garlic powder
- 1 tbsp onion powder
- 1 tsp black pepper
- 1 tsp crushed red pepper

Optional Sides

- Salad (2 cups greens, 1 tbsp extra virgin olive oil, 2 tbsp balsamic - 307c, 4P, 11C, 27F)
- Protein shake (2 cups almond milk, 1 scoop Dummy Supps - 190c, 26P, 9C, 6F)

Instructions

1. Dice parsley.
2. Spray a pan with cooking spray and heat to medium-high. Add minced garlic and sauté for 2 minutes.
3. Add ground turkey/beef with listed seasonings. Cook for 10-12 minutes, until fully cooked.
4. Add marinara sauce, ricotta cheese, and parmesan cheese to meat. Simmer for 5 minutes.
5. Boil pasta for 9-11 minutes. Drain.
6. Mix pasta into the pan with the meat mixture and stir well.
7. Top with mozzarella cheese and bake at 375°F for 20 minutes.

MULTIPLE MEAL PREPS

PROTEIN GOULASH

Calories: 530 **Protein: 46** **Carbs: 40** **Fat: 17**

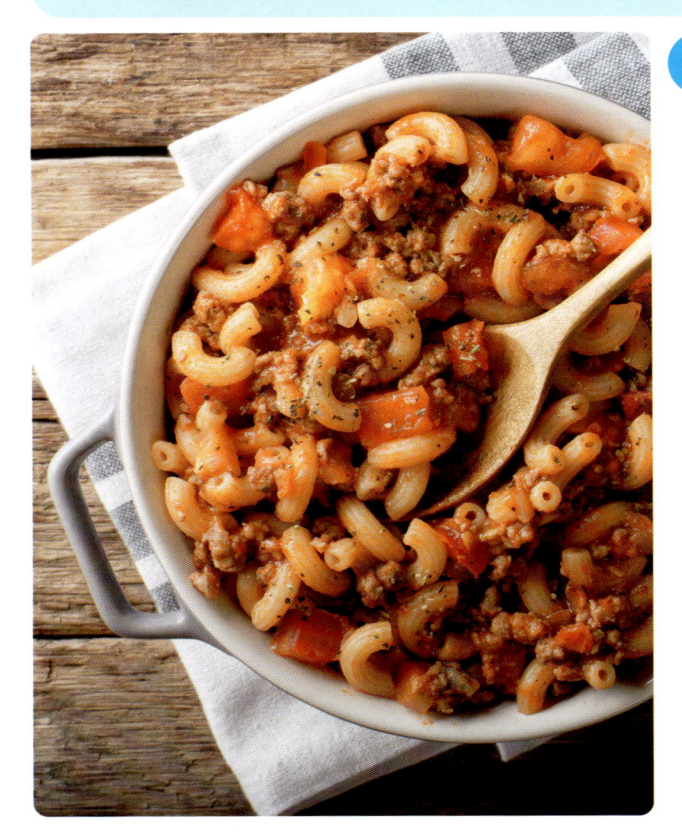

Ingredients — Servings: 8 (1 1/2 CUP)

Pasta:
- 3 lb lean ground beef/turkey
- 1 (14.5 oz.) box protein pasta
- 2 tbsp minced garlic
- 1 sweet onion
- 2 bell peppers
- 1 (30 oz.) can diced tomatoes
- 1 (15 oz.) can tomato sauce
- 2 tbsp tomato paste
- 2 tbsp garlic powder
- 1 tbsp onion powder
- 1 tsp chili powder
- 1 tsp Italian seasoning
- 1/2 tsp black pepper

Optional Sides
- Salad (2 cups greens, 1 tbsp extra virgin olive oil, 2 tbsp balsamic - 307c, 4P, 11C, 27F)
- Protein shake (2 cups almond milk, 1 scoop Dummy Supps - 190c, 26P, 9C, 6F)

Instructions
1. Dice onion and bell peppers.
2. Heat a pan over medium heat. Add onion, bell peppers, minced garlic cooking for 4-5 minutes until softened.
3. Add ground beef/turkey and cook for 10-12 minutes until browned.
4. Add drained diced tomatoes, tomato sauce, tomato paste, and listed seasonings. Simmer for 10-15 minutes.
5. Boil pasta for 9-11 minutes. Drain.
6. Add pasta to meat sauce.

MULTIPLE MEAL PREPS

CREAMY PROTEIN PASTA

Calories: 590 **Protein: 53** **Carbs: 40** **Fat: 23**

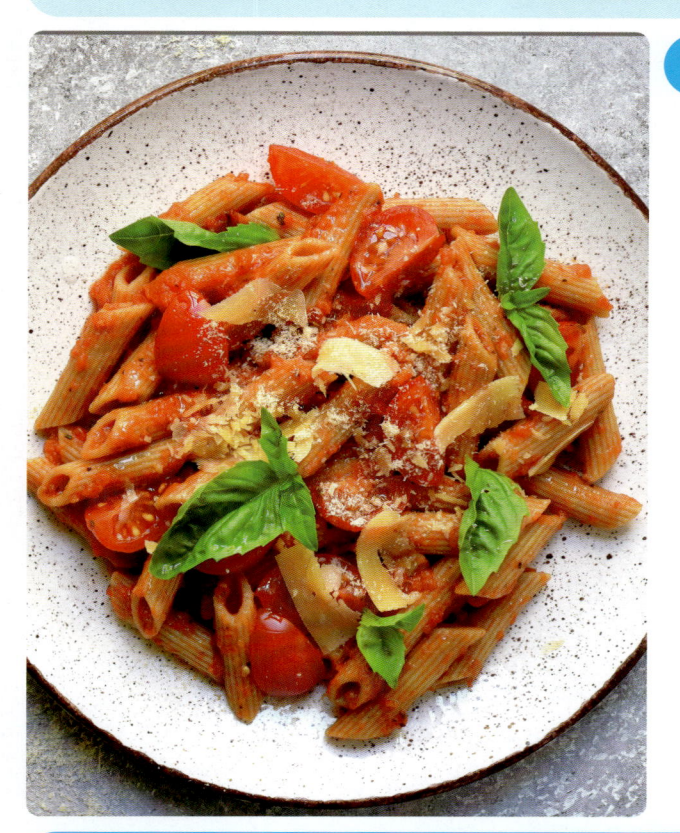

Ingredients — Servings: 8 (1 1/2 CUP)

Pasta:
- 3 lb lean ground beef/turkey
- 1 (14.5 oz.) box protein pasta
- 2 tbsp minced garlic
- 1 (15 oz.) container part-skim ricotta
- 1 (24 oz.) marinara sauce
- 1/2 cup low fat mozzarella cheese
- 2 tbsp garlic powder
- 1 tbsp onion powder
- 1 tbsp Italian seasoning
- 1 tsp black pepper
- 1 bunch Italian parsley

Optional Sides

- Salad (2 cups greens, 1 tbsp extra virgin olive oil, 2 tbsp balsamic - 307c, 4P, 11C, 27F)
- Protein shake (2 cups almond milk, 1 scoop Dummy Supps - 190c, 26P, 9C, 6F)

Instructions

1. Heat a pan over medium heat. Add ground beef/turkey and cook for 5-7 minutes until browned.
2. Stir in minced garlic, garlic powder, onion powder, Italian seasoning, and black pepper. Cook for 1 minute.
3. Add marinara sauce and simmer for 5 minutes.
4. Stir in ricotta cheese and mozzarella cheese until fully combined and creamy.
5. Boil pasta for 9-11 minutes. Drain.
6. Add cooked pasta to the pan and toss until well coated.
7. Top with chopped Italian parsley.

MULTIPLE MEAL PREPS

CHICKEN RIGGIES

Calories: 570 **Protein: 54** **Carbs: 40** **Fat: 20**

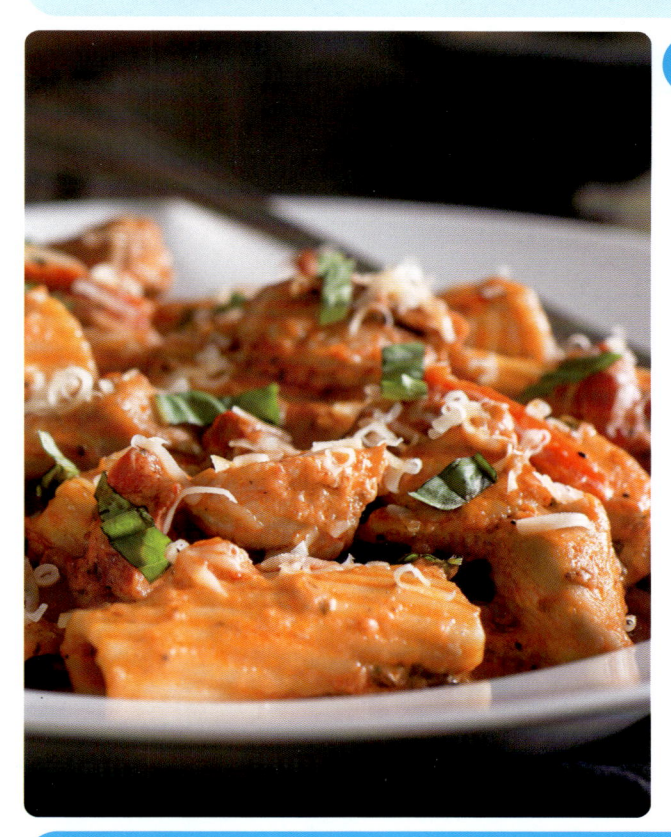

Ingredients   Servings: 10 (1 1/2 CUP)

Pasta:
- 3 lb chicken breast
- 1 (14.5 oz.) box protein pasta
- 1 yellow onion
- 2 bell peppers
- 1 cup hot cherry peppers
- 2 (24 oz.) containers It's a Utica Thing! Riggies
- 1 cup parmesan cheese
- 2 tbsp minced garlic
- 2 tbsp garlic powder
- 1 tbsp onion powder
- 1/2 tsp black pepper
- 2 tsp crushed red pepper flakes

Optional Sides
- Salad (2 cups greens, 1 tbsp extra virgin olive oil, 2 tbsp balsamic - 307c, 4P, 11C, 27F)
- Protein shake (2 cups almond milk, 1 scoop Dummy Supps - 190c, 26P, 9C, 6F)

Instructions
1. Dice onion and bell peppers. Chop hot cherry peppers.
2. Heat a pan over medium heat. Add onion, bell peppers, and minced garlic. Sauté for 4-5 minutes until softened.
3. Add chicken, garlic powder, onion powder, black pepper, and crushed red pepper flakes. Cook for 10-12 minutes until browned.
4. Stir in hot cherry peppers and cook for 2 minutes.
5. Pour in Riggies sauce and let simmer for 5 minutes.
6. Boil pasta for 9-11 minutes. Drain.
7. Add cooked pasta to the pan and toss until well coated.
8. Stir in parmesan cheese and serve warm.

MULTIPLE MEAL PREPS

PENNE ALLA VODKA

Calories: 550 **Protein: 54** **Carbs: 45** **Fat: 25**

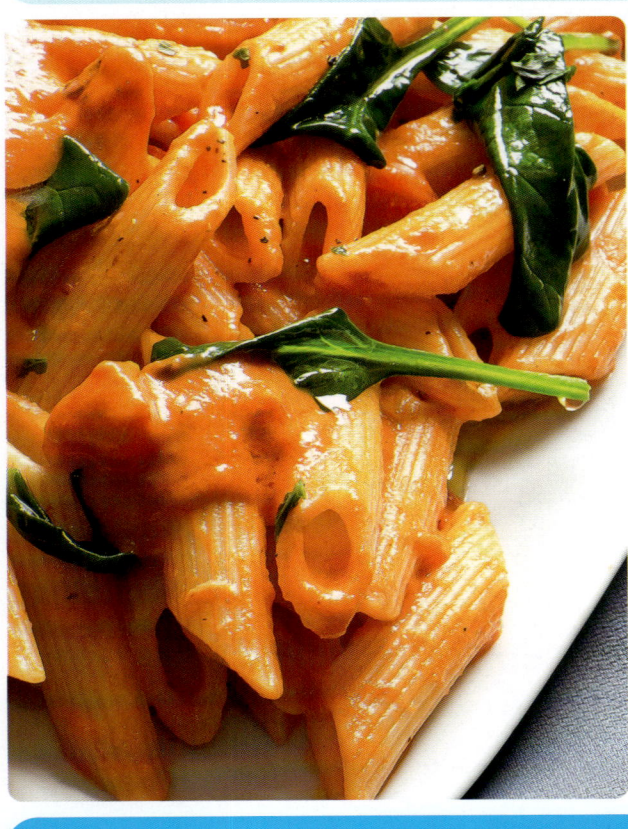

Ingredients **Servings: 8 (1 1/2 CUP)**

Pasta:
- 3 lb chicken breast
- 1 (14.5 oz.) box protein pasta
- 2 tbsp minced garlic
- 1 (10 oz.) container baby spinach
- 1/2 cup low fat mozzarella cheese
- 1/4 cup parmesan cheese
- 1 (24 oz.) container vodka sauce
- 2 tbsp garlic powder
- 1 tbsp onion powder
- 1 tsp Italian seasoning
- 1 tsp black pepper
- 1 bunch Italian parsley

Optional Sides

- Salad (2 cups greens, 1 tbsp extra virgin olive oil, 2 tbsp balsamic - 307c, 4P, 11C, 27F)
- Protein shake (2 cups almond milk, 1 scoop Dummy Supps - 190c, 26P, 9C, 6F)

Instructions

1. Dice chicken into bite-sized pieces.
2. Heat a pan over medium heat with cooking spray. Add chicken, garlic powder, onion powder, Italian seasoning, and black pepper. Cook for 6-8 minutes until fully cooked.
3. Stir in minced garlic and cook for 1 minute.
4. Add vodka sauce and simmer for 5 minutes.
5. Stir in baby spinach and cook until wilted.
6. Mix in mozzarella and parmesan cheese until melted and creamy.
7. Boil pasta for 9-11 minutes. Drain.
8. Add cooked pasta to the pan and toss until well coated.
9. Top with chopped Italian parsley.

MULTIPLE MEAL PREPS

SPICY RIGGATONI

Calories: 630   **Protein: 47**   **Carbs: 40**   **Fat: 31**

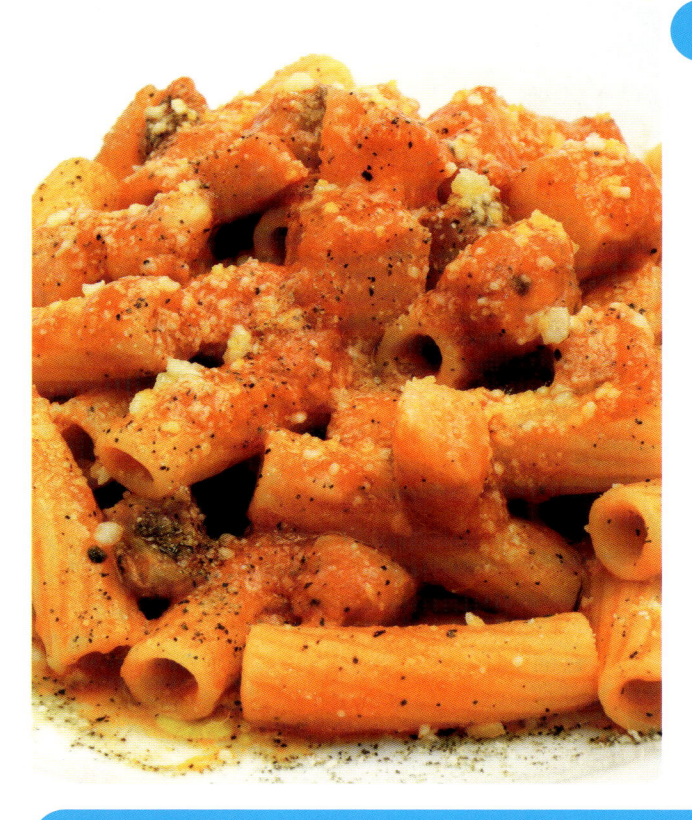

Ingredients   Servings: 10 (1 1/2 CUP)

Pasta:
- 3 lb ground turkey/beef
- 1 (14.5 oz.) box protein/chickpea pasta
- 2 tbsp minced garlic
- 1 (24 oz.) bottle fra diavolo sauce
- 1 (15 oz.) container part skim ricotta cheese
- 1/4 cup parmesan cheese
- 1 bunch parsley
- 1 tbsp Italian seasoning
- 1 tbsp garlic powder
- 1 tbsp onion powder
- 1 tsp black pepper
- 1 tsp crushed red pepper

Optional Sides
- Salad (2 cups greens, 1 tbsp extra virgin olive oil, 2 tbsp balsamic - 307c, 4P, 11C, 27F)
- Protein shake (2 cups almond milk, 1 scoop Dummy Supps - 190c, 26P, 9C, 6F)

Instructions
1. Dice parsley.
2. Spray a pan with cooking spray and heat to medium-high. Add minced garlic and sauté for 2 minutes.
3. Add ground turkey/beef with listed seasonings. Cook for 10-12 minutes, until fully cooked.
4. Add fra diavolo sauce, ricotta cheese, and parmesan cheese to meat. Simmer for 5 minutes.
5. Boil pasta for 9-11 minutes. Drain.
6. Mix pasta into the pan with the meat mixture and stir well.
7. Top with mozzarella cheese and bake at 375°F for 20 minutes.

MULTIPLE MEAL PREPS

PASTA BOLOGNESE

Calories: 560 **Protein: 52** **Carbs: 45** **Fat: 20**

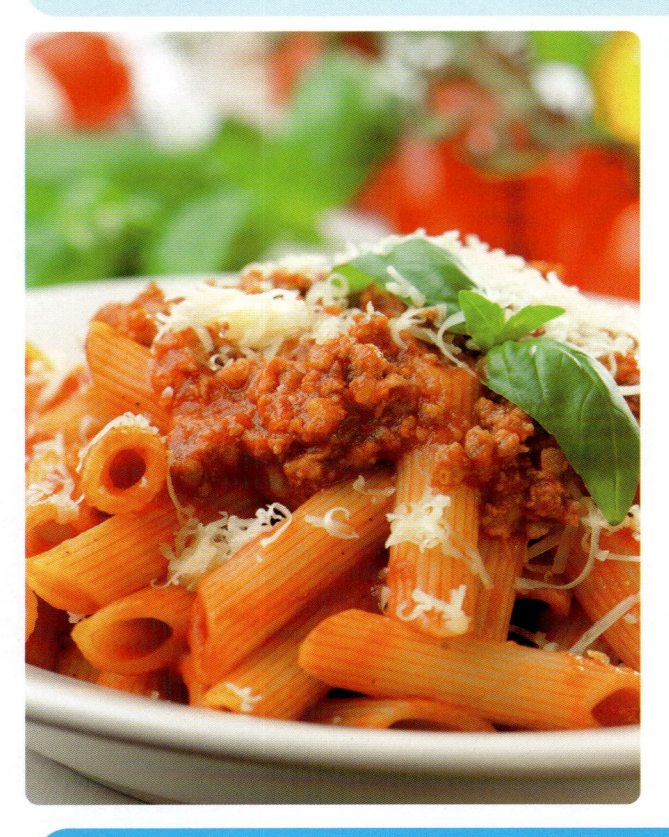

Ingredients — Servings: 8 (1 1/2 CUP)

Pasta:
- 3 lb ground beef/turkey
- 1 (14.5 oz) box protein pasta
- 1 sweet onion
- 1 (28 oz.) can crushed tomatoes
- 1 cup marinara sauce
- 2 tbsp minced garlic
- 2 tbsp tomato paste
- 1 cup parmesan cheese
- 2 tbsp Italian seasoning
- 1/2 tsp black pepper
- 1/4 tsp salt
- 1/2 tsp red pepper flakes

Optional Sides

- Salad (2 cups greens, 1 tbsp extra virgin olive oil, 2 tbsp balsamic - 307c, 4P, 11C, 27F)
- Protein shake (2 cups almond milk, 1 scoop Dummy Supps - 190c, 26P, 9C, 6F)

Instructions

1. Dice sweet onion.
2. Heat a pan over medium heat. Add onion and minced garlic. Cook for 3-4 minutes until softened.
3. Add ground beef/turkey, Italian seasoning, black pepper, salt, and red pepper flakes. Cook for 10-12 minutes until browned.
4. Stir in tomato paste, crushed tomatoes, and marinara sauce. Simmer for 15-20 minutes, stirring occasionally.
5. Cook pasta for 9-11 minutes. Drain and set aside.
6. Stir parmesan cheese into the sauce until melted and combined.
7. Toss pasta with the sauce.

MULTIPLE MEAL PREPS

CHIPOTLE MAC + CHEESE

Calories: 610 **Protein: 54** **Carbs: 42** **Fat: 34**

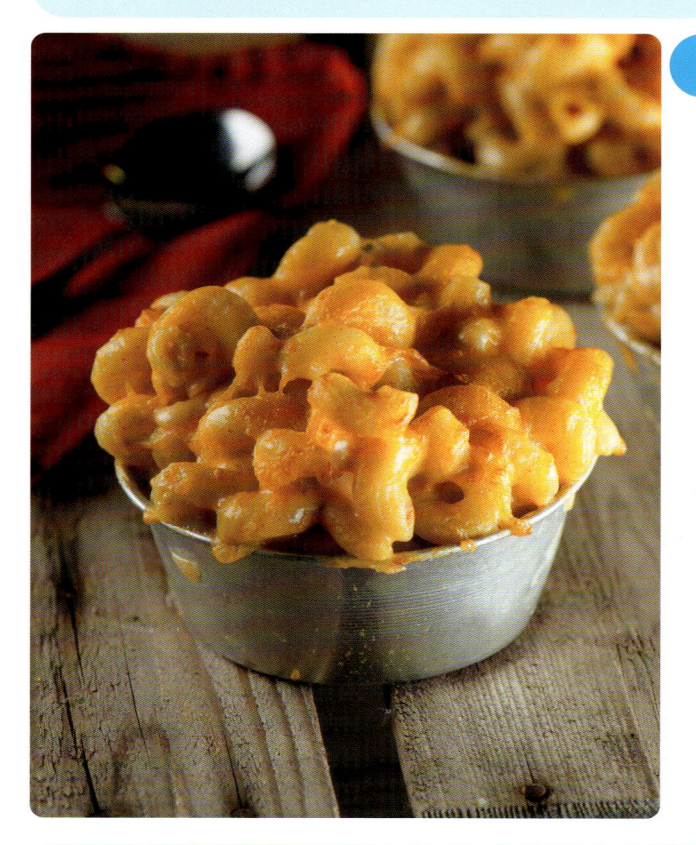

Ingredients Servings: 10 (1 1/2 CUP)

Pasta:
- 3 lb ground turkey/beef
- 1 (14.5 oz.) box protein/chickpea pasta
- 2 bell peppers
- 1 sweet onion
- 2 jalapeno peppers
- 2 (1 oz.) packets taco seasoning

Cheese Sauce:
- 3 cups low fat cottage cheese
- 2 cup shredded cheddar cheese
- 1 (7 oz.) can chipotle peppers in adobo sauce
- 1 lime
- 1/4 cup 1% milk

Optional Sides

- Salad (2 cups greens, 1 tbsp extra virgin olive oil, 2 tbsp balsamic - 307c, 4P, 11C, 27F)
- Protein shake (2 cups almond milk, 1 scoop Dummy Supps - 190c, 26P, 9C, 6F)

Instructions

1. Dice bell peppers, onion, and jalapeños.
2. Spray a pan with cooking spray and heat to medium-high. Add vegetables, salt, and pepper. Sauté for 5 minutes.
3. Add ground turkey and taco seasoning. Cook for 10-12 minutes until done.
4. Boil pasta for 9-11 minutes. Drain.
5. Blend cheese sauce ingredients until smooth.
6. Combine pasta with turkey and vegetables.
7. Stir in cheese sauce and heat for 2-3 minutes.

MULTIPLE MEAL PREPS

SPAGHETTI AND MEATBALLS

Calories: 590 **Protein: 52** **Carbs: 48** **Fat: 23**

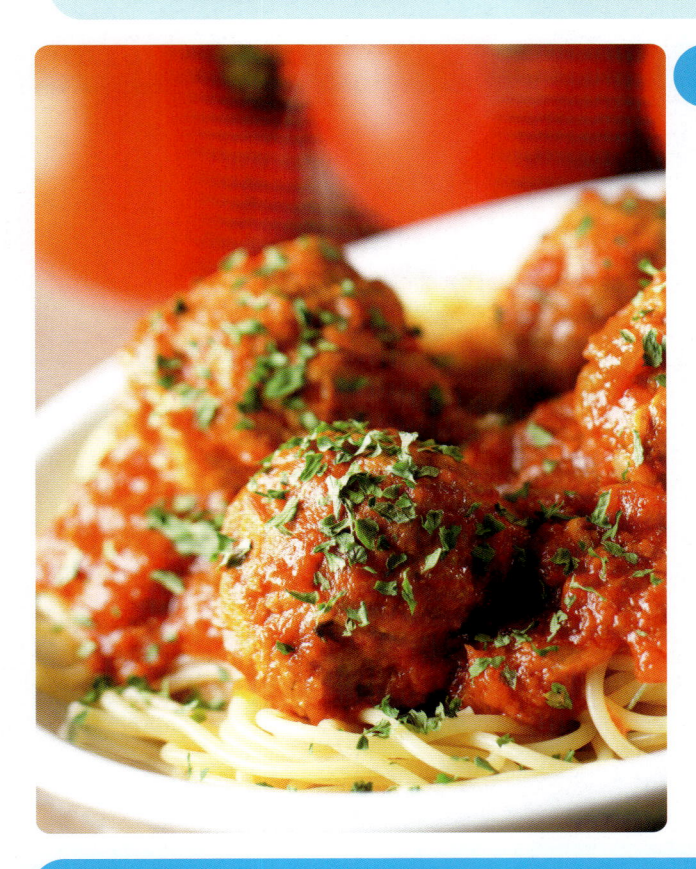

Ingredients   Servings: 8 (1 1/2 CUP)

Pasta:
- 3 lb lean ground bee/ground turkey
- 1 (14.5 oz.) box of protein pasta
- 2 large eggs
- 1/2 cup bread crumbs
- 1/4 cup 1% milk
- 1 cup parmesan cheese
- 2 tbsp Italian seasoning
- 2 tbsp garlic powder
- 1 tbsp onion powder
- 1/2 tsp salt
- 1 tsp black pepper
- 1 (24 oz.) container marinara
- 1 (15 oz.) can crushed tomatoes
- 1 bunch parsley

Optional Sides

- Salad (2 cups greens, 1 tbsp extra virgin olive oil, 2 tbsp balsamic - 307c, 4P, 11C, 27F)
- Protein shake (2 cups almond milk, 1 scoop Dummy Supps - 190c, 26P, 9C, 6F)

Instructions

1. Preheat oven to 400°F.
2. In a bowl, mix ground beef, eggs, bread crumbs, milk, 1/2 cup parmesan cheese, Italian seasoning, garlic powder, onion powder, salt, and black pepper.
3. Roll into 8 meatballs and place on a lined baking sheet.
4. Bake for 15-20 minutes until browned and cooked through.
5. Boil pasta for 9-11 minutes. Drain.
6. Heat marinara sauce in a pan over medium heat. Add meatballs and simmer for 5 minutes.
7. Toss pasta with sauce and meatballs. Top with 1/2 cup parmesan cheese and chopped parsley.

MULTIPLE MEAL PREPS

POPCORN CHICKEN MAC & CHEESE

Calories: 600 **Protein: 63** **Carbs: 42** **Fat: 18**

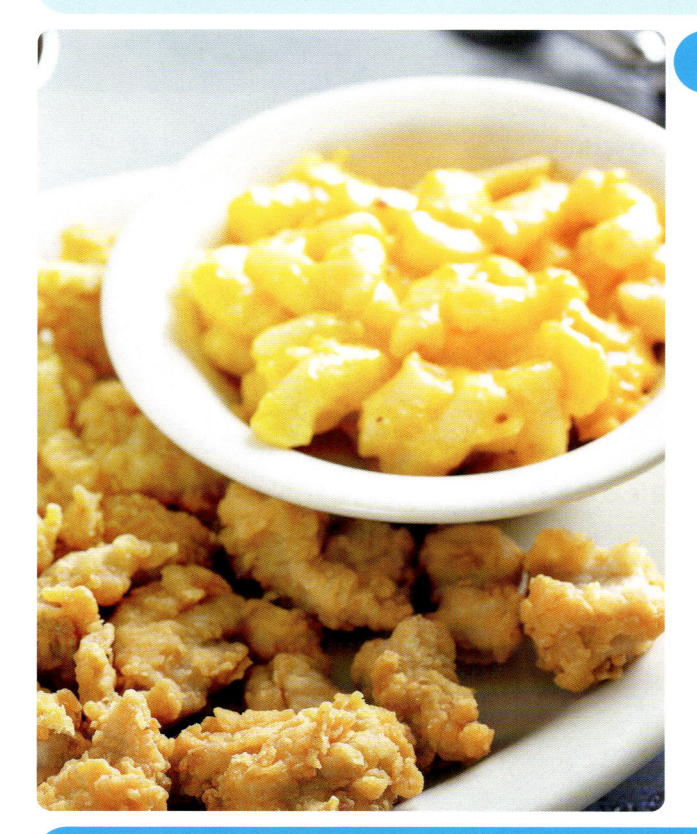

Ingredients — Servings: 10 (1 1/2 CUP)

Pasta:
- 3 lbs chicken breast
- 3/4 cup egg whites
- 2 tbsp cornstarch
- 1/4 cup all purpose flour
- 1 1/2 cups panko bread crumbs
- 1 (14.5 oz.) container protein pasta
- 2 tbsp garlic powder
- 1 tbsp onion powder
- 1 tsp paprika
- 1 tsp Italian seasoning
- ½ tsp salt
- 1 tsp pepper

Cheese Sauce:
- 3 cups low fat cottage cheese
- ½ cup whipped cream cheese
- 2 cups shredded cheddar cheese
- ¼ cup 1% milk

Optional Sides
- Salad (2 cups greens, 1 tbsp extra virgin olive oil, 2 tbsp balsamic - 307c, 4P, 11C, 27F)
- Protein shake (2 cups almond milk, 1 scoop Dummy Supps - 190c, 26P, 9C, 6F)

Instructions
1. Dice chicken into bite-sized pieces.
2. In one bowl, whisk egg whites and cornstarch. In another, mix flour, panko, garlic powder, onion powder, paprika, Italian seasoning, salt, and pepper.
3. Dip chicken into the egg mixture, then coat in seasoned panko.
4. Air Fryer: Cook at 400°F for 10-12 minutes, flipping halfway.
5. Oven: Bake at 400°F for 20-25 minutes until crispy.
6. Cook pasta for 9-11 minutes. Drain and set aside.
7. Blend cottage cheese, whipped cream cheese, cheddar cheese, and milk until smooth. Heat in a pan over low heat until warm.
8. Mix pasta with cheese sauce until fully coated.
9. Top with crispy popcorn chicken and serve.

MULTIPLE MEAL PREPS

BEEF BURRITO BOWLS

Calories: 590 **Protein: 43** **Carbs: 38** **Fat: 29**

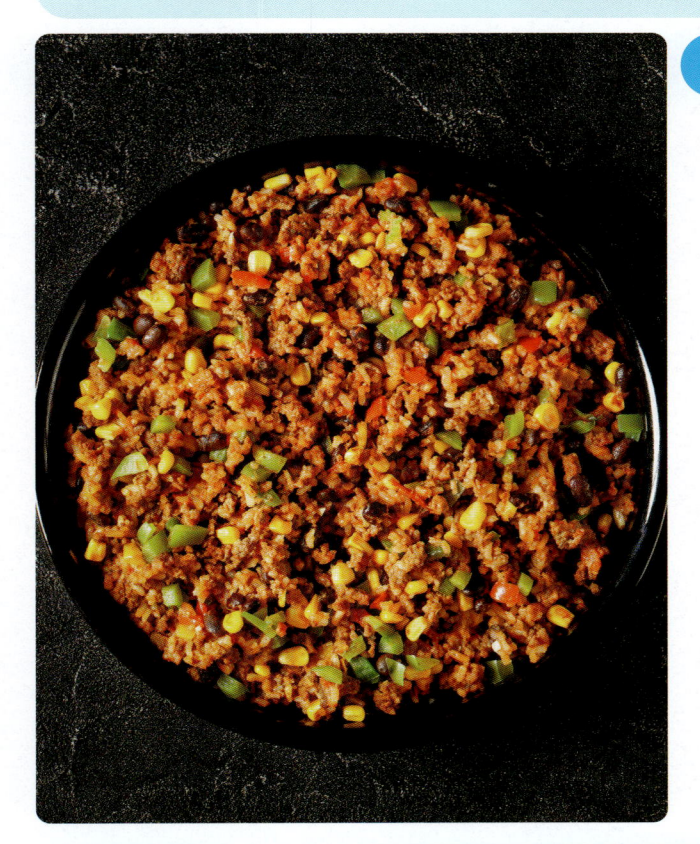

Ingredients — Servings: 6 (1 1/2 CUP)

Bowls:
- 3 lb ground turkey/beef
- 1 cup dry rice
- 1 red onion
- 2 bell peppers
- 2 jalapeno peppers
- 1 bunch cilantro
- 2 (1 oz.) packets taco seasoning

Pico De Gallo:
- 5 roma tomatoes
- 1 red onion
- 2 jalapeno peppers
- 1 bunch cilantro
- 1 lime
- 1 tsp garlic powder
- 1/2 tsp salt

Optional Sides

- Salad (2 cups greens, 1 tbsp extra virgin olive oil, 2 tbsp balsamic - 307c, 4P, 11C, 27F)
- Protein shake (2 cups almond milk, 1 scoop Dummy Supps - 190c, 26P, 9C, 6F)
- Avocado (1/2 whole - 120c, 2P, 6C, 11F)
- Shredded cheese (1/4 cup - 80c, 8P, 2C, 6F)

Instructions

1. Dice bell peppers, onion, and jalapeños.
2. Spray a pan with cooking spray and heat to medium-high. Add diced vegetables, salt, and pepper. Sauté for 5 minutes.
3. Add ground beef/turkey and taco seasoning. Cook for 10-12 minutes until done.
4. Add 2 cups water and rice in pot, bring to boil on high heat, turn to low, cover, and cook for 10 minutes.
5. Dice roma tomatoes, red onion, jalapeños, and cilantro. Mix with lime juice and seasonings.
6. Serve rice topped with cooked meat, sautéed veggies, fresh pico, and chopped cilantro.

MULTIPLE MEAL PREPS

CHICKEN BURRITO BOWLS

Calories: 550 **Protein: 55** **Carbs: 38** **Fat: 24**

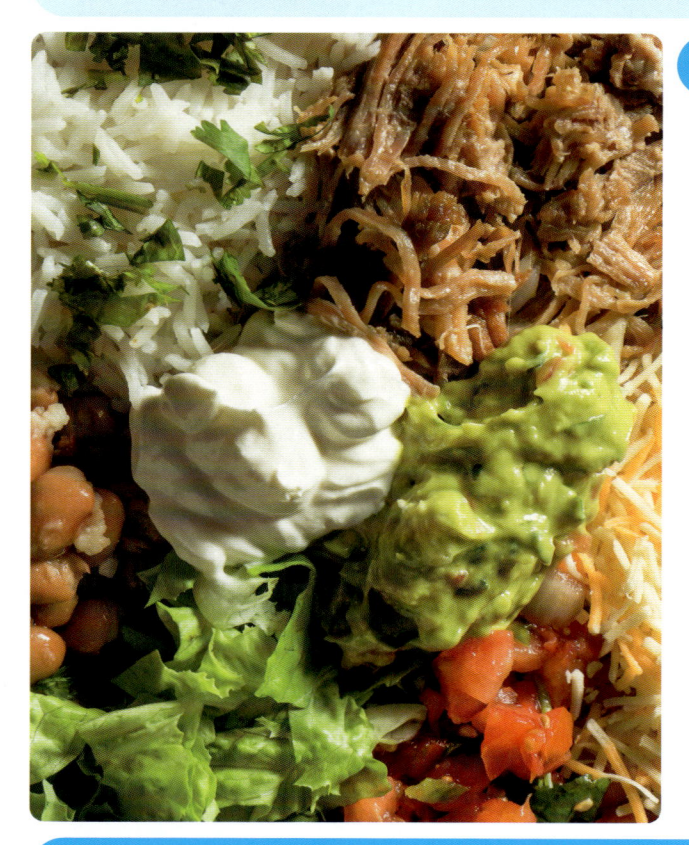

Ingredients   Servings: 6 (1 1/2 CUP)

Bowls:
- 3 lb chicken breast
- 1 cup dry rice
- 1 red onion
- 2 bell peppers
- 2 jalapeno peppers
- 1 bunch cilantro
- 2 (1 oz.) packets taco seasoning

Pico De Gallo:
- 5 roma tomatoes
- 1 red onion
- 2 jalapeno peppers
- 1 bunch cilantro
- 1 lime
- 1 tsp garlic powder
- 1/2 tsp salt

Optional Sides
- Salad (2 cups greens, 1 tbsp extra virgin olive oil, 2 tbsp balsamic - 307c, 4P, 11C, 27F)
- Protein shake (2 cups almond milk, 1 scoop Dummy Supps - 190c, 26P, 9C, 6F)
- Avocado (1/2 whole - 120c, 2P, 6C, 11F)
- Shredded cheese (1/4 cup - 80c, 8P, 2C, 6F)

Instructions
1. Dice bell peppers, onion, and jalapeños. Dice chicken into bite sized pieces.
2. Spray a pan with cooking spray and heat to medium-high. Add diced vegetables, salt, and pepper. Sauté for 5 minutes.
3. Add diced chicken and taco seasoning. Cook for 10-12 minutes until done.
4. Add 2 cups water and rice in pot, bring to boil on high heat, turn to low, cover, and cook for 10 minutes.
5. Dice roma tomatoes, red onion, jalapeños, and cilantro. Mix with lime juice and seasonings.
6. Serve rice topped with cooked chicken, sautéed veggies, fresh pico, and chopped cilantro.

MULTIPLE MEAL PREPS

CHEESY LASAGNA BAKE

Calories: 600 **Protein: 53** **Carbs: 42** **Fat: 10**

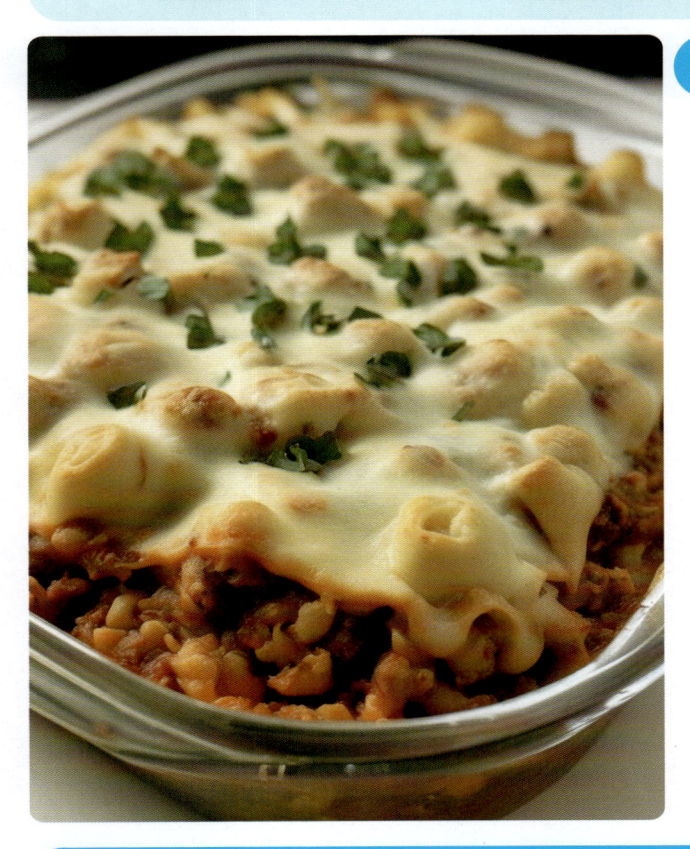

Ingredients Servings: 6 (1 SLICE)

Pasta:
- 2 lbs ground beef
- 1 (9 oz.) box no bake lasagna noodles
- 2 tbsp minced garlic
- 1 cup tomato sauce
- 1 1/2 cup marinara sauce
- 1 (15 oz.) container low fat ricotta cheese
- 1 cup low-fat mozzarella cheese
- 1/2 cup parmesan cheese
- 1 tbsp Italian seasoning
- 1 tsp crushed red pepper flakes
- 1 tbsp garlic powder
- 1 tsp onion powder
- 1 tsp black pepper

Optional Sides

- Salad (2 cups greens, 1 tbsp extra virgin olive oil, 2 tbsp balsamic - 307c, 4P, 11C, 27F)
- Protein shake (2 cups almond milk, 1 scoop Dummy Supps - 190c, 26P, 9C, 6F)

Instructions

1. Preheat oven to 375°F.
2. Cook ground beef in a pan over medium heat with minced garlic and listed seasonings for 5-7 minutes until browned.
3. Stir in tomato sauce and marinara sauce. Simmer for 2-3 minutes.
4. In 6 individual glass containers, spread a thin layer of meat sauce on the bottom.
5. Break lasagna noodles in half to fit the containers. Layer 2.5 noodles per layer, followed by ricotta cheese, meat sauce, mozzarella, and parmesan. Repeat layers until ingredients are used, ending with cheese on top.
6. Cover with tin foil and bake for 20 minutes. Remove foil and bake uncovered for an additional 5 minutes.
7. Let cool for 5 minutes before serving.

MULTIPLE MEAL PREPS

CHICKEN STIR FRY BOWLS

Calories: 500   **Protein: 56**   **Carbs: 33**   **Fat: 13**

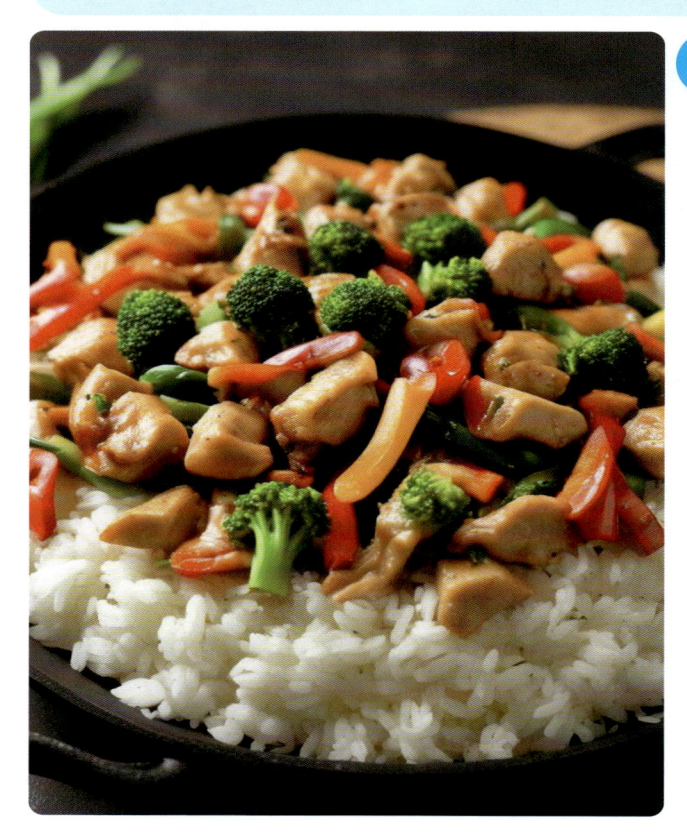

Ingredients   Servings: 8 (1 1/2 CUP)

Stir Fry:
- 3 lb chicken breast
- 1 cup dry rice
- 2 eggs
- 2 (10 oz.) bags frozen stir fry vegetables
- 2 tbsp minced garlic
- 1 tbsp minced ginger
- 1 (12 oz.) container G Hughes sweet chili
- 2 tbsp low sodium soy sauce
- 1 tbsp sriracha
- 1 tbsp sesame oil
- 1 tbsp onion powder
- 1 tsp black pepper
- 1/2 tsp red pepper flakes

Optional Sides

- Salad (2 cups greens, 1 tbsp extra virgin olive oil, 2 tbsp balsamic - 307c, 4P, 11C, 27F)
- Protein shake (2 cups almond milk, 1 scoop Dummy Supps - 190c, 26P, 9C, 6F)

Instructions

1. Dice chicken into bite-sized pieces.
2. Heat sesame oil in a large pan over medium-high heat. Add chicken and cook for 5-7 minutes until browned.
3. Add garlic, ginger, and listed ingredients. Stir and cook for 1-2 minutes.
4. Push chicken to one side of the pan. Crack eggs into the empty side and scramble until cooked. Mix with chicken.
5. Add frozen stir-fry vegetables and cook for 5-7 minutes until tender.
6. Add 2 cups water and rice in pot, bring to boil on high heat, turn to low, cover, and cook for 10 minutes.
7. Stir in sweet chili sauce, soy sauce, and sriracha. Cook for 2-3 minutes until well combined.
8. Serve the stir-fry over rice.

MULTIPLE MEAL PREPS

CHICKEN FAJITA BOWLS

Calories: 550 **Protein: 55** **Carbs: 38** **Fat: 24**

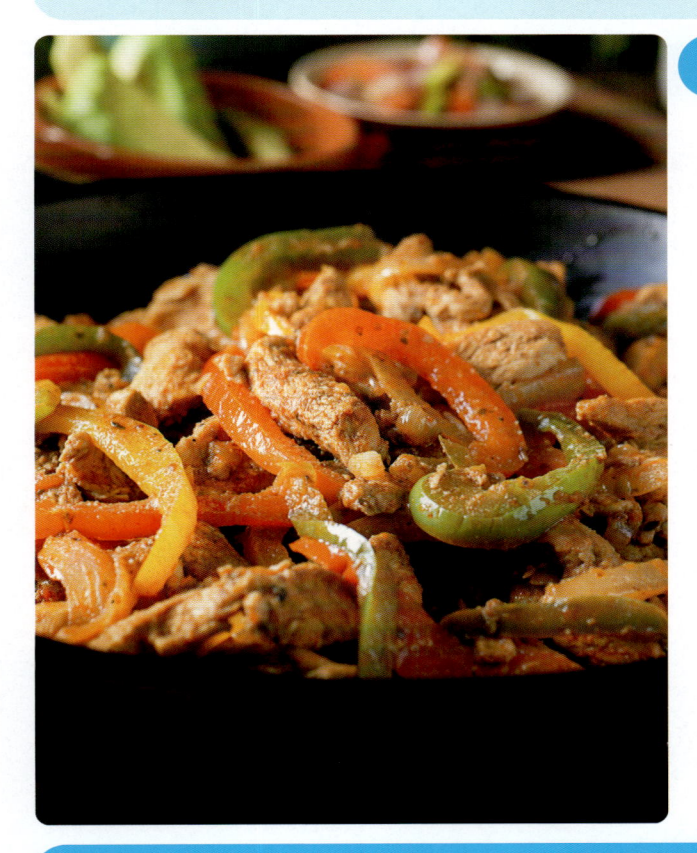

Ingredients Servings: 6 (1 1/2 CUP)

Bowls:
- 3 lb chicken breast
- 1 cup dry rice
- 1 red onion
- 2 bell peppers
- 1 bunch cilantro
- 1 lime
- 1 cup shredded cheese
- 1 (1 oz.) packet taco seasoning
- 1/2 teaspoon black pepper
- 1/4 teaspoon salt

Optional Sides

- Salad (2 cups greens, 1 tbsp extra virgin olive oil, 2 tbsp balsamic - 307c, 4P, 11C, 27F)
- Protein shake (2 cups almond milk, 1 scoop Dummy Supps - 190c, 26P, 9C, 6F)
- Avocado (1/2 whole - 120c, 2P, 6C, 11F)
- Mission low carb tortilla (12 oz. - 70c, 5P, 4C, 3F)

Instructions

1. Slice bell peppers and red onion into thin strips. Dice chicken into bite-sized pieces.
2. Heat a large pan over medium-high heat and spray with cooking spray. Add bell peppers, onions, salt and pepper to the pan. Sauté for 4-5 minutes until vegetables are tender.
3. Add chicken and taco seasoning to the pan. Cook for 8-10 minutes until chicken is browned and cooked through.
4. Add 2 cups water and rice in pot, bring to boil on high heat, turn to low, cover, and cook for 10 minutes.
5. Serve chicken and vegetables over rice.
6. Top with shredded cheese, chopped cilantro, and a squeeze of lime.

MULTIPLE MEAL PREPS

CHICKEN TACOS & CILANTRO LIME CREMA

Calories: 350 **Protein: 46** **Carbs: 10** **Fat: 11**

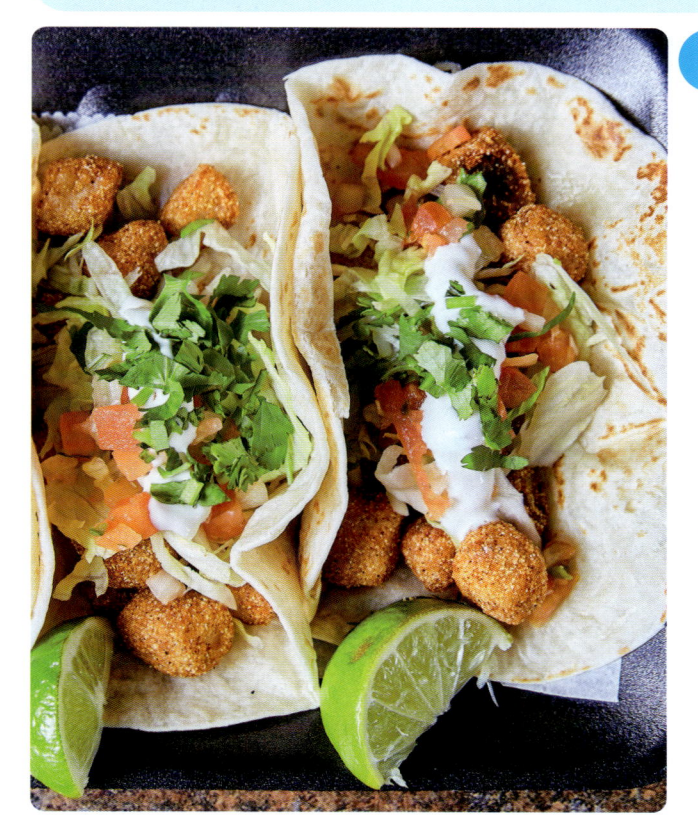

Ingredients   Servings: 6 (1 BURRITO)

Tacos:
- 2 lb chicken breast
- 1 (10 oz.) can of green chilis
- 8 (12 oz.) mission low carb tortillas
- 1 white onion
- 1 bunch cilantro
- 1 lime
- 1 cup shredded cheese
- 1 (1 oz.) packet taco seasoning

Crema:
- 1/4 cup nonfat plain greek yogurt
- 1/4 cup lite sour cream
- 1/2 bunch cilantro
- 1 tbsp minced garlic
- 1 lime
- 1/4 tsp salt

Optional Sides

- Salad (2 cups greens, 1 tbsp extra virgin olive oil, 2 tbsp balsamic - 307c, 4P, 11C, 27F)
- Protein shake (2 cups almond milk, 1 scoop Dummy Supps - 190c, 26P, 9C, 6F)
- Avocado (1/2 whole - 120c, 2P, 6C, 11F)
- Salsa (2 tbsp - 10c, 0P, 2C, 0F)

Instructions

1. Dice white onion and chop cilantro. Dice chicken into bite sized pieces.
2. Heat a pan over medium heat with cooking spray. Cook chicken for 8-10 minutes until fully cooked.
3. Add green chilies and taco seasoning to pan with chicken on low heat. Stir and cook for 2-3 minutes.
4. Blend Greek yogurt, sour cream, cilantro, minced garlic, lime juice, and salt until smooth to make the cilantro lime crema.
5. Warm tortillas in a dry pan or microwave.
6. Fill tortillas with chicken, shredded cheese, white onion, and cilantro.
7. Drizzle with cilantro lime crema and serve with a squeeze of lime.

MULTIPLE MEAL PREPS

CHICKEN PARM BOWLS

Calories: 490 **Protein: 53** **Carbs: 50** **Fat: 10**

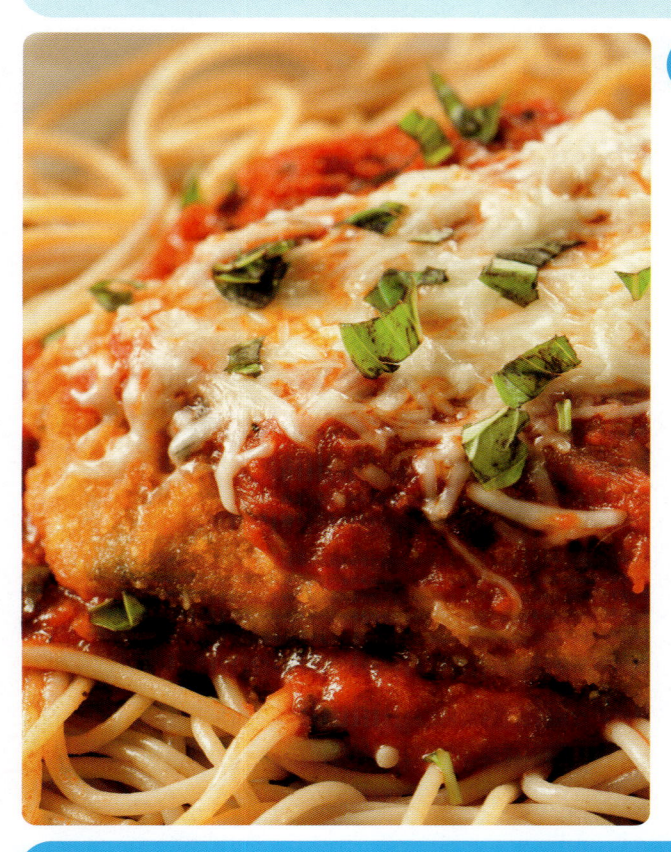

Ingredients   Servings: 6 (1 1/2 CUP)

Bowls:
- 2 lb chicken breast
- 1/2 (14.5 oz.) box protein pasta
- 1/2 cup egg whites
- 1 cup panko bread crumbs
- 1 cup low-fat mozzarella cheese
- 1/2 cup parmesan cheese
- 2 cups marinara sauce
- 2 tbsp garlic powder
- 1 tbsp onion powder
- 1 tbsp Italian seasoning
- 1/2 tsp black pepper
- 1/2 cup red pepper flakes

Optional Sides

- Salad (2 cups greens, 1 tbsp extra virgin olive oil, 2 tbsp balsamic - 307c, 4P, 11C, 27F)
- Protein shake (2 cups almond milk, 1 scoop Dummy Supps - 190c, 26P, 9C, 6F)

Instructions

1. Preheat oven to 400°F or air fryer to 375°F.
2. Dice chicken into bite sized pieces.
3. In one bowl, whisk egg whites. In another, mix panko with garlic powder, onion powder, Italian seasoning, black pepper, and red pepper flakes.
4. Dip chicken into egg whites, then coat with seasoned panko.
5. Air Fryer: Cook for 10-12 minutes, flipping halfway.
6. Oven: Bake on a lined sheet for 12-15 minutes until golden brown.
7. Boil pasta for 9-11 minutes. Drain.
8. Warm marinara sauce in a pan.
9. Divide pasta, chicken, and marinara into meal prep containers.
10. Top each with mozzarella and parmesan cheese and bake on low for 5 minutes until cheese is melted.

MULTIPLE MEAL PREPS

CHICKEN ALFREDO BOWLS

Calories: 480 **Protein: 54** **Carbs: 48** **Fat: 10**

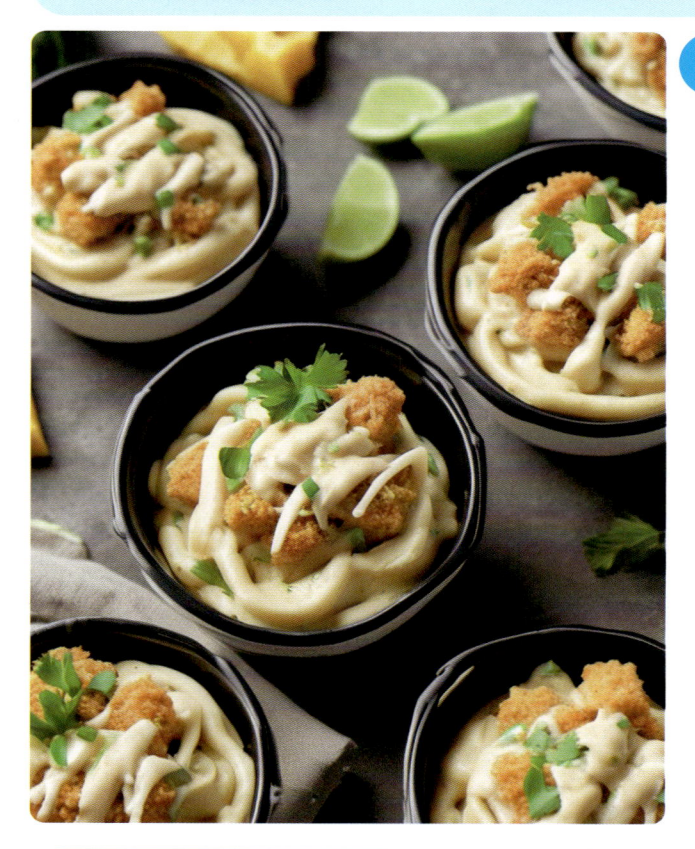

Ingredients   Servings: 8 (1 1/2 CUP)

Bowls:
- 2 lb chicken breast
- 1/2 (14.5 oz.) box protein pasta
- 1/2 cup egg whites
- 1 cup panko bread crumbs
- 2 tbsp garlic powder
- 1 tbsp onion powder
- 1 tbsp Italian seasoning
- 1/2 tsp black pepper

Alfredo sauce:
- 2 cups low-fat cottage cheese
- 2 tbsp minced garlic
- 1/2 cup low-fat mozzarella cheese
- 1/4 cup parmesan cheese
- 1/4 cup 1% milk
- 1 tablespoon Italian seasoning
- 1 tablespoon black pepper

Optional Sides

- Salad (2 cups greens, 1 tbsp extra virgin olive oil, 2 tbsp balsamic - 307c, 4P, 11C, 27F)
- Protein shake (2 cups almond milk, 1 scoop Dummy Supps - 190c, 26P, 9C, 6F)

Instructions

1. Preheat oven to 400°F or air fryer to 375°F.
2. Dice chicken into bite sized pieces.
3. In one bowl, whisk egg whites. In another, mix panko with garlic powder, onion powder, Italian seasoning, black pepper, and red pepper flakes.
4. Dip chicken into egg whites, then coat with seasoned panko.
5. Air Fryer: Cook for 10-12 minutes, flipping halfway.
6. Oven: Bake on a lined sheet for 12-15 minutes until golden brown.
7. Boil pasta for 9-11 minutes. Drain.
8. Warm marinara sauce in a pan.
9. Divide pasta, chicken, and marinara into meal prep containers.
10. Top each with mozzarella and parmesan cheese.

MULTIPLE MEAL PREPS

STEAK STIR FRY BOWLS

Calories: 490 **Protein: 41** **Carbs: 35** **Fat: 21**

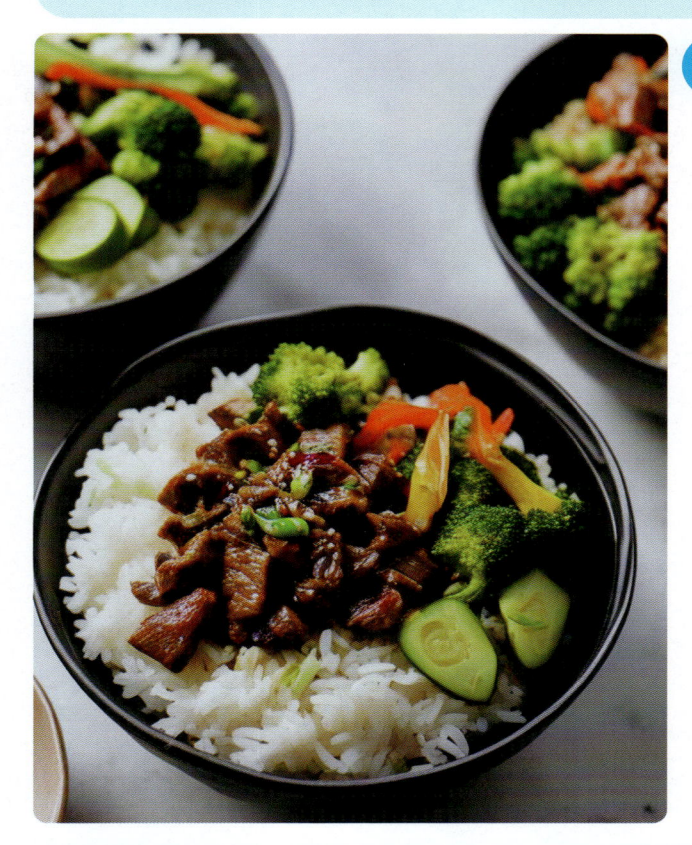

Ingredients — Servings: 8 (1 1/2 CUP)

Stir Fry:
- 3 lb carne asada/shaved beef
- 1 cup dry rice
- 2 eggs
- 2 (10 oz.) bags frozen stir fry vegetables
- 2 tbsp minced garlic
- 1 tbsp minced ginger
- 1 (12 oz.) container G Hughes sweet chili
- 2 tbsp low sodium soy sauce
- 1 tbsp sriracha
- 1 tbsp sesame oil
- 1 tbsp onion powder
- 1 tsp black pepper
- 1/2 tsp red pepper flakes

Optional Sides
- Salad (2 cups greens, 1 tbsp extra virgin olive oil, 2 tbsp balsamic - 307c, 4P, 11C, 27F)
- Protein shake (2 cups almond milk, 1 scoop Dummy Supps - 190c, 26P, 9C, 6F)

Instructions

1. Heat sesame oil in a large pan over medium-high heat. Add steak and cook for 5-7 minutes until browned.
2. Add garlic, ginger, and listed ingredients. Stir and cook for 1-2 minutes.
3. Push steak to one side of the pan. Crack eggs into the empty side and scramble until cooked. Mix with chicken.
4. Add frozen stir-fry vegetables and cook for 5-7 minutes until tender.
5. Add 2 cups water and rice in pot, bring to boil on high heat, turn to low, cover, and cook for 10 minutes.
6. Stir in sweet chili sauce, soy sauce, and sriracha. Cook for 2-3 minutes until well combined.
7. Serve the stir-fry over rice.

MULTIPLE MEAL PREPS

STEAK FAJITA BOWLS

Calories: 600   **Protein: 52**   **Carbs: 33**   **Fat: 28**

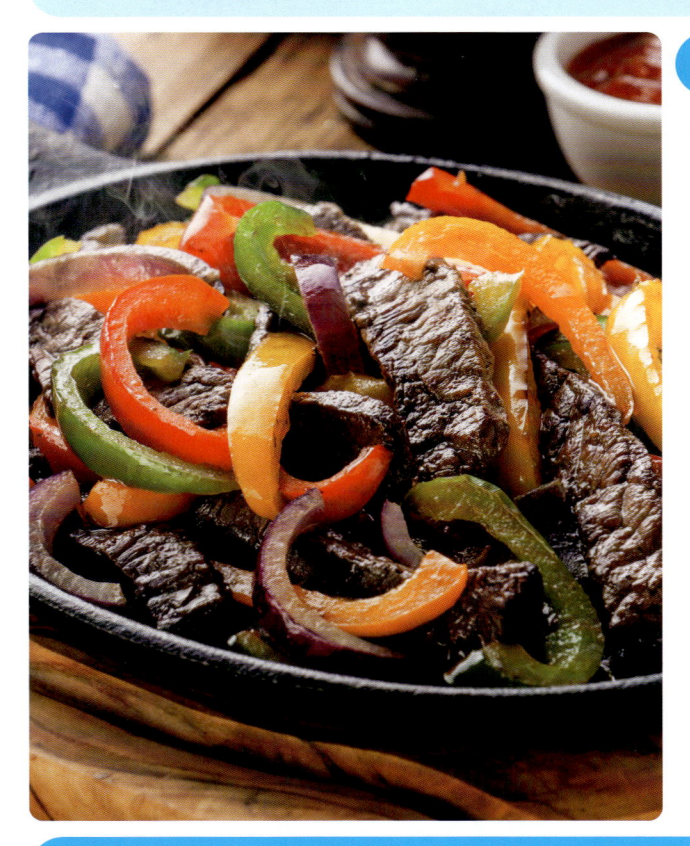

Ingredients — Servings: 6 (1 1/2 CUP)

Bowls:
- 3 lb carne asada/shaved beef
- 1 cup dry rice
- 1 red onion
- 2 bell peppers
- 1 bunch cilantro
- 1 lime
- 1 cup shredded cheese
- 1 (1 oz.) packet taco seasoning
- 1/2 teaspoon black pepper
- 1/4 teaspoon salt

Optional Sides
- Salad (2 cups greens, 1 tbsp extra virgin olive oil, 2 tbsp balsamic - 307c, 4P, 11C, 27F)
- Protein shake (2 cups almond milk, 1 scoop Dummy Supps - 190c, 26P, 9C, 6F)
- Avocado (1/2 whole - 120c, 2P, 6C, 11F)
- Mission low carb tortilla (12 oz. - 70c, 5P, 4C, 3F)

Instructions
1. Slice bell peppers and red onion into thin strips.
2. Heat a large pan over medium-high heat and spray with cooking spray. Add bell peppers, onions, salt and pepper to the pan. Sauté for 4-5 minutes until vegetables are tender.
3. Add carne asada/shaved and taco seasoning to the pan. Cook for 5-7 minutes until steak is browned and cooked through.
4. Add 2 cups water and rice in pot, bring to boil on high heat, turn to low, cover, and cook for 10 minutes.
5. Serve chicken and vegetables over rice.
6. Top with shredded cheese, chopped cilantro, and a squeeze of lime.

MULTIPLE MEAL PREPS

BEEF TACOS & SPICY CHIPOTLE CREMA

Calories: 450 **Protein: 42** **Carbs: 10** **Fat: 21**

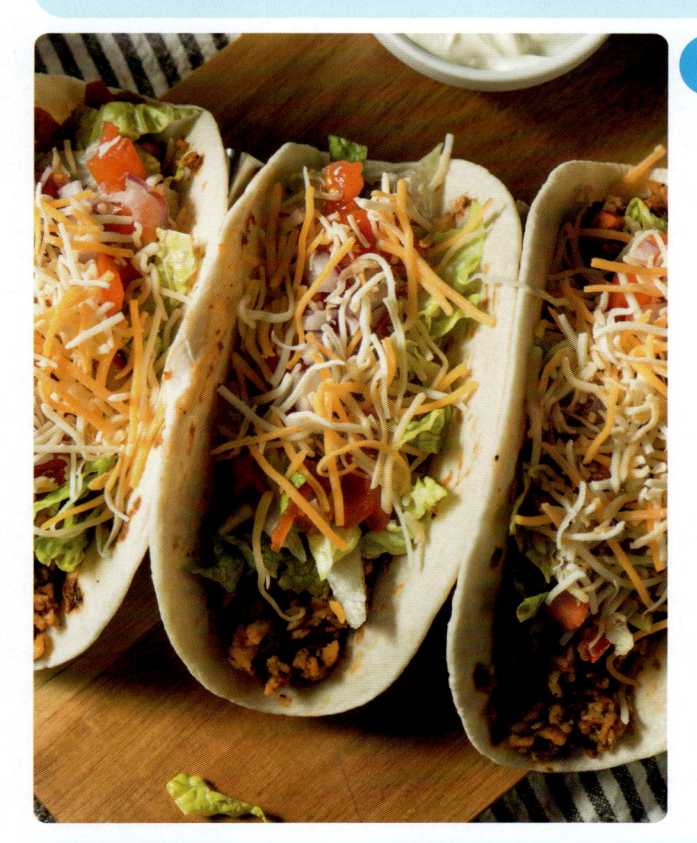

Ingredients — Servings: 6 (1 TACO)

Tacos:
- 2 lb ground beef/turkey
- 1 (10 oz.) can of green chilis
- 8 (12 oz.) mission low carb tortillas
- 1 white onion
- 1/2 bunch cilantro
- 1 lime
- 1 cup shredded cheese
- 1 (1 oz.) packet taco seasoning

Crema:
- 1/4 cup nonfat plain greek yogurt
- 1/4 cup lite sour cream
- 4 tbsp chipotle peppers in adobo sauce
- 1 tbsp minced garlic
- 1 lime
- 1/4 tsp salt

Optional Sides
- Salad (2 cups greens, 1 tbsp extra virgin olive oil, 2 tbsp balsamic - 307c, 4P, 11C, 27F)
- Protein shake (2 cups almond milk, 1 scoop Dummy Supps - 190c, 26P, 9C, 6F)
- Avocado (1/2 whole - 120c, 2P, 6C, 11F)
- Salsa (2 tbsp - 10c, 0P, 2C, 0F)

Instructions
1. Dice white onion and chop cilantro.
2. Heat a pan over medium heat. Cook ground beef/turkey for 5-7 minutes until browned.
3. Stir in green chilies and taco seasoning to pan on low heat. Cook for 2-3 minutes.
4. Blend Greek yogurt, sour cream, chipotle peppers, minced garlic, lime juice, and salt until smooth to make the spicy chipotle crema.
5. Warm tortillas in a dry pan or microwave.
6. Fill tortillas with beef, shredded cheese, white onion, and cilantro.
7. Drizzle with chipotle crema and serve with a squeeze of lime.

MULTIPLE MEAL PREPS

STEAK TACOS & GUACAMOLE

Calories: 520 **Protein: 43** **Carbs: 11** **Fat: 30**

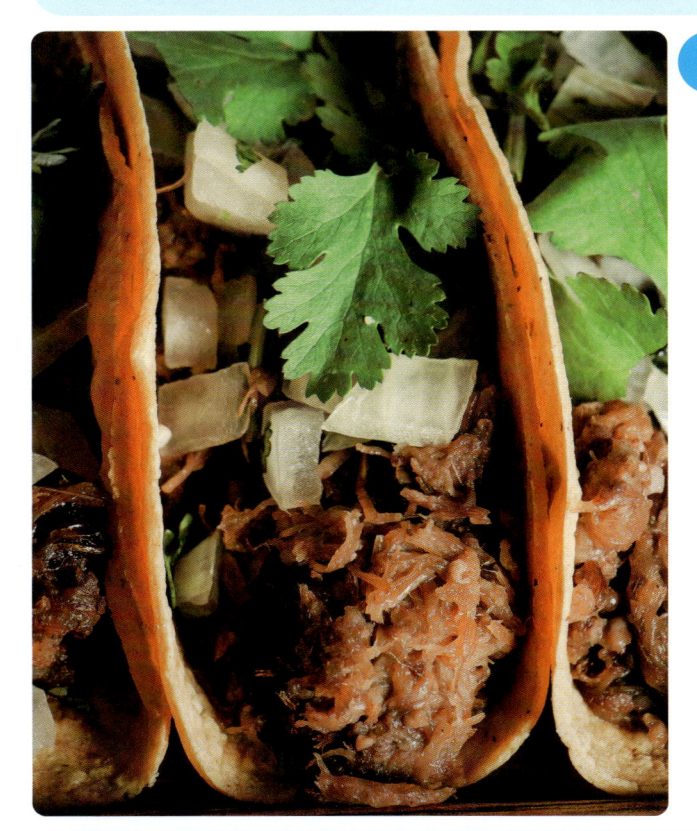

Ingredients   Servings: 6 (1 BURRITO)

Tacos:
- 2 lb sirloin steak
- 1 (10 oz.) can of green chilis
- 8 (12 oz.) mission low carb tortillas
- 1 white onion
- 1/2 bunch cilantro
- 1 lime
- 1 cup shredded cheese
- 1 (1 oz.) packet taco seasoning

Guacamole:
- 1 avocado
- 1 roma tomato
- 1/2 bunch cilantro
- 2 tbsp lime juice
- 1 jalapeno pepper
- 1 tsp garlic powder
- 1/4 tsp salt

Optional Sides

- Salad (2 cups greens, 1 tbsp extra virgin olive oil, 2 tbsp balsamic - 307c, 4P, 11C, 27F)
- Protein shake (2 cups almond milk, 1 scoop Dummy Supps - 190c, 26P, 9C, 6F)
- Lite sour cream (2 tbsp - 3
- Salsa (2 tbsp - 10c, 0P, 2C, 0F)

Instructions

1. Dice white onion and chop cilantro.
2. Heat a pan over medium-high heat with cooking spray. Sear sirloin steak for 3-4 minutes per side until browned.
3. Remove steak, let rest for 5 minutes, then slice thinly.
4. Add sliced steak back to the pan with green chilies and taco seasoning on low heat. Stir and cook for 2-3 minutes.
5. Warm tortillas in a dry pan or microwave.
6. Mash avocado in a bowl. Dice tomato and jalapeño, then mix with avocado, cilantro, lime juice, garlic powder, and salt to make guacamole.
7. Fill tortillas with steak, shredded cheese, white onion, and cilantro.
8. Serve tacos with guacamole and a squeeze of lime.

MULTIPLE MEAL PREPS

CHICKEN NOODLE SOUP

Calories: 450 **Protein: 41** **Carbs: 19** **Fat: 23**

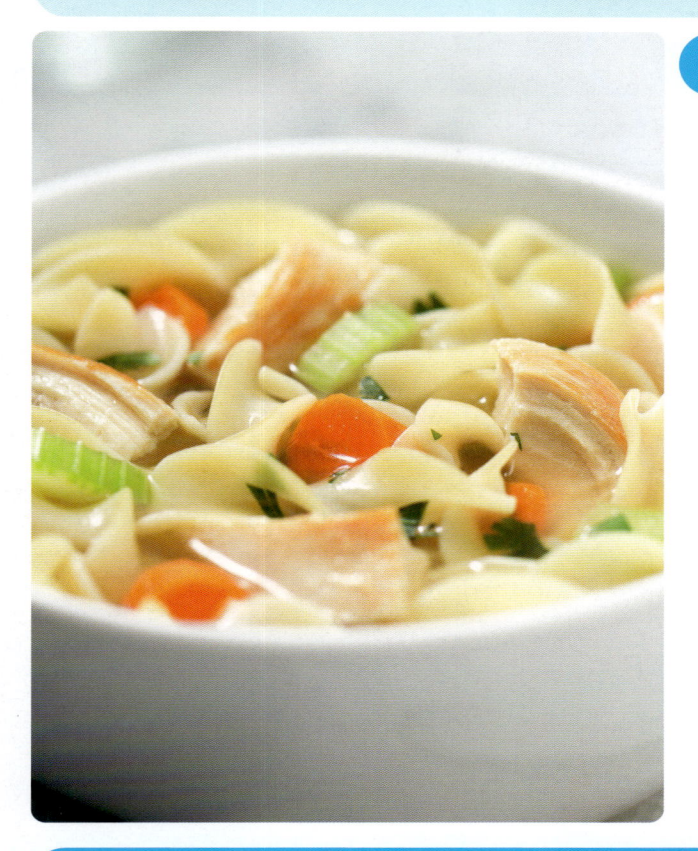

Ingredients **Servings: 8 (1 1/2 CUP)**

Soup:
- 1 (36 oz.) rotisserie chicken
- 1 (14.5 oz.) box protein pasta
- 1 lb baby carrots
- 1 lb celery
- 2 yellow onions
- 3 tablespoons minced garlic
- 6 cups bone broth
- 4 teaspoons chicken bouillon
- 1 tablespoon rosemary
- 2 teaspoons sage
- 2 teaspoons crushed red pepper flakes
- 2 teaspoons black pepper

Optional Sides

- Salad (2 cups greens, 1 tbsp extra virgin olive oil, 2 tbsp balsamic - 307c, 4P, 11C, 27F)
- Protein shake (2 cups almond milk, 1 scoop Dummy Supps - 190c, 26P, 9C, 6F)

Instructions

1. Dice onions and celery. Slice baby carrots.
2. Shred rotisserie chicken and set aside.
3. Heat a large pot over medium heat. Add onions, celery, carrots, and minced garlic. Sauté for 5 minutes until softened.
4. Pour in bone broth and add chicken bouillon, rosemary, sage, crushed red pepper flakes, and black pepper. Stir well.
5. Bring to a boil, then reduce heat and simmer for 15 minutes.
6. Add protein pasta and cook for 9-11 minutes until tender.
7. Stir in shredded rotisserie chicken and cook for 2-3 more minutes until heated through.

MULTIPLE MEAL PREPS

BEEF AND BEAN TACO SOUP

Calories: 480 **Protein: 51** **Carbs: 21** **Fat: 22**

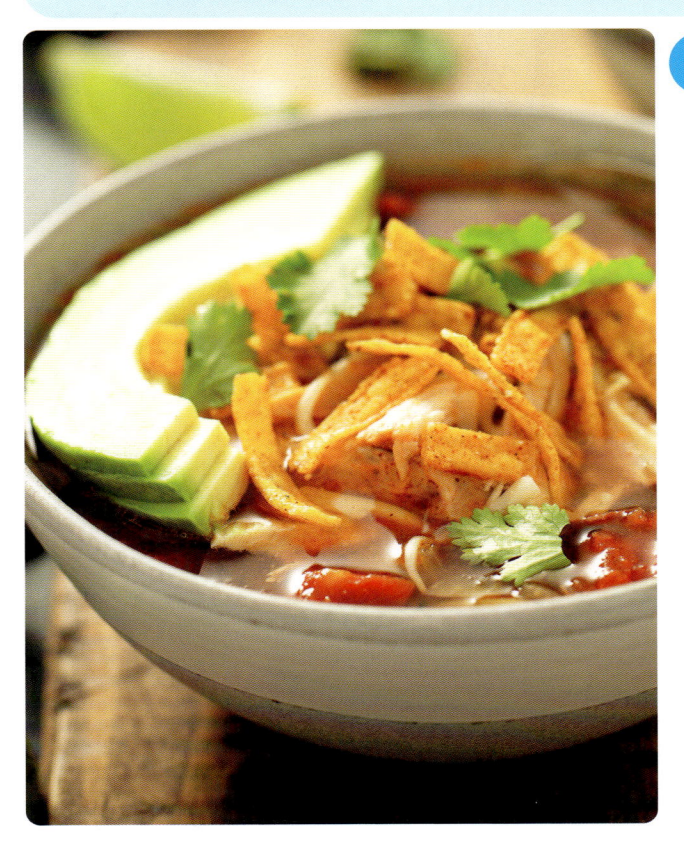

Ingredients   Servings: 8 (1 1/2 CUP)

Soup:
- 3 lb ground beef/turkey
- 1 yellow onion
- 2 bell peppers
- 2 jalapeno peppers
- 3 tablespoons minced garlic
- 1 (15 oz.) can tomato sauce
- 1 (15 oz.) can black beans
- 1 (15 oz) can diced tomatoes
- 6 cups bone broth
- 1 1/2 cups shredded cheese
- 2 (1 oz.) taco seasoning packets

Optional Sides

- Lite sour cream (2 tbsp - 35c, 1P, 2C, 3F)
- Avocado (1/2 whole - 120c, 2P, 6C, 11F)
- Tortilla strips (1/4 cup - 30c, 0P, 4C, 2F)

Instructions

1. Dice onion, bell peppers, and jalapeños.
2. Heat a large pot over medium heat. Add onion, bell peppers, and jalapeños. Cook for 4-5 minutes until softened.
3. Add ground beef/turkey and cook for 8-10 minutes until browned. Stir in minced garlic and cook for 1 more minute.
4. Add tomato sauce, diced tomatoes, black beans, bone broth, and taco seasoning packets. Stir well and bring to a boil.
5. Reduce heat and simmer for 20-25 minutes, stirring occasionally.
6. Stir in shredded cheese until melted.

MULTIPLE MEAL PREPS

ROTISSERIE CHICKEN SALAD SANDWICHES

Calories: 570   **Protein: 50**   **Carbs: 33**   **Fat: 31**

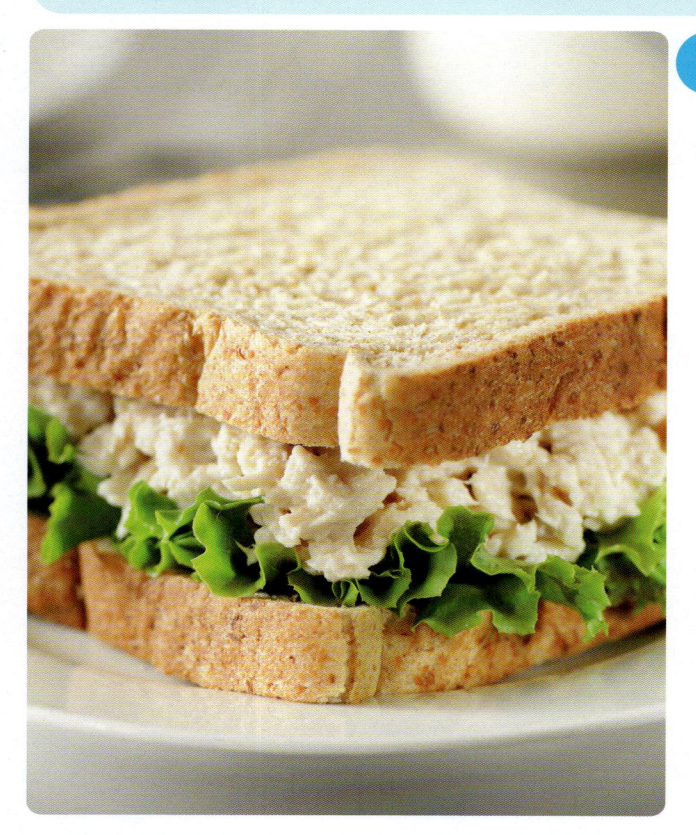

Ingredients   Servings: 6 (1 SANDWICH)

Sandwiches:
- 1 (36 oz.) rotisserie chicken
- 6 647 low carb buns
- 6 stalks celery
- 1/2 red onion
- 1 cup lite mayonnaise
- 1/4 cup nonfat plain greek yogurt
- 2 tsp dijon mustard
- 1 lemon
- 1/2 cup dill pickles
- 1/4 cup dried cranberries
- 1 tablespoon garlic powder
- 1 teaspoon chili powder
- 1/2 teaspoon black pepper

Optional Sides

- Salad (2 cups greens, 1 tbsp extra virgin olive oil, 2 tbsp balsamic - 307c, 4P, 11C, 27F)
- Protein shake (2 cups almond milk, 1 scoop Dummy Supps - 190c, 26P, 9C, 6F)

Instructions

1. Shred rotisserie chicken and place in a large bowl.
2. Dice celery, red onion, and pickles.
3. Add celery, red onion, mayonnaise, Greek yogurt, dijon mustard, juice from the lemon, dill pickles dried cranberries, garlic powder, chili powder, and black pepper to the bowl.
4. Mix until well combined.
5. Toast buns if desired.
6. Serve chicken salad on buns and enjoy.

MULTIPLE MEAL PREPS

ROTISSERIE BUFFALO SALAD SANDWICHES

Calories: 560 **Protein: 52** **Carbs: 29** **Fat: 31**

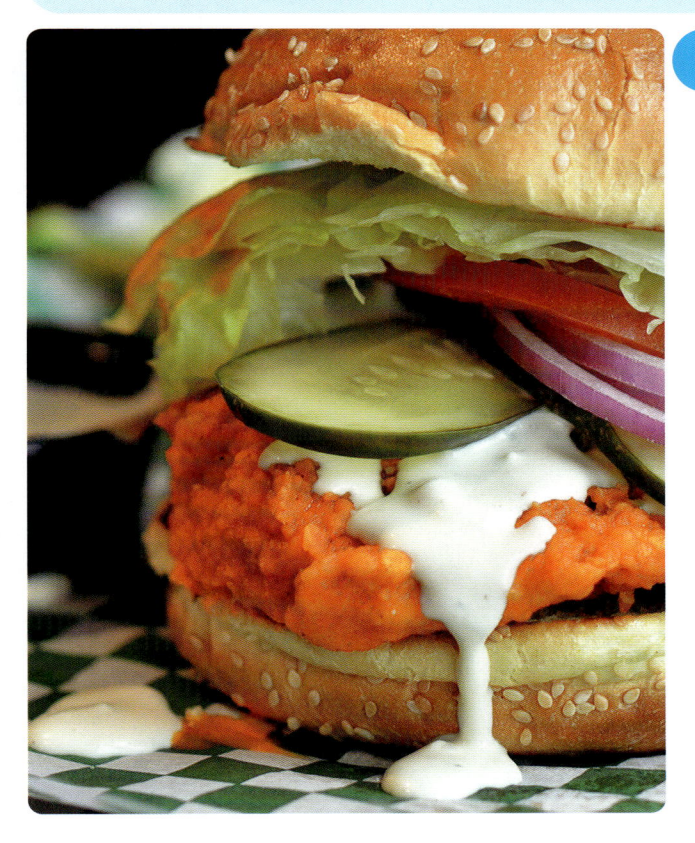

Ingredients   Servings: 6 (1 SANDWICH)

Sandwiches:
- 1 (36 oz.) rotisserie chicken
- 6 low-carb buns
- 6 stalks celery
- 1/2 red onion
- 1/2 cup lite mayonnaise
- 1/4 cup nonfat plain Greek yogurt
- 1/2 cup buffalo sauce
- 1 tbsp lemon juice
- 1 bunch green onions
- 1 tbsp garlic powder
- 1 tsp onion powder
- ½ tsp black pepper
- ½ tsp cayenne pepper
- 1 tbsp ranch seasoning

Protein Ranch:
- 1 cup nonfat plain greek yogurt
- 1 tbsp ranch seasoning
- 2 tsp lime juice

Optional Sides

- Salad (2 cups greens, 1 tbsp extra virgin olive oil, 2 tbsp balsamic - 307c, 4P, 11C, 27F)
- Protein shake (2 cups almond milk, 1 scoop Dummy Supps - 190c, 26P, 9C, 6F)

Instructions

1. Shred rotisserie chicken and place in a large bowl.
2. Dice celery and red onion.
3. Add celery, red onion, mayonnaise, Greek yogurt, juice from the lemon, dried cranberries, garlic powder, chili powder, and black pepper to the bowl.
4. Mix until well combined.
5. Toast buns if desired.
6. In a small bowl, mix ingredients for the protein ranch.
7. Serve chicken salad on buns and top with protein ranch.

MULTIPLE MEAL PREPS

ROTISSERIE BBQ CHICKEN SANDWICHES

Calories: 550 **Protein: 50** **Carbs: 28** **Fat: 31**

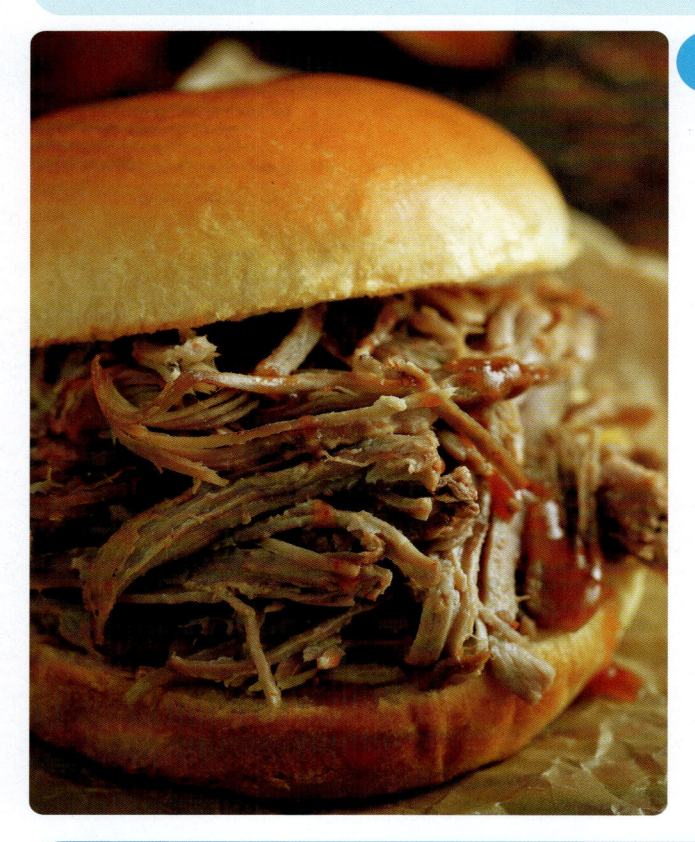

Ingredients   Servings: 6 (1 SANDWICH)

Sandwiches:
- 1 (36 oz.) rotisserie chicken
- 6 low-carb buns
- 6 stalks celery, diced
- 1/2 red onion, diced
- 1/2 cup lite mayonnaise
- 1/4 cup nonfat plain Greek yogurt
- 1/2 cup BBQ sauce
- 1 tbsp garlic powder
- 1 tsp onion powder
- ½ tsp black pepper
- ½ tsp cayenne pepper
- 1 tbsp ranch seasoning
- 1 tablespoon lemon juice
- 1 bunch green onions

Optional Sides

- Salad (2 cups greens, 1 tbsp extra virgin olive oil, 2 tbsp balsamic - 307c, 4P, 11C, 27F)
- Protein shake (2 cups almond milk, 1 scoop Dummy Supps - 190c, 26P, 9C, 6F)

Instructions

1. Shred rotisserie chicken and place in a large bowl.
2. Dice celery and red onion.
3. Add celery, red onion, mayonnaise, Greek yogurt, juice from the lemon, dried cranberries, garlic powder, chili powder, and black pepper to the bowl.
4. Mix until well combined.
5. Toast buns if desired.
6. Serve chicken salad on buns and enjoy.

MULTIPLE MEAL PREPS

CHICKEN PATTIES

Calories: 410   **Protein: 46**   **Carbs: 40**   **Fat: 10**

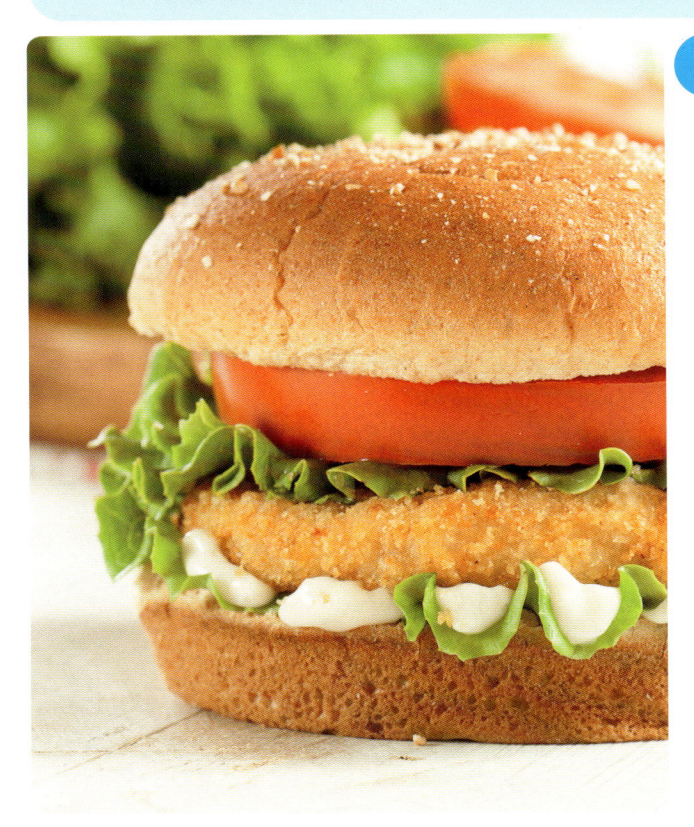

Ingredients   Servings: 6 (1 SANDWICH)

Sandwiches:
- 2 lb ground chicken
- 6 low calorie brioche buns
- 1 egg
- 1 cup egg whites
- 1/4 cup flour
- 1 cup Italian bread crumbs
- 1/2 cup parmesan cheese
- 1 tbsp garlic powder
- 1 tbsp onion powder
- 1 tbsp Italian seasoning
- 1/4 tsp salt
- 1/2 tsp black pepper

Optional Sides
- Salad (2 cups greens, 1 tbsp extra virgin olive oil, 2 tbsp balsamic - 307c, 4P, 11C, 27F)
- Protein shake (2 cups almond milk, 1 scoop Dummy Supps - 190c, 26P, 9C, 6F)
- Lettuce (2 slices, 5c, 0P, 0C, 0F)
- Tomato (2 slices, 9c, 0P, 6C, 0F)
- Lite mayo (2 tbsp, 50c, 0P, 4C, 2F)

Instructions
1. Preheat oven to 400°F.
2. In a bowl, mix ground chicken, egg, parmesan cheese, flour, garlic powder, onion powder, Italian seasoning, salt, and black pepper until combined.
3. Divide mixture into 6 equal portions and shape into patties.
4. In one bowl, whisk egg whites. In another, add Italian bread crumbs.
5. Dip each patty into egg whites, then coat with bread crumbs.
6. Air Fryer: Cook at 400°F for 12-15 minutes, flipping halfway.
7. Oven: Bake at 400°F for 15 minutes flip and cook for additional 15 minutes, until golden and cooked through.

MULTIPLE MEAL PREPS

BUFFALO CHICKEN PATTIES

Calories: 420 **Protein: 45** **Carbs: 42** **Fat: 11**

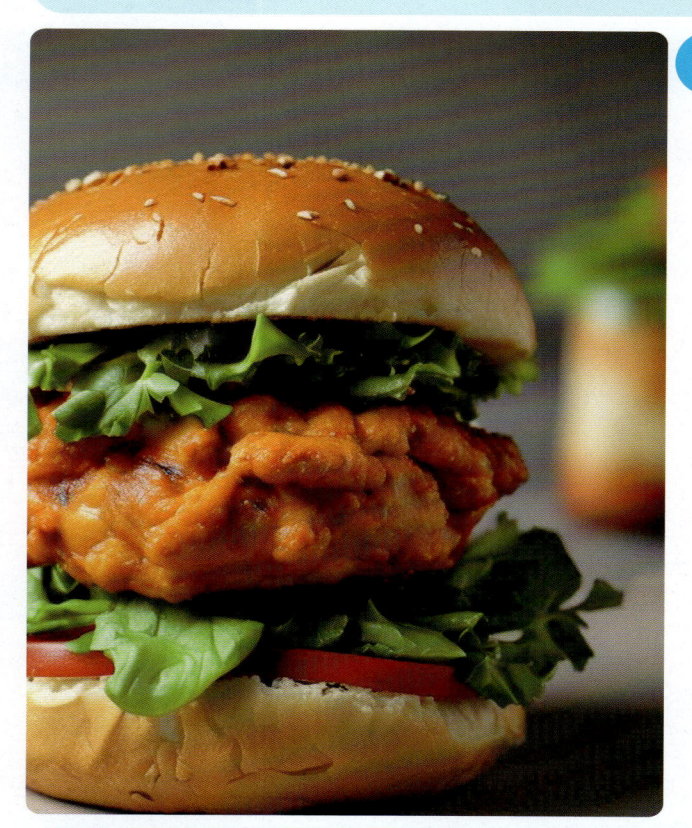

Ingredients   Servings: 6 (1 SANDWICH)

Sandwiches:
- 2 lb ground chicken
- 6 low calorie brioche buns
- 1 egg
- 1 cup egg whites
- 1/4 cup flour
- 1 cup Italian bread crumbs
- 1/2 cup parmesan cheese
- 1 tbsp garlic powder
- 1 tbsp onion powder
- 1 tbsp Italian seasoning
- 1/4 tsp salt
- 1/2 tsp black pepper

Buffalo Sauce:
- 1/2 cup buffalo wing sauce
- 1 tsp butter

Optional Sides

- Salad (2 cups greens, 1 tbsp extra virgin olive oil, 2 tbsp balsamic - 307c, 4P, 11C, 27F)
- Protein shake (2 cups almond milk, 1 scoop Dummy Supps - 190c, 26P, 9C, 6F)
- Lettuce (2 slices, 5c, 0P, 0C, 0F)
- Crumbled blue cheese (2 tbsp -
- Lite mayo (2 tbsp, 50c, 0P, 4C, 2F)

Instructions

1. Preheat oven to 400°F.
2. In a bowl, mix ground chicken, egg, parmesan cheese, garlic powder, onion powder, Italian seasoning, salt, and black pepper until combined.
3. Divide mixture into 6 equal portions and shape into patties.
4. In one bowl, whisk egg whites. In another, add flour. In a third, add Italian bread crumbs.
5. Dredge each patty in egg whites, then coat with flour, then coat with bread crumbs.
6. Air Fryer: Cook at 400°F for 12-15 minutes, flipping halfway.
7. Oven: Bake at 400°F for 20-25 minutes until golden and cooked through.
8. Melt butter and mix with buffalo wing sauce.
9. Toss cooked patties in buffalo sauce until fully coated.

MULTIPLE MEAL PREPS

CHICKEN PARM PATTIES

Calories: 510 **Protein: 53** **Carbs: 44** **Fat: 18**

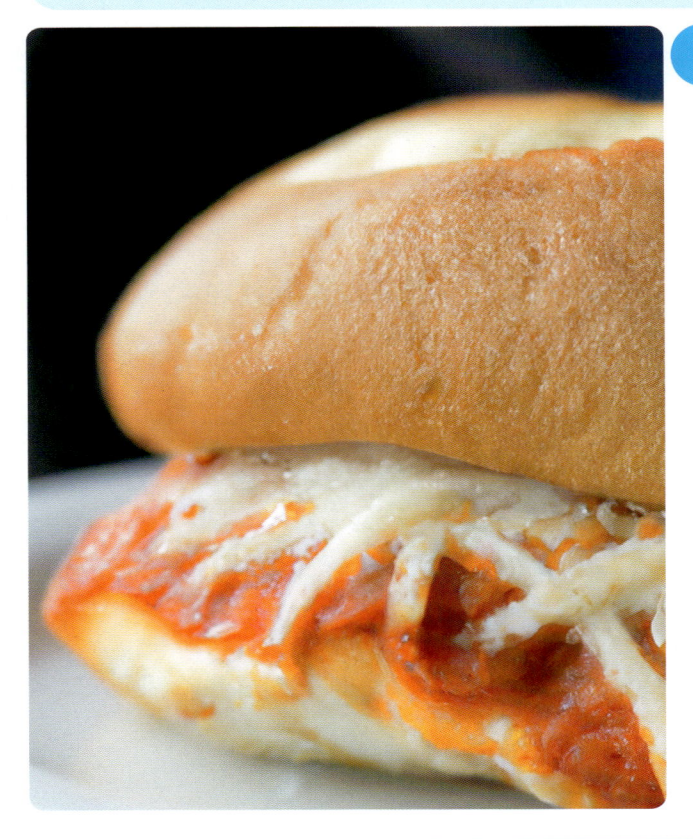

Ingredients   Servings: 6 (1 SANDWICH)

Sandwiches:
- 2 lb ground chicken
- 6 low calorie brioche buns
- 1 egg
- 1 cup egg whites
- 1/4 cup flour
- 1 cup Italian bread crumbs
- 1/2 cup parmesan cheese
- 6 slices mozzarella
- 1 tbsp garlic powder
- 1 tbsp onion powder
- 1 tbsp Italian seasoning
- 1/4 tsp salt
- 1/2 tsp black pepper

Optional Sides

- Salad (2 cups greens, 1 tbsp extra virgin olive oil, 2 tbsp balsamic - 307c, 4P, 11C, 27F)
- Protein shake (2 cups almond milk, 1 scoop Dummy Supps - 190c, 26P, 9C, 6F)

Instructions

1. Preheat oven to 400°F.
2. In a bowl, mix ground chicken, egg, parmesan cheese, flour, garlic powder, onion powder, Italian seasoning, salt, and black pepper until combined.
3. Divide mixture into 6 equal portions and shape into patties.
4. In one bowl, whisk egg whites. In another, add Italian bread crumbs.
5. Dip each patty into egg whites, then coat with bread crumbs.
6. Air Fryer: Cook at 400°F for 12-15 minutes, flipping halfway.
7. Oven: Bake at 400°F for 15 minutes flip and cook for additional 15 minutes, until golden and cooked through.
8. Top with mozzarella cheese slices and marinara sauce.

MULTIPLE MEAL PREPS

ROTISSERIE BBQ CHICKEN STUFFED SWEET POTATOES

Calories: 600 **Protein: 47** **Carbs: 35** **Fat: 31**

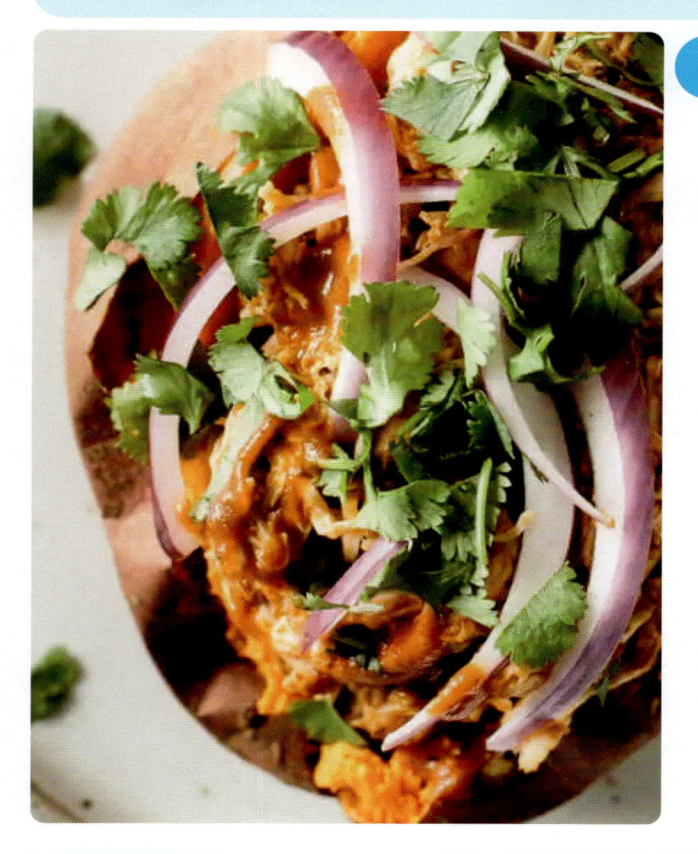

Ingredients Servings: 6 (1 1/2 CUP)

Bowls:
- 1 (36 oz.) rotisserie chicken
- 1 (12 oz.) container G Hughes BBQ sauce
- 6 sweet potatoes
- 1/2 red onion
- 1 tbsp garlic powder
- 1 tsp onion powder
- 1 tsp chili powder
- 1/2 tsp black pepper
- 1 bunch parsley

Optional Sides

- Salad (2 cups greens, 1 tbsp extra virgin olive oil, 2 tbsp balsamic - 307c, 4P, 11C, 27F)
- Protein shake (2 cups almond milk, 1 scoop Dummy Supps - 190c, 26P, 9C, 6F)

Instructions

1. Preheat oven to 400°F.
2. Pierce sweet potatoes with a fork and bake for 40-45 minutes until soft.
3. Shred rotisserie chicken and place in a bowl.
4. Dice red onion and chop parsley.
5. Mix chicken with BBQ sauce, garlic powder, onion powder, chili powder, and black pepper.
6. Slice open baked sweet potatoes and stuff with BBQ chicken mixture.
7. Top with diced red onion and chopped parsley before serving.

MULTIPLE MEAL PREPS

ROTISSERIE CHICKEN GREEK BOWLS

Calories: 550   **Protein: 54**   **Carbs: 30**   **Fat: 23**

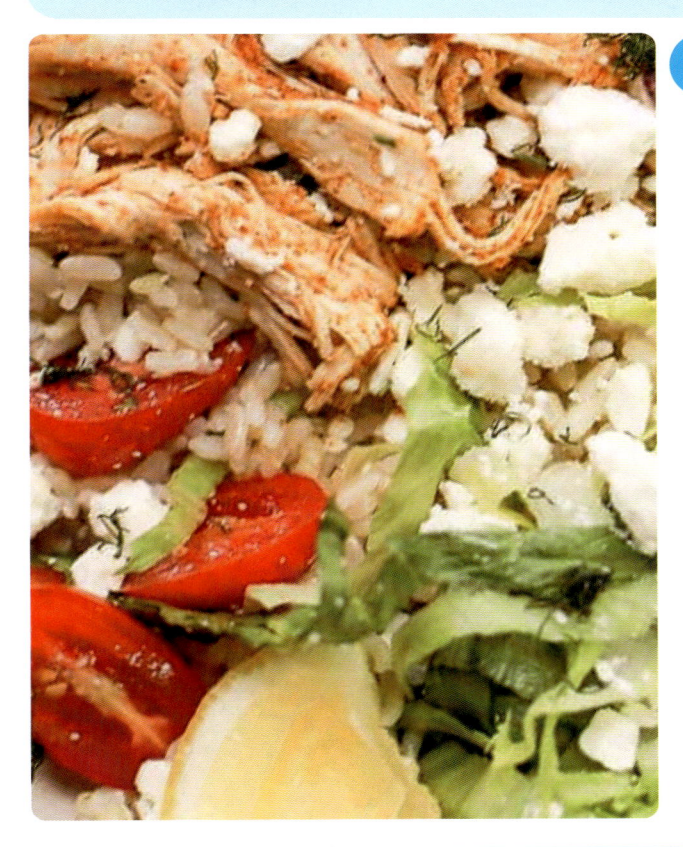

Ingredients   Servings: 6 (1 1/2 CUP)

Bowls:
- 1 (36 oz.) rotisserie chicken
- 1 cup dry rice
- 1 cucumber
- 1 red onion
- 1 (10 oz.) container cherry tomatoes
- 1 cup lowfat feta cheese
- 1 tbsp lemon juice

Tzatziki:
- 1 cup nonfat plain greek yogurt
- 1/2 cup cucumber
- 1 tbsp lemon juice
- 1/4 tsp salt
- 1/2 tsp black pepper
- 1 tsp dill

Optional Sides

- Salad (2 cups greens, 1 tbsp extra virgin olive oil, 2 tbsp balsamic - 307c, 4P, 11C, 27F)
- Protein shake (2 cups almond milk, 1 scoop Dummy Supps - 190c, 26P, 9C, 6F)

Instructions

1. Shred rotisserie chicken and place in a large bowl.
2. Dice cucumber and halve cherry tomatoes.
3. Blend Greek yogurt, cucumber, lemon juice, salt, black pepper, and dill to make tzatziki.
4. Add 2 cups water and rice in pot, bring to boil on high heat, turn to low, cover, and cook for 10 minutes.
5. Assemble bowls with rice, chicken, cucumbers, tomatoes, and feta cheese.
6. Drizzle tzatziki before serving.

MULTIPLE MEAL PREPS

ROTISSERIE CHICKEN ENCHILADAS

Calories: 600   **Protein: 61**   **Carbs: 26**   **Fat: 28**

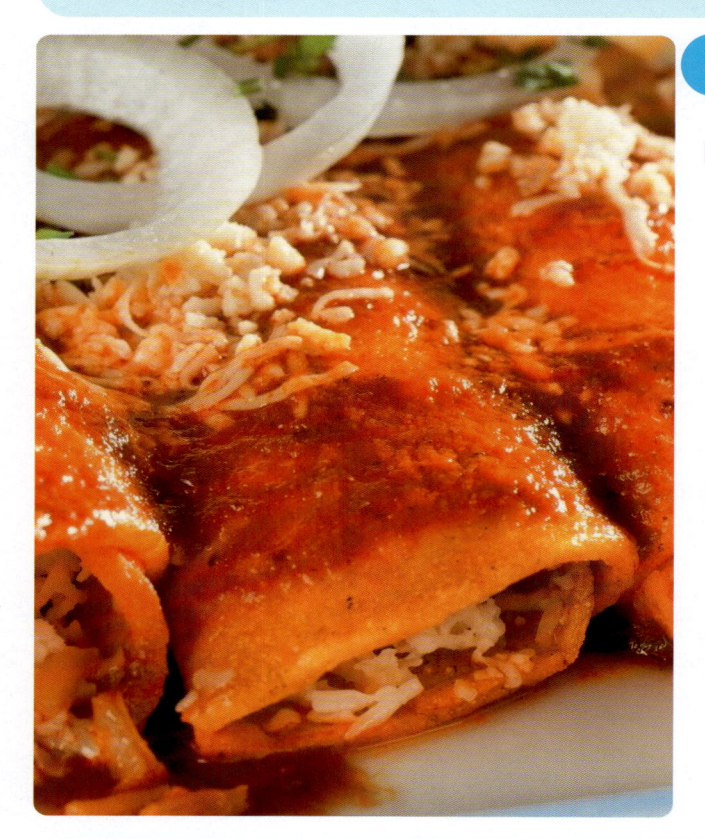

Ingredients Servings: 6 (1 ENCHILADA)

Enchiladas:
- 1 (36 oz.) rotisserie chicken
- 6 (12 oz.) Mission low carb tortillas
- 1 (15 oz.) can black beans
- 1 (10 oz.) can diced tomatoes
- 1/2 cup nonfat plain greek yogurt
- 1 cup enchilada sauce
- 1 cup shredded Mexican cheese

Pico De Gallo:
- 5 roma tomatoes
- 1 red onion
- 2 jalapeno peppers
- 1 bunch cilantro
- 1 lime
- 1 tsp garlic powder
- 1/2 tsp salt

Optional Sides

- Salad (2 cups greens, 1 tbsp extra virgin olive oil, 2 tbsp balsamic - 307c, 4P, 11C, 27F)
- Protein shake (2 cups almond milk, 1 scoop Dummy Supps - 190c, 26P, 9C, 6F)

Instructions

1. Shred rotisserie chicken and mix with black beans, diced tomatoes, greek yogurt, and 1/4 cup enchilada sauce.
2. Fill tortillas with the chicken mixture, roll tightly, and place seam-side down in a baking dish.
3. Pour remaining enchilada sauce over the tortillas and sprinkle with shredded Mexican cheese.
4. Bake at 375°F for 20 minutes until cheese is melted and bubbly.
5. Dice tomatoes, red onion, and jalapeños. Mix with chopped cilantro, lime juice, garlic powder, and salt to make pico de gallo.
6. Serve enchiladas topped with fresh pico de gallo.

MULTIPLE MEAL PREPS

STUFFED PEPPERS

Calories: 460 **Protein: 41** **Carbs: 37** **Fat: 18**

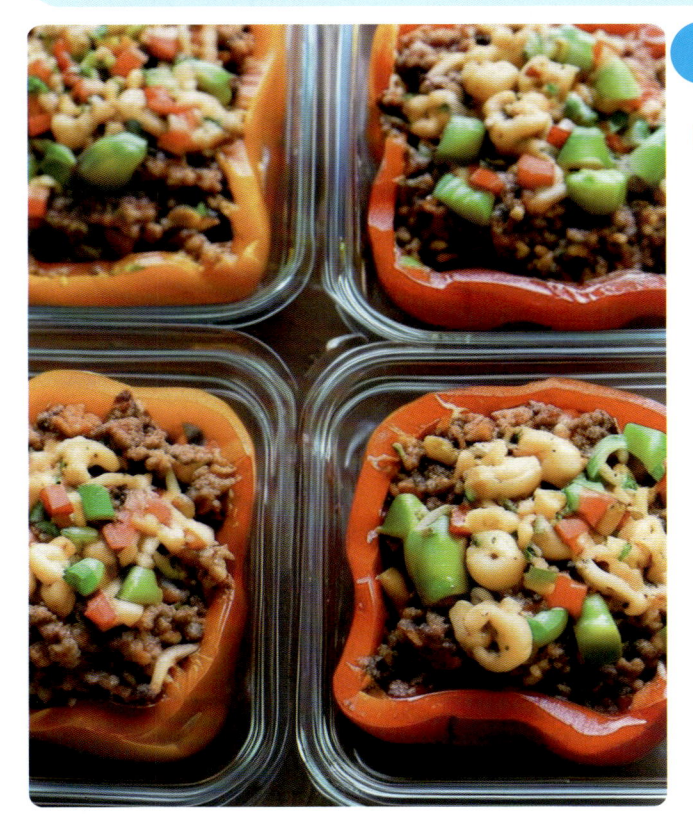

Ingredients Servings: 6 (1 PEPPER)

Peppers:
- 2 lb ground beef/turkey
- 1 cup dry rice
- 6 bell peppers
- 1 yellow onion
- 1 cup low-fat mozzarella cheese
- 1 (15 oz.) can tomato sauce
- 2 tbsp garlic powder
- 1 tbsp onion powder
- 1 tsp chili powder
- 1/4 tsp salt
- 1/2 tsp black pepper

Optional Sides

- Salad (2 cups greens, 1 tbsp extra virgin olive oil, 2 tbsp balsamic - 307c, 4P, 11C, 27F)
- Protein shake (2 cups almond milk, 1 scoop Dummy Supps - 190c, 26P, 9C, 6F)

Instructions

1. Preheat oven to 350°F.
2. Cut tops off bell peppers and remove seeds. Place in the oven for 20 minutes while cooking the beef.
3. Dice onion.
4. Heat a pan over medium heat. Add ground beef/turkey, onion, garlic powder, onion powder, chili powder, salt, and black pepper. Cook for 8-10 minutes until browned.
5. Add 2 cups water and rice in pot, bring to boil on high heat, turn to low, cover, and cook for 10 minutes.
6. Add tomato sauce and cooked rice to the pan. Stir until combined.
7. Remove peppers from the oven and fill each with the beef mixture.
8. Top with mozzarella cheese.
9. Bake for 20 minutes until peppers are tender and cheese is melted.

MULTIPLE MEAL PREPS

ITALIAN STUFFED PEPPERS

Calories: 420   **Protein: 48**   **Carbs: 16**   **Fat: 17**

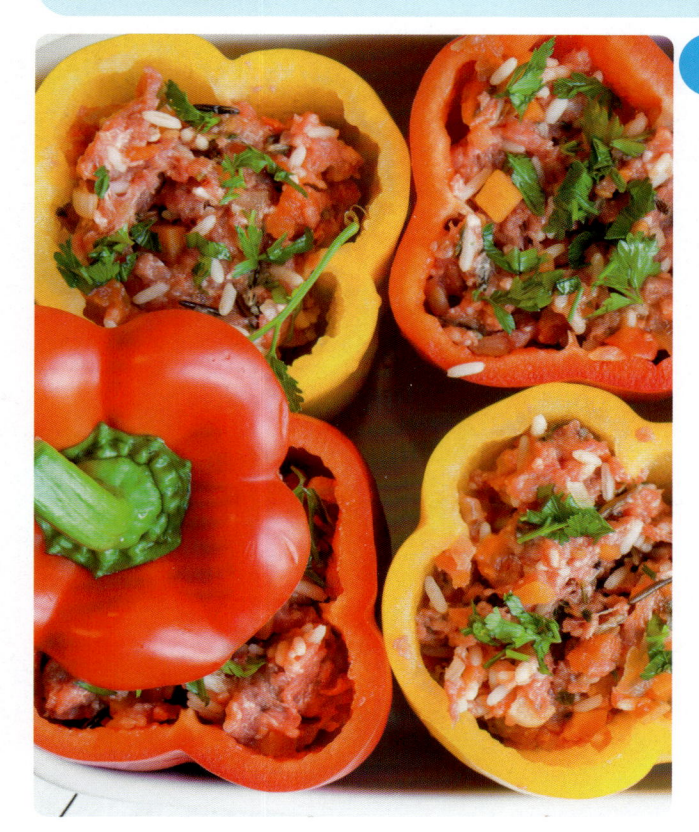

Ingredients Servings: 6 (1 PEPPER)

Peppers:
- 2 lb lean ground beef/turkey
- 6 bell peppers
- 1 sweet onion
- 4 tbsp minced garlic
- 1 (15 oz.) container low-fat ricotta cheese
- 1 cup low-fat mozzarella cheese
- 1 (15 oz.) can tomato sauce
- 1 bunch Italian parsley
- 1 tbsp garlic powder
- 1 tbsp onion powder
- 1 tbsp italian seasoning
- 1 tsp chili powder
- 1/2 tsp black pepper

Optional Sides

- Salad (2 cups greens, 1 tbsp extra virgin olive oil, 2 tbsp balsamic - 307c, 4P, 11C, 27F)
- Protein shake (2 cups almond milk, 1 scoop Dummy Supps - 190c, 26P, 9C, 6F)

Instructions

1. Preheat oven to 350°F.
2. Cut tops off bell peppers and remove seeds. Place in the oven for 20 minutes while cooking the beef.
3. Dice onion.
4. Heat a pan over medium heat. Add ground beef/turkey, onion, minced garlic, garlic powder, onion powder, Italian seasoning, chili powder, and black pepper. Cook for 8-10 minutes until browned.
5. Stir in tomato sauce and ricotta cheese until fully combined.
6. Remove peppers from the oven and fill each with the beef mixture.
7. Top with mozzarella cheese.
8. Bake for 20 minutes until peppers are tender and cheese is melted.
9. Garnish with chopped Italian parsley before serving.

MULTIPLE MEAL PREPS

AVOCADO CHICKEN SALAD

Calories: 460   **Protein: 53**   **Carbs: 34**   **Fat: 20**

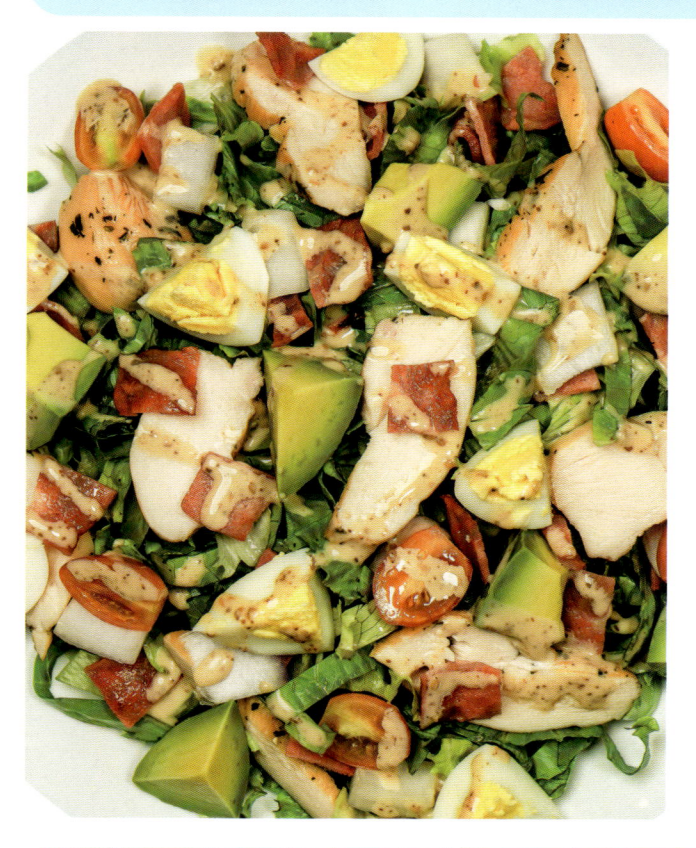

Ingredients   **Servings: 6**

Salad:
- 2 lbs chicken breast
- 4 avocados
- 4 hard boiled eggs
- 1 (10 oz.) container cherry tomatoes
- 1/2 cup corn
- 2 jalapeno peppers
- 1 red onion

Dressing:
- 1 cup nonfat plain greek yogurt
- 1/4 cup lime juice
- 1 tbsp extra virgin olive oil
- 4 tbsp cilantro
- 2 tsp honey
- 1/4 tsp salt
- 1/2 tsp pepper

Optional Sides

- Salad (2 cups greens, 1 tbsp extra virgin olive oil, 2 tbsp balsamic - 307c, 4P, 11C, 27F)
- Protein shake (2 cups almond milk, 1 scoop Dummy Supps - 190c, 26P, 9C, 6F)

Instructions

1. Dice chicken into bite-sized pieces.
2. Heat a pan over medium heat with cooking spray. Cook chicken for 8-10 minutes until browned and fully cooked.
3. Dice red onion, jalapeño, cherry tomatoes, and hard-boiled eggs. Cut avocados into chunks.
4. Blend Greek yogurt, lime juice, olive oil, cilantro, honey, salt, and pepper to make the dressing.
5. In a large bowl, combine cooked chicken, avocados, eggs, tomatoes, corn, jalapeño, and red onion.
6. Pour dressing over the salad and mix until evenly coated.

MULTIPLE MEAL PREPS

ASIAN CHICKEN SLAW SALAD

Calories: 490 **Protein: 55** **Carbs: 10** **Fat: 25**

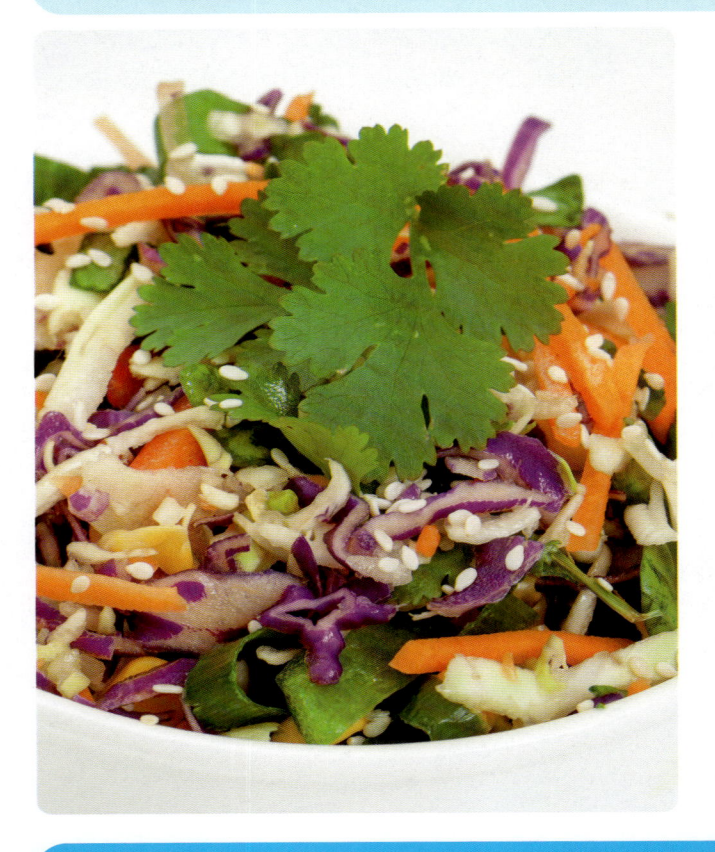

Ingredients Servings: 6

Salad:
- 3 lb chicken breast
- 2 (16 oz.) bags asian slaw mix
- 1 bunch cilantro
- 1/2 cup sliced cashews
- 2 tbsp rice vinegar
- 2 tbsp minced garlic
- 1 tbsp minced ginger
- 1 tbsp onion powder
- 1/2 tsp black pepper
- 1/4 tsp salt
- 1 (12 oz.) container G Hughes Asian Miso
- 6 tsp sesame seeds

Optional Sides

- Salad (2 cups greens, 1 tbsp extra virgin olive oil, 2 tbsp balsamic - 307c, 4P, 11C, 27F)
- Protein shake (2 cups almond milk, 1 scoop Dummy Supps - 190c, 26P, 9C, 6F)

Instructions

1. Dice chicken into bite-sized pieces.
2. Heat a pan over medium heat with cooking spray. Add chicken, minced garlic, minced ginger, onion powder, salt, and black pepper. Cook for 10-12 minutes until fully cooked.
3. In a large bowl, add Asian slaw mix, chopped cilantro, sliced cashews, and sesame seeds.
4. Drizzle rice vinegar and Asian miso dressing over the slaw. Toss until evenly coated.
5. Add cooked chicken and mix well.

MULTIPLE MEAL PREPS

BEEF TACO SALAD

Calories: 470   **Protein: 45**   **Carbs: 18**   **Fat: 20**

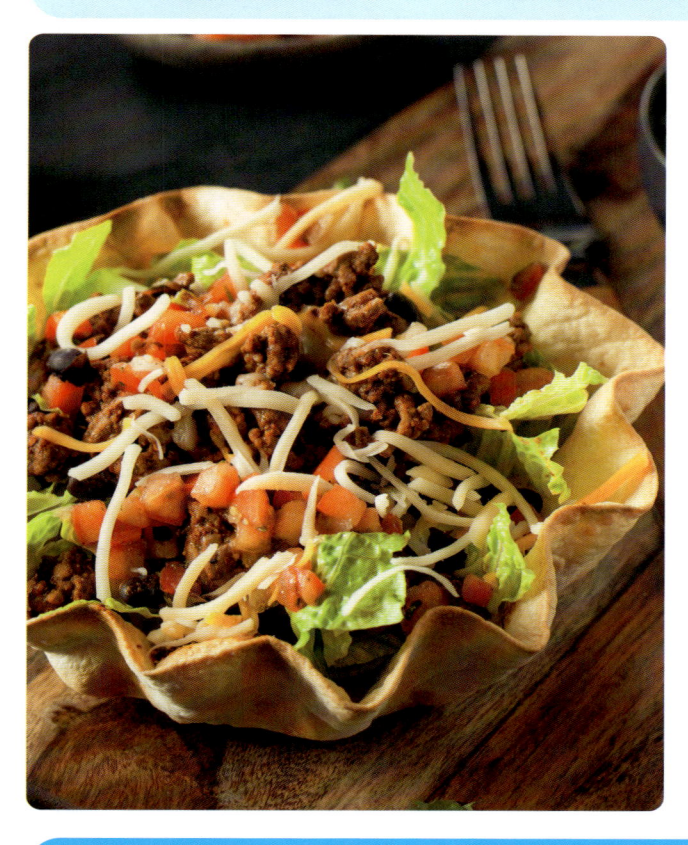

Ingredients   **Servings: 8**

Salad:
- 3 lb lean ground beef
- 8 (12 oz.) Mission low carb tortillas
- 8 cups shredded lettuce
- 1 red onion
- 6 roma tomatoes
- 1 (15 oz.) can black beans
- 1 1/2 cups shredded cheese
- 2 (1 oz.) packets taco seasoning

Optional Sides

- Lite sour cream (2 tbsp - 35c, 1P, 2C, 3F)
- Avocado (1/2 whole - 120c, 2P, 6C, 11F)
- Salsa (1/2 cup - 44c, 2P, 9C, 0F)

Instructions

1. Preheat air fryer to 375°F. Place tortillas in an oven-safe bowl or taco shell mold. Air fry for 6-8 minutes until crispy.
2. Dice red onion and roma tomatoes. Drain and rinse black beans.
3. Heat a pan over medium heat. Add ground beef and taco seasoning. Cook for 10-12 minutes until browned.
4. Divide shredded lettuce into tortillas.
5. Top with cooked beef, black beans, diced red onion, and roma tomatoes.
6. Sprinkle with shredded cheese.
7. Serve in crispy tortilla shells.

MULTIPLE MEAL PREPS

CHICKEN COBB SALAD

Calories: 620   **Protein: 64**   **Carbs: 18**   **Fat: 33**

Ingredients   Servings: 6

Salad:
- 2 lb chicken breast
- 6 slices turkey bacon
- 8 cups romaine lettuce
- 1 red onion
- 1 (10 oz.) container cherry tomatoes
- 6 hard boiled eggs
- 2 avocados
- 6 tbsp crumbled blue cheese
- 2 tbsp garlic powder
- 1 tbsp onion powder
- 1 tsp black pepper

Green Dressing:
- 2 cups nonfat plain Greek yogurt
- 1 bunch cilantro
- 4 tbsp fresh lemon juice
- 2 tbsp extra-virgin olive oil
- 4 tbsp minced garlic
- ¼ teaspoon sea salt
- 1/2 tsp black pepper

Optional Sides

- Salad (2 cups greens, 1 tbsp extra virgin olive oil, 2 tbsp balsamic - 307c, 4P, 11C, 27F)
- Protein shake (2 cups almond milk, 1 scoop Dummy Supps - 190c, 26P, 9C, 6F)

Instructions

1. Dice red onion, halve cherry tomatoes, and slice avocados.
2. Cook turkey bacon in a pan over medium heat for 6-8 minutes until crispy. Let cool and chop into pieces.
3. Add eggs to a pot, cover with water, and bring to a boil. Turn off heat, cover, and let sit for 10 minutes. Drain and cool. Peel and slice.
4. Dice chicken into bite-sized pieces. Season with garlic powder, onion powder, and black pepper. Cook in a pan over medium heat for 10-12 minutes until fully cooked.
5. In a blender, combine Greek yogurt, parsley, cilantro, lemon juice, olive oil, capers, minced garlic, sea salt, and black pepper. Blend until smooth.
6. Divide romaine lettuce into bowls.
7. Top with chicken, turkey bacon, red onion, cherry tomatoes, hard-boiled eggs, avocado, and blue cheese.
8. Drizzle with green dressing before serving.

MULTIPLE MEAL PREPS

CHICKEN CAESAR SALAD

Calories: 600 **Protein: 52** **Carbs: 10** **Fat: 32**

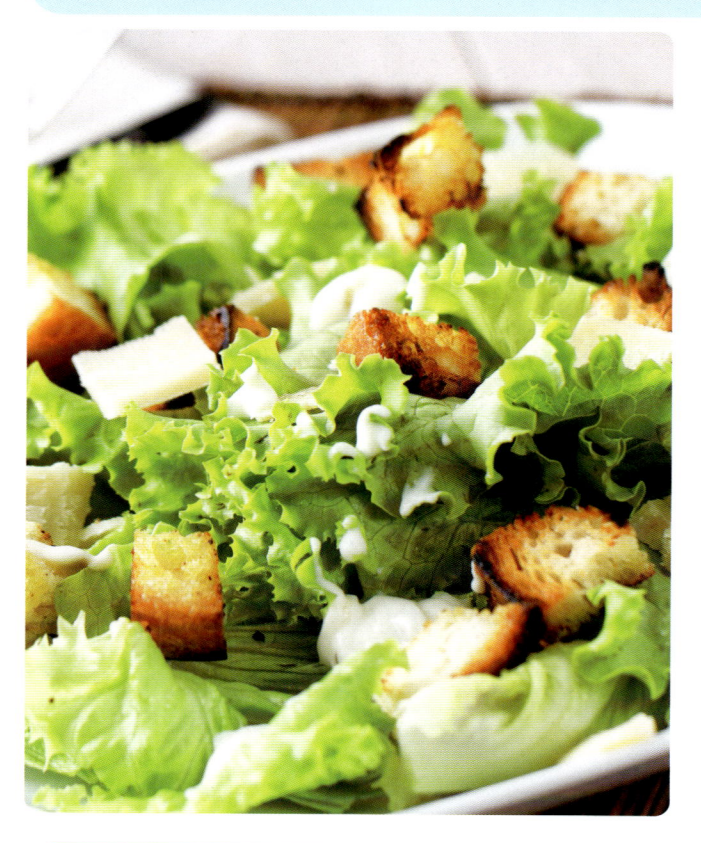

Ingredients — Servings: 6

Salad:
- 2 lb chicken breast
- 6 cups romaine lettuce
- 2 tbsp dijon mustard
- 1 tbsp extra virgin olive oil
- 2 tbsp garlic powder
- 1 tbsp onion powder
- 1 tsp black pepper
- 1/2 tsp salt
- 1 cup Parmesan cheese
- 2 cups croutons

Dressing:
- 1/2 cup olive oil
- 1 cup nonfat plain greek yogurt
- 2 large egg yolks
- 2 tbsp minced garlic
- 1 lemon
- 2 tbsp dijon mustard
- 1/2 tsp black pepper

Optional Sides

- Salad (2 cups greens, 1 tbsp extra virgin olive oil, 2 tbsp balsamic - 307c, 4P, 11C, 27F)
- Protein shake (2 cups almond milk, 1 scoop Dummy Supps - 190c, 26P, 9C, 6F)

Instructions

1. Chop romaine lettuce and set aside.
2. Dice chicken into bite-sized pieces.
3. Heat a pan over medium heat with olive oil. Add chicken, Dijon mustard, garlic powder, onion powder, black pepper, and salt. Cook for 10-12 minutes until fully cooked.
4. Blend olive oil, yogurt, egg yolks, minced garlic, lemon juice, Dijon mustard, and black pepper until smooth to make the dressing.
5. Divide romaine lettuce into bowls.
6. Top with cooked chicken, Parmesan cheese, and croutons.
7. Drizzle with Caesar dressing before serving.

MULTIPLE MEAL PREPS

BUFFALO CHICKEN SALAD

Calories: 440 **Protein: 54** **Carbs: 14** **Fat: 18**

Ingredients Servings: 6

Salad:
- 2 lb chicken breast
- 6 cups romaine lettuce
- 1 red onion
- 1 (10 oz.) container cherry tomatoes
- 6 tbsp crumbled blue cheese
- 1/2 cup buffalo wing sauce
- 2 tbsp garlic powder
- 1 tbsp onion powder
- 1 tsp black pepper

Ranch Dressing:
- 2 cups nonfat plain Greek yogurt
- 1 bunch cilantro
- 1 lemon
- 1 tbsp extra-virgin olive oil
- 1 (1 oz.) packet ranch dressing seasoning

Optional Sides

- Salad (2 cups greens, 1 tbsp extra virgin olive oil, 2 tbsp balsamic - 307c, 4P, 11C, 27F)
- Protein shake (2 cups almond milk, 1 scoop Dummy Supps - 190c, 26P, 9C, 6F)

Instructions

1. Chop romaine lettuce. Dice red onion and halve cherry tomatoes.
2. Dice chicken into bite-sized pieces.
3. Heat a pan over medium heat with cooking spray. Add chicken, buffalo wing sauce, garlic powder, onion powder, and black pepper. Cook for 10-12 minutes until fully cooked.
4. Blend Greek yogurt, cilantro, lemon juice, olive oil, and ranch seasoning until smooth to make the dressing.
5. Divide romaine lettuce into bowls.
6. Top with cooked buffalo chicken, red onion, cherry tomatoes, and crumbled blue cheese.
7. Drizzle with ranch dressing before serving.

MULTIPLE MEAL PREPS

CHICKEN BACON RANCH PIZZA

Calories: 600 **Protein: 57** **Carbs: 33** **Fat: 30**

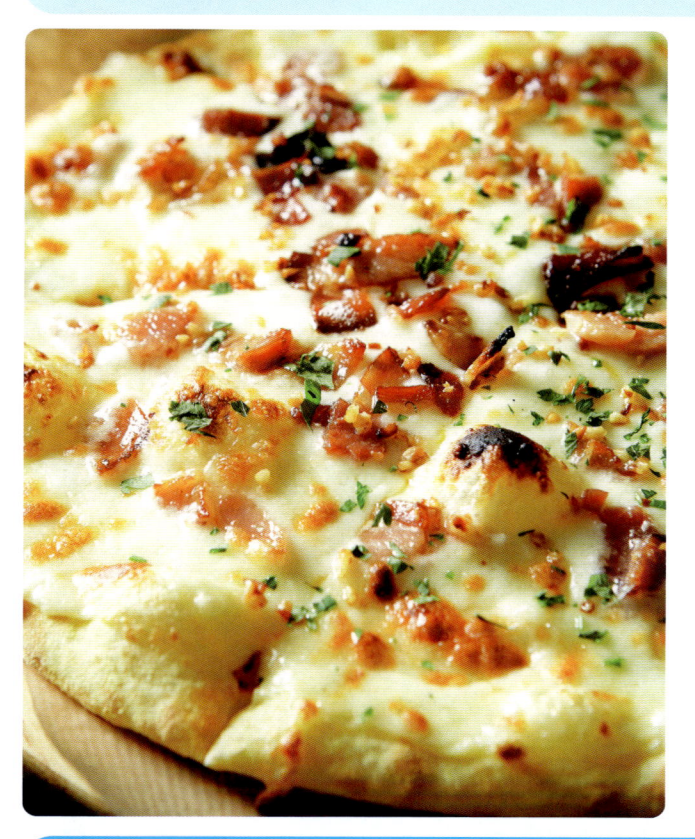

Ingredients Servings: 2

Pizza:
- 1/2 cup all purpose flour
- 3/4 cup nonfat plain greek yogurt
- 1/2 cup part skim mozzarella cheese
- 1 cup shredded chicken
- 12 slices turkey bacon
- 1/2 cup nonfat plain greek yogurt
- 1 tsp baking powder

Ranch Dressing:
- 1 cup nonfat plain Greek yogurt
- 2 tbsp bunch cilantro
- 2 tbsp lemon
- 1 tsp extra-virgin olive oil
- 1 tbsp ranch dressing seasoning

Optional Sides

- Salad (2 cups greens, 1 tbsp extra virgin olive oil, 2 tbsp balsamic - 307c, 4P, 11C, 27F)
- Protein shake (2 cups almond milk, 1 scoop Dummy Supps - 190c, 26P, 9C, 6F)

Instructions

1. Preheat oven to 425°F.
2. Mix flour, Greek yogurt, and baking powder in a bowl until a dough forms.
3. Roll out dough on a floured surface and shape into a pizza crust.
4. Place crust on a parchment-lined baking sheet or pizza stone.
5. Cook turkey bacon in a pan over medium heat until crispy, then chop into pieces.
6. Blend Greek yogurt, cilantro, lemon juice, olive oil, and ranch seasoning until smooth to make the ranch dressing.
7. Spread ranch dressing over the pizza crust.
8. Top with shredded chicken, chopped turkey bacon, and mozzarella cheese.
9. Bake for 15-20 minutes until cheese is melted and crust is golden.
10. Drizzle with ranch dressing before serving.

MULTIPLE MEAL PREPS

BUFFALO CHICKEN PIZZA

Calories: 610   **Protein: 57**   **Carbs: 33**   **Fat: 32**

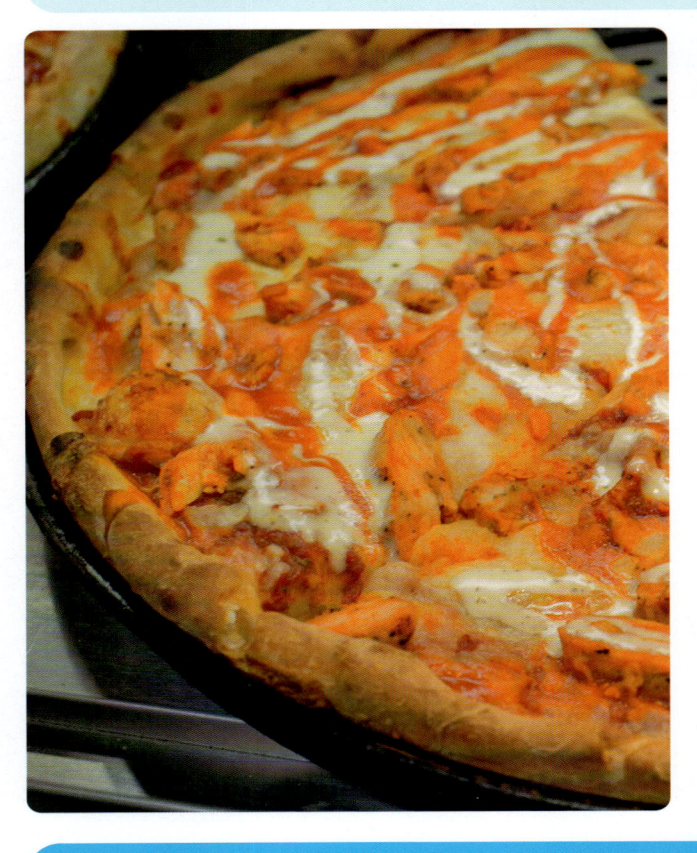

Ingredients   Servings: 2

Pizza:
- 1/2 cup all purpose flour
- 3/4 cup nonfat plain greek yogurt
- 1/4 cup franks red hot
- 1 tbsp butter
- 1/2 cup part skim mozzarella cheese
- 1 cup shredded chicken
- 1/2 cup nonfat plain greek yogurt
- 1 tsp baking powder

Ranch Dressing:
- 1 cup nonfat plain Greek yogurt
- 2 tbsp bunch cilantro
- 2 tbsp lemon
- 1 tsp extra-virgin olive oil
- 1 tbsp ranch dressing seasoning

Optional Sides

- Salad (2 cups greens, 1 tbsp extra virgin olive oil, 2 tbsp balsamic - 307c, 4P, 11C, 27F)
- Protein shake (2 cups almond milk, 1 scoop Dummy Supps - 190c, 26P, 9C, 6F)

Instructions

1. Preheat oven to 425°F.
2. Mix flour, Greek yogurt, and baking powder in a bowl until a dough forms.
3. Roll out dough on a floured surface and shape into a pizza crust.
4. Place crust on a parchment-lined baking sheet or pizza stone.
5. Melt butter and mix with Frank's Red Hot to make buffalo sauce.
6. Toss shredded chicken in buffalo sauce until evenly coated.
7. Blend Greek yogurt, cilantro, lemon juice, olive oil, and ranch seasoning until smooth to make the ranch dressing.
8. Spread ranch dressing over the pizza crust.
9. Top with buffalo chicken and mozzarella cheese.
10. Bake for 15-20 minutes until cheese is melted and crust is golden.
11. Drizzle with ranch dressing before serving.

MULTIPLE MEAL PREPS

BBQ CHICKEN PIZZA

Calories: 400 **Protein: 46** **Carbs: 35** **Fat: 13**

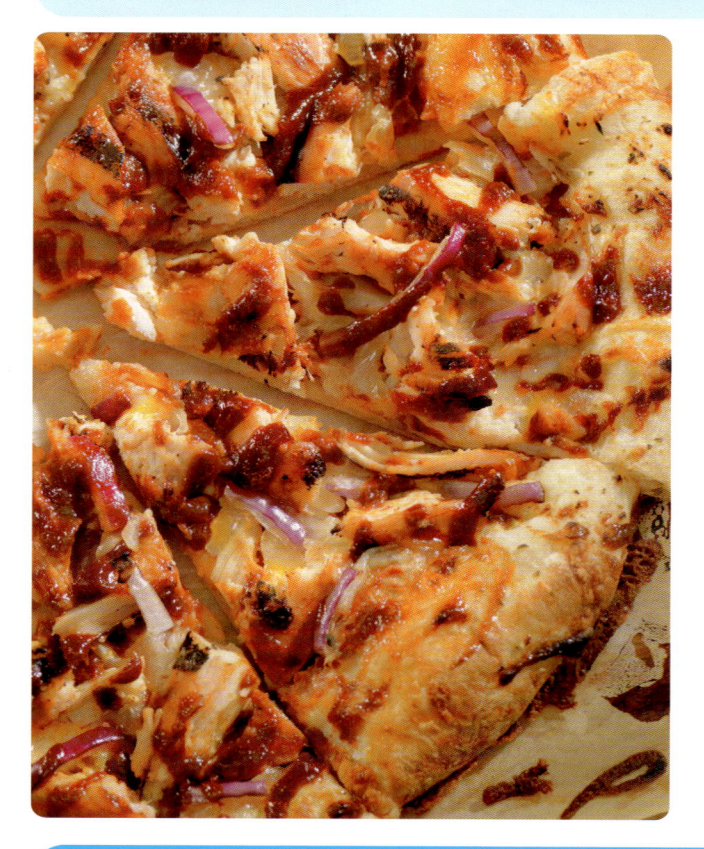

Ingredients **Servings: 2**

Pizza:
- 1/2 cup all purpose flour
- 3/4 cup nonfat plain greek yogurt
- 1/2 cup G Hughes BBQ sauce
- 1/2 cup part skim mozzarella cheese
- 1 cup shredded chicken
- 1/4 cup red onion
- 1 tsp baking powder

Optional Sides

- Salad (2 cups greens, 1 tbsp extra virgin olive oil, 2 tbsp balsamic - 307c, 4P, 11C, 27F)
- Protein shake (2 cups almond milk, 1 scoop Dummy Supps - 190c, 26P, 9C, 6F)

Instructions

1. Preheat oven to 425°F.
2. Mix flour, Greek yogurt, and baking powder in a bowl until a dough forms.
3. Roll out dough on a floured surface and shape into a pizza crust.
4. Place crust on a parchment-lined baking sheet or pizza stone.
5. Toss shredded chicken in BBQ sauce until evenly coated.
6. Spread a thin layer of BBQ sauce over the pizza crust.
7. Top with BBQ chicken, mozzarella cheese, and sliced red onion.
8. Bake for 15-20 minutes until cheese is melted and crust is golden.

INDIVIDUAL MEAL PREP

OPTIONAL ADD ON'S

SNACKS

- **Protein Shake:** 1 scoop Dummy Supps Whey, 2 cups almond milk (190c, 26P, 9C, 6F)
- **Chocolate PB Shake:** 1 scoop Dummy Supps Chocolate Whey, 2 cups almond milk (190c, 26P, 9C, 6F)
- **Side Salad:** 2 cups greens, 2 tbsp olive oil, 2 tbsp balsamic: (307c, 4P, 11C, 27F)
- **PB&J Sandwich:** 2 slices 647 bread, 2 tbsp PB2, 1 tbsp water, 2 tbsp SF jam (160c, 9P, 31C, 3F)
- **PB & Banana Sandwich:** 2 slices 647 bread, 2 tbsp PB2, 1 tbsp water, 1 banana, 1 tsp cinnamon (235c, 10P, 50C, 3F)
- **Hard Boiled Eggs:** 2 eggs (144c, 12P, 0C, 10F)
- **Turkey Rice Cake:** 2 salted rice cakes, 2 slices turkey breast, 1 slice cheese, 1 tbsp lite mayo (220c, 16P, 25C, 8F)
- **Turkey Roll Ups:** 4 slices turkey breast (119c, 17P, 2C, 4F)
- **Mixed nuts:** 1/4 cup (217c, 7P, 21C, 21F)

- **Raspberries:** 1 cup (80c, 1P, 18C, 1F)
- **Blackberries:** 1 cup (80c, 1P, 18C, 1F)
- **Apple:** 1 whole (100c, 1P, 28C, 0F)
- **Strawberries:** 2 cups diced (100c, 1P, 23C, 1F)
- **Grapes:** 2 cups (200c, 1P, 54C, 0F)
- **Apple & PB:** 1 whole apple, 2 tbsp PB2, 1 tbsp water (154c, 6P, 33C, 2F)
- **Blueberries:** 1 cup (80c, 1P, 22C, 0F)
- **Clementines:** 2 whole (70c, 1P, 18C, 0F)
- **Veggies & Ranch:** 1 cup nonfat plain greek yogurt, 2 tsp ranch seasoning, 5 stalks celery/10 baby carrots (250c, 22P, 9C, 0F)
- **Veggies & Taco Dip:** 1 cup nonfat plain greek yogurt, 2 tsp taco seasoning, 5 stalks celery/10 baby carrots (250c, 22P, 9C, 0F)
- **Lite Popcorn:** 2 cups (150c, 2P, 15C, 10F)
- **Greek Yogurt:** 3/4 cup non fat plain, 1/2 cup berries (150c, 25P, 30C, 1F)

INDIVIDUAL MEAL PREP

OPTIONAL ADD ON'S

SAUCES

- **Tzatziki Sauce:** 1/2 cup nonfat plain greek yogurt, 1/4 cup grated cucumber, 1 tbsp dill, 2 tsp lemon juice, 1/2 tsp olive oil. 1/4 tsp salt (100c, 11P, 11C, 2F)
- **Protein Ranch:** 1/2 cup nonfat plain greek yogurt, 2 tsp ranch dressing seasoning (80c, 11P, 4C, 2F)
- **Protein Taco Dip:** 1/2 cup nonfat plain greek yogurt, 2 tsp taco dressing seasoning (80c, 11P, 4C, 2F)
- **Hot Sauce:** 2 tbsp (0c, 0P, 0C, 0F)
- **Salsa:** 2 tbsp (10c, 0P, 3C, 0F)
- **Lite Sour Cream:** 2 tbsp (35c, 2P, 2C, 3F)
- **Marinara:** 1/2 cup (50c, 2P, 11C, 1F)
- **Yellow Mustard:** 2 tbsp (1P, 0C, 0F)
- **Low Sodium Soy Sauce:** 1 tbsp (10c, 1P, 1C, 0F)
- **Hummus:** 1 tbsp (36c, 1P, 2C, 3F)
- **Balsamic Glaze:** 1 tbsp (25c, 0P, 6C, 0F)
- **Olive Oil:** 1 tbsp (120c, 0P, 0C, 14F)
- **Balsamic Vinegar:** 1 tbsp (14c, 0P, 3C, 0F)
- **G Hughes Teriyaki:** 2 tbsp (10c, 0P, 2C, 0F)
- **G Hughes Thai Chili:** 2 tbsp (10c, 0P, 2C, 0F)
- **G Hughes Burger Sauce:** 2 tbsp (100c, 0P, 2C, 10F)
- **G Hughes Stir Fry:** 2 tbsp (10c, 0P, 2C, 0F)
- **G Hughes BBQ:** 2 tbsp (10c, 0P, 2C, 0F)
- **G Hughes Sweet & Spicy:** 2 tbsp (10c, 0P, 2C, 0F)
- **G Hughes Ketchup:** 2 tbsp (5c, 0P, 2C, 0F)
- **G Hughes Sweet Chili Sauce:** 2 tbsp (100c, 0P, 2C, 10F)

CHEESECAKES

PROTEIN CHEESECAKES

DESSERT RECIPES

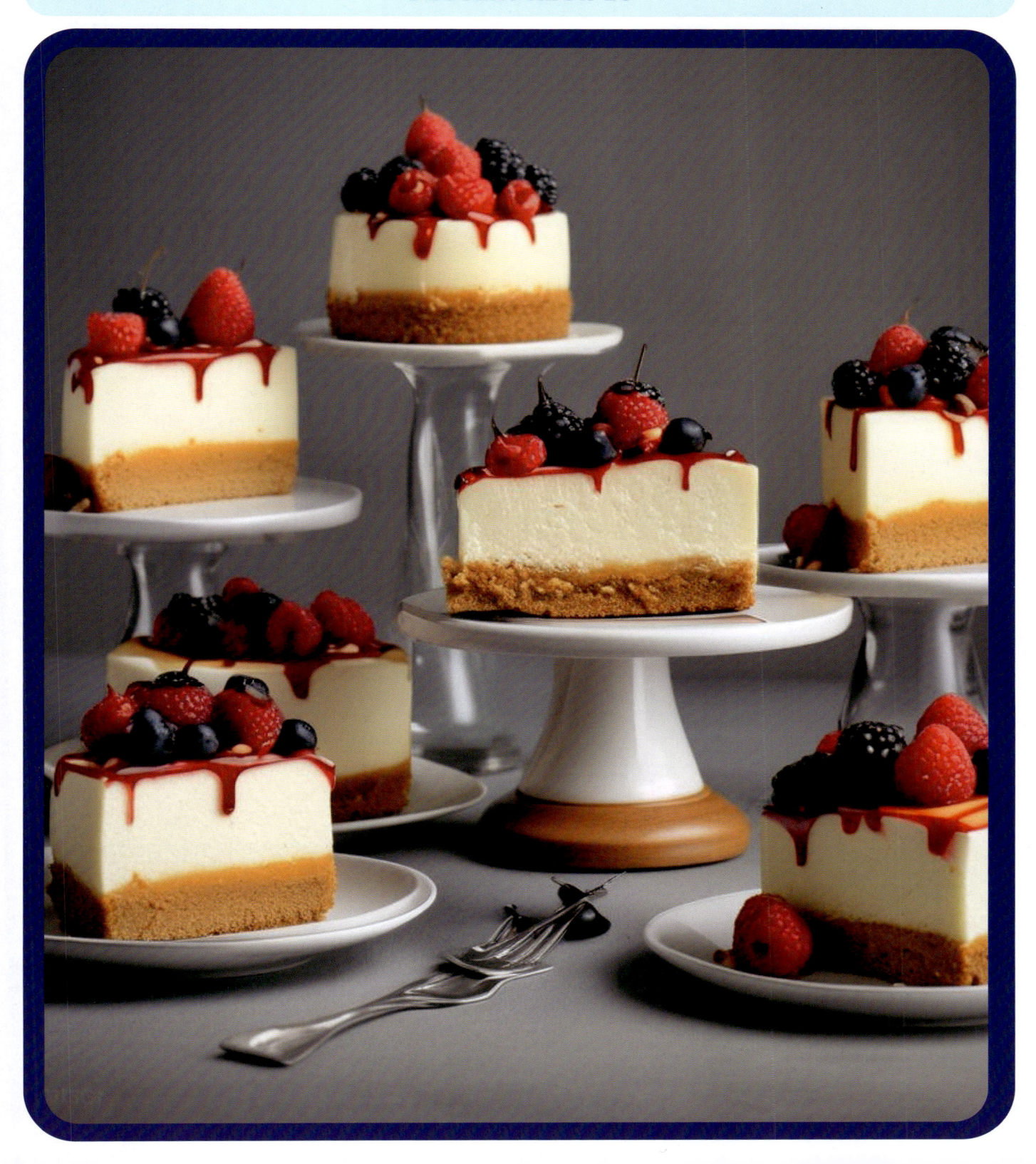

CHEESECAKES

CHOCOLATE

Calories: 430 **Protein: 44** **Carbs: 34** **Fat: 13**

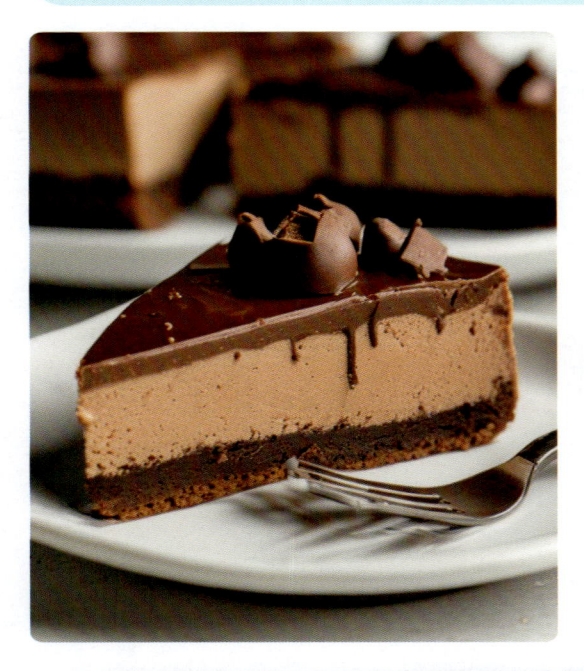

Ingredients — Servings: 1

- 3/4 cup nonfat plain Greek yogurt
- 1 scoop Dummy Supps Chocolate Whey
- 2 tbsp whipped cream cheese
- 1 tbsp cocoa powder
- 1 graham cracker

Dummy Supps Whey Protein — SCAN ME

Instructions

1. In a bowl, mix Greek yogurt, chocolate whey, whipped cream cheese, and cocoa powder until smooth.
2. Crush the graham cracker and sprinkle on top.
3. Set in fridge for 10 minutes or overnight.

VANILLA

Calories: 410 **Protein: 43** **Carbs: 31** **Fat: 12**

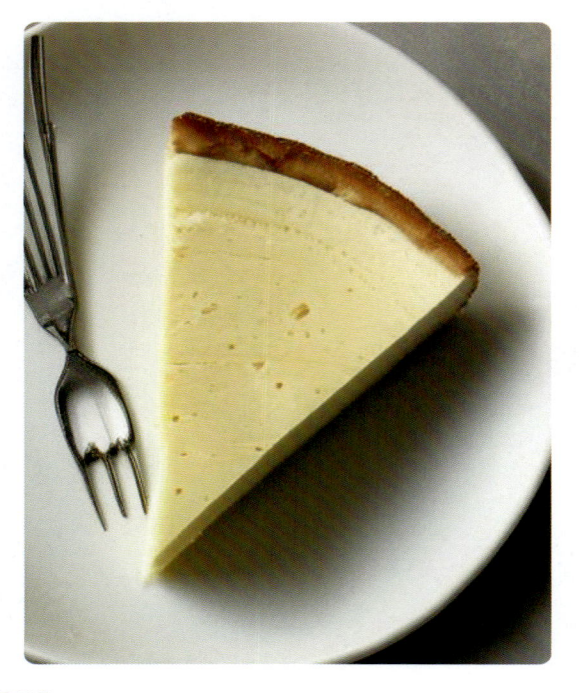

Ingredients — Servings: 1

- 3/4 cup nonfat vanilla Greek yogurt
- 1 scoop Dummy Supps Vanilla Whey
- 2 tbsp whipped cream cheese
- 2 tbsp Lilly's White Chocolate Chips
- 1/2 tsp vanilla extract
- 1 graham cracker

Dummy Supps Whey Protein — SCAN ME

Instructions

1. In a bowl, mix nonfat vanilla Greek yogurt, vanilla whey, whipped cream cheese, and vanilla extract until smooth.
2. Fold in Lilly's White Chocolate Chips.
3. Crush the graham cracker and fold it into the mixture.
4. Set in the fridge for 10 minutes or overnight.

CHEESECAKES

CHOCOLATE CHIP

Calories: 430 **Protein: 44** **Carbs: 28** **Fat: 20**

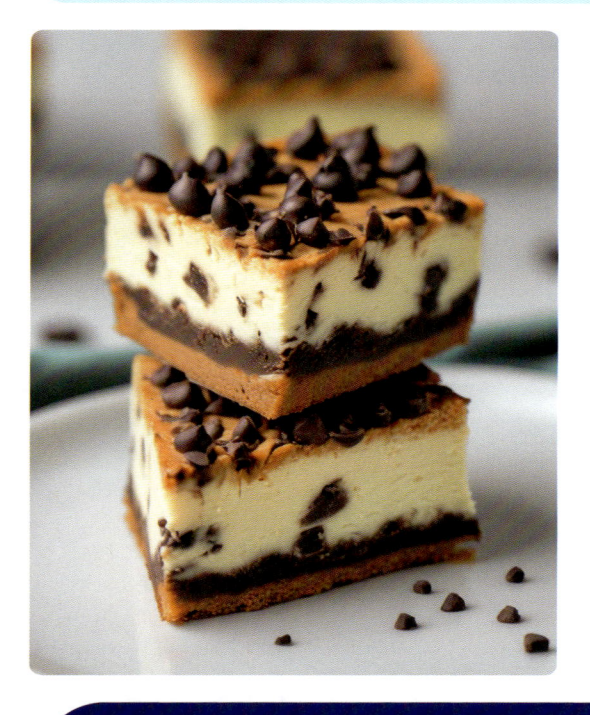

Ingredients — Servings: 1

- 3/4 cup nonfat vanilla Greek yogurt
- 1/2 scoop Dummy Supps Chocolate Whey
- 1/2 scoop Dummy Supps Vanilla Whey
- 2 tbsp Lilly's Dark Chocolate Chips
- 2 tbsp whipped cream cheese
- 2 Simple Mills Chocolate Chip Crunchy Cookies

Dummy Supps Whey Protein — SCAN ME

Instructions

1. In a bowl, mix 3/4 cup nonfat vanilla Greek yogurt, 1/2 scoop Dummy Supps Chocolate Whey, 1/2 scoop Dummy Supps Vanilla Whey, and 2 tbsp whipped cream cheese until smooth.
2. Fold in 2 tbsp Lilly's Dark Chocolate Chips.
3. Crush the 2 Simple Mills Chocolate Chip Crunchy Cookies and fold them into the mixture.
4. Refrigerate for at least 10 minutes or overnight.

CHOCOLATE PEANUT BUTTER

Calories: 410 **Protein: 48** **Carbs: 28** **Fat: 14**

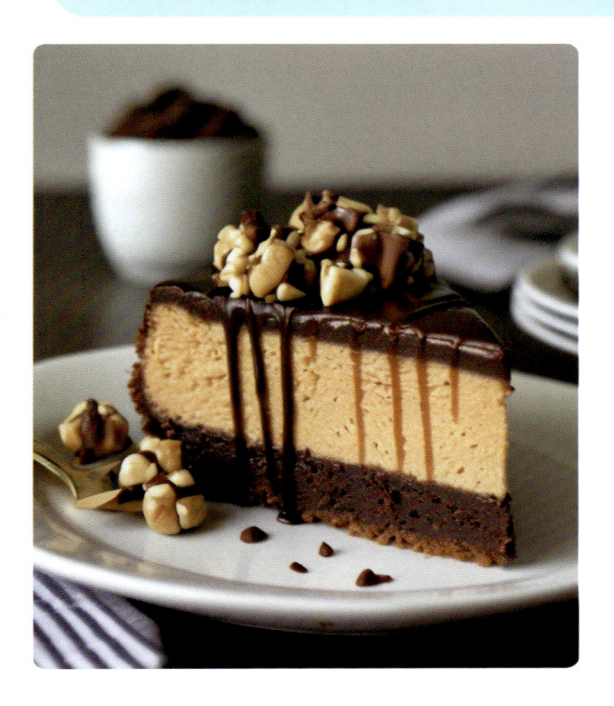

Ingredients — Servings: 1

- 3/4 cup nonfat plain Greek yogurt
- 1 scoop Dummy Supps Chocolate PB whey
- 2 tbsp whipped cream cheese
- 2 tbsp powdered peanut butter
- 1 graham cracker

Dummy Supps Whey Protein — SCAN ME

Instructions

1. In a bowl, mix Greek yogurt, chocolate PB whey, whipped cream cheese, and powdered peanut butter until smooth.
2. Crush the graham cracker and sprinkle on top.
3. Set in fridge for 10 minutes or overnight.

CHEESECAKES

APPLE PIE

Calories: 410 **Protein: 43** **Carbs: 36** **Fat: 12**

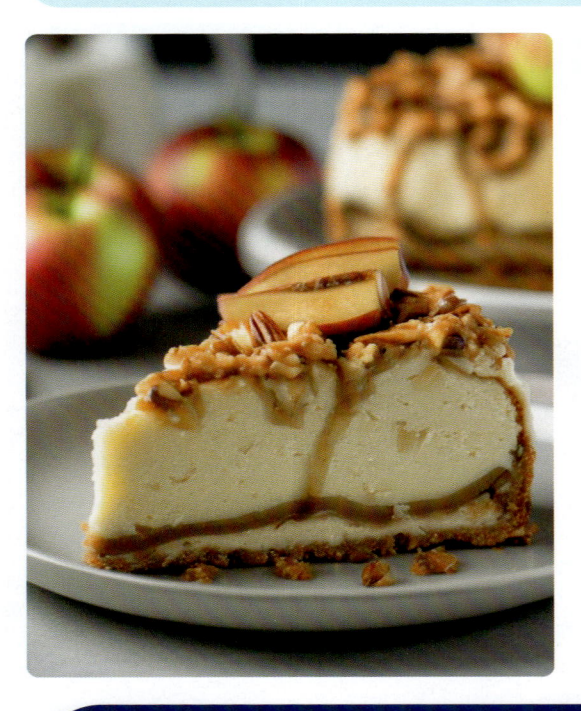

Ingredients — Servings: 1

- 3/4 cup nonfat vanilla Greek yogurt
- 1 scoop Dummy Supps Vanilla Whey
- 2 tbsp whipped cream cheese
- 1/2 chopped apple
- 1 tsp lemon juice
- 1 tbsp zero-calorie brown sugar
- 1 tsp cinnamon
- 1 graham cracker

Dummy Supps Whey Protein — SCAN ME

Instructions

1. In a bowl, mix Greek yogurt, vanilla whey, and whipped cream cheese until smooth. Chop the apple into small pieces.
2. Set in fridge for 10 minutes or overnight.
3. Heat a pan over medium heat and add apple, lemon juice, cinnamon, and brown sugar. Sauté for 3-4 minutes until softened.
4. Top cheesecake with sautéed apples and crushed graham cracker.

SALTED CARAMEL

Calories: 410 **Protein: 43** **Carbs: 29** **Fat: 16**

Ingredients — Servings: 1

- 3/4 cup nonfat plain Greek yogurt
- 1 scoop Dummy Supps Salted Caramel Whey
- 2 tbsp whipped cream cheese
- 2 tbsp Lilly's Salted Caramel Chips
- 1 graham cracker
- 1/4 tsp salt

Dummy Supps Whey Protein — SCAN ME

Instructions

1. In a bowl, mix Greek yogurt, salted caramel whey, and whipped cream cheese until smooth.
2. Stir in Lilly's Salted Caramel Chips.
3. Crush the graham cracker and sprinkle on top with salt.
4. Set in fridge for 10 minutes or overnight.

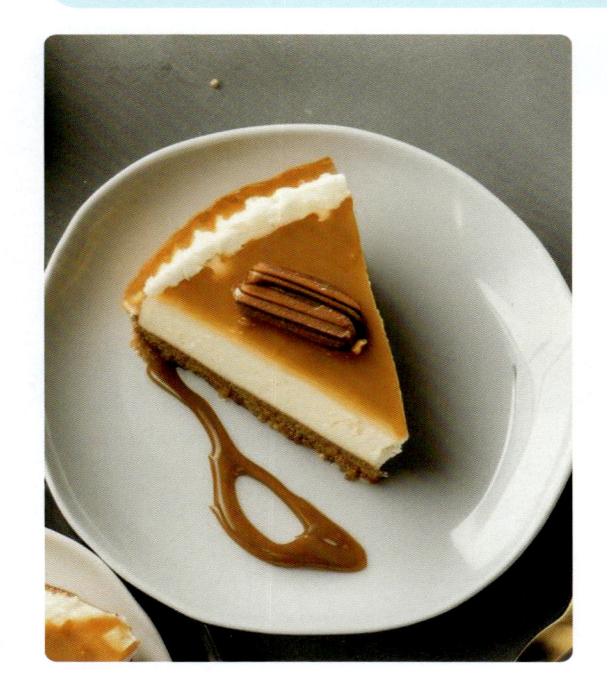

CHEESECAKES

TIRAMISU

Calories: 380 **Protein: 44** **Carbs: 24** **Fat: 14**

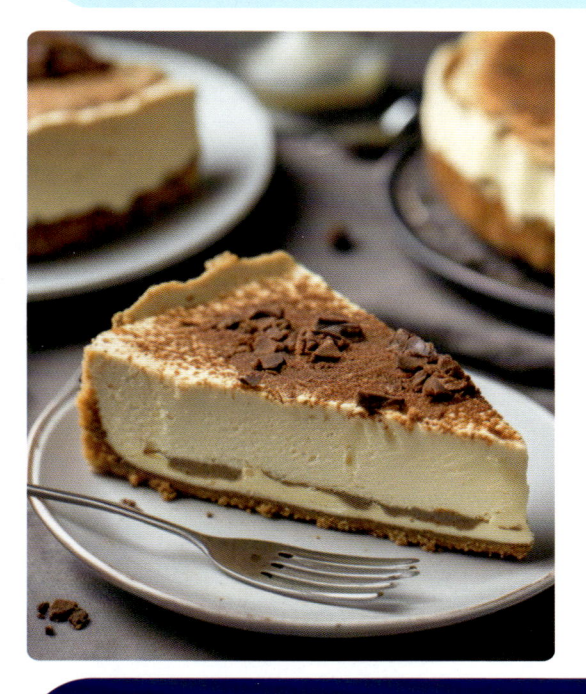

Ingredients — Servings: 1

- 3/4 cup nonfat plain Greek yogurt
- 1 scoop Dummy Supps Chocolate Whey
- 2 tbsp whipped cream cheese
- 1 tsp instant espresso
- 1 tbsp cocoa powder
- 1 graham cracker

Dummy Supps Whey Protein (SCAN ME)

Instructions

1. In a bowl, mix Greek yogurt, chocolate whey, whipped cream cheese, instant espresso, and cocoa powder until smooth.
2. Crush the graham cracker and sprinkle on top.
3. Set in fridge for 10 minutes or overnight.

MINT CHOCOLATE

Calories: 430 **Protein: 45** **Carbs: 31** **Fat: 18**

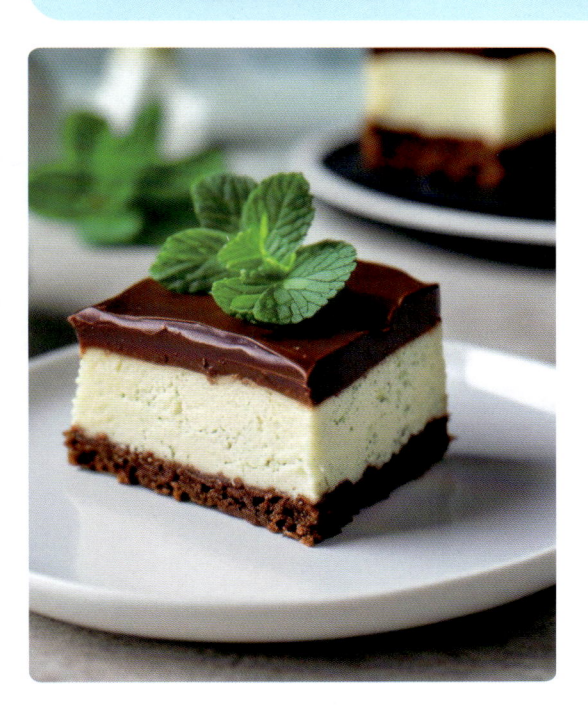

Ingredients — Servings: 1

- 3/4 cup nonfat plain Greek yogurt
- 1 scoop Dummy Supps Chocolate Whey
- 1 tsp instant espresso
- 2 tbsp whipped cream cheese
- 1/2 tsp spearmint extract
- 1 tbsp cocoa powder
- 2 tbsp Lilly's Mint Chocolate Chips
- 2 Simple Mills Chocolate Mint Thins

Dummy Supps Whey Protein (SCAN ME)

Instructions

1. In a bowl, mix nonfat plain Greek yogurt, chocolate whey, instant espresso, whipped cream cheese, spearmint extract, and cocoa powder until smooth.
2. Crush the Simple Mills Chocolate Mint Thins and fold them into the mixture.
3. Set in the fridge for 10 minutes or overnight.

CHEESECAKES

PEANUT BUTTER AND JELLY

Calories: 570 **Protein: 53** **Carbs: 39** **Fat: 25**

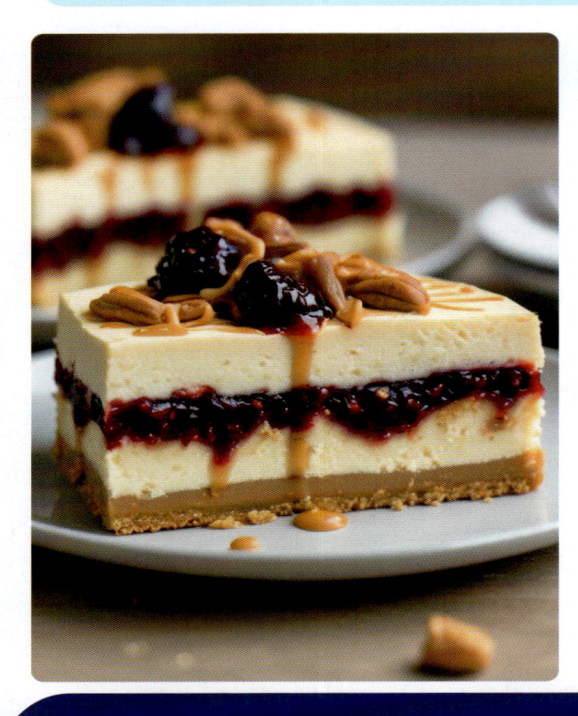

Ingredients — Servings: 1

- 3/4 cup nonfat plain Greek yogurt
- 1 scoop Dummy Supps Berry Whey
- 2 tbsp whipped cream cheese
- 1 cup strawberries
- 1 tbsp zero calorie sugar
- 1 tsp lemon juice
- 1 tbsp PB&J Dummy Butter
- 1 graham cracker

Dummy Supps Whey Protein — SCAN ME

Instructions

1. In a bowl, mix Greek yogurt, vanilla whey protein, and whipped cream cheese until smooth.
2. Refrigerate for at least 10 minutes or overnight.
3. In a pan over medium heat, add strawberries, zero-calorie sweetener, and lemon juice. Sauté for 3-4 minutes until softened.
4. Top the chilled yogurt mixture with the sautéed strawberries and sprinkle with crushed graham cracker.

MOCHA

Calories: 510 **Protein: 52** **Carbs: 28** **Fat: 25**

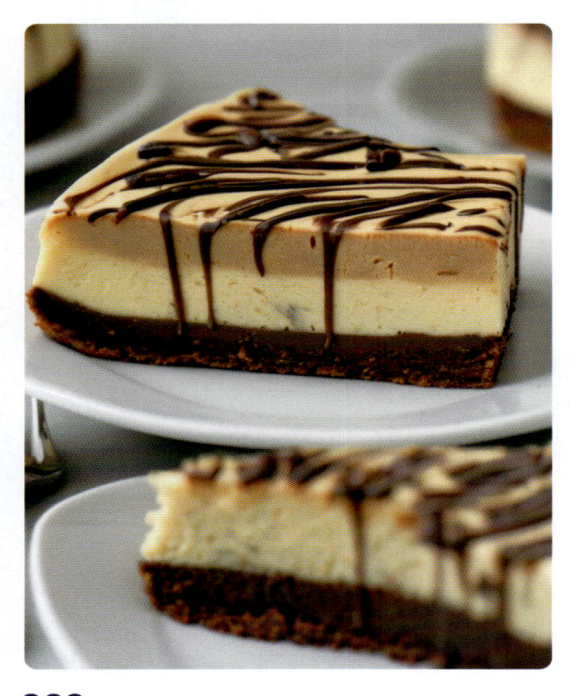

Ingredients — Servings: 1

- 3/4 cup nonfat plain Greek yogurt
- 1 scoop Dummy Supps Chocolate Whey Protein
- 1 tsp instant espresso
- 2 tbsp whipped cream cheese
- 1 tbsp Mocha Peanut Dummy Butter
- 1 graham cracker

Dummy Supps Whey Protein — SCAN ME

Instructions

1. In a bowl, mix nonfat plain Greek yogurt, Dummy Supps Chocolate Whey Protein, instant espresso whipped cream cheese, and Mocha Peanut Dummy Butter until smooth.
2. Crush the graham cracker and sprinkle on top.
3. Set in the fridge for 10 minutes or overnight.

CHEESECAKES

BERRY BLAST

Calories: 560 **Protein: 53** **Carbs: 40** **Fat: 25**

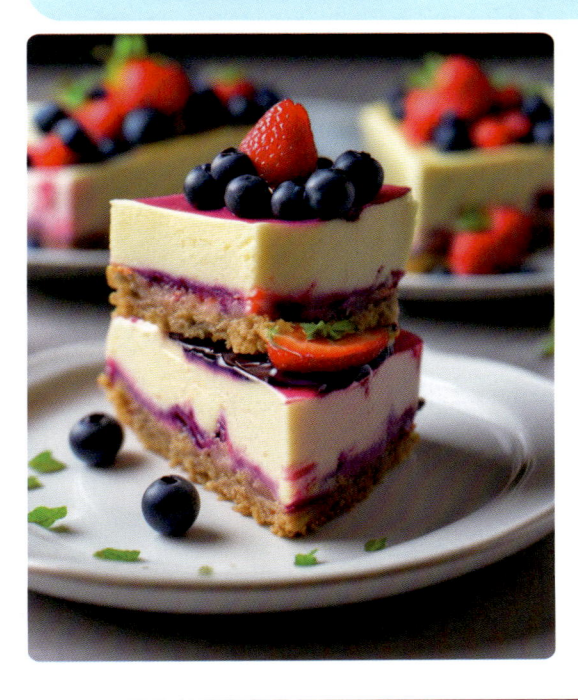

Ingredients Servings: 1

- 3/4 cup nonfat plain Greek yogurt
- 1 scoop Dummy Supps Berry Whey Protein
- 2 tbsp whipped cream cheese
- 1 cup mixed berries
- 1 tbsp PB&J Dummy Butter
- 1 graham cracker

Dummy Supps Whey Protein — SCAN ME

Instructions

1. In a bowl, mix nonfat plain Greek yogurt, Dummy Supps Berry Whey Protein, whipped cream cheese, and PB&J Dummy Butter until smooth.
2. Crush the graham cracker and sprinkle on top.
3. Set in the fridge for 10 minutes or overnight.

KEY LIME PIE

Calories: 350 **Protein: 43** **Carbs: 22** **Fat: 12**

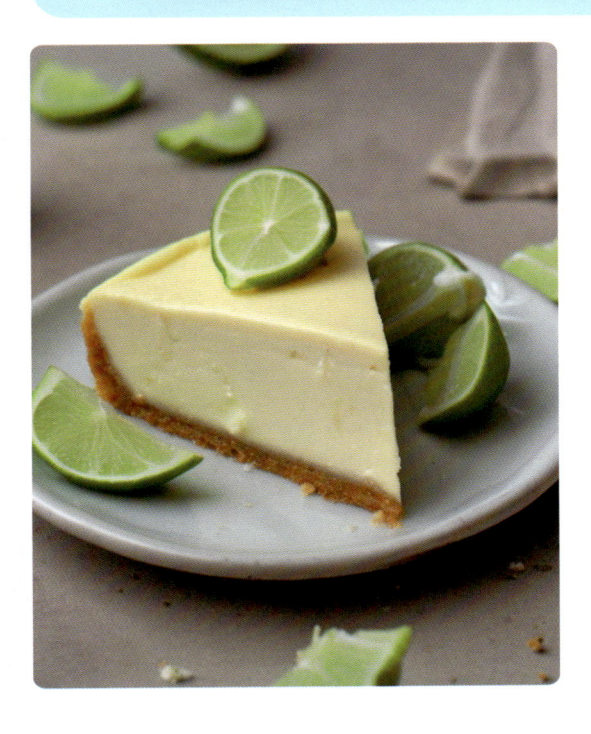

Ingredients Servings: 1

- 3/4 cup nonfat plain Greek yogurt
- 1 scoop Dummy Supps Vanilla Whey Protein
- 2 tbsp whipped cream cheese
- 1 tsp lime juice
- 1 tablespoon lime zest

Dummy Supps Whey Protein — SCAN ME

Instructions

1. In a bowl, mix nonfat plain Greek yogurt, Dummy Supps Vanilla Whey Protein, whipped cream cheese, lime juice, and lime zest until smooth.
2. Crush the graham cracker and sprinkle on top.
3. Set in the fridge for 10 minutes or overnight.

CHEESECAKES

MAPLE PECAN

Calories: 400   **Protein: 44**   **Carbs: 17**   **Fat: 23**

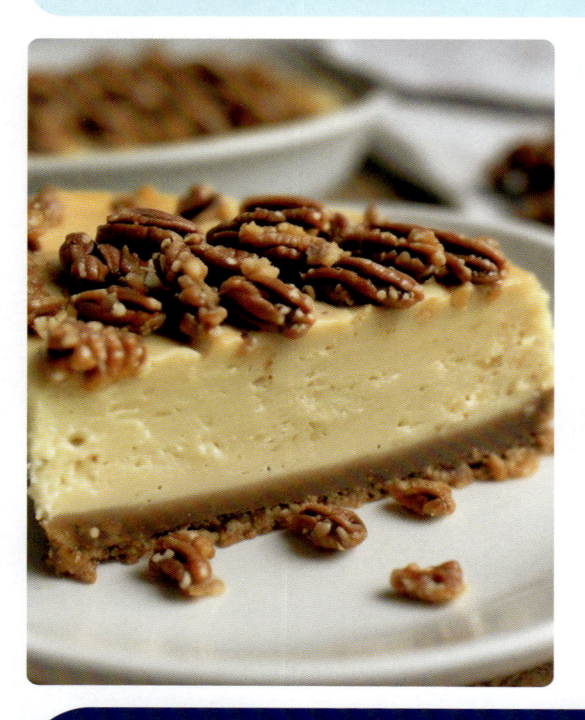

Ingredients   Servings: 1

- 3/4 cup nonfat plain Greek yogurt
- 1 scoop Dummy Supps Cinnamon Bun Whey Protein
- 2 tbsp whipped cream cheese
- 1 tbsp chopped pecans
- 1 graham cracker

Dummy Supps Whey Protein — SCAN ME

Instructions

1. In a bowl, mix nonfat plain Greek yogurt, Dummy Supps Cinnamon Bun Whey Protein, whipped cream cheese, and Maple Pecan Dummy Butter until smooth.
2. Crush the graham cracker and sprinkle on top.
3. Set in the fridge for 10 minutes or overnight.

ALMOND JOY

Calories: 550   **Protein: 52**   **Carbs: 29**   **Fat: 28**

Ingredients   Servings: 1

- 3/4 cup nonfat plain Greek yogurt
- 1 scoop Dummy Supps Chocolate Whey Protein
- 1 tsp instant espresso
- 2 tbsp whipped cream cheese
- 1 tbsp unsweetened coconut shreds
- 1 tbsp Mocha Peanut Dummy Butter

Dummy Supps Whey Protein — SCAN ME

Instructions

1. In a bowl, mix nonfat plain Greek yogurt, Dummy Supps Chocolate Whey Protein, instant espresso, whipped cream cheese, and Mocha Peanut Dummy Butter until smooth.
2. Crush the graham cracker and sprinkle on top.
3. Set in the fridge for 10 minutes or overnight.

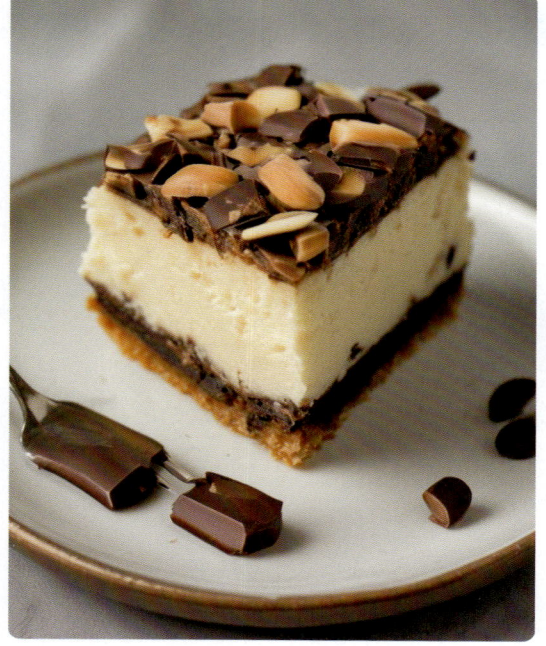

CHEESECAKES

MOCHA PEANUT BUTTER

Calories: 570 **Protein: 53** **Carbs: 37** **Fat: 30**

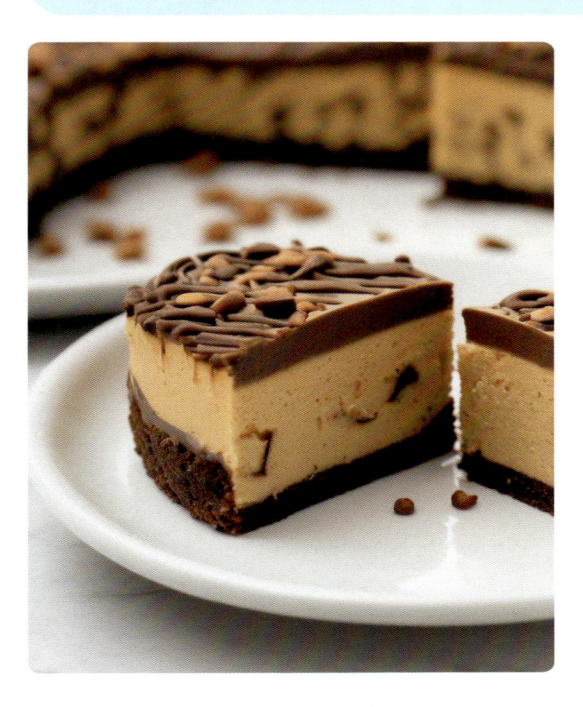

Ingredients — Servings: 1

- 3/4 cup nonfat plain Greek yogurt
- 1 scoop Dummy Supps Chocolate Whey Protein
- 1 tsp instant espresso
- 2 tbsp whipped cream cheese
- 1 tbsp Mocha Dummy Butter
- 2 tbsp Lilly's Dark Chocolate Chips
- 1 graham cracker

Dummy Supps Whey Protein — SCAN ME

Instructions

1. In a bowl, mix nonfat plain Greek yogurt, Dummy Supps Chocolate Protein, instant espresso, whipped cream cheese, and PB&J Dummy Butter until smooth.
2. Crush the graham cracker and sprinkle on top.
3. Set in the fridge for 10 minutes or overnight.

MIXED BERRY

Calories: 420 **Protein: 44** **Carbs: 39** **Fat: 18**

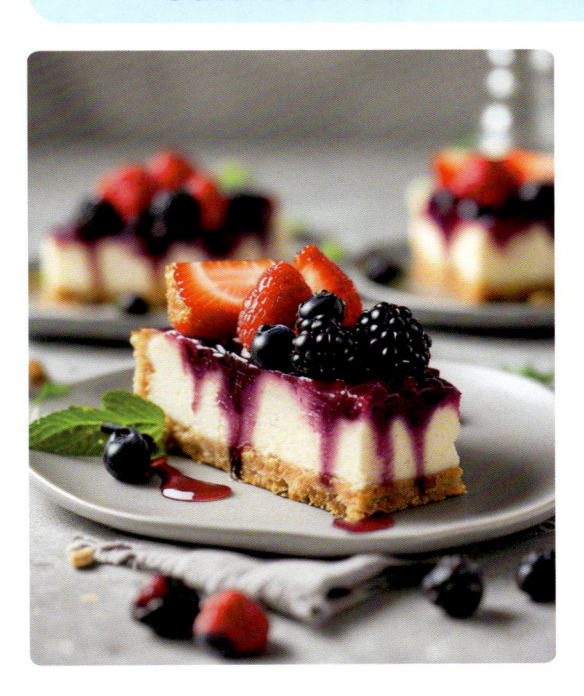

Ingredients — Servings: 1

- 3/4 cup nonfat plain Greek yogurt
- 1 scoop Dummy Supps Berry Whey Protein
- 2 tbsp whipped cream cheese
- 1 cup mixed berries
- 1 graham cracker

Dummy Supps Whey Protein — SCAN ME

Instructions

1. In a bowl, mix nonfat plain Greek yogurt, Dummy Supps Berry Whey Protein, whipped cream cheese, and Mocha Peanut Dummy Butter until smooth.
2. Crush the graham cracker and sprinkle on top.
3. Set in the fridge for 10 minutes or overnight.

CHEESECAKES

VANILLA PEANUT BUTTER

Calories: 370 **Protein: 48** **Carbs: 26** **Fat: 9**

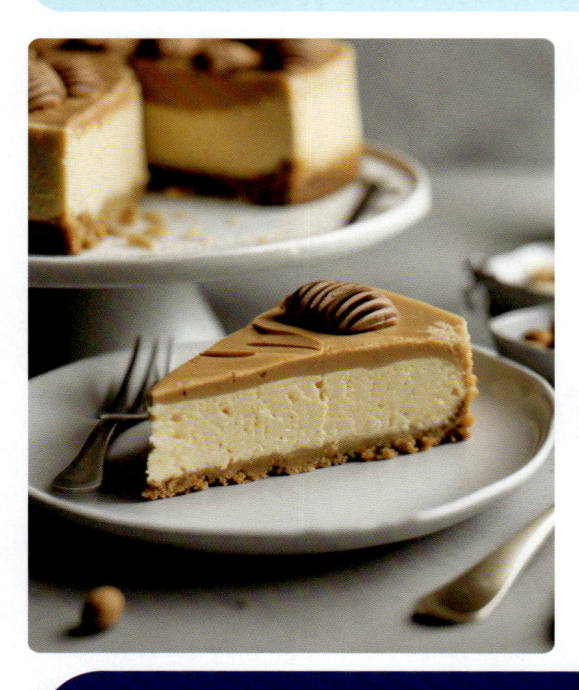

Ingredients Servings: 1

- 3/4 cup nonfat plain Greek yogurt
- 1 scoop Dummy Supps Vanilla Whey
- 2 tbsp powdered peanut butter
- 1 graham cracker
- 1/4 tsp salt

Dummy Supps Whey Protein
SCAN ME

Instructions

1. In a bowl, mix Greek yogurt, vanilla whey, powdered peanut butter, and salt until smooth.
2. Crush the graham cracker and sprinkle on top.
3. Set in fridge for 10 minutes or overnight.

CINNAMON SWIRL

Calories: 370 **Protein: 43** **Carbs: 37** **Fat: 12**

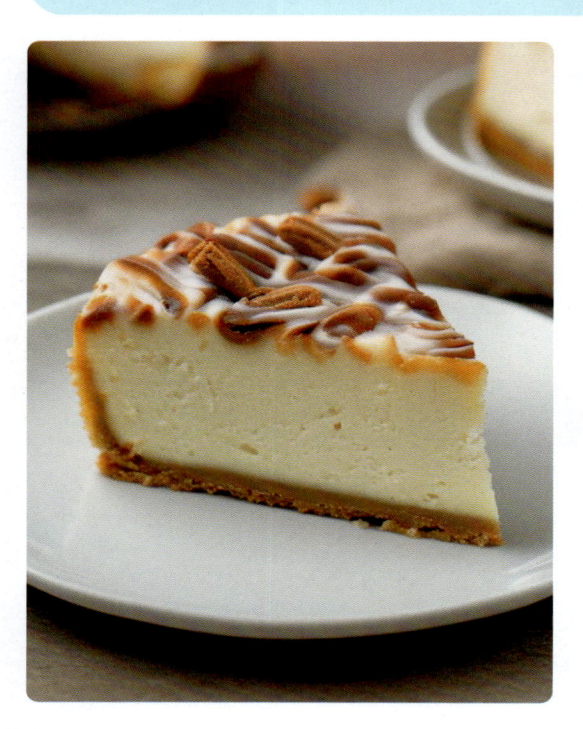

Ingredients Servings: 1

- 3/4 cup nonfat vanilla Greek yogurt
- 1 scoop Dummy Supps Cinnamon Swirl Whey
- 2 tbsp whipped cream cheese
- 1/2 tsp cinnamon
- 2 tbsp zero-calorie brown sugar
- 2 tbsp Lilly's Cinnamon Chocolate Chips
- 1 graham cracker

Dummy Supps Whey Protein
SCAN ME

Instructions

1. In a bowl, mix 3/4 cup nonfat vanilla Greek yogurt, 1 scoop Dummy Supps Cinnamon Swirl Whey, 2 tbsp whipped cream cheese, 1 tbsp cinnamon, and 2 tbsp zero-calorie brown sugar until smooth.
2. Crush the graham cracker and fold it into the mixture.
3. Refrigerate for at least 10 minutes or overnight.

CHEESECAKES

BANANA CREAM PIE

Calories: 420　　**Protein: 44**　　**Carbs: 38**　　**Fat: 14**

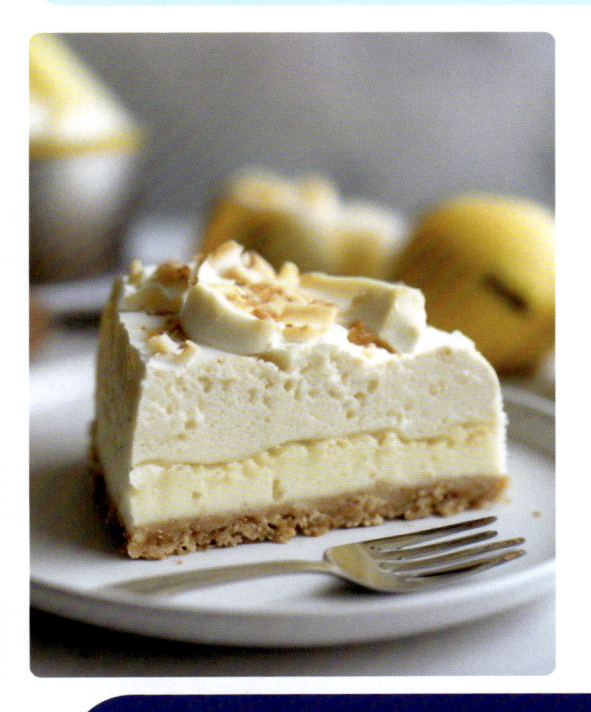

Ingredients　　Servings: 1

- 3/4 cup nonfat vanilla Greek yogurt
- 1 scoop Dummy Supps Vanilla Whey
- 2 tbsp whipped cream cheese
- 1/2 banana
- 2 tbsp Lite Cool Whip®
- 1 graham cracker

Dummy Supps Whey Protein

Instructions

1. In a bowl, mix Greek yogurt, vanilla whey, and whipped cream cheese until smooth.
2. Fold in Lite Cool Whip.
3. Slice the banana and stir it into the mixture.
4. Crush the graham cracker and sprinkle on top.
5. Set in the fridge for 10 minutes or overnight.

STRAWBERRY SHORTCAKE

Calories: 420　　**Protein: 44**　　**Carbs: 36**　　**Fat: 13**

Ingredients　　Servings: 1

- 3/4 cup nonfat vanilla Greek yogurt
- 1 scoop Dummy Supps vanilla whey
- 2 tbsp whipped cream cheese
- 1 cup fresh strawberries
- 2 tbsp Lite Cool Whip®
- 1 graham cracker

Dummy Supps Whey Protein

Instructions

1. In a bowl, mix 3/4 cup nonfat vanilla Greek yogurt, 1 scoop Dummy Supps vanilla whey, and 2 tbsp whipped cream cheese until smooth.
2. Fold in 1 cup fresh strawberries, chopped.
3. Crush the graham cracker and fold it into the mixture.
4. Top with 2 tbsp Lite Cool Whip®.
5. Refrigerate for at least 10 minutes or overnight.

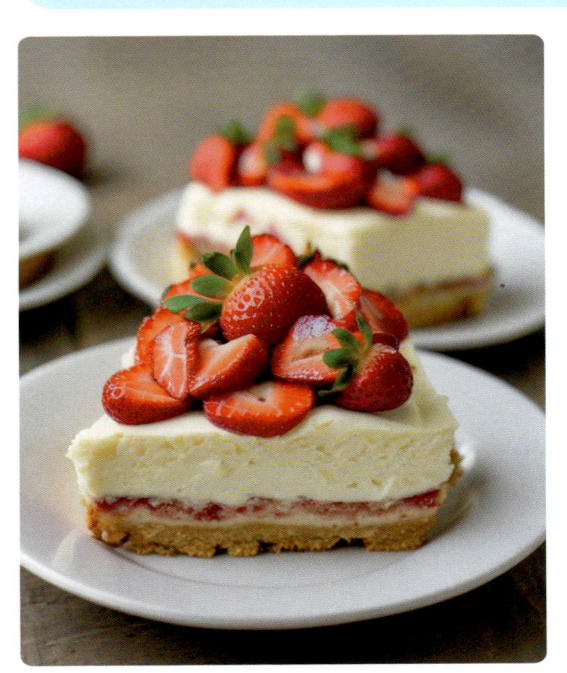

CHEESECAKES

COCONUT CREAM PIE

Calories: 400 **Protein: 44** **Carbs: 24** **Fat: 13**

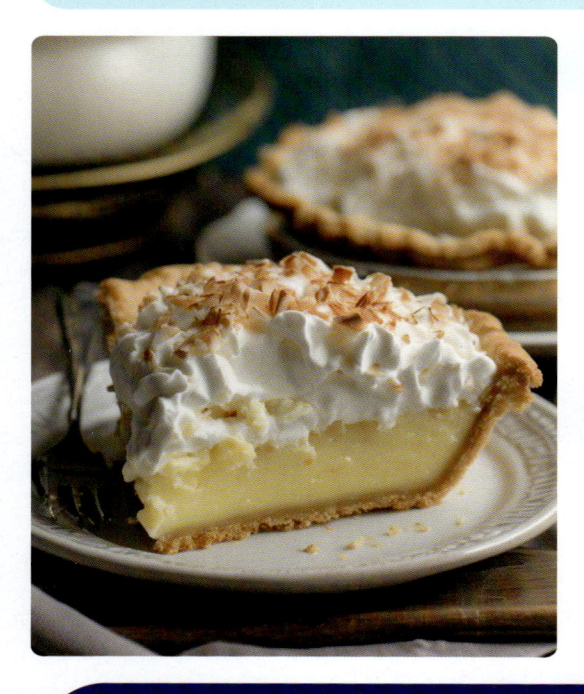

Ingredients — Servings: 1

- 3/4 cup nonfat vanilla Greek yogurt
- 1 scoop Dummy Supps Vanilla whey
- 2 tbsp whipped cream cheese
- 1 tbsp unsweetened coconut flakes
- 1/2 tsp vanilla extract
- 1 graham cracker

Dummy Supps Whey Protein — SCAN ME

Instructions

1. In a bowl, mix Greek yogurt, vanilla whey, whipped cream cheese, unsweetened coconut flakes, and vanilla extract until smooth.
2. Crush the graham cracker and sprinkle on top.
3. Set in fridge for 10 minutes or overnight.

S'MORES CHEESECAKE

Calories: 456 **Protein: 45** **Carbs: 44** **Fat: 18**

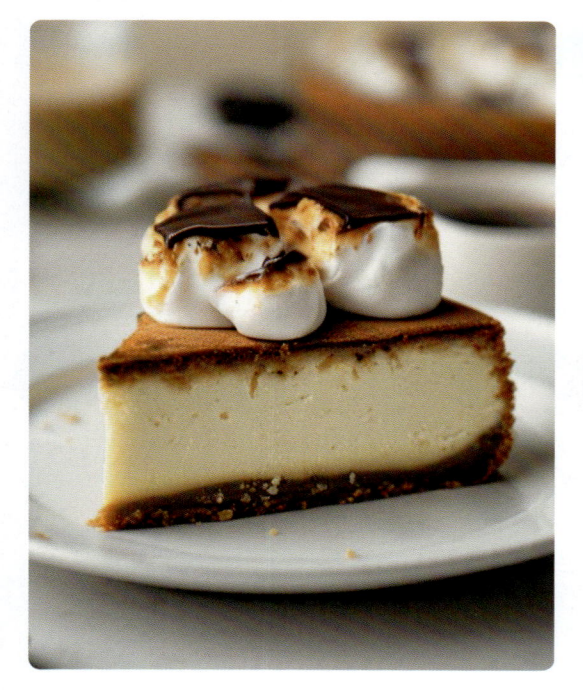

Ingredients — Servings: 1

- 3/4 cup nonfat vanilla Greek yogurt
- 1 scoop Dummy Supps Mocha/Chocolate whey
- 2 tbsp whipped cream cheese
- 2 tbsp marshmallow spread
- 1 tbsp cocoa powder
- 2 tbsp Lily's dark chocolate chips
- 1 graham cracker

Dummy Supps Whey Protein — SCAN ME

Instructions

1. In a bowl, mix Greek yogurt, mocha/chocolate whey, whipped cream cheese, marshmallow spread, and cocoa powder until smooth.
2. Stir in Lily's dark chocolate chips.
3. Crush the graham cracker and sprinkle on top.
4. Set in fridge for 10 minutes or overnight.

CHEESECAKES

CINNAMON ROLL

Calories: 374   **Protein: 43**   **Carbs: 29**   **Fat: 12**

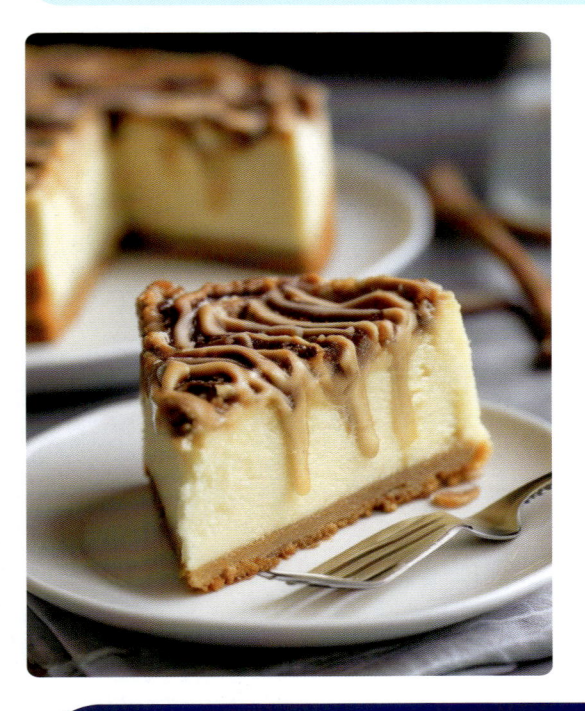

Ingredients — Servings: 1

- 3/4 cup nonfat plain Greek yogurt
- 1 scoop Dummy Supps Cinnamon Swirl whey
- 2 tbsp whipped cream cheese
- 1 graham cracker
- 1 tbsp brown sugar zero-calorie sweetener
- 1 tsp cinnamon

Dummy Supps Whey Protein (SCAN ME)

Instructions

1. In a mixing bowl, combine Greek yogurt, cinnamon swirl whey protein, whipped cream cheese, cinnamon, and brown sugar.
2. Mix until well combined and smooth.
3. Set in fridge for 10 minutes.
4. Top with crushed graham cracker.

PUMPKIN ROLL

Calories: 361   **Protein: 43**   **Carbs: 25**   **Fat: 12**

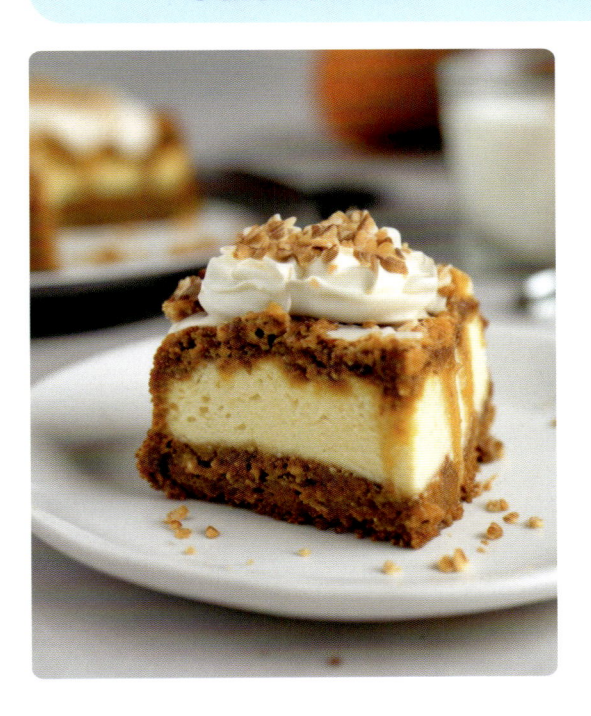

Ingredients — Servings: 1

- 3/4 cup nonfat vanilla Greek yogurt
- 1 scoop Dummy Supps cinnamon swirl whey
- 2 tbsp whipped cream cheese
- 2 tbsp pumpkin puree
- 1 tsp pumpkin spice
- 1 graham cracker

Instructions

1. In a bowl, mix 3/4 cup nonfat vanilla Greek yogurt, 1 scoop Dummy Supps cinnamon swirl whey, 2 tbsp whipped cream cheese, 2 tbsp pumpkin puree, and 1 tsp pumpkin spice until smooth.
2. Crush the graham cracker and fold it into the mixture.
3. Refrigerate for at least 10 minutes or overnight.

CHEESECAKES

PINEAPPLE UPSIDE DOWN CAKE

Calories: 440 **Protein: 43** **Carbs: 33** **Fat: 12**

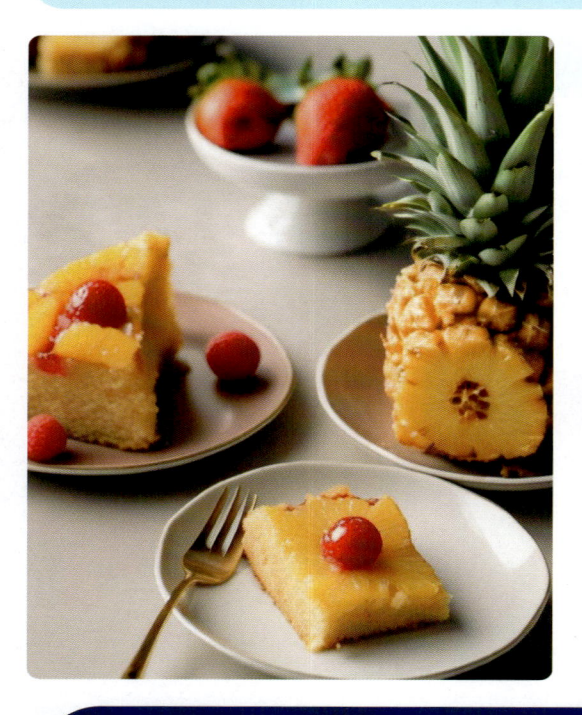

Ingredients — Servings: 1

- 3/4 cup nonfat vanilla Greek yogurt
- 1 scoop Dummy Supps Cinnamon Swirl Whey
- 2 tbsp whipped cream cheese
- 1/2 cup unsweetened pineapple chunks
- 2 maraschino cherries
- 1 graham cracker

Dummy Supps Whey Protein — SCAN ME

Instructions

1. In a bowl, mix Greek yogurt, vanilla whey, and whipped cream cheese until smooth.
2. Dice pineapple and stir it into the mixture.
3. Chop maraschino cherries and mix them in.
4. Crush the graham cracker and sprinkle on top.
5. Set in fridge for 10 minutes or overnight.

BANANAS FOSTER

Calories: 460 **Protein: 44** **Carbs: 49** **Fat: 12**

Ingredients — Servings: 1

- 3/4 cup nonfat vanilla Greek yogurt
- 1 scoop Dummy Supps Cinnamon Swirl Whey
- 2 tbsp whipped cream cheese
- 1/2 banana
- 1 tsp maple syrup
- 1/2 tsp cinnamon
- 1 graham cracker

Dummy Supps Whey Protein — SCAN ME

Instructions

1. In a bowl, mix Greek yogurt, cinnamon swirl whey, whipped cream cheese, and maple syrup until smooth.
2. Slice the banana and fold it into the mixture.
3. Crush the graham cracker and stir it in.
4. Sprinkle cinnamon on top.
5. Set in the fridge for 10 minutes or overnight.

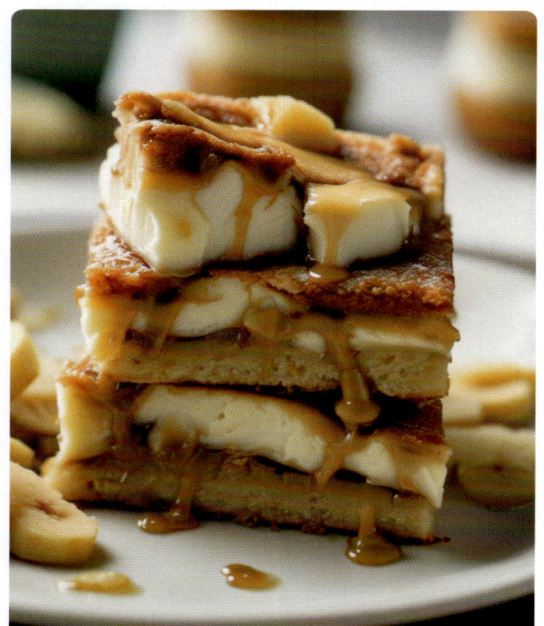

CHEESECAKES

VANILLA ALMOND

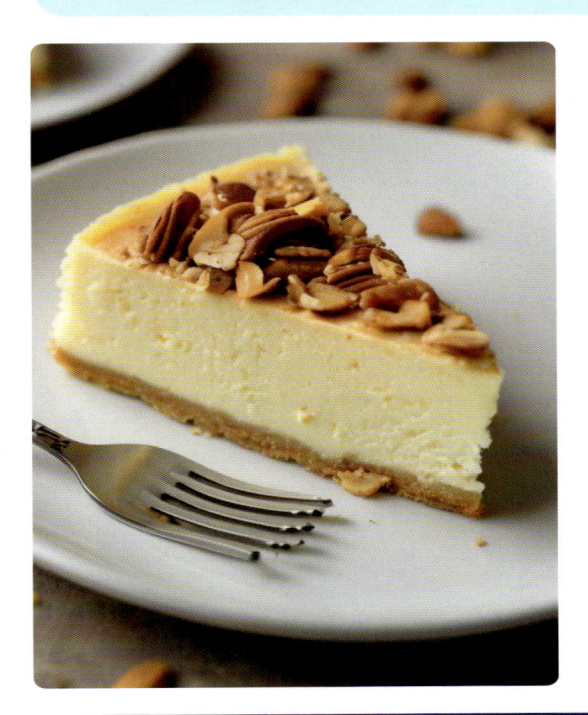

Calories: 370 **Protein: 44** **Carbs: 26** **Fat: 14**

Ingredients — Servings: 1

- 3/4 cup nonfat vanilla Greek yogurt
- 1 scoop Dummy Supps Vanilla Whey
- 2 tbsp whipped cream cheese
- 1/2 tsp almond extract
- 1 tbsp sliced almonds
- 1 graham cracker

Dummy Supps Whey Protein
SCAN ME

Instructions

1. In a bowl, mix Greek yogurt, vanilla whey, whipped cream cheese, and almond extract until smooth.
2. Crush the graham cracker, almonds, and sprinkle on top.
3. Add sliced almonds and serve.

CHOCOLATE ALMOND

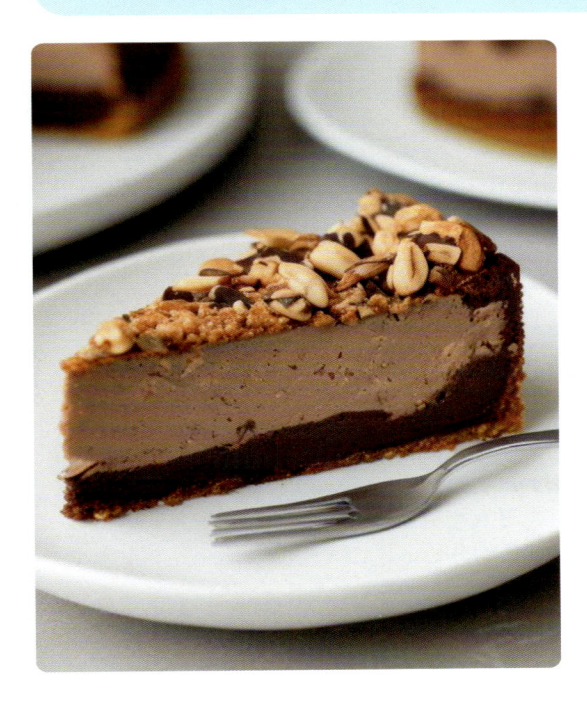

Calories: 370 **Protein: 44** **Carbs: 26** **Fat: 14**

Ingredients — Servings: 1

- 3/4 cup nonfat vanilla Greek yogurt
- 1 scoop Dummy Supps Chocolate Whey
- 2 tbsp whipped cream cheese
- 1/2 tsp almond extract
- 1 tbsp sliced almonds
- 1 graham cracker

Dummy Supps Whey Protein
SCAN ME

Instructions

1. In a bowl, mix Greek yogurt, chocolate whey, whipped cream cheese, and cocoa powder until smooth.
2. Crush the graham cracker, almonds, and sprinkle on top.
3. Set in fridge for 10 minutes or overnight.

CHEESECAKES

VANILLA COFFEE

Calories: 370 **Protein: 43** **Carbs: 23** **Fat: 13**

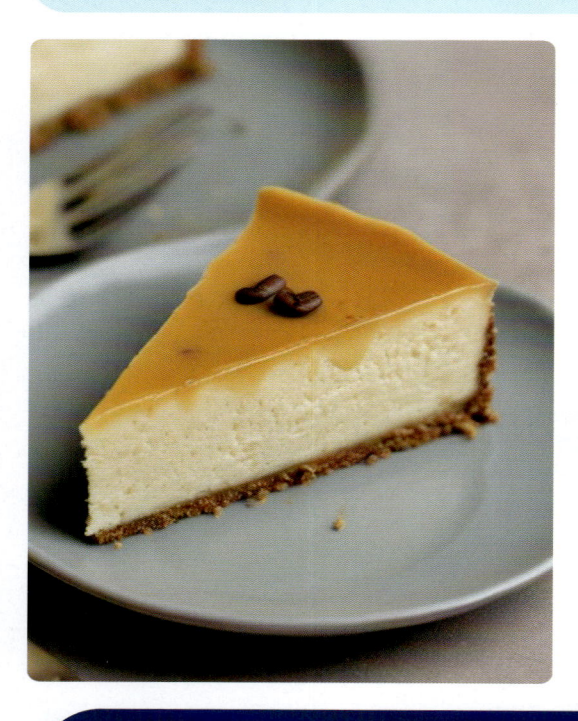

Ingredients — Servings: 1

- 3/4 cup nonfat vanilla Greek yogurt
- 1 scoop Dummy Supps Mocha Whey
- 2 tbsp whipped cream cheese
- 1/2 tsp instant espresso
- 1/2 tsp vanilla extract
- 1 graham cracker

Dummy Supps Whey Protein — SCAN ME

Instructions

1. In a bowl, mix Greek yogurt, mocha whey, whipped cream cheese, instant espresso, and vanilla extract until smooth.
2. Crush the graham cracker and sprinkle on top.
3. Set in fridge for 10 minutes or overnight.

CHOCOLATE COFFEE

Calories: 370 **Protein: 44** **Carbs: 26** **Fat: 13**

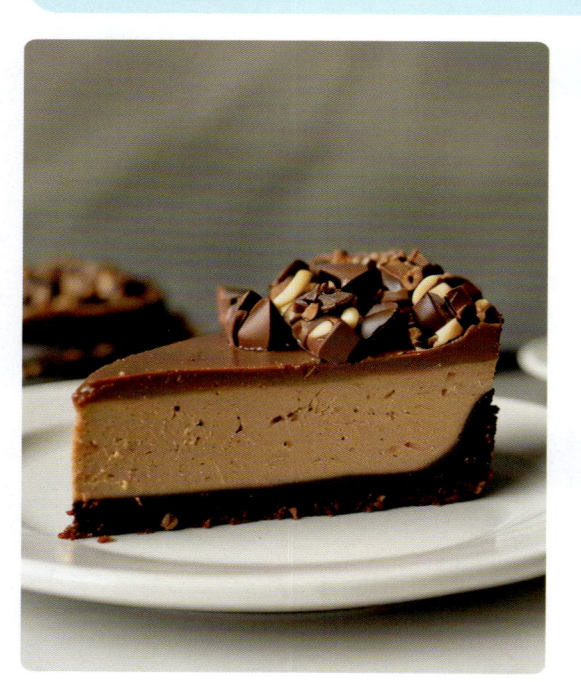

Ingredients — Servings: 1

- 3/4 cup nonfat plain Greek yogurt
- 1 scoop Dummy Supps Mocha Whey protein
- 2 tbsp whipped cream cheese
- 1 tsp instant espresso
- 1 tbsp cocoa powder
- 1 graham cracker

Dummy Supps Whey Protein — SCAN ME

Instructions

1. In a bowl, mix Greek yogurt, mocha whey protein, whipped cream cheese, instant espresso, and cocoa powder until smooth.
2. Crush the graham cracker and sprinkle on top.
3. Set in fridge for 10 minutes or overnight.

CHEESECAKES

STRAWBERRY

Calories: 410 **Protein: 44** **Carbs: 37** **Fat: 12**

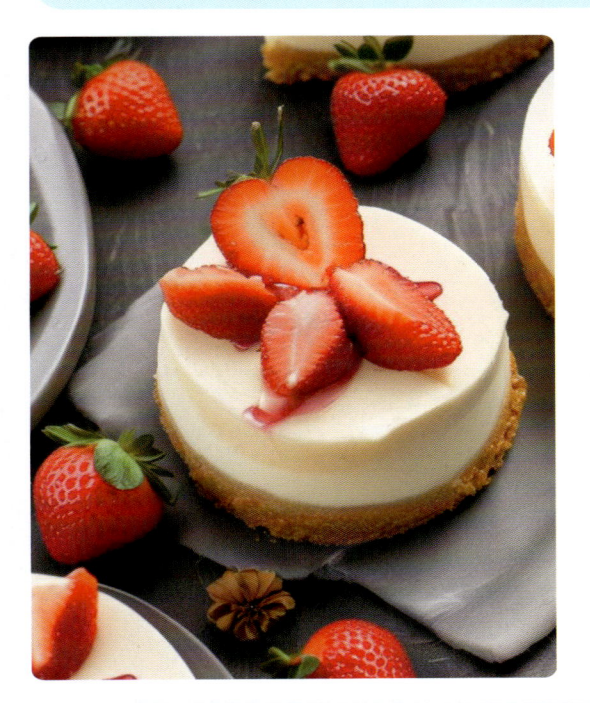

Ingredients — Servings: 1

- 3/4 cup nonfat vanilla Greek yogurt
- 1 scoop Dummy Supps Vanilla Whey protein
- 2 tbsp whipped cream cheese
- 1 cup fresh strawberries
- 1 tbsp zero-calorie sugar
- 1 tsp lemon juice
- 1 graham cracker

Dummy Supps Whey Protein — SCAN ME

Instructions

1. In a bowl, mix Greek yogurt, vanilla whey protein, and whipped cream cheese until smooth.
2. Set in fridge for 10 minutes or overnight.
3. Slice strawberries and add them to a pan over medium heat.
4. Add zero-calorie sugar and lemon juice, then sauté for 3-4 minutes until softened.
5. Top with sautéed strawberries and crushed graham cracker.

CHOCOLATE COVERED STRAWBERRY

Calories: 470 **Protein: 46** **Carbs: 45** **Fat: 18**

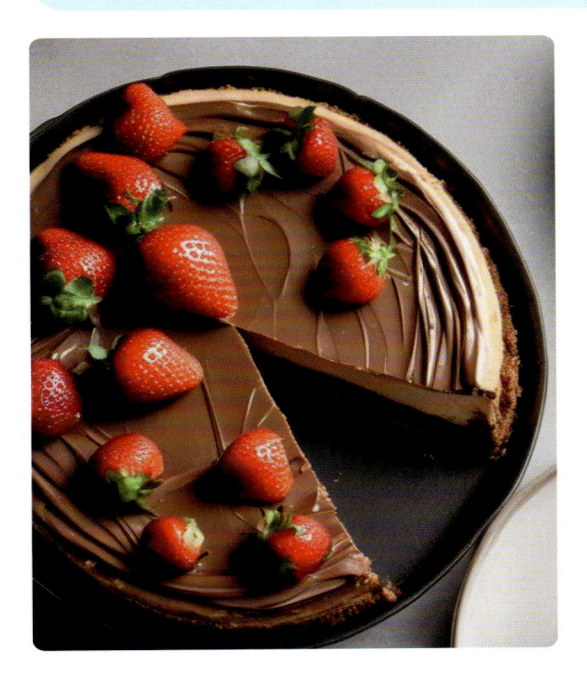

Ingredients — Servings: 1

- 3/4 cup nonfat vanilla Greek yogurt
- 1 scoop Dummy Supps Chocolate Whey
- 2 tbsp whipped cream cheese
- 1 cup fresh strawberries
- 1 tbsp cocoa powder
- 2 tbsp Lily's chocolate chips
- 1 graham cracker

Dummy Supps Whey Protein — SCAN ME

Instructions

1. In a bowl, mix Greek yogurt, chocolate whey, whipped cream cheese, and cocoa powder until smooth.
2. Slice strawberries and stir them into the mixture.
3. Add Lily's chocolate chips and mix gently.
4. Crush the graham cracker and sprinkle on top.
5. Set in fridge for 10 minutes or overnight.

CHEESECAKES

BLUEBERRY

Calories: 400 **Protein: 44** **Carbs: 34** **Fat: 12**

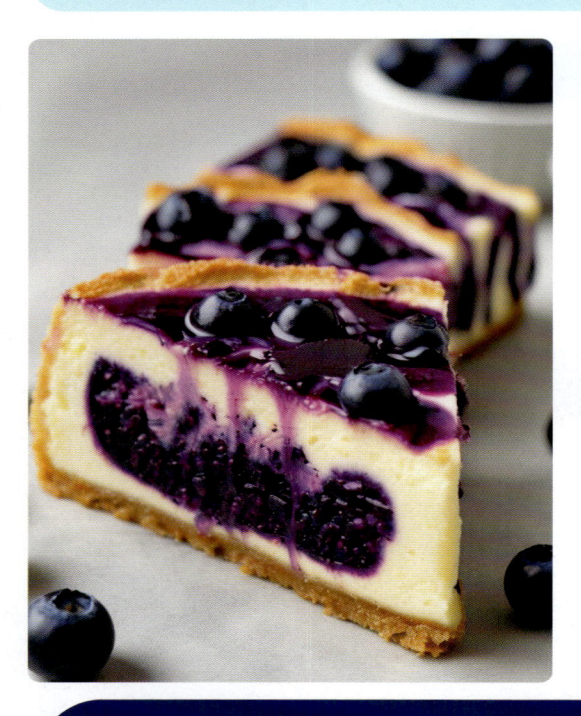

Ingredients — Servings: 1

- 3/4 cup nonfat vanilla Greek yogurt
- 1 scoop Dummy Supps Berry/Vanilla Whey
- 2 tbsp whipped cream cheese
- 1 cup fresh blueberries
- 1 tbsp zero-calorie sugar
- 1 tsp lemon juice
- 1 graham cracker

Dummy Supps Whey Protein — SCAN ME

Instructions

1. In a bowl, mix Greek yogurt, berry whey, and whipped cream cheese until smooth.
2. Set in fridge for 10 minutes or overnight.
3. Add blueberries to a pan over medium heat.
4. Stir in zero-calorie sugar and lemon juice, then sauté for 3-4 minutes until softened and slightly syrupy.
5. Top with sautéed blueberries and crushed graham cracker.

RASPBERRY

Calories: 430 **Protein: 45** **Carbs: 41** **Fat: 13**

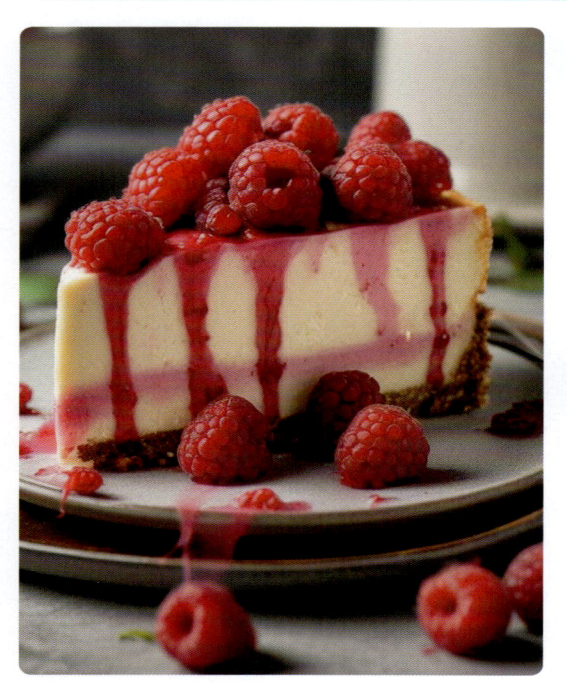

Ingredients — Servings: 1

- 3/4 cup mixed berry Greek yogurt
- 1 scoop Dummy Supps Berry/Vanilla whey
- 2 tbsp whipped cream cheese
- 1 cup fresh raspberries
- 1 tbsp zero-calorie sugar
- 1 tsp lemon juice
- 1 graham cracker

Dummy Supps Whey Protein — SCAN ME

Instructions

1. In a bowl, mix 3/4 cup mixed berry Greek yogurt, 1 scoop Dummy Supps Berry/Vanilla whey, and 2 tbsp whipped cream cheese until smooth.
2. Refrigerate for at least 10 minutes or overnight.
3. In a pan over medium heat, add 1 cup fresh raspberries.
4. Stir in 1 tbsp zero-calorie sugar and 1 tsp lemon juice; sauté for 3-4 minutes until softened and slightly syrupy.
5. Top the chilled yogurt mixture with the warm raspberry compote and sprinkle with crushed graham cracker.

CHEESECAKES

LEMON VANILLA

Calories: 360 **Protein: 43** **Carbs: 24** **Fat: 12**

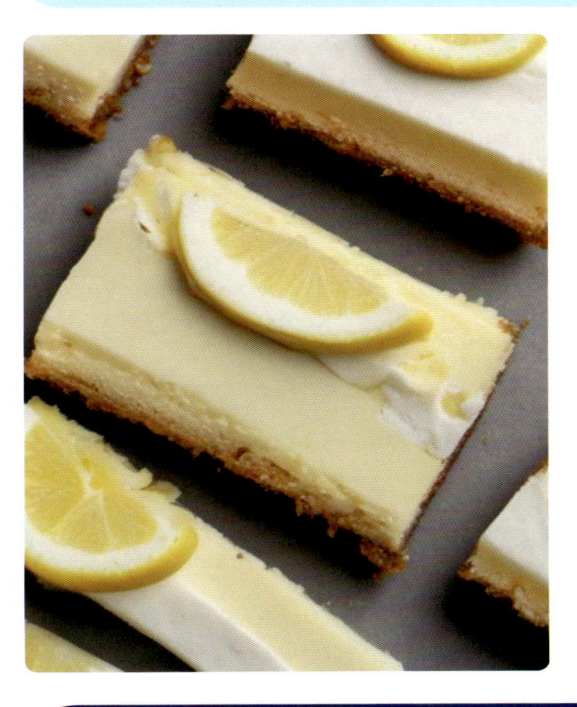

Ingredients — Servings: 1

- 3/4 cup nonfat vanilla Greek yogurt
- 1 scoop Dummy Supps Vanilla Whey
- 2 tbsp whipped cream cheese
- 1 tsp lemon juice
- 1/2 tsp lemon zest
- 1 graham cracker

Dummy Supps Whey Protein — SCAN ME

Instructions

1. In a bowl, mix nonfat vanilla Greek yogurt, vanilla whey, whipped cream cheese, lemon juice, and lemon zest until smooth.
2. Crush the graham cracker and fold it into the mixture.
3. Set in the fridge for 10 minutes or overnight.

VANILLA BANANA

Calories: 460 **Protein: 45** **Carbs: 44** **Fat: 18**

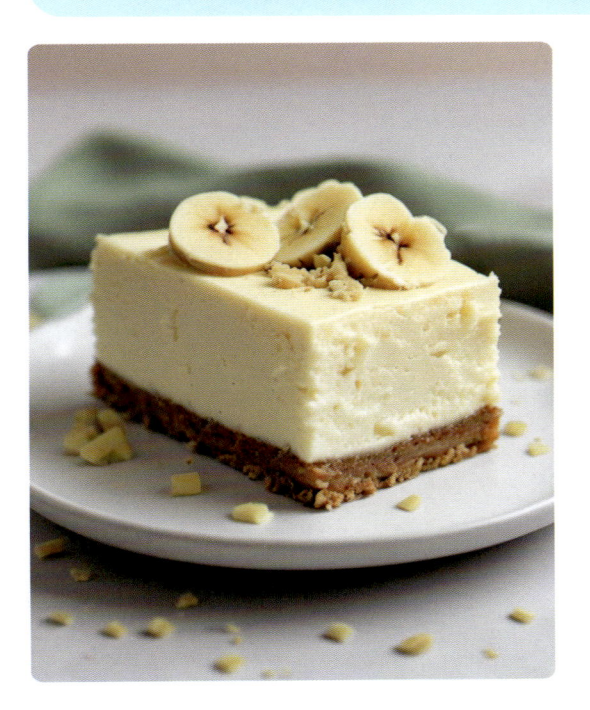

Ingredients — Servings: 1

- 3/4 cup nonfat vanilla Greek yogurt
- 1 scoop Dummy Supps Vanilla Whey
- 2 tbsp whipped cream cheese
- 1/2 banana
- 2 tbsp Lilly's White Chocolate Chips
- 1/2 tsp vanilla extract
- 1 graham cracker

Dummy Supps Whey Protein — SCAN ME

Instructions

1. In a bowl, mix Greek yogurt, vanilla whey, whipped cream cheese, and vanilla extract until smooth.
2. Stir in Lilly's White Chocolate Chips.
3. Slice the banana and fold it into the mixture.
4. Crush the graham cracker and sprinkle on top.
5. Set in the fridge for 10 minutes or overnight.

CHEESECAKES

LEMON COCONUT

Calories: 370 **Protein: 43** **Carbs: 26** **Fat: 13**

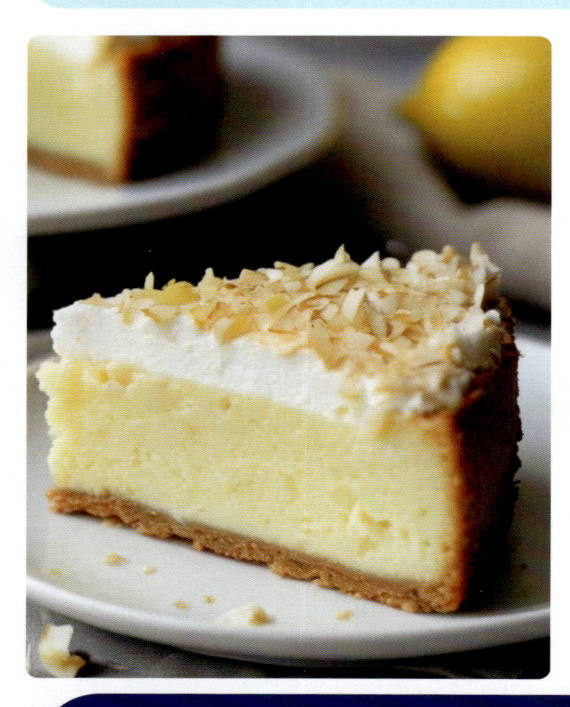

Ingredients — Servings: 1

- 3/4 cup nonfat vanilla Greek yogurt
- 1 scoop Dummy Supps Vanilla Whey
- 2 tbsp whipped cream cheese
- 1 tbsp unsweetened coconut flakes
- 1 tsp lemon juice
- 1/2 lemon zest
- 1 graham cracker

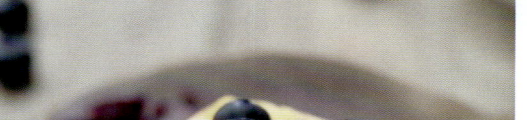

Dummy Supps Whey Protein — SCAN ME

Instructions

1. In a bowl, mix nonfat vanilla Greek yogurt, vanilla whey protein powder, whipped cream cheese, lemon juice, and unsweetened coconut flakes until smooth.
2. Crush the graham cracker and fold it into the mixture.
3. Refrigerate for at least 10 minutes or overnight.

LEMON BLUEBERRY

Calories: 380 **Protein: 43** **Carbs: 29** **Fat: 12**

Ingredients — Servings: 1

- 3/4 cup nonfat vanilla Greek yogurt
- 1 scoop Dummy Supps Vanilla Whey
- 2 tbsp whipped cream cheese
- 1 tsp lemon juice
- 1/2 cup fresh or frozen blueberries
- 1 graham cracker

Dummy Supps Whey Protein — SCAN ME

Instructions

1. In a bowl, mix nonfat vanilla Greek yogurt, vanilla whey, whipped cream cheese, and lemon juice until smooth.
2. Fold in frozen blueberries.
3. Crush the graham cracker and fold it into the mixture.
4. Set in the fridge for 10 minutes or overnight.

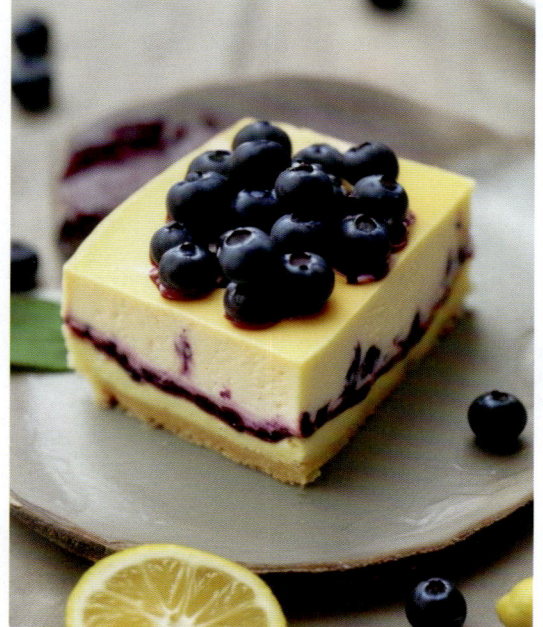

ICE CREAM

PROTEIN ICE CREAM

DESSERT RECIPES

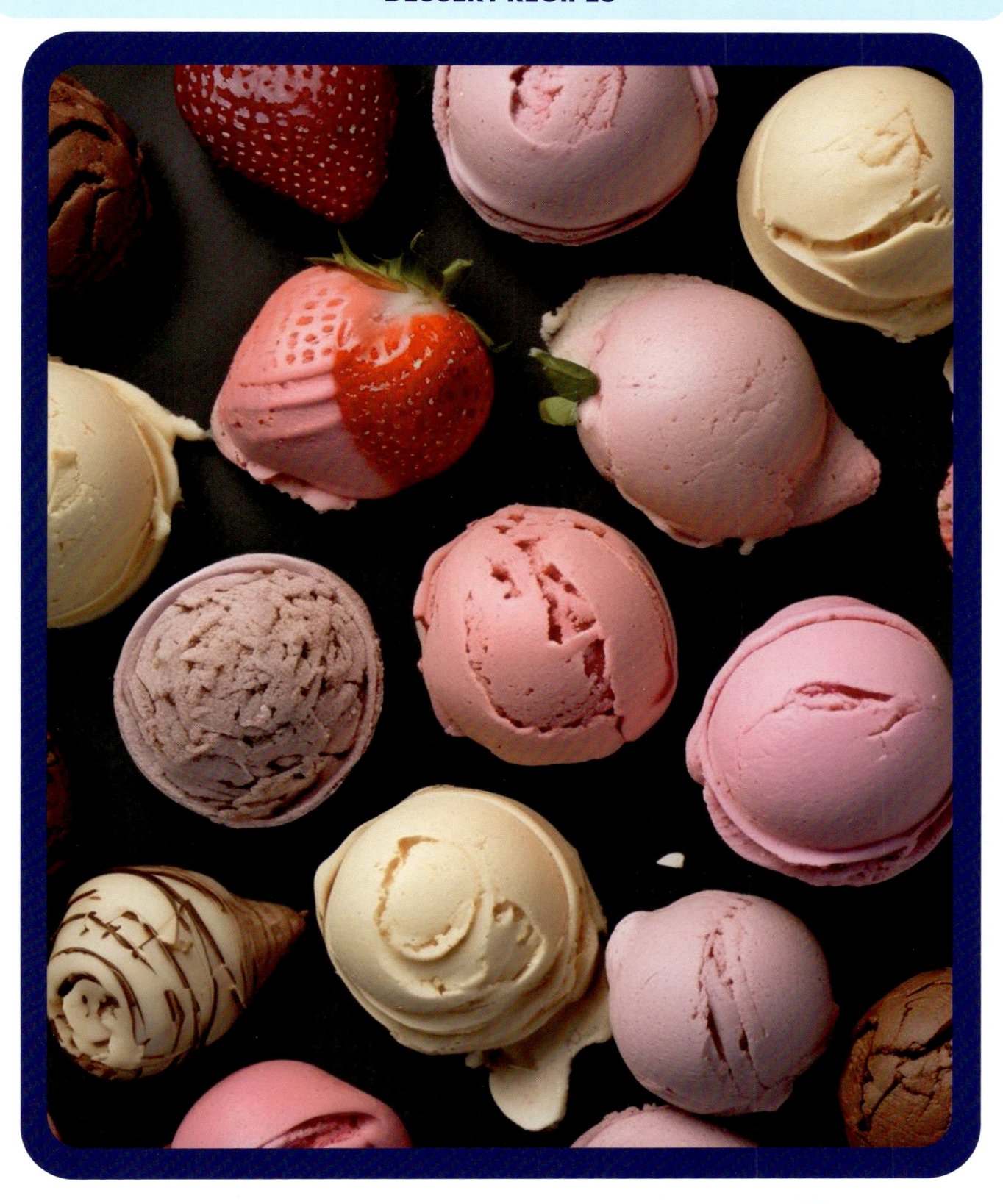

ICE CREAM

CHOCOLATE

Calories: 330   **Protein: 65**   **Carbs: 32**   **Fat: 16**

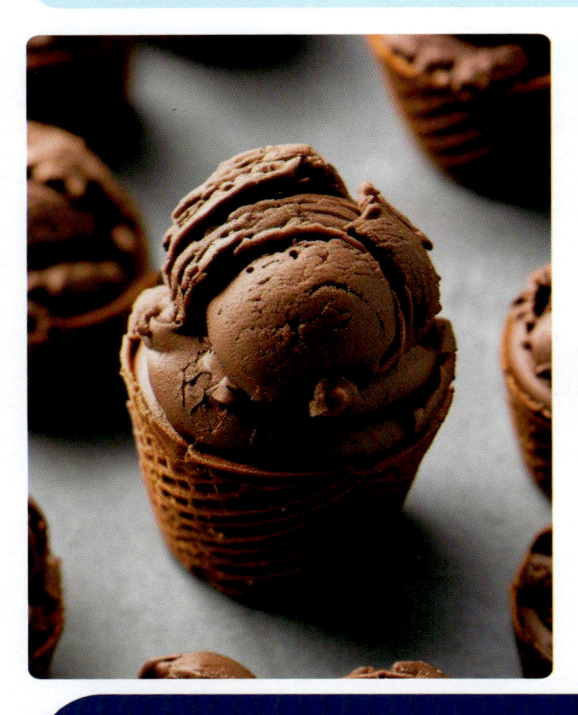

Ingredients — Servings: 1

- 1 cup low-fat cottage cheese
- 1 scoop Dummy Supps Chocolate Whey
- 1 tbsp cocoa powder
- 1 tbsp Mocha Dummy Butter
- 2 tbsp Lily's Dark Chocolate Chips

Dummy Supps Whey Protein — SCAN ME

Instructions

1. In a blender, combine cottage cheese, Dummy Supps Chocolate Whey, cocoa powder, and Mocha Dummy Butter.
2. Blend until smooth.
3. Pour mixture into a freezer-safe bowl.
4. Stir in Lily's Dark Chocolate Chips.
5. Freeze for at least 20 minutes until the ice cream has set.

CLASSIC VANILLA

Calories: 320   **Protein: 50**   **Carbs: 15**   **Fat: 1**

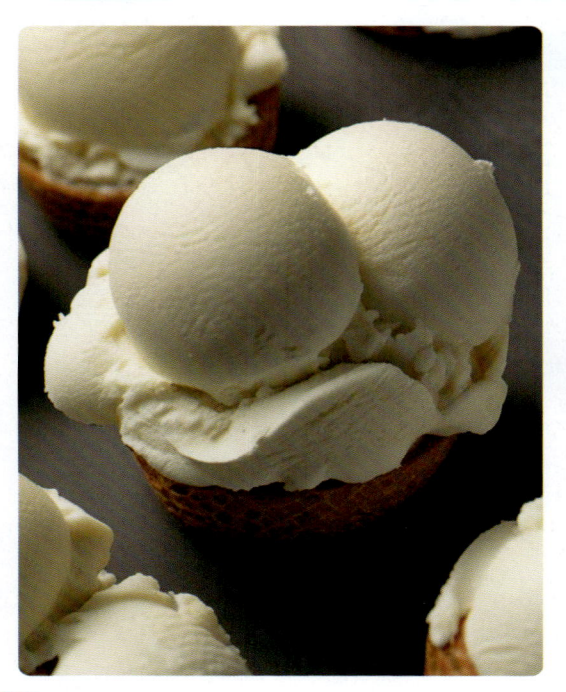

Ingredients — Servings: 1

- 1 cup low-fat cottage cheese
- 1 scoop Dummy Supps vanilla whey
- 1/2 tsp vanilla extract
- 2 tbsp Lilly's White Chocolate Chips

Dummy Supps Whey Protein — SCAN ME

Instructions

1. In a blender, combine cottage cheese, Dummy Supps Vanilla Whey, and vanilla extract.
2. Blend until smooth.
3. Pour mixture into a freezer-safe bowl.
4. Stir in Lily's White Chocolate Chips.
5. Freeze for at least 20 minutes until the ice cream has set.

ICE CREAM

CHOCOLATE PEANUT BUTTER

Calories: 520 | **Protein: 65** | **Carbs: 32** | **Fat: 16**

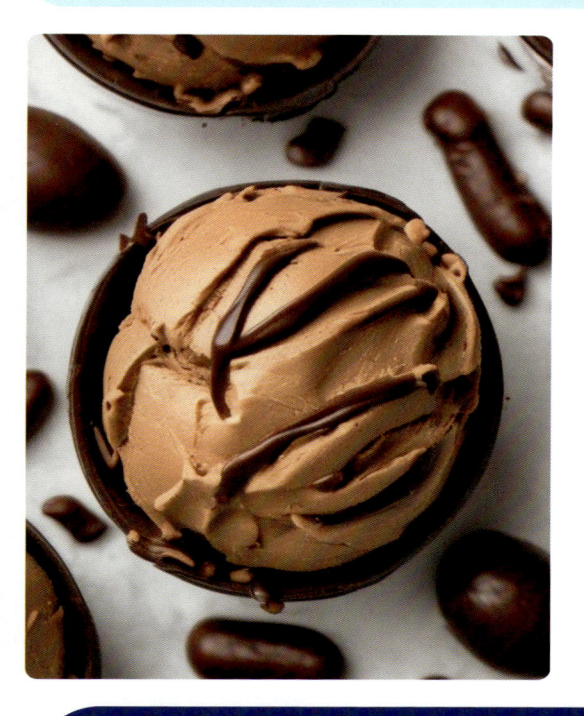

Ingredients — Servings: 1

- 1 cup low-fat cottage cheese
- 1 scoop Dummy Supps Chocolate PB whey
- 2 tbsp powdered peanut butter
- 1 tbsp Mocha Dummy Butter
- 2 tbsp Lily's Dark Chocolate Chips

Dummy Supps Whey Protein — SCAN ME

Instructions

1. In a blender, combine cottage cheese, Dummy Supps Chocolate PB Whey, powdered peanut butter, and Mocha Dummy Butter.
2. Blend until smooth.
3. Pour mixture into a freezer-safe bowl.
4. Stir in Lily's Dark Chocolate Chips.
5. Freeze for at least 20 minutes until the ice cream has set.

CHOCOLATE ESPRESSO

Calories: 420 | **Protein: 58** | **Carbs: 36** | **Fat: 13**

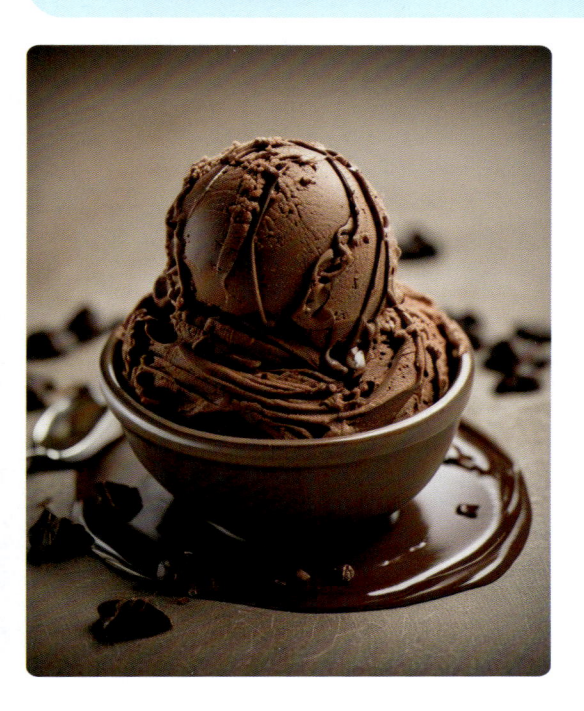

Ingredients — Servings: 1

- 1 cup low-fat cottage cheese
- 1 scoop Dummy Supps Mocha Whey
- 1 tsp instant espresso
- 1 tsp cocoa powder
- 1 tbsp Mocha Dummy Butter
- 1 serving Lily's dark chocolate chips

Dummy Supps Whey Protein — SCAN ME

Instructions

1. In a blender, combine cottage cheese, Dummy Supps Mocha Whey, instant espresso, cocoa powder, and Mocha Dummy Butter.
2. Blend until smooth.
3. Pour mixture into a freezer-safe bowl.
4. Stir in Lily's Dark Chocolate Chips.
5. Freeze for at least 20 minutes until the ice cream has set.

ICE CREAM

PB&J

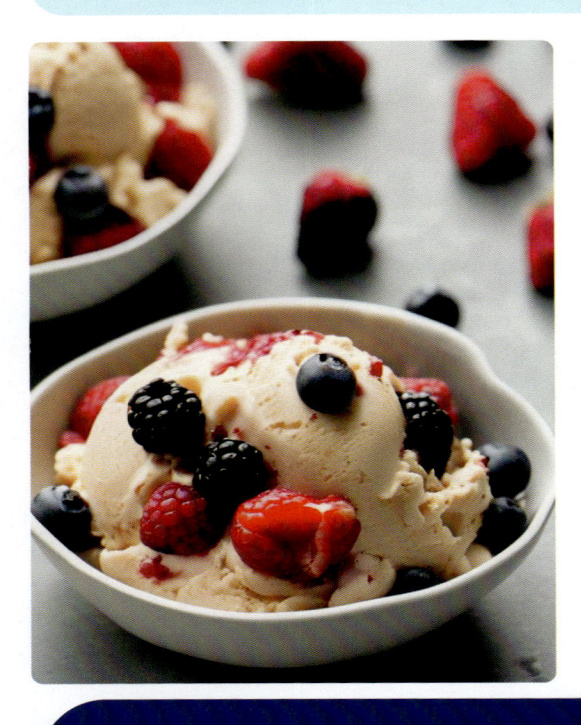

Calories: 520   **Protein: 60**   **Carbs: 32**   **Fat: 16**

Ingredients   Servings: 1

- 1 cup low-fat cottage cheese
- 1 scoop Dummy Supps Berry Whey Protein
- 1 tbsp PB&J Dummy Butter
- 1/2 cup frozen mixed berries
- 1 tsp sugar free strawberry jam

Dummy Supps Whey Protein — SCAN ME

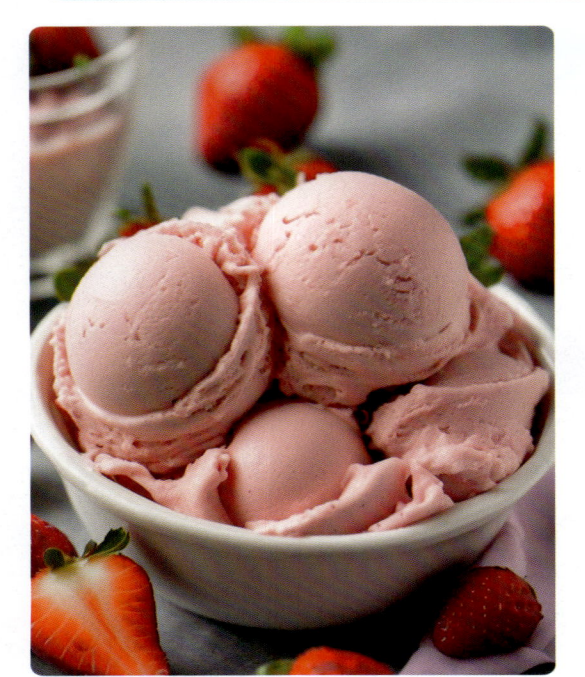

Instructions

1. In a blender, combine cottage cheese, Dummy Supps Berry Whey Protein, PB&J Dummy Butter, and sugar-free strawberry jam.
2. Blend until smooth.
3. Pour mixture into a freezer-safe bowl.
4. Stir in frozen mixed berries.
5. Freeze for at least 20 minutes until the ice cream has set.

STRAWBERRY

Calories: 520   **Protein: 60**   **Carbs: 32**   **Fat: 16**

Ingredients   Servings: 1

- 1 cup frozen strawberries
- 1 cup low-fat cottage cheese
- 1 scoop Dummy Supps Berry Whey
- 1 tbsp PB&J Dummy Butter
- 1/2 tsp vanilla extract

Dummy Supps Whey Protein — SCAN ME

Instructions

1. In a blender, combine frozen strawberries, cottage cheese, Dummy Supps Berry Whey, PB&J Dummy Butter, and vanilla extract.
2. Blend until smooth and creamy.
3. Pour mixture into a freezer-safe bowl.
4. Freeze for at least 20 minutes until the ice cream has set.

ICE CREAM

MINT CHOCOLATE

Calories: 571   **Protein: 63**   **Carbs: 36**   **Fat: 23**

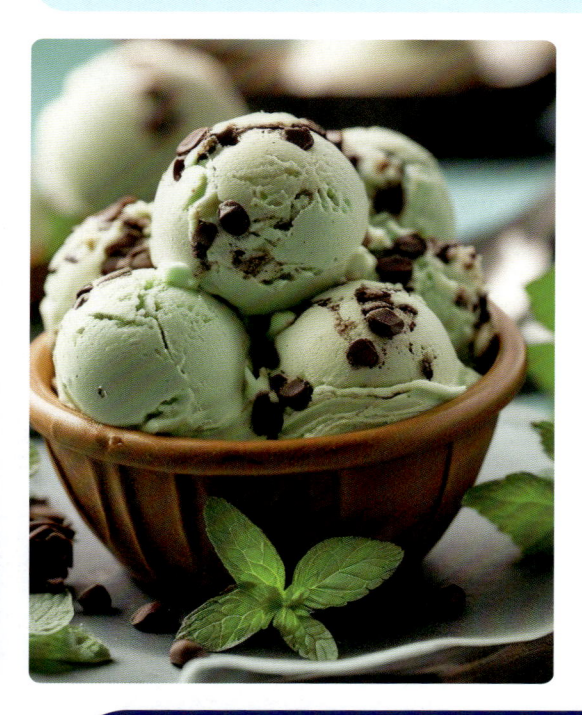

Ingredients   Servings: 1

- 1 cup low-fat cottage cheese
- 1/2 scoop Dummy Supps Vanilla Whey
- 1/2 scoop Dummy Supps Chocolate Whey
- 1/2 tsp spearmint extract
- 2 tbsp Lily's dark chocolate chips
- 1 tbsp Mocha Dummy Butter
- 4 Simple Mills Chocolate Brownie Sweet Thins

Dummy Supps Whey Protein
SCAN ME

Instructions

1. In a blender, combine cottage cheese, Dummy Supps Vanilla Whey, Dummy Supps Chocolate Whey, spearmint extract, and Mocha Dummy Butter.
2. Blend until smooth.
3. Pour mixture into a freezer-safe bowl.
4. Stir in Lily's Dark Chocolate Chips and crushed Simple Mills Chocolate Brownie Sweet Thins.
5. Freeze for at least 20 minutes until the ice cream has set.

SALTED CARAMEL PRETZEL

Calories: 510   **Protein: 60**   **Carbs: 31**   **Fat: 17**

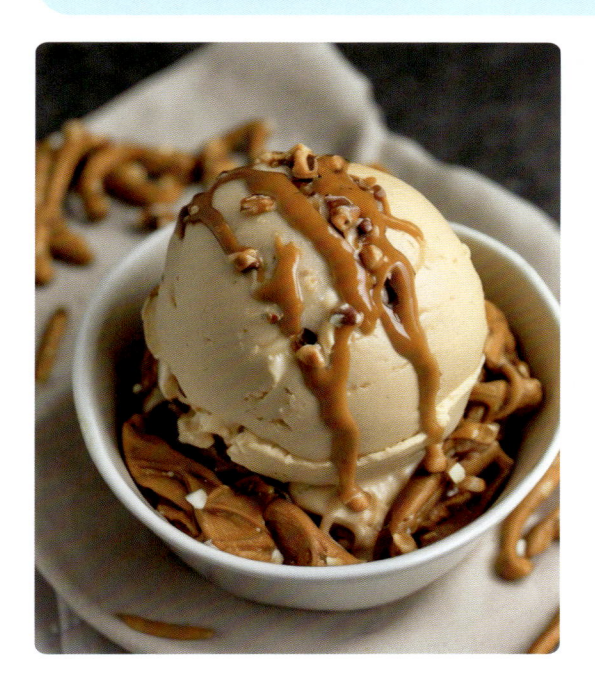

Ingredients   Servings: 1

- 1 cup low-fat cottage cheese
- 1 scoop Dummy Supps Salted Caramel Whey
- 2 tbsp instant espresso
- 1 tbsp Mocha Dummy Butter
- 5 pretzel thins
- 1/4 tsp salt

Dummy Supps Whey Protein
SCAN ME

Instructions

1. In a blender, combine cottage cheese, Dummy Supps Salted Caramel Whey, instant espresso, Mocha Dummy Butter, and salt.
2. Blend until smooth.
3. Pour mixture into a freezer-safe bowl.
4. Crush pretzel thins and stir them into the mixture.
5. Freeze for at least 20 minutes until the ice cream has set.

ICE CREAM

CINNAMON SWIRL

Calories: 520 **Protein: 57** **Carbs: 32** **Fat: 18**

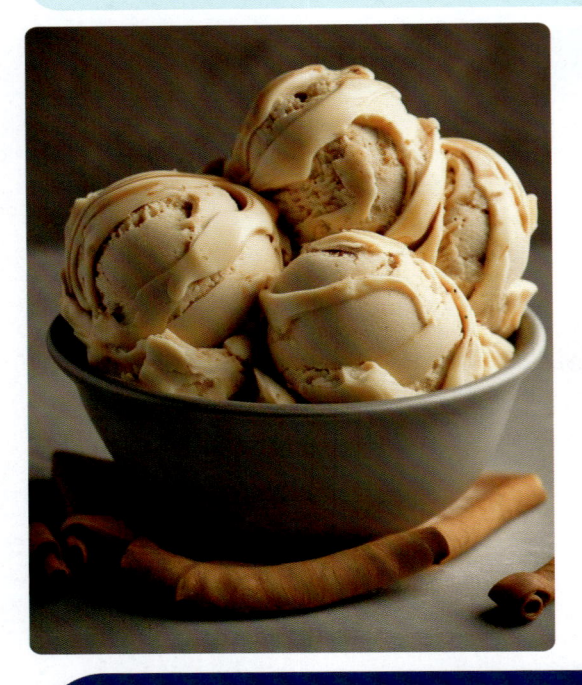

Ingredients — Servings: 1

- 1 cup low-fat cottage cheese
- 1 scoop Dummy Supps Cinnamon Bun Whey
- 1 tbsp Mocha Dummy Butter
- 1/2 tsp ground cinnamon
- 1 graham cracker

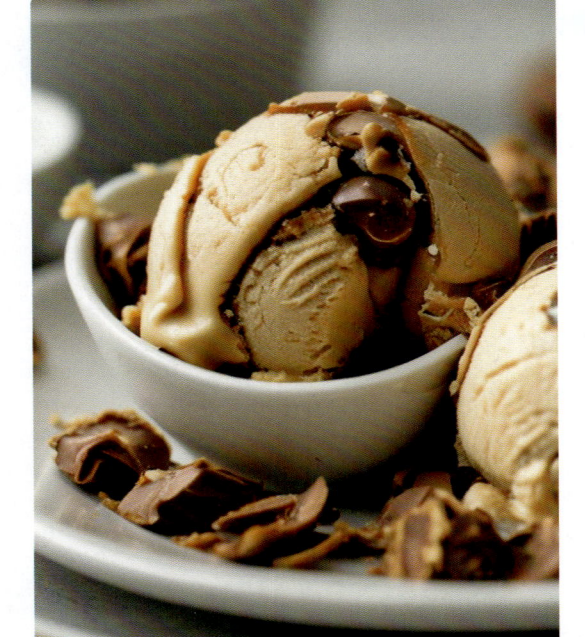

Dummy Supps Whey Protein — SCAN ME

Instructions

1. In a blender, combine cottage cheese, Dummy Supps Cinnamon Bun Whey, Mocha Dummy Butter, and ground cinnamon.
2. Blend until smooth.
3. Pour mixture into a freezer-safe bowl.
4. Crush graham cracker and stir it into the mixture.
5. Freeze for at least 20 minutes until the ice cream has set.

PEANUT BUTTER CUP

Calories: 470 **Protein: 55** **Carbs: 28** **Fat: 16**

Ingredients — Servings: 1

- 1 cup low-fat cottage cheese
- 1 scoop Dummy Supps Chocolate PB Whey
- 2 tbsp powdered peanut butter
- 1 tbsp peanut butter
- 2 tbsp Lily's Dark Chocolate Chips

Dummy Supps Whey Protein — SCAN ME

Instructions

1. In a blender, combine cottage cheese, Dummy Supps Chocolate PB Whey, powdered peanut butter, and peanut butter.
2. Blend until smooth.
3. Pour mixture into a freezer-safe bowl.
4. Stir in Lily's Dark Chocolate Chips.
5. Freeze for at least 20 minutes until the ice cream has set.

DONUTS

PROTEIN DONUTS

DESSERT RECIPES

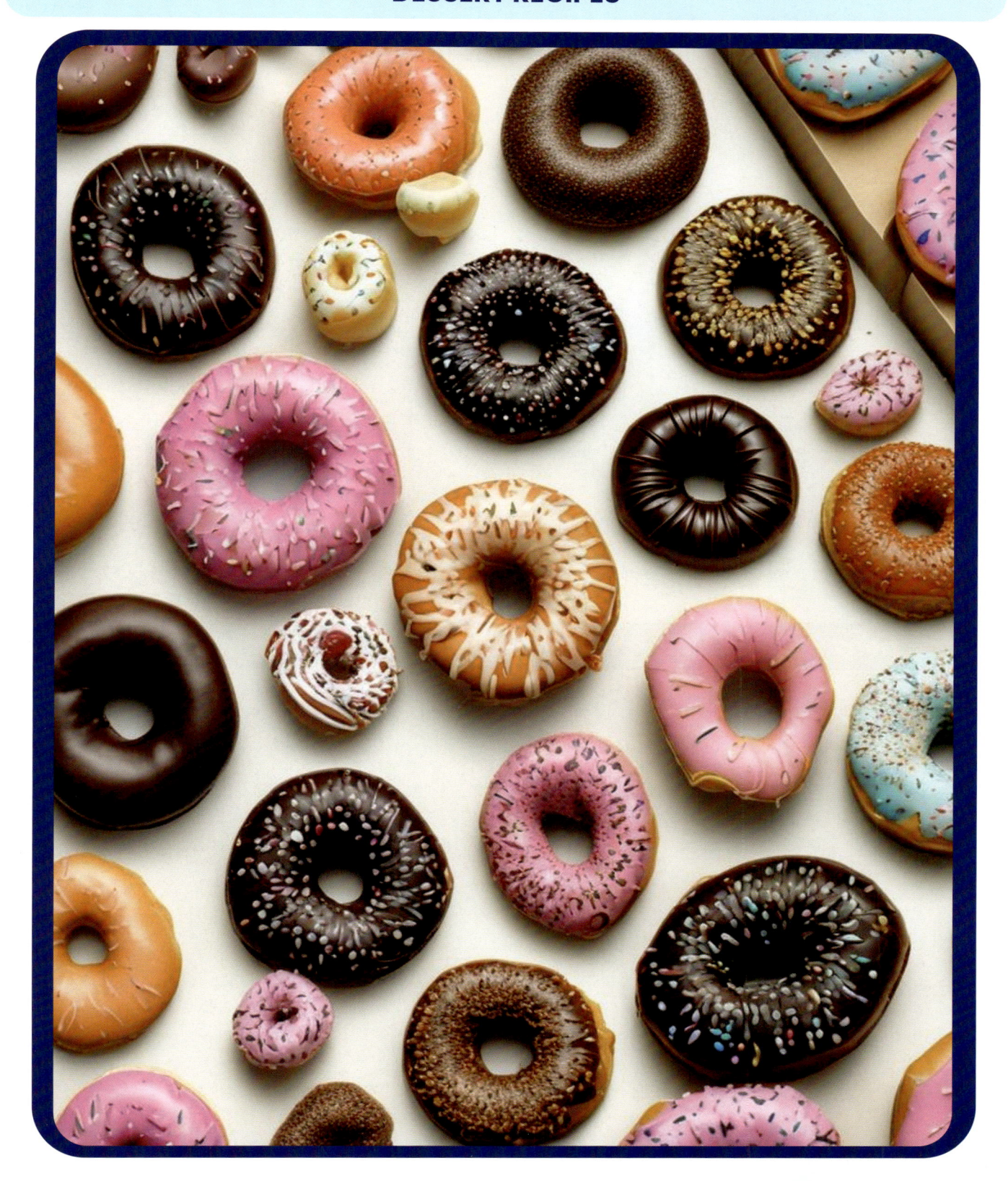

DONUTS

CHOCOLATE FROSTED DONUT

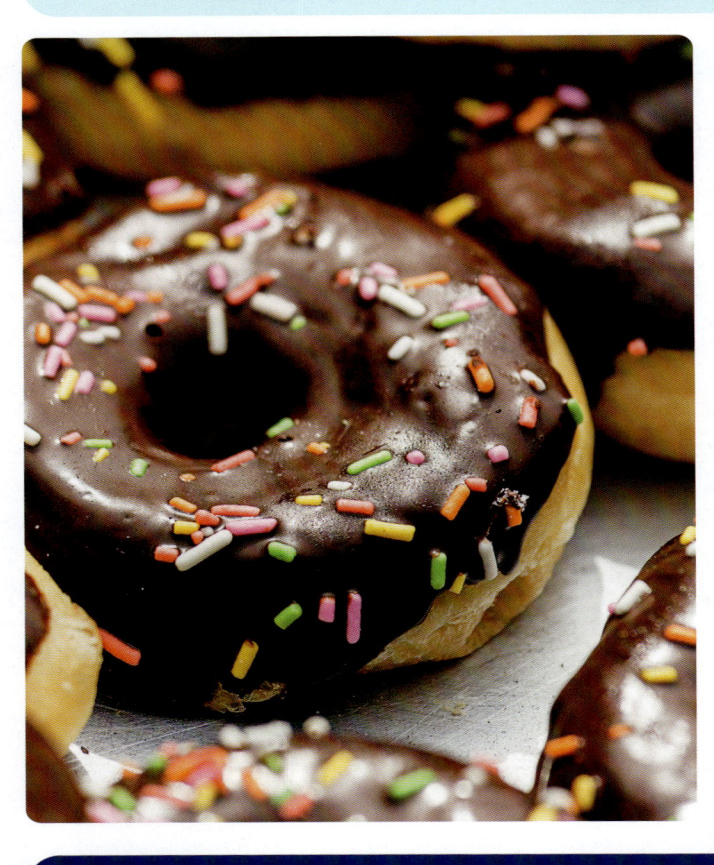

Calories: 210 **Protein: 15** **Carbs: 29** **Fat: 9**

Ingredients   Servings: 6

- 1 cup nonfat plain Greek yogurt
- 1 egg
- 2 tbsp softened butter
- 2 tsp vanilla extract
- 1/4 cup almond flour
- 3 scoops Dummy Supps Vanilla Whey
- 1 1/2 tsp baking powder
- 2 tbsp cane sugar
- 1/2 cup Lilly's Dark Chocolate Chips
- 2 tsp coconut oil

Dummy Supps Whey Protein

Instructions

1. Preheat oven to 350°F.
2. In a large mixing bowl, whisk Greek yogurt, egg, butter, and vanilla extract until well combined.
3. Add flour, whey protein, baking powder, sugar, and combine ingredients until batter is formed.
4. Add donut batter to donut pan and bake for 10-12 minutes.
5. To a small mixing bowl, combine chocolate chips and coconut oil and microwave for 30 seconds at a time until completely melted.
6. Remove donuts from pan and add frosting to each.

DONUTS

APPLE FRITTER

Calories: 160 **Protein: 14** **Carbs: 17** **Fat: 5**

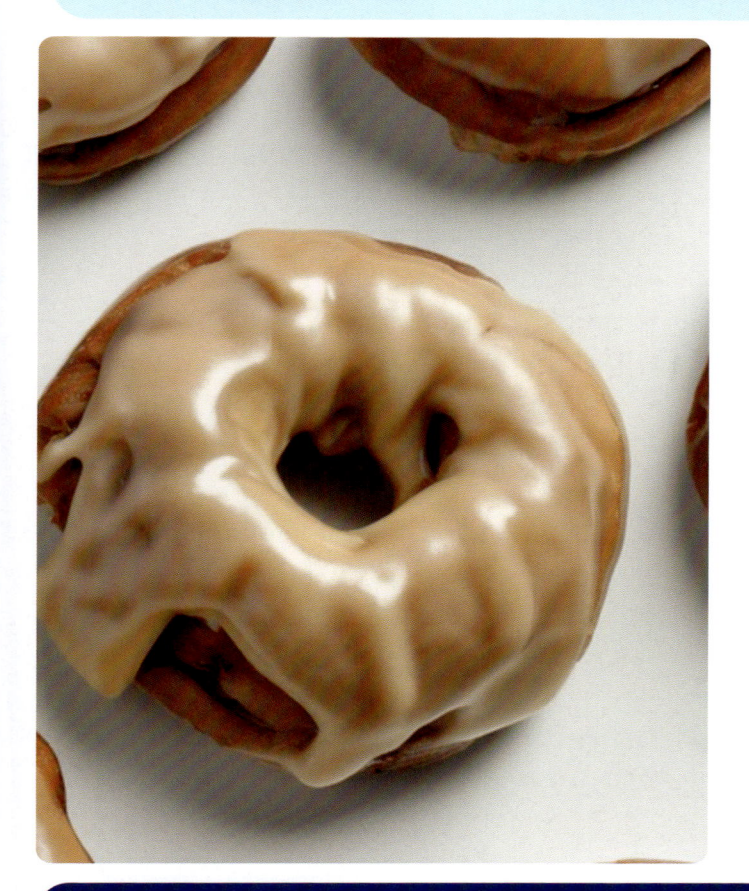

Ingredients — Servings: 6

- 2 apples
- 1 container unsweetened applesauce
- 1 egg
- 1/2 cup unsweetened almond milk
- 1 tsp vanilla extract
- 2 tbsp butter
- 1/2 cup almond flour
- 4 scoops Dummy Supps Cinnamon Swirl Whey
- 2 tbsp zero calorie granulated sugar
- 2 tsp baking powder
- 4 tsp apple pie spice
- 2 tsp unsweetened almond milk
- 1/4 cup zero calorie confectioners sugar
- 1/2 tsp vanilla extract
- 2 tsp unsweetened almond milk

Dummy Supps Whey Protein

Instructions

1. Preheat oven to 350°F.
2. Dice apples into small bite sized pieces.
3. Add apples to baking sheet, season with 2 tsp apple pie spice, and place into oven for 10 minutes to soften.
4. To large mixing bowl add applesauce, egg, vanilla extract, butter, almond milk and mix well.
5. Add flour, cinnamon swirl whey protein, zero calorie sugar, 2 tsp apple pie spice, 2 tsp baking powder, and mix until well combined.
6. Add 2 tsp of almond milk to thin out batter if necessary.
7. Add batter to donut tin and bake for 10-12 minutes.
8. For glaze, add zero calorie confectioners sugar, almond milk, vanilla extract, and top each donut.

DONUTS

BLUEBERRY GLAZED DONUT

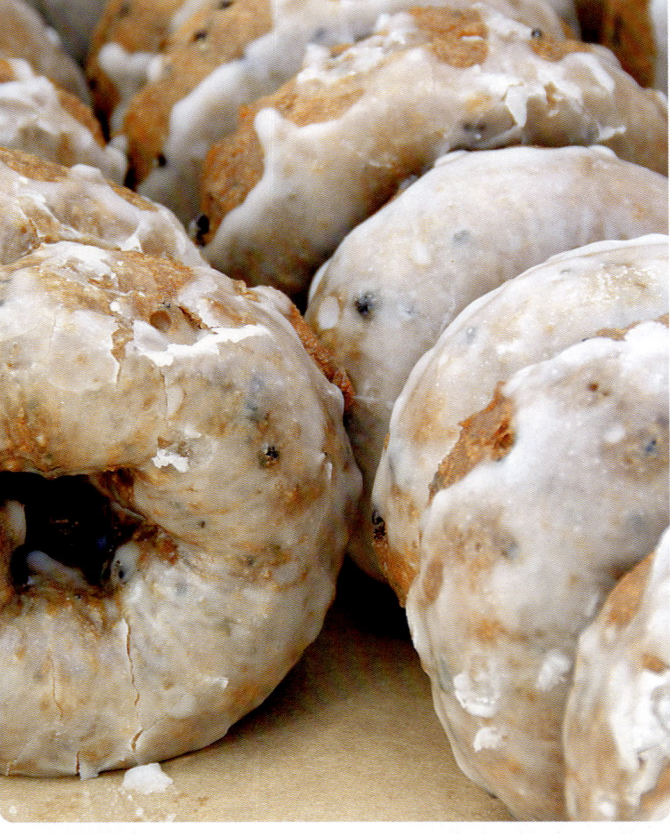

Calories: 190 **Protein: 18** **Carbs: 13** **Fat: 6**

Ingredients   Servings: 6

- 1 cup nonfat plain Greek yogurt
- 1 egg
- 2 tbsp softened butter
- 2 tsp vanilla extract
- 1 cup fresh blueberries
- 1/4 cup almond flour
- 3 scoops Dummy Supps Vanilla Whey
- 1 1/2 tsp baking powder
- 2 tbsp cane sugar
- 1/4 cup zero calorie confectioners sugar
- 2 tsp unsweetened almond milk

Dummy Supps Whey Protein

Instructions

1. Preheat oven to 350°F.
2. In a large mixing bowl, whisk Greek yogurt, egg, butter, vanilla extract, and blueberries until well combined.
3. Add flour, whey protein, baking powder, sugar, and combine ingredients until batter is formed.
4. Add donut batter to donut pan and bake for 10-12 minutes.
5. To a small mixing bowl, combine confectioners sugar and almond milk and mix.
6. Remove donuts from pan and add glaze to each.

DONUTS

CHOCOLATE GLAZED DONUT

Calories: 210 **Protein: 16** **Carbs: 29** **Fat: 9**

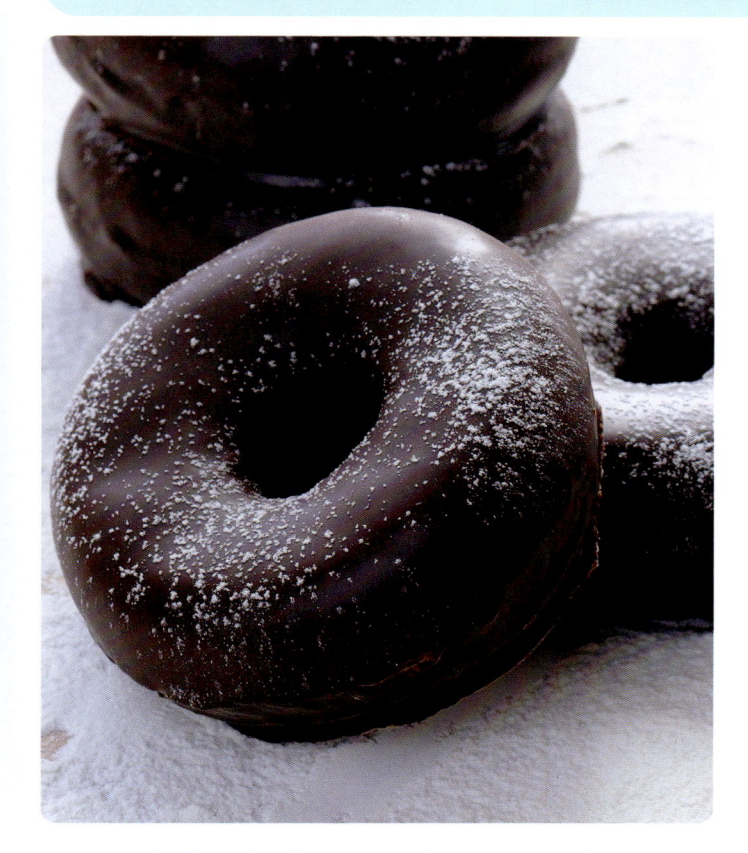

Ingredients Servings: 6

- 1 cup nonfat plain Greek yogurt
- 1 egg
- 2 tbsp softened butter
- 1/4 cup almond flour
- 3 scoops Dummy Supps Chocolate Whey
- 1/4 cup unsweetened almond milk
- 1 1/2 tsp baking powder
- 2 tbsp cane sugar
- 2 tbsp cocoa powder
- 1/2 cup Lilly's Dark Chocolate Chips
- 2 tsp coconut oil

Dummy Supps Whey Protein

Instructions

1. Preheat oven to 350°F.
2. In a large mixing bowl, whisk Greek yogurt, egg, and butter until well combined.
3. Add flour, whey protein, baking powder, sugar, cocoa powder, and combine ingredients until batter is formed.
4. Add almond milk to thin the batter if necessary.
5. Add donut batter to donut pan and bake for 10-12 minutes.
6. To a small mixing bowl, combine chocolate chips and coconut oil and microwave for 30 seconds at a time until completely melted.
7. Remove donuts from pan and add frosting to each.

DONUTS

CINNAMON BUN DONUTS

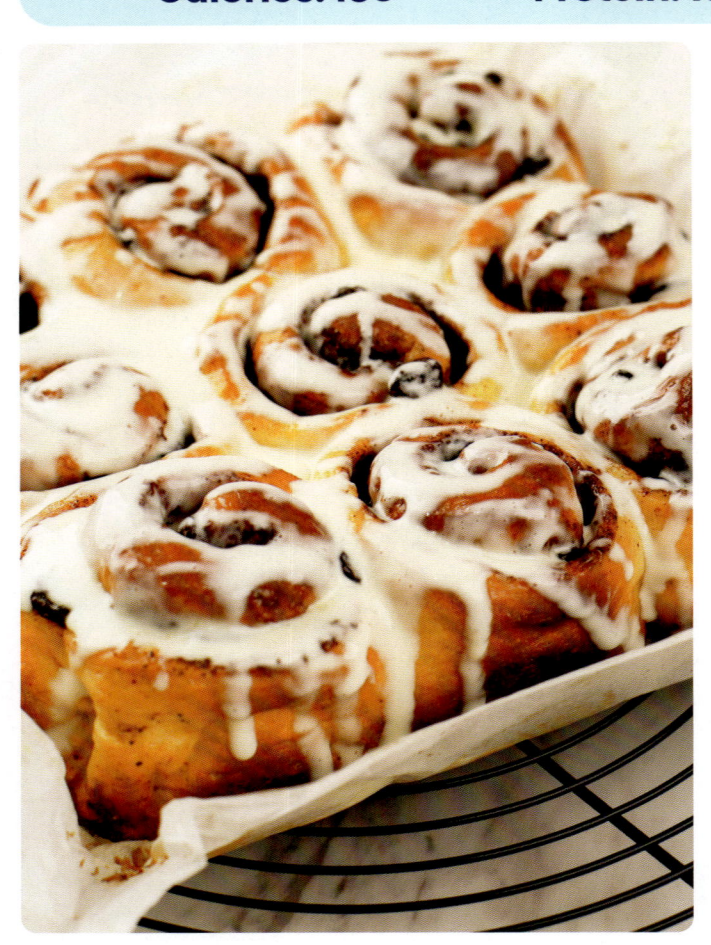

Calories: 180 **Protein: 18** **Carbs: 13** **Fat: 6**

Ingredients — Servings: 6

- 1 cup nonfat plain Greek yogurt
- 1 egg
- 2 tbsp softened butter
- 2 tsp vanilla extract
- 1/4 cup almond flour
- 3 scoops Dummy Supps Cinnamon Swirl Whey
- 1 1/2 tsp baking powder
- 2 tbsp cane sugar
- 1 tbsp ground cinnamon
- 1/2 cup whipped cream cheese
- 1 tsp cinnamon
- 2 tbsp zero calorie confectioners sugar
- 2 tsp unsweetened almond milk

Dummy Supps Whey Protein

Instructions

1. Preheat oven to 350°F.
2. In a large mixing bowl, whisk Greek yogurt, egg, butter, and vanilla extract until well combined.
3. Add flour, whey protein, baking powder, sugar, cinnamon, and combine ingredients until batter is formed.
4. Add donut batter to donut pan and bake for 10-12 minutes.
5. To a small mixing bowl, combine whipped cream cheese, cinnamon, confectioners sugar and mix until completely mixed.
6. Remove donuts from pan and add frosting to each.

DONUTS

PUMPKIN GLAZED DONUTS

Calories: 200 **Protein: 18** **Carbs: 16** **Fat: 8**

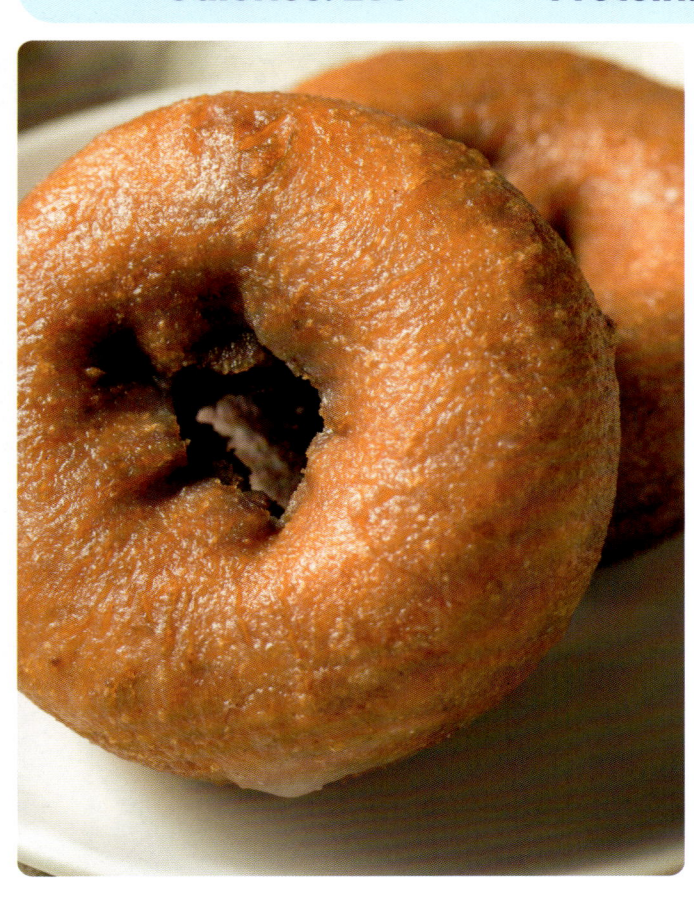

Ingredients   Servings: 6

- 1 cup pumpkin puree
- 1 egg
- 2 tbsp softened butter
- 2 tsp vanilla extract
- 2 tbsp maple syrup
- 1/4 cup almond flour
- 3 scoops Dummy Supps Cinnamon Swirl Whey
- 1 1/2 tsp baking powder
- 1 tbsp ground cinnamon
- 1 tsp nutmeg
- 1 tsp pumpkin pie spice
- 1/2 cup whipped cream cheese
- 1 tsp cinnamon
- 1 tsp pumpkin pie spice
- 2 tbsp zero calorie confectioners sugar

Dummy Supps Whey Protein

Instructions

1. Preheat oven to 350°F.
2. In a large mixing bowl, whisk pumpkin puree, egg, butter, vanilla extract, and maple syrup until well combined.
3. Add flour, whey protein, baking powder, cinnamon, nutmeg, pumpkin pie spice, and combine ingredients until batter is formed.
4. Add donut batter to donut pan and bake for 10-12 minutes.
5. To a small mixing bowl, combine whipped cream cheese, cinnamon, pumpkin pie spice, confectioners sugar and mix until completely mixed.
6. Remove donuts from pan and add frosting to each.

DONUTS

PUMPKIN SPICED DONUTS

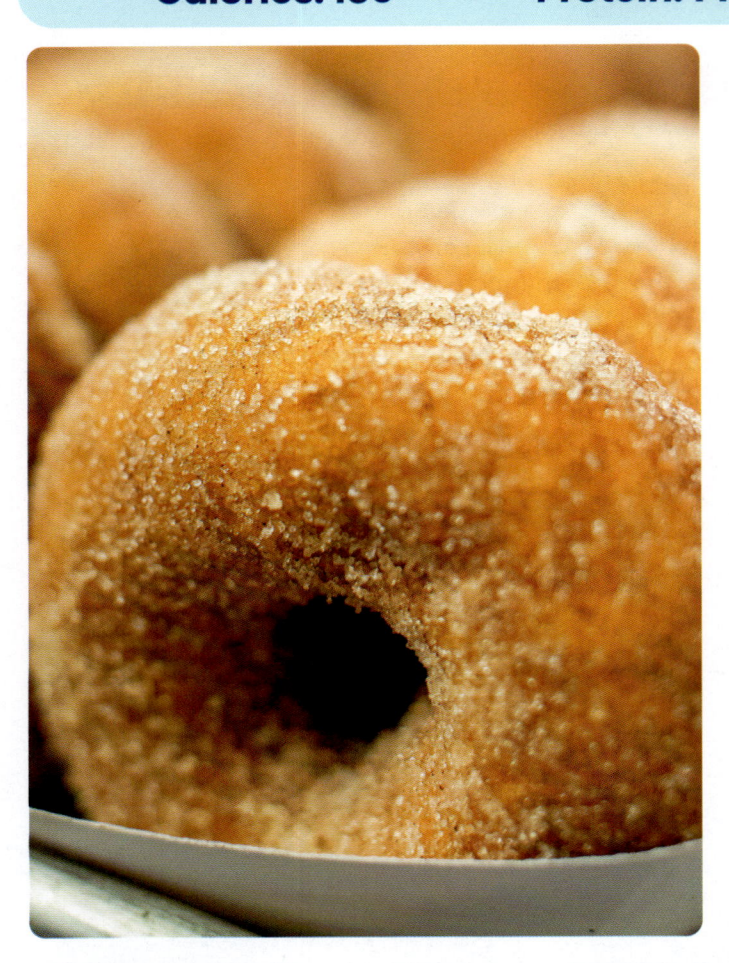

Calories: 180 **Protein: 14** **Carbs: 14** **Fat: 7**

Ingredients Servings: 6

- 1 cup pumpkin puree
- 1 egg
- 2 tbsp softened butter
- 2 tsp vanilla extract
- 2 tbsp maple syrup
- 1/4 cup almond flour
- 3 scoops Dummy Supps Cinnamon Swirl Whey
- 1 1/2 tsp baking powder
- 2 tbsp ground cinnamon
- 1 tsp nutmeg
- 4 tbsp zero calorie sugar
- 1 tsp pumpkin pie spice
- 1 tbsp butter
- 1 tsp cinnamon

Dummy Supps Whey Protein

Instructions

1. Preheat oven to 350°F.
2. In a large mixing bowl, whisk pumpkin puree, egg, butter, vanilla extract, and maple syrup until well combined.
3. Add flour, whey protein, baking powder, cinnamon, nutmeg, pumpkin pie spice, and combine ingredients until batter is formed.
4. Add donut batter to donut pan and bake for 10-12 minutes.
5. To a small mixing bowl, combine zero calorie sugar, cinnamon, and pumpkin pie spice.
6. Melt butter, brush over donuts, and add pumpkin spice.

DONUTS

MAPLE BACON DONUT

Calories: 260 **Protein: 21** **Carbs: 18** **Fat: 11**

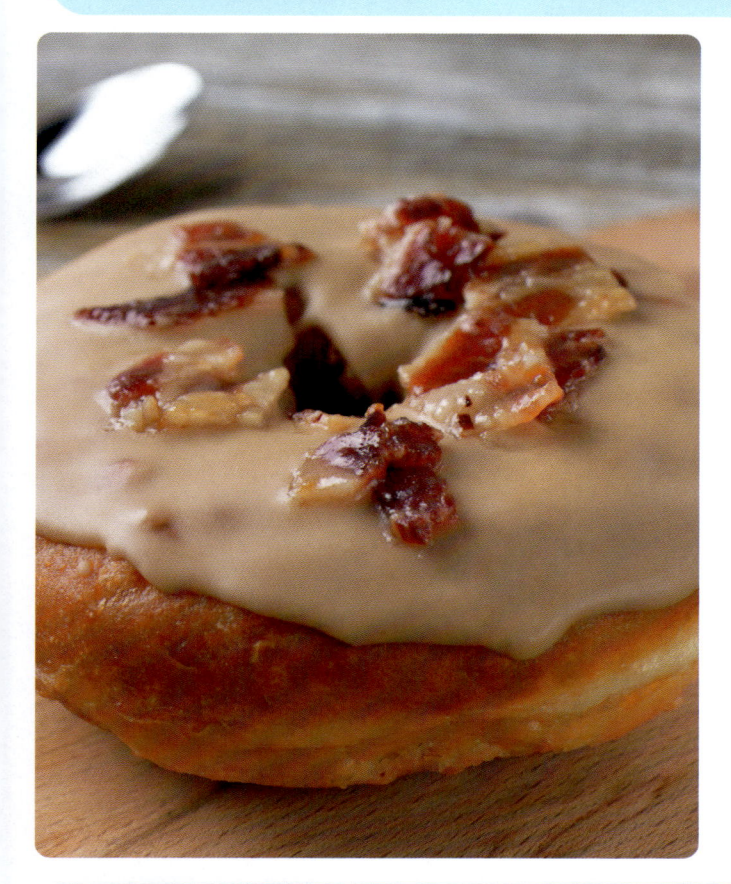

Ingredients Servings: 6

- 6 slices turkey bacon
- 1 cup nonfat plain Greek yogurt
- 1 egg
- 2 tbsp softened butter
- 2 tsp maple extract
- 2 tbsp maple syrup
- 1/4 cup almond flour
- 3 scoops Dummy Supps Cinnamon Swirl Whey
- 1 1/2 tsp baking powder
- 1 tbsp ground cinnamon
- 1/2 cup whipped cream cheese
- 1 tsp cinnamon
- 1 tbsp maple syrup
- 2 tbsp zero calorie confectioners sugar

Dummy Supps Whey Protein

Instructions

1. Preheat oven to 350°F.
2. Add turkey bacon to pan on medium high heat with cooking spray for 5 minutes, flip, and cook for additional 5 minutes or until crisp or place into microwave for 2-3 minutes until crisp.
3. In a large mixing bowl whisk: yogurt, egg, butter, maple extract, and maple syrup until well combined.
4. Add flour, whey protein, baking powder, cinnamon, and combine ingredients until batter is formed.
5. Add donut batter to donut pan and bake for 10-12 minutes.
6. To a small mixing bowl, combine whipped cream cheese, cinnamon, maple syrup, confectioners sugar and mix until completely mixed.
7. Remove donuts from pan and add frosting to each.

OTHER DESSERTS

OTHER DESSERT OPTIONS

DESSERT RECIPES

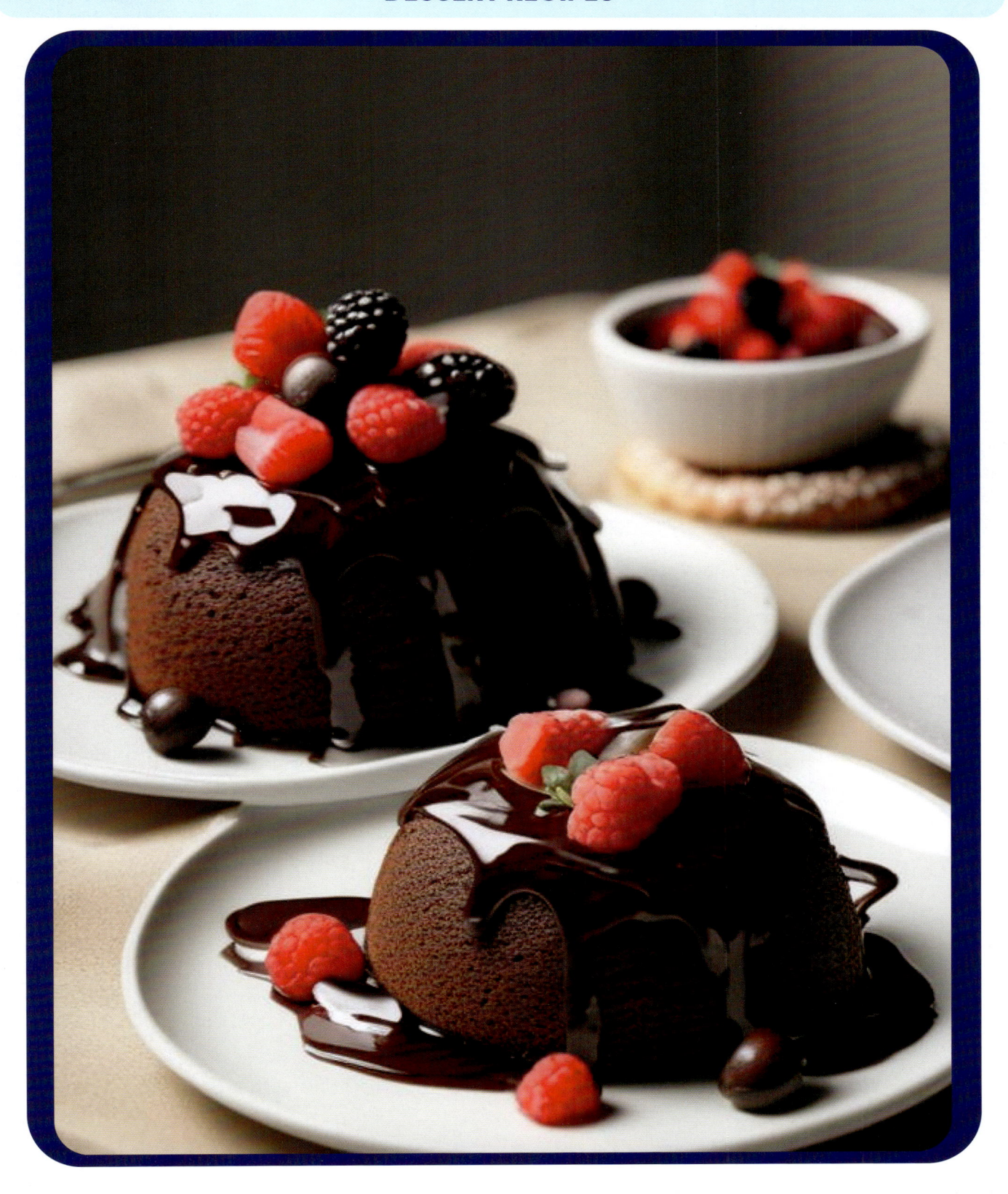

OTHER DESSERTS

CHEWY PROTEIN BARS

Calories: 170 **Protein: 9** **Carbs: 17** **Fat: 8**

Ingredients — Servings: 10

- 1/2 cup peanut butter powder
- 1/2 cup Mocha Dummy Butter/Peanut Butter
- 1/4 cup sugar-free maple syrup
- 2 scoops Dummy Supps vanilla whey
- 3 cups Rice Krispies
- 2 tbsp Lily's Dark chocolate chips
- 1/2 tsp coconut oil

Dummy Supps Whey Protein

Instructions

1. Melt peanut butter in the microwave for 30 seconds.
2. In a mixing bowl, combine peanut butter powder, melted peanut butter, sugar-free maple syrup, vanilla whey protein and mix well.
3. Add Rice Krispies and stir until the cereal is fully coated.
4. Pour the mixture into a baking dish and firmly press down to fill out the container evenly.
5. Add Lily's dark chocolate chips and coconut oil to a bowl and microwave for 1 minute until melted.
6. Drizzle chocolate over the top of pan.
7. Refrigerate for 1 hour until the chocolate has set then slice into 12 bars.

OTHER DESSERTS

CHOCOLATE CHIP COOKIES

Calories: 190 **Protein: 9** **Carbs: 10** **Fat: 13**

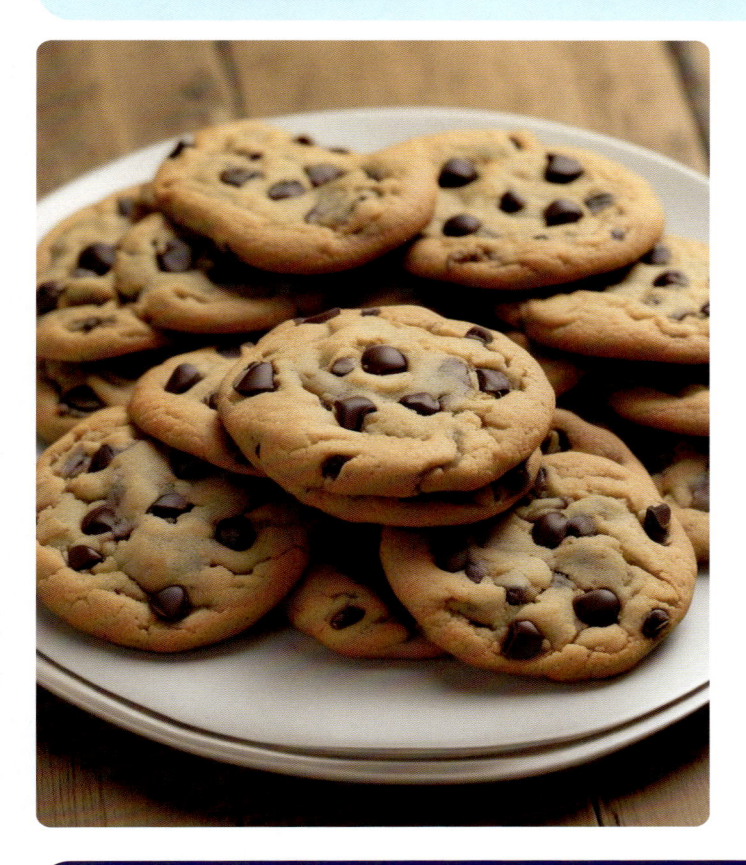

Ingredients   Servings: 8

- 1 banana
- 1 egg
- 1/2 cup peanut butter
- 1 tsp vanilla extract
- 1 scoop Dummy Supps vanilla whey
- 1/2 cup almond flour
- 1 tsp baking powder
- 2 tbsp Lily's Dark Chocolate Chips
- 1/4 tsp salt

Dummy Supps Whey Protein

Instructions

1. Preheat the oven to 350°F.
2. Melt peanut butter in the microwave for 30 seconds.
3. In a mixing bowl, mash banana until smooth, then add egg, vanilla extract, and melted peanut butter and whisk until combined.
4. Add whey protein, almond flour, and baking powder, then mix well.
5. Fold in Lily's dark chocolate chips.
6. Chill the dough in the fridge for 15–20 minutes.
7. Scoop 9 cookie dough balls onto a baking sheet.
8. Bake for 9–11 minutes until the edges are golden brown.
9. Transfer to a wire rack to cool completely.

OTHER DESSERTS

BULK PROTEIN BROWNIES

Calories: 260 **Protein: 13** **Carbs: 15** **Fat: 17**

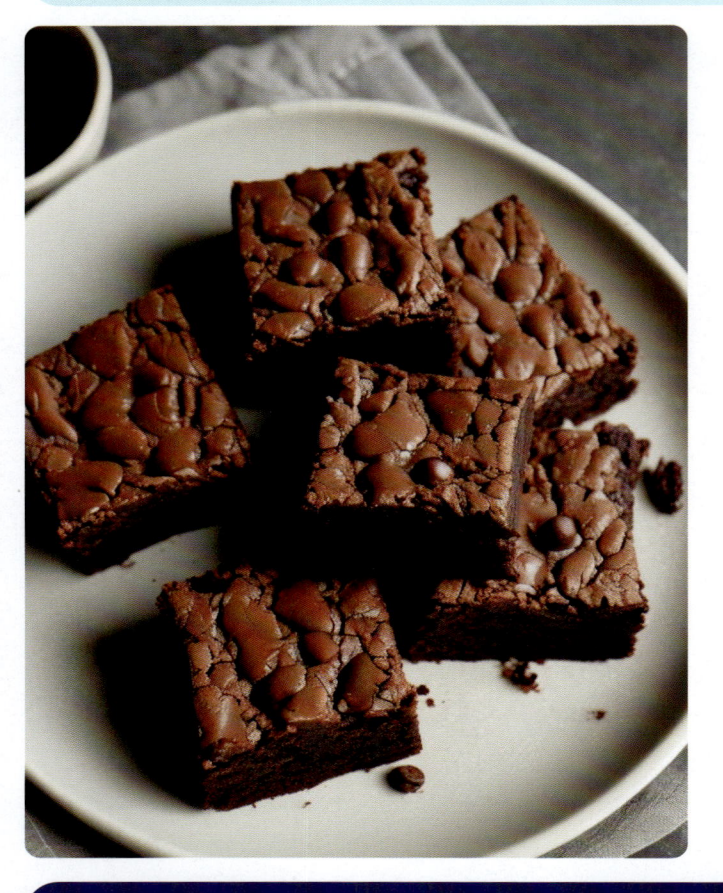

Ingredients Servings: 9

- 1 cup Mocha Dummy Butter/peanut butter
- 2 eggs
- 1/2 cup maple syrup
- 1/2 tsp vanilla extract
- 2 scoops Dummy Supps Chocolate Whey
- 1/4 cup cocoa powder
- 1/2 tsp salt
- 1/2 cup unsweetened almond milk (as needed to thin batter)
- 4 tbsp Lily's Dark Chocolate Chips

Dummy Supps Whey Protein

Instructions

1. Preheat oven to 350°F.
2. Melt peanut butter in the microwave for 30 seconds.
3. In a mixing bowl, add melted peanut butter, eggs, maple syrup, and vanilla extract and whisk until well combined.
4. Add whey, cocoa powder, and salt, and mix well.
5. Use almond milk to thin the batter if necessary.
6. Fold in Lily's dark chocolate chips.
7. Drop the batter into a baking pan lined with cooking spray and bake for 25-30 minutes.
8. Let the brownies cool, then slice.

OTHER DESSERTS

CHOCOLATE PB BROWNIES

Calories: 220 **Protein: 12** **Carbs: 21** **Fat: 12**

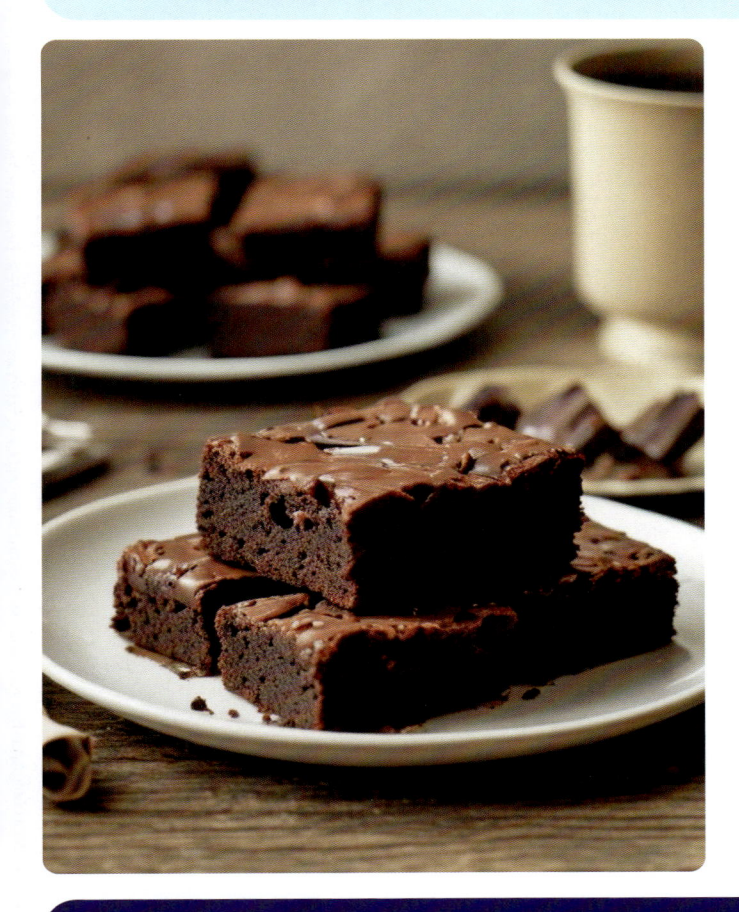

Ingredients Servings: 9

- 3 bananas
- 2 eggs
- 1/2 cup Mocha Dummy Butter/almond butter
- 3 scoops Dummy Supps Chocolate PB Whey
- 1/4 cup cocoa powder
- 1/2 tsp salt
- 1 tsp baking powder
- 4 tbsp Lilly's chocolate chips

Dummy Supps Whey Protein

Instructions

1. Preheat oven to 350 degrees.
2. To a large mixing bowl, mash bananas, then add peanut/almond butter, whey protein, cocoa powder, salt, baking powder, chocolate chips, and blend until well combined.
3. Add ingredients to a baking pan with cooking spray and bake for 15-20 minutes or until the top is firm to the touch.
4. Split into 9 brownied.

OTHER DESSERTS

CHOCOLATE PB LAVA CAKE

Calories: 470 **Protein: 43** **Carbs: 34** **Fat: 27**

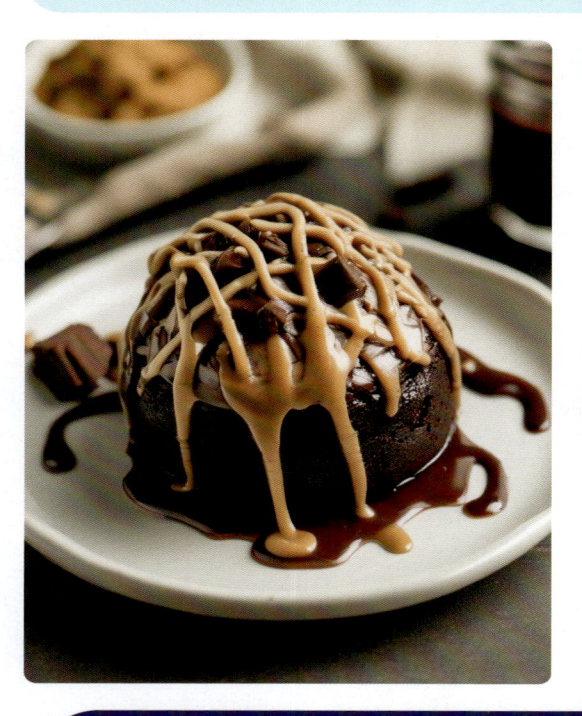

Ingredients — Servings: 1

- 1/2 cup cottage cheese
- 2 tbsp cocoa powder
- 2 tbsp Dummy Supps Chocolate PB Whey
- 1 egg
- 2 tbsp Lilly's Dark Chocolate Chips
- 1/4 tsp salt
- 1 tbsp Mocha Dummy Butter/Almond Butter

Dummy Supps Whey Protein — SCAN ME

Instructions

1. Blend cottage cheese, cocoa powder, Dummy Supps Chocolate PB Whey, egg, and Mocha Dummy Butter/Almond Butter until smooth.
2. Microwave for 90-120 seconds until desired firmness.
3. Top with Lily's Dark Chocolate Chips, salt, and drizzle with extra Mocha Dummy Butter/Almond Butter.

CHOCOLATE BERRY LAVA CAKE

Calories: 510 **Protein: 44** **Carbs: 43** **Fat: 27**

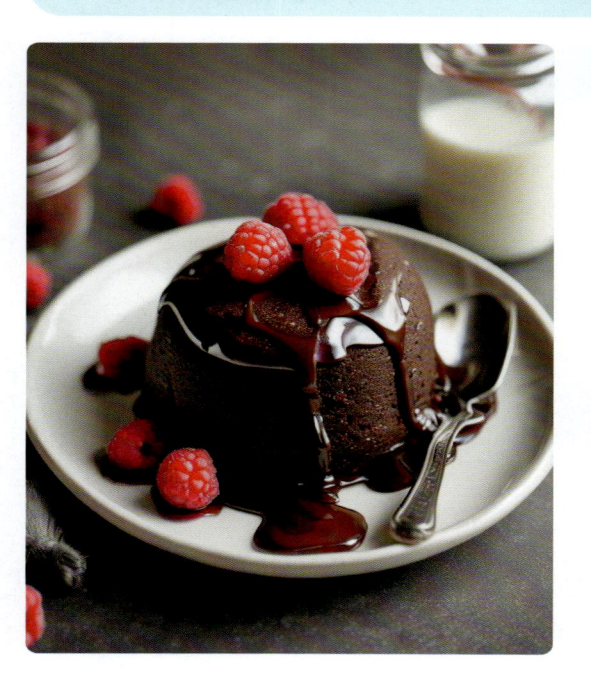

Ingredients — Servings: 1

- 1/2 cup cottage cheese
- 2 tbsp cocoa powder
- 2 tbsp Dummy Supps Chocolate Whey
- 1 egg
- 2 tbsp Lilly's Dark Chocolate Chips
- 1/4 tsp salt
- 1 tbsp PB&J Dummy Butter/Almond Butter
- 1/2 cup raspberries

Dummy Supps Whey Protein — SCAN ME

Instructions

1. Blend cottage cheese, cocoa powder, Dummy Supps Chocolate PB Whey, egg, salt, and PB&J/Almond Butter until smooth.
2. Stir in raspberries and Lily's White Chocolate Chips.
3. Microwave for 90-120 seconds until desired firmness.
4. Top with extra raspberries, salt, and a drizzle of PB&J Dummy Butter/Almond Butter.

OTHER DESSERTS

CHOCOLATE STRAWBERRY LAVA CAKE

Calories: 500 **Protein: 44** **Carbs: 40** **Fat: 27**

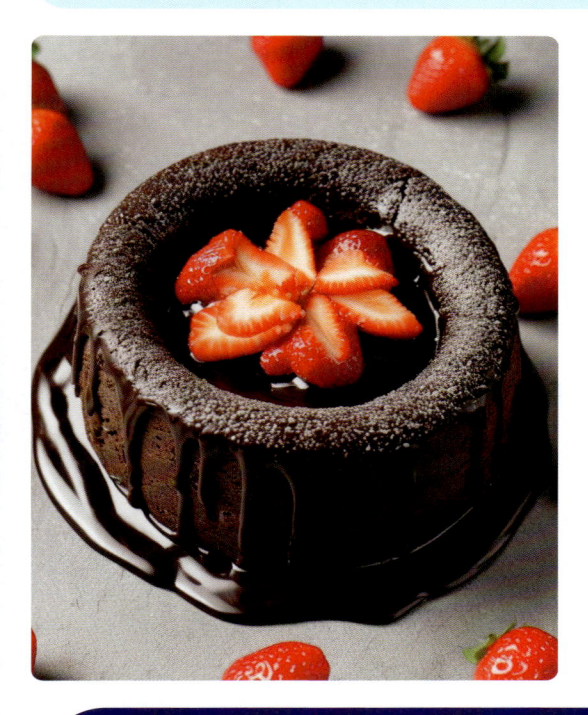

Ingredients — Servings: 1

- 1/2 cup cottage cheese
- 2 tbsp cocoa powder
- 2 tbsp Dummy Supps Chocolate Whey
- 1 egg
- 2 tbsp Lilly's Dark Chocolate Chips
- 1/4 tsp salt
- 1 tbsp PB&J Dummy Butter/Almond Butter
- 1/2 cup strawberries

Dummy Supps Whey Protein (SCAN ME)

Instructions

1. Blend cottage cheese, cocoa powder, Dummy Supps Chocolate PB Whey, egg, salt, and PB&J/Almond Butter until smooth.
2. Stir in chopped strawberries and Lily's White Chocolate Chips.
3. Microwave for 90-120 seconds until desired firmness.
4. Top with extra strawberries, a drizzle of PB&J Dummy Butter/Almond Butter, and a pinch of salt.

MOCHA LAVA CAKE

Calories: 480 **Protein: 44** **Carbs: 34** **Fat: 27**

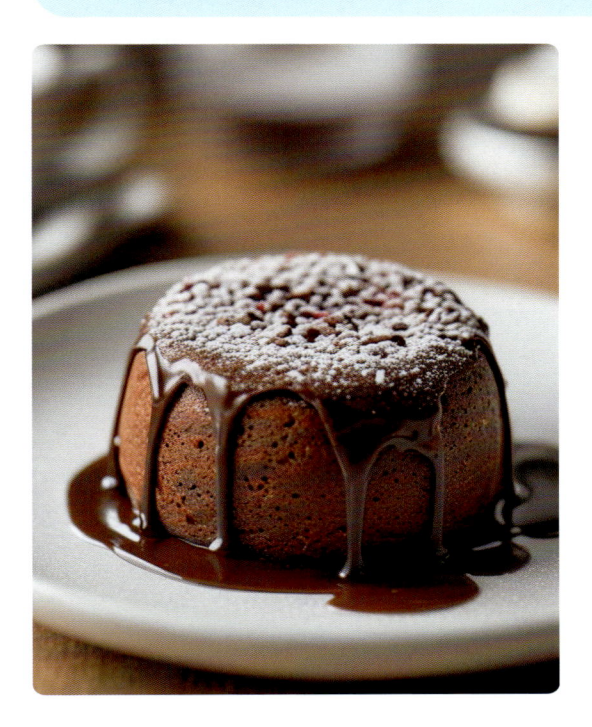

Ingredients — Servings: 1

- 1/2 cup cottage cheese
- 2 tbsp cocoa powder
- 1 tsp instant coffee
- 2 tbsp Dummy Supps Mocha Whey
- 1 egg
- 2 tbsp Lilly's Dark Chocolate Chips
- 1/4 tsp salt
- 1 tbsp Mocha Dummy Butter/Almond Butter

Dummy Supps Whey Protein (SCAN ME)

Instructions

1. Blend cottage cheese, cocoa powder, instant coffee, Dummy Supps Mocha Whey, egg, salt, and Mocha Dummy Butter/Almond Butter until smooth.
2. Microwave for 90-120 seconds until desired firmness.
3. Top with Lily's Dark Chocolate Chips, a drizzle of Mocha Dummy Butter/Almond Butter, and a pinch of salt.

OTHER DESSERTS

CHOCOLATE LAVA CAKE

Calories: 310   **Protein: 34**   **Carbs: 28**   **Fat: 14**

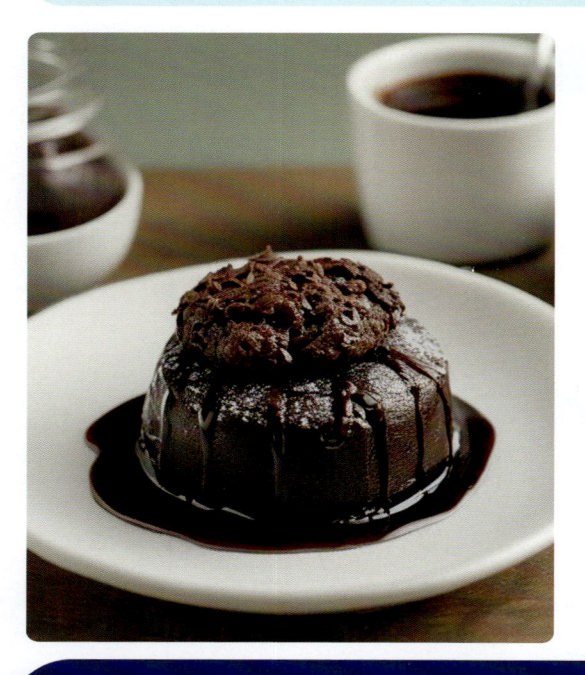

Ingredients   Servings: 1

- 1/2 cup cottage cheese
- 3 tbsp cocoa powder
- 1 egg
- 2 tbsp monk fruit
- 2 tbsp Lilly's Dark Chocolate Chips
- 1/4 tsp salt

Dummy Supps Whey Protein — SCAN ME

Instructions

1. Blend cottage cheese, cocoa powder, egg, and maple syrup until smooth.
2. Microwave for 90-120 seconds until desired firmness.
3. Top with Lily's Dark Chocolate Chips and salt.

BLUEBERRY MUFFINS

Calories: 230   **Protein: 20**   **Carbs: 18**   **Fat: 10**

Ingredients   Servings: 6

- 2 bananas
- 3/4 cup nonfat Greek yogurt
- 1 egg
- 1/4 cup sugar-free maple syrup
- 1 tsp vanilla extract
- 1 tsp coconut oil
- 3/4 cup almond flour
- 3 scoops Dummy Supps Vanilla Whey
- 1 tsp baking powder
- 1 1/2 cups blueberries
- 1/2 tsp salt

Dummy Supps Whey Protein — SCAN ME

Instructions

1. Preheat oven to 350ºF.
2. In a large mixing bowl, mash bananas, then add Greek yogurt, egg, sugar-free maple syrup, vanilla extract, and coconut oil. Whisk until smooth.
3. Add almond flour, Dummy Supps Vanilla Whey, baking powder, and salt, then mix well.
4. Gently fold in blueberries.
5. Grease the muffin tins and pour in the batter.
6. Bake for 25-30 minutes, or until a toothpick comes out clean.

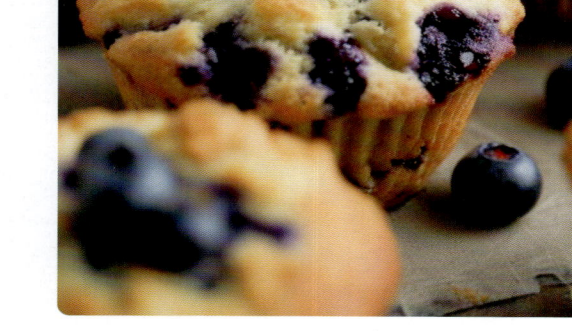

OTHER DESSERTS

MIXED BERRY MUFFINS

Calories: 240   **Protein: 20**   **Carbs: 18**   **Fat: 10**

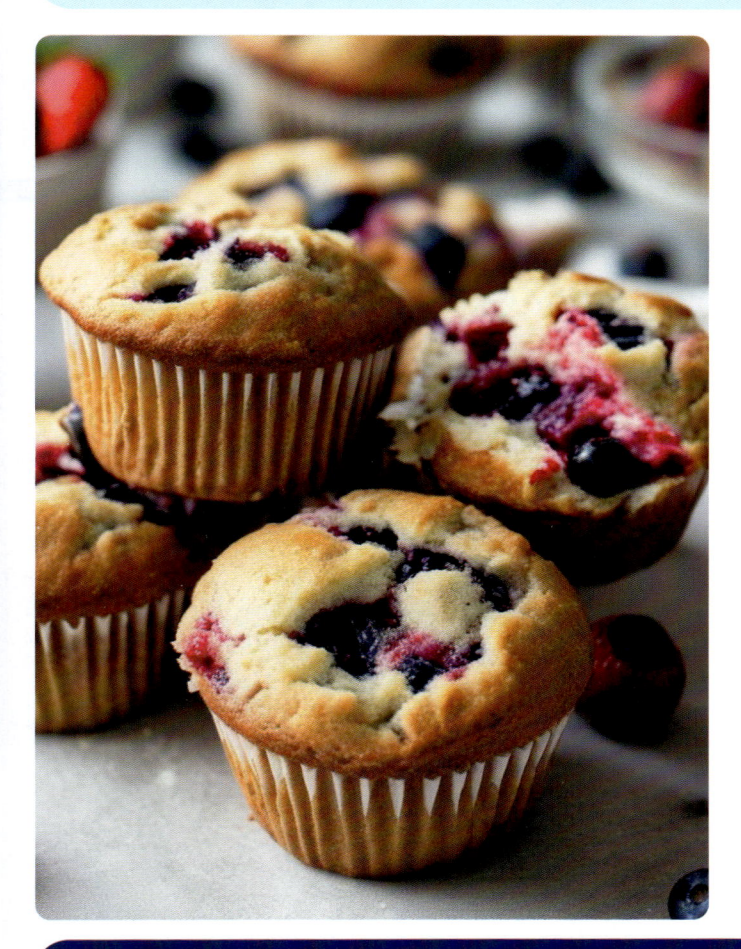

Ingredients   Servings: 6

- 2 bananas
- 3/4 cup nonfat plain Greek yogurt
- 1 egg
- 1/4 cup sugar-free maple syrup
- 1 tsp vanilla extract
- 3 scoops Muscle Dummies Berry Whey
- 3/4 cup almond flour
- 1 tsp and baking powder
- 1/4 tsp salt
- 1 1/2 cups mixed berries (blueberries, raspberries, strawberries)

Dummy Supps Whey Protein

Instructions

1. Preheat oven to 350°F.
2. In a large mixing bowl, mash bananas, then add Greek yogurt, egg, sugar-free maple syrup, and vanilla extract. Whisk until smooth.
3. Add Muscle Dummies Vanilla Whey, almond flour, baking powder, and salt, then mix well.
4. Gently fold in mixed berries, ensuring they are evenly distributed.
5. Grease the muffin tins and pour in the batter.
6. Bake for 25-30 minutes, or until a toothpick comes out clean.

OTHER DESSERTS

CHOCOLATE MOCHA MUFFINS

Calories: 260   **Protein: 20**   **Carbs: 22**   **Fat: 11**

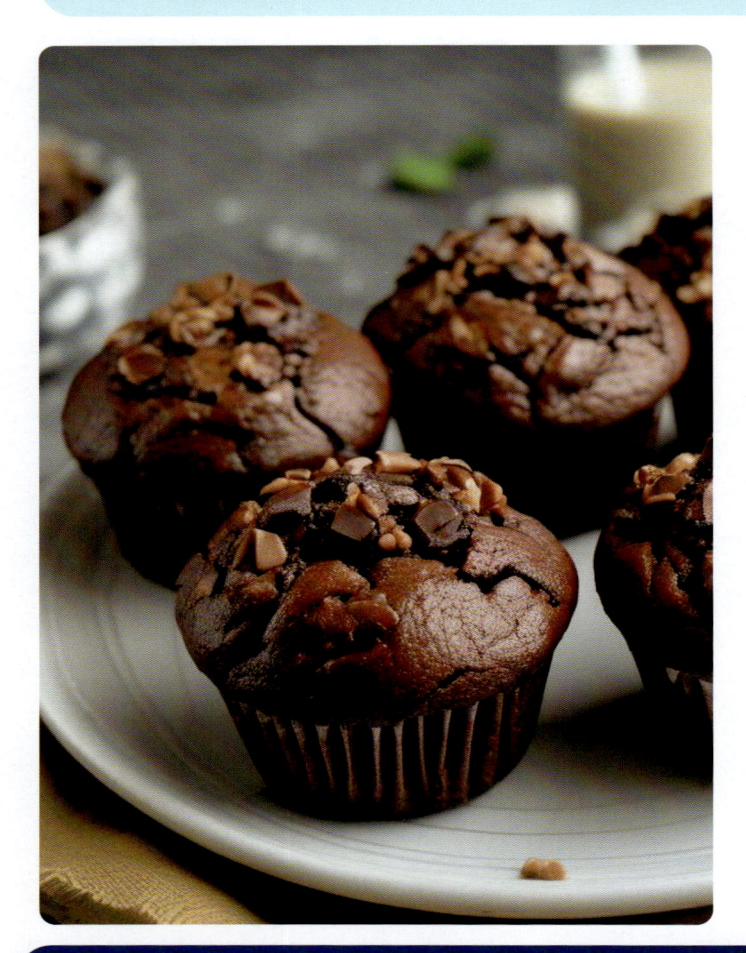

Ingredients   Servings: 6

- 2 bananas
- 3/4 cup nonfat plain Greek yogurt
- 1 egg
- 1/4 cup sugar-free maple syrup
- 1 tsp vanilla extract
- 2 tbsp cocoa powder
- 2 tbsp instant coffee or espresso powder
- 3 scoops Muscle Dummies Mocha Whey
- 1/2 cup almond flour
- 1 tsp and baking powder
- 1/4 tsp salt
- 4 tbsp Lily's Dark Chocolate Chips

Dummy Supps Whey Protein

Instructions

1. Preheat oven to 350°F.
2. In a large mixing bowl, mash bananas, then add Greek yogurt, egg, sugar-free maple syrup, and vanilla extract. Whisk until smooth.
3. Add Muscle Dummies Mocha Whey, cocoa powder, instant coffee, almond flour, baking powder, and salt, then mix well.
4. Fold in Lily's Dark Chocolate Chips.
5. Grease the muffin tins and pour in the batter.
6. Bake for 25-30 minutes, or until a toothpick comes out clean.

OTHER DESSERTS

CHOCOLATE CHIP MUFFINS

Calories: 260   **Protein: 20**   **Carbs: 22**   **Fat: 11**

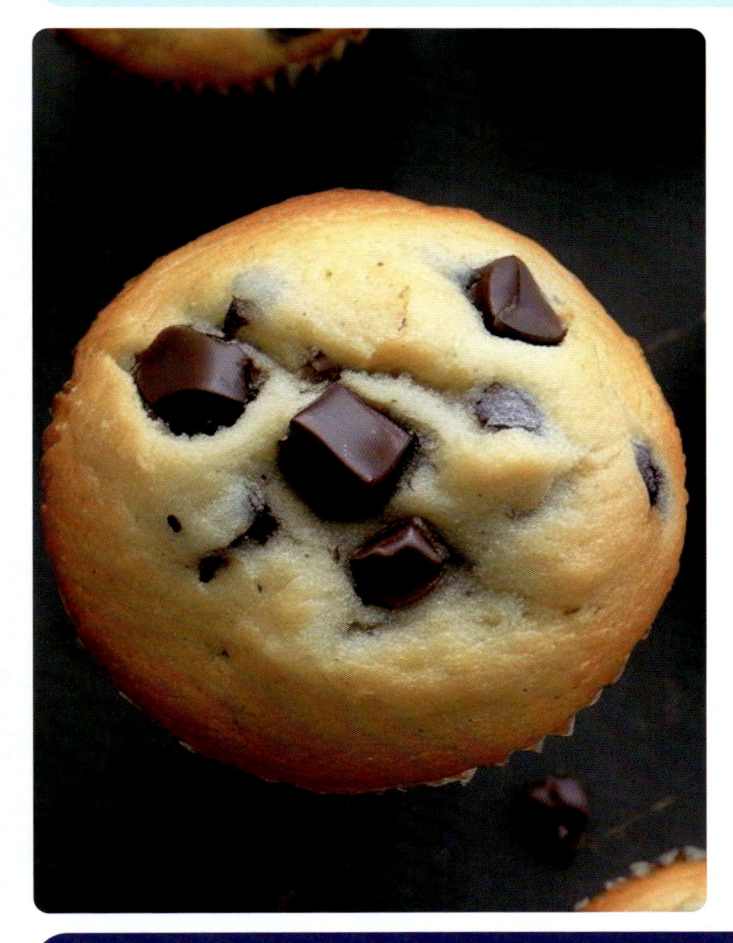

Ingredients   **Servings: 6**

- 2 bananas
- 3/4 cup nonfat Greek yogurt
- 1 egg
- 1/4 cup sugar-free maple syrup
- 1 tsp vanilla extract
- 1 tsp coconut oil
- 3/4 cup almond flour
- 3 scoops Dummy Supps Vanilla Whey
- 1 tsp baking powder
- 4 tbsp Lily's dark chocolate chips
- 1/2 tsp salt

Dummy Supps Whey Protein

Instructions

1. Preheat oven to 350°F.
2. In a large mixing bowl, mash bananas, then add Greek yogurt, egg, sugar-free maple syrup, vanilla extract, and coconut oil. Whisk until smooth.
3. Add almond flour, Dummy Supps Vanilla Whey, baking powder, and salt, then mix well.
4. Fold in Lily's dark chocolate chips.
5. Grease the muffin tins and pour in the batter.
6. Bake for 25-30 minutes, or until a toothpick comes out clean.

OTHER DESSERTS

PUMPKIN SPICE MUFFINS

Calories: 300 **Protein: 20** **Carbs: 29** **Fat: 13**

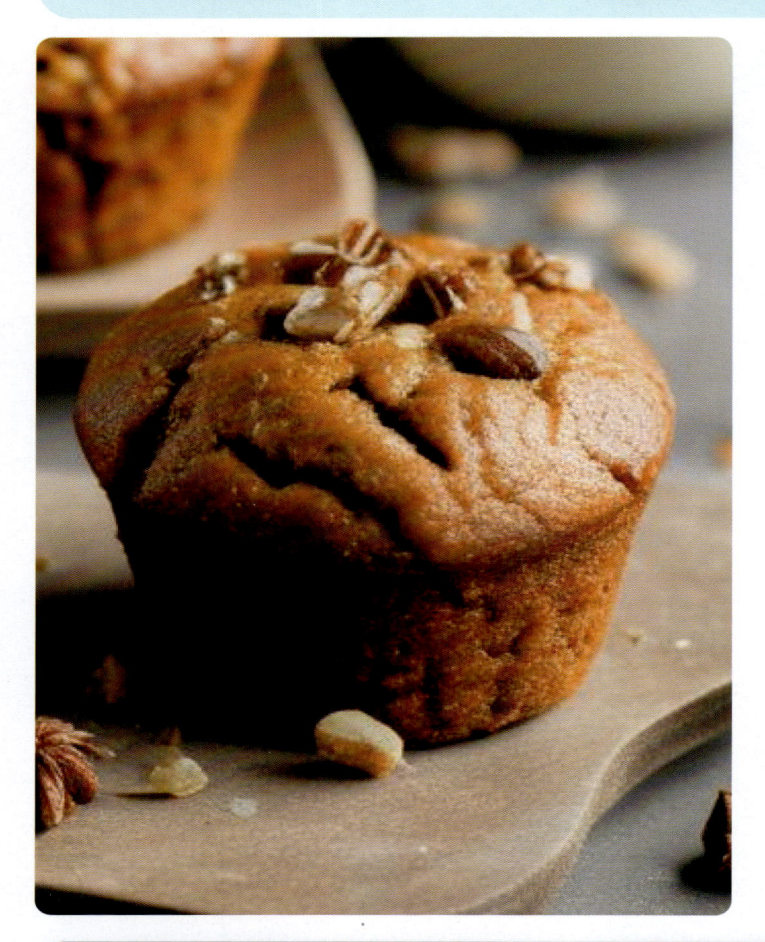

Ingredients   Servings: 6

- 1 cup pumpkin puree
- 1/2 cup nonfat plain Greek yogurt
- 1 egg
- 1/4 cup sugar-free maple syrup
- 1 tsp vanilla extract
- 3 scoops Muscle Dummies Cinnamon Swirl whey
- 3/4 cup almond flour
- 1 tsp coconut oil
- 4 tbsp Lilly's dark chocolate chips
- 1 tbsp pumpkin pie spice
- 1 tsp baking powder
- 1/2 tsp salt

Dummy Supps Whey Protein

Instructions

1. Preheat oven to 350°F.
2. In a large mixing bowl, combine pumpkin puree, Greek yogurt, egg, sugar-free maple syrup, vanilla extract, and coconut oil. Whisk until smooth.
3. Add almond flour, Muscle Dummies Cinnamon Swirl Whey, pumpkin pie spice, baking powder, and salt, then mix well.
4. Fold in Lily's dark chocolate chips.
5. Grease the muffin tins and pour in the batter.
6. Bake for 25-30 minutes, or until a toothpick comes out clean.

OTHER DESSERTS

DOUBLE CHUNK CHOCOLATE MUFFINS

Calories: 250   **Protein: 20**   **Carbs: 26**   **Fat: 10**

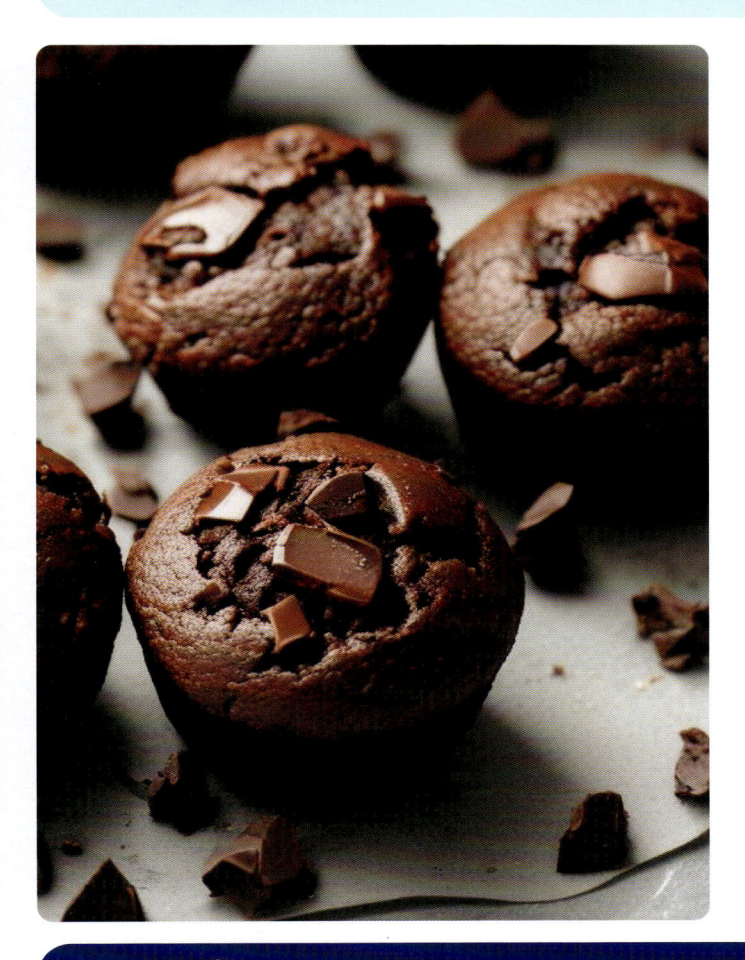

Ingredients   **Servings: 6**

- 4 bananas
- 3/4 cup nonfat plain Greek yogurt
- 1 egg
- 1/4 cup sugar-free maple syrup
- 1 tsp vanilla extract
- 3 scoops Muscle Dummies Chocolate Whey
- 1/2 cup almond flour
- 4 tbsp Lilly's Dark Chocolate Chips
- 2 tbsp cocoa powder
- 1 tsp baking soda and powder
- 1/4 tsp salt

Dummy Supps Whey Protein

SCAN ME

Instructions

1. Preheat oven to 350°F.
2. In a large mixing bowl, mash bananas, then add Greek yogurt, egg, sugar-free maple syrup, and vanilla extract. Whisk until smooth.
3. Add Muscle Dummies Chocolate Whey, almond flour, cocoa powder, baking soda, baking powder, and salt, then mix well.
4. Fold in Lily's dark chocolate chips.
5. Grease the muffin tins and pour in the batter.
6. Bake for 25-30 minutes, or until a toothpick comes out clean.

OTHER DESSERTS

CHOCOLATE BANANA BREAD

Calories: 270 **Protein: 20** **Carbs: 30** **Fat: 13**

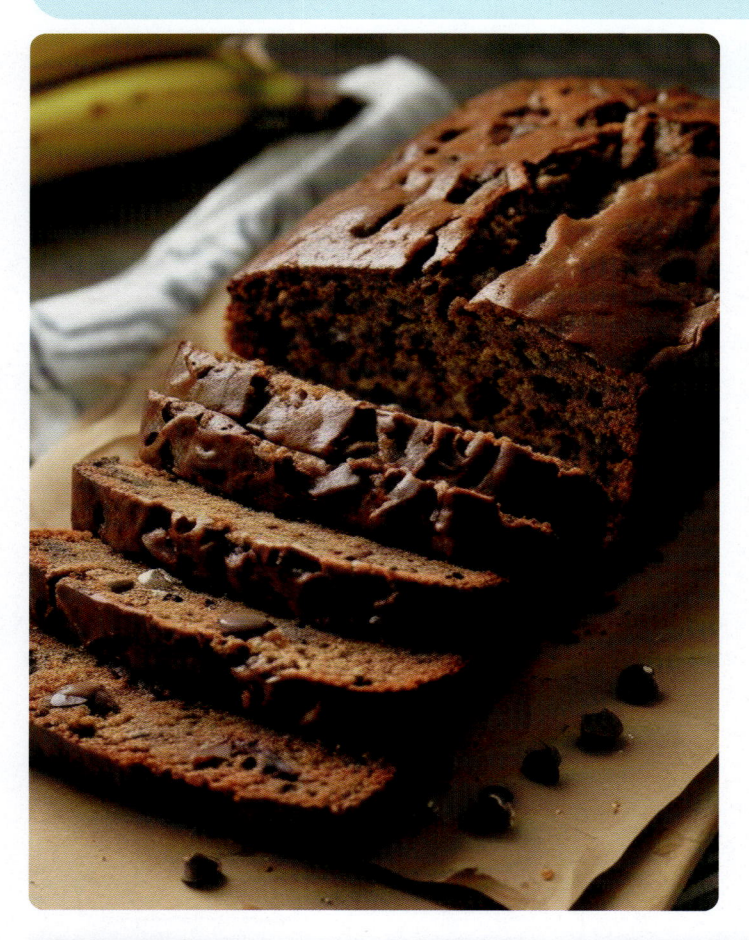

Ingredients — Servings: 9

- 4 bananas
- 2 eggs
- 1/4 cup maple syrup
- 1 cup nonfat plain Greek yogurt
- 1 tsp vanilla extract
- 1 cup almond flour
- 3 scoops Dummy Supps Chocolate whey
- 2 tbsp cocoa powder
- 1 tsp baking powder
- 1/2 tsp salt
- 1/2 cup Lily's dark chocolate chips
- 1 tbsp melted coconut oil

Dummy Supps Whey Protein

Instructions

1. Preheat oven to 325°F.
2. In a large mixing bowl, mash bananas, then add eggs, maple syrup, Greek yogurt, and vanilla extract. Whisk until smooth.
3. Add almond flour, Dummy Supps Vanilla Whey, cocoa powder, baking powder, and salt, then mix until fully combined.
4. Fold in Lily's dark chocolate chips, ensuring even distribution.
5. Grease a 9x5-inch loaf pan and pour in the batter, spreading evenly.
6. Bake for 40-50 minutes (check at 35 minutes, or until a toothpick inserted in the center comes out clean.

OTHER DESSERTS

PUMPKIN BANANA BREAD

Calories: 250 **Protein: 18** **Carbs: 16** **Fat: 13**

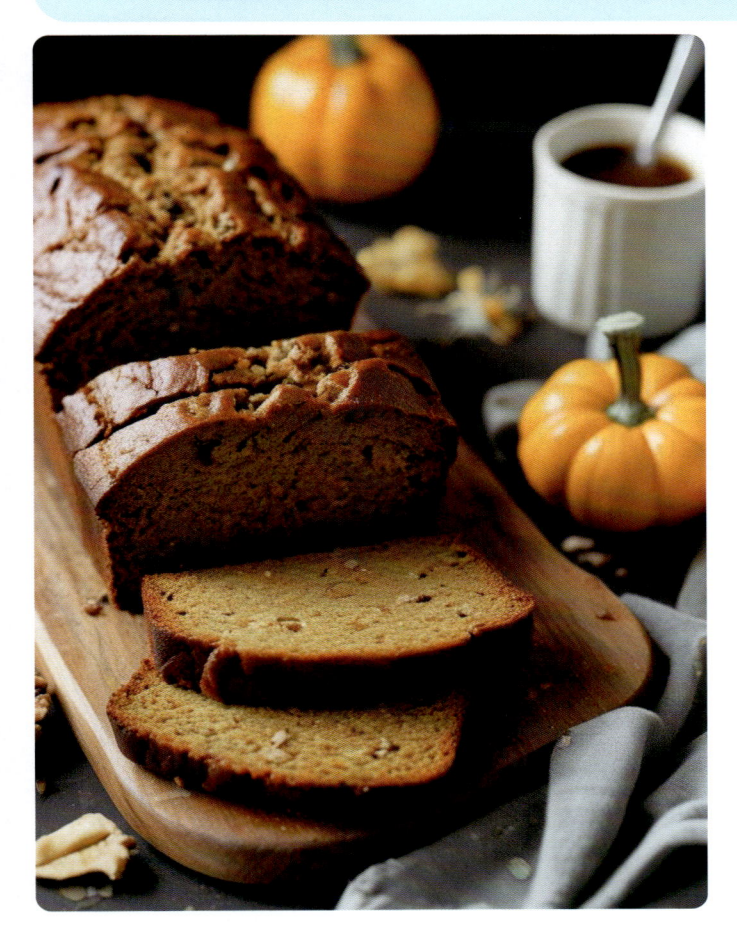

Ingredients **Servings: 9**

- 1 cup pumpkin puree
- 3/4 cup non fat plain Greek yogurt
- 2 eggs
- 1 tsp vanilla extract
- 3 scoops Dummy Supps Cinnamon Swirl Whey
- 1 cup almond/oat flour
- 1 tbsp pumpkin pie spice
- 1 tsp baking powder
- 1/2 tsp salt
- 1/2 cup Lilly's dark chocolate chips
- 1 tbsp melted coconut oil

Dummy Supps Whey Protein

Instructions

1. Preheat oven to 325°F.
2. In a large mixing bowl, combine pumpkin puree, Greek yogurt, eggs, and vanilla extract. Whisk until smooth.
3. Add Dummy Supps Cinnamon Swirl Whey, almond/oat flour, pumpkin pie spice, baking powder, and salt, then mix until fully combined.
4. Fold in Lily's dark chocolate chips, ensuring even distribution.
5. Grease a 9x5-inch loaf pan and pour in the batter, spreading evenly.
6. Bake for 40-50 minutes, or until a toothpick inserted in the center comes out clean.

OTHER DESSERTS

BERRY BANANA BREAD

Calories: 250 **Protein: 19** **Carbs: 32** **Fat: 9**

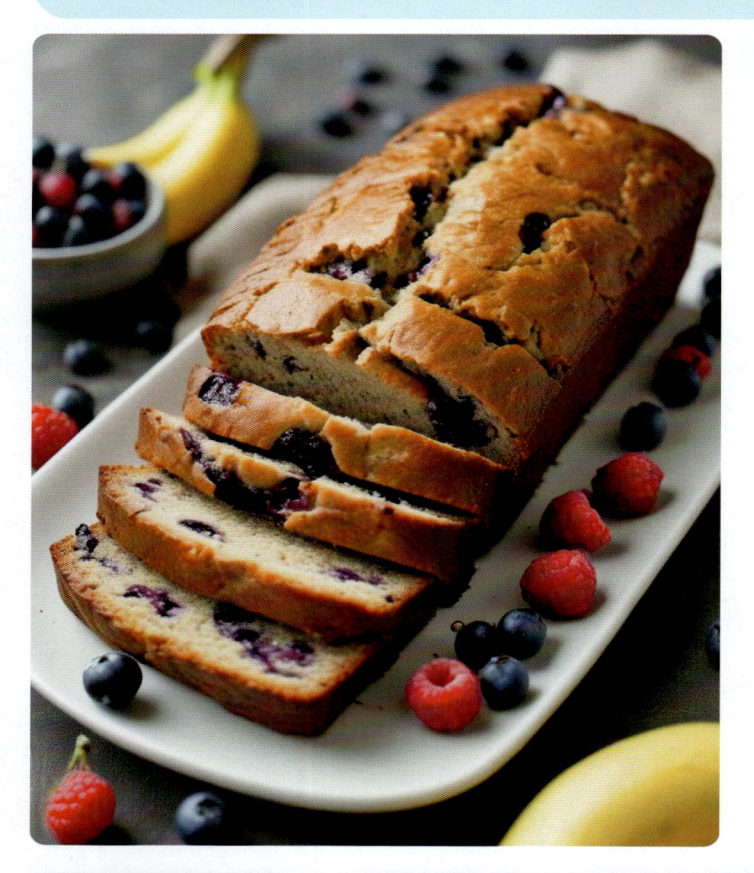

Ingredients   Servings: 9

- 4 bananas
- 2 eggs
- 1/4 cup maple syrup
- 1 cup nonfat plain Greek yogurt
- 1 tsp vanilla extract
- 1 cup almond flour
- 3 scoops Dummy Supps Berry Whey
- 1 tsp baking powder
- 1/2 tsp salt
- 1 1/2 cups mixed berries (blueberries, raspberries, strawberries)
- 1 tbsp melted coconut oil

Dummy Supps Whey Protein

Instructions

1. Preheat oven to 325°F.
2. In a large mixing bowl, mash bananas, then add eggs, maple syrup, Greek yogurt, and vanilla extract. Whisk until smooth.
3. Add almond flour, Dummy Supps Berry Whey, baking powder, and salt, then mix well.
4. Gently fold in mixed berries to prevent them from breaking too much.
5. Grease a loaf pan and pour in the batter, spreading evenly.
6. Bake for 40-45 minutes (check at 35 minutes), or until a toothpick comes out clean.

OTHER DESSERTS

CHOCOLATE MOCHA BANANA BREAD

Calories: 280 **Protein: 20** **Carbs: 25** **Fat: 14**

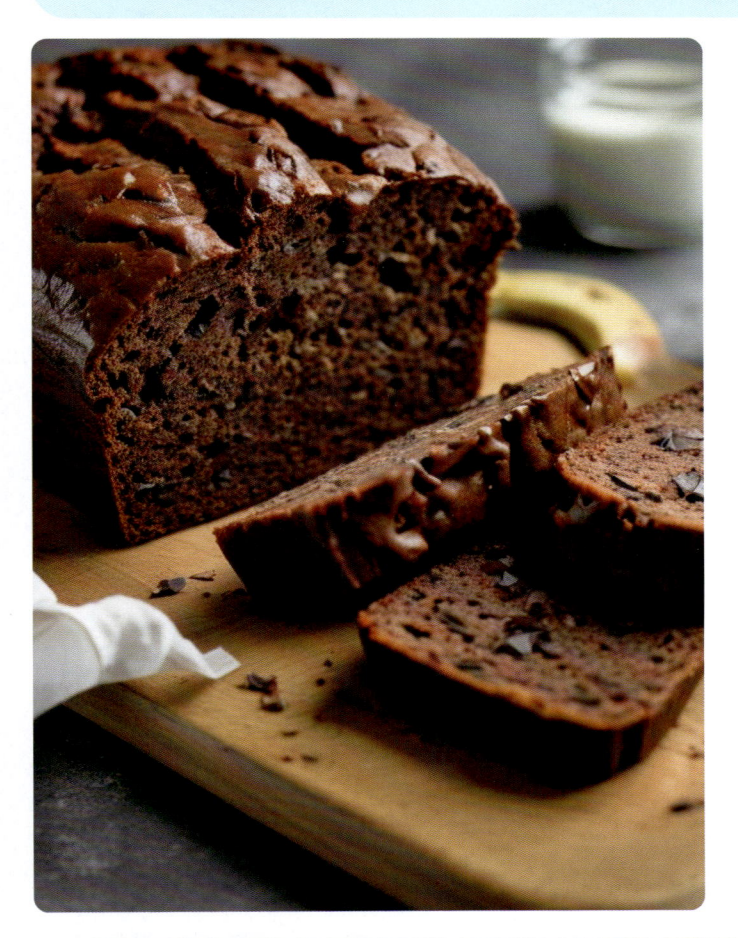

Ingredients   Servings: 9

- 4 bananas
- 2 eggs
- 1/4 cup maple syrup
- 1 cup nonfat plain Greek yogurt
- 1 tsp vanilla extract
- 1 cup almond flour
- 3 scoops Dummy Supps Mocha Whey
- 1/4 cup cocoa powder
- 1 tbsp instant coffee or espresso powder
- 1 tsp baking powder
- 1/2 tsp salt
- 1/2 cup Lily's dark chocolate chips
- 1 tbsp melted coconut oil

Dummy Supps Whey Protein

Instructions

1. Preheat oven to 325°F.
2. In a large mixing bowl, mash bananas, then add eggs, maple syrup, Greek yogurt, and vanilla extract. Whisk until smooth.
3. Add almond flour, Dummy Supps Mocha Whey, cocoa powder, instant coffee, baking powder, and salt, then mix until fully combined.
4. Fold in Lily's dark chocolate chips, ensuring even distribution.
5. Grease a 9x5-inch loaf pan and pour in the batter, spreading evenly.
6. Bake for 40-50 minutes (check at 35 minutes), or until a toothpick inserted in the center comes out clean.

OTHER DESSERTS

CHOCOLATE CHIP BANANA BREAD

Calories: 270 **Protein: 20** **Carbs: 25** **Fat: 13**

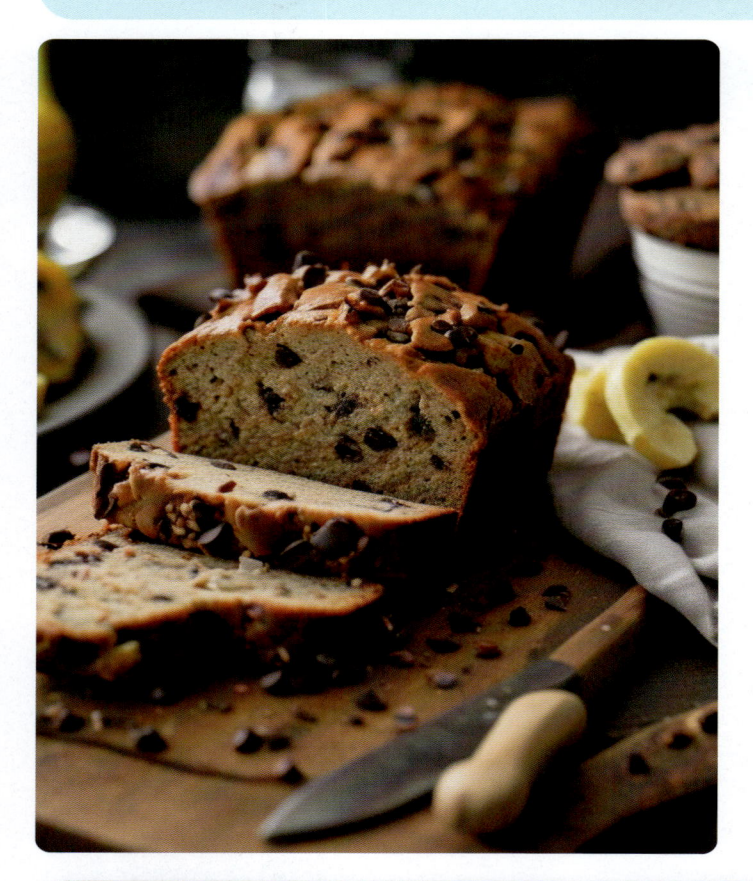

Ingredients **Servings: 9**

- 4 bananas
- 2 eggs
- 1/4 cup maple syrup
- 1 cup nonfat plain Greek yogurt
- 1 tsp vanilla extract
- 1 cup almond flour
- 3 scoops Dummy Supps Vanilla whey
- 1 tsp baking powder
- 1/2 tsp salt
- 1/2 cup Lily's dark chocolate chips
- 1 tbsp melted coconut oil

Dummy Supps Whey Protein

Instructions

1. Preheat oven to 325°F.
2. In a large mixing bowl, mash bananas, then add eggs, maple syrup, Greek yogurt, and vanilla extract. Whisk until smooth.
3. Add almond flour, Dummy Supps Berry Whey, baking powder, and salt, then mix well.
4. Gently fold in mixed berries to prevent them from breaking too much.
5. Grease a loaf pan and pour in the batter, spreading evenly.
6. Bake for 40-45 minutes (check at 35 minutes), or until a toothpick comes out clean.

OTHER DESSERTS

CINNAMON ROLLS

Calories: 250 **Protein: 24** **Carbs: 11** **Fat: 7**

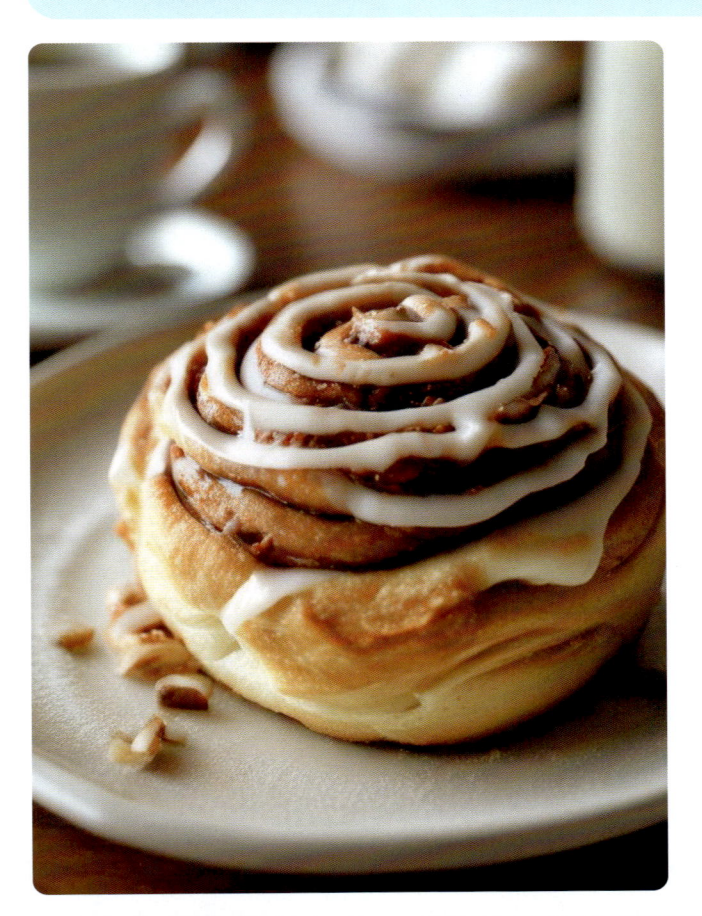

Ingredients — Servings: 8

- 1 cup Kodiak Cinnamon Pancake Mix
- 4 scoops Dummy Supps Cinnamon Swirl Whey
- 1 tsp baking powder
- 2 cups nonfat plain Greek yogurt
- 3 tbsp cinnamon
- 2 tbsp flour
- 1 (12 oz.) container whipped cream cheese
- 1/2 cup whipped cream cheese
- 1 scoop Dummy Supps Cinnamon Swirl Whey
- 1 tsp cinnamon
- 1 tsp unsweetened almond milk
- 2 tbsp zero calorie confectioners sugar

Dummy Supps Whey Protein

Instructions

1. Preheat oven to 350°F.
2. In a mixing bowl, combine pancake mix, 3 scoops of whey, baking powder, Greek yogurt, 1 tbsp of cinnamon, and roll until all ingredients are combined into a dough.
3. Add dough onto large cutting board with 2 tbsp of flour covering the board and roll out until flat.
4. In a large mixing bowl add whipped cream cheese, 1 tbsp cinnamon, 1 scoop of whey, and mix until well combined.
5. Add filling mix and spread thin layer on top of rolled out dough.
6. Top filling with 1 tbsp of cinnamon.
7. Roll dough on top of itself lengthwise creating a layered cylinder.
8. Cut into 10 separate rolls.
9. Add rolls into baking dish with cooking spray and cook for 35-40 minutes.
10. Add icing ingredients into mixing bowl, stir well, and top each cinnamon roll.

OTHER DESSERTS

OATMEAL CREAM PIES

Calories: 380   **Protein: 29**   **Carbs: 41**   **Fat: 11**

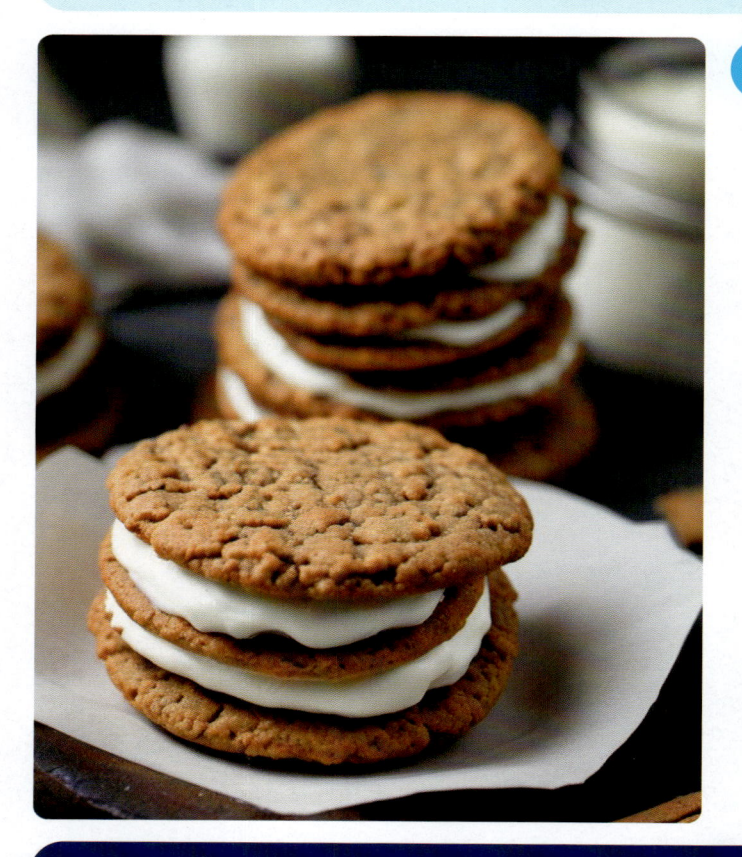

Ingredients   Servings: 1

- 1/2 cup oat flour
- 1/2 cup steel cut oats
- 3 scoops Dummy Supps vanilla whey
- 1/2 tsp baking soda
- 2 tbsp melted butter
- 1 tsp molasses
- 1/2 tsp vanilla extract
- 1/4 cup light brown sugar
- 1/4 cup unsweetened almond milk
- 1 tbsp cinnamon

Dummy Supps Whey Protein

Instructions

1. Preheat oven to 350°F.
2. In a small mixing bowl, whisk cream cheese, whey protein, vanilla extract, and cinnamon into frosting, add to small sandwich pag, then add to fridge.
3. In a mixing bowl, add oat flour, oats, whey protein, baking soda, melted butter, molasses, vanilla extract, brown sugar, cinnamon, almond milk, and combine ingredients until dough is formed.
4. Form dough into cookies and add on baking sheet with parchment paper or cooking spray and gently press down with a fork.
5. Bake for 5-6 minutes.
6. Let cookies cool for 10 minutes.
7. Cut corner of sandwich bag with frosting and add frosting to each cookie.

SMOOTHIES & SHAKES

PROTEIN SHAKES

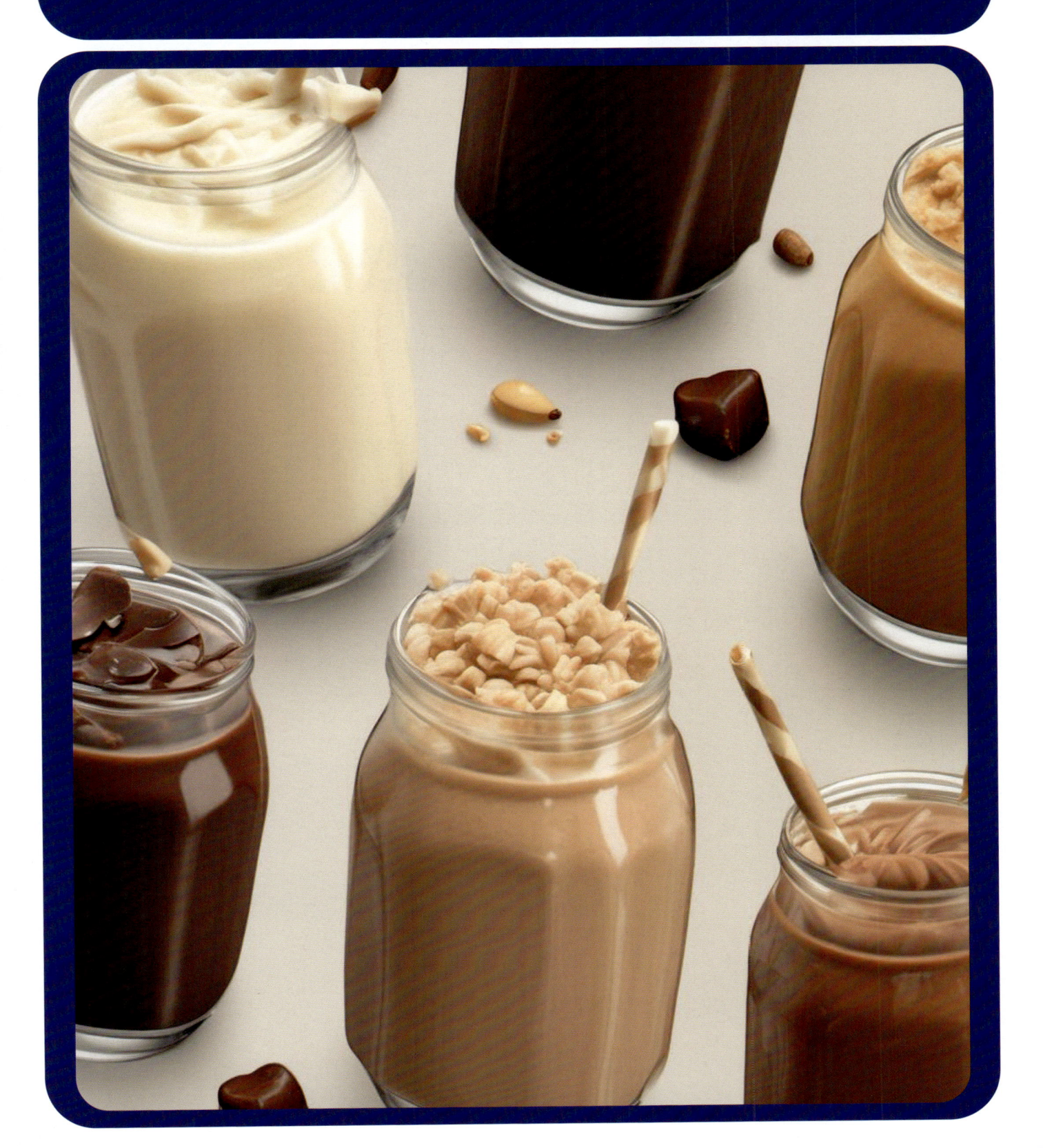

SMOOTHIES & SHAKES

CLASSIC CHOCOLATE

Calories: 490   **Protein: 44**   **Carbs: 30**   **Fat: 21**

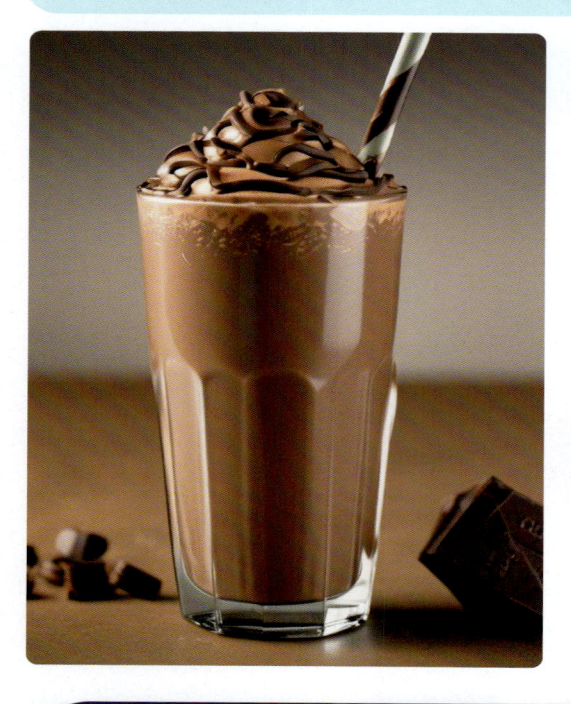

Ingredients   Servings: 1

- 1 scoop Dummy Supps Chocolate Whey
- 1 cup unsweetened almond milk
- 1/2 cup nonfat plain Greek yogurt
- 1/2 cup frozen sliced banana
- 2 tbsp Lilly's Dark Chocolate Chips
- 1 tbsp cocoa powder
- 1 tbsp Mocha Dummy Butter
- 1/2 cup ice

Dummy Supps Whey Protein
Dummy Butter Peanut Butter

Instructions

1. Add all ingredients to a blender.
2. Blend until smooth.
3. Pour into a glass and enjoy!

CLASSIC VANILLA

Calories: 480   **Protein: 44**   **Carbs: 30**   **Fat: 21**

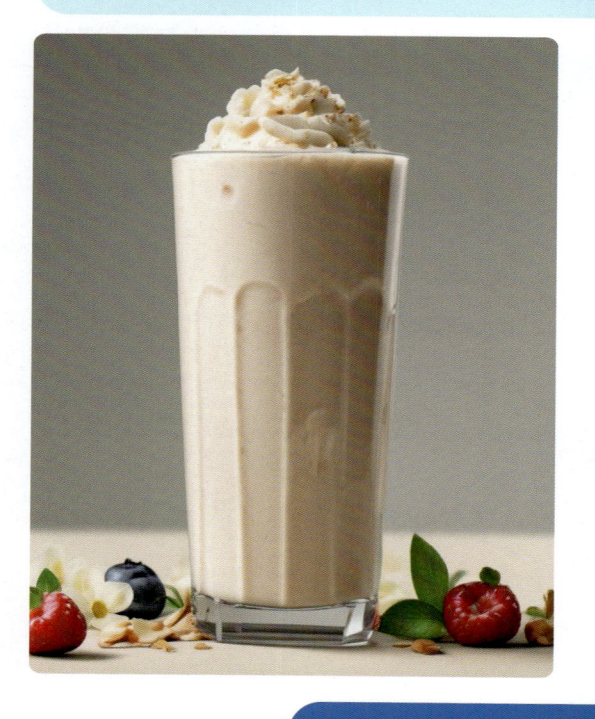

Ingredients   Servings: 1

- 1 scoop Dummy Supps Vanilla Whey
- 1 cup unsweetened almond milk
- 1/2 cup nonfat plain Greek yogurt
- 1/2 cup frozen sliced banana
- 2 tbsp Lilly's White Chocolate Chips
- 1/2 tsp vanilla extract
- 2 tbsp Lily's white chocolate chips
- 1/2 cup ice

Dummy Supps Whey Protein
Dummy Butter Peanut Butter

Instructions

1. Add all ingredients to a blender.
2. Blend until smooth.
3. Pour into a glass and enjoy!

Optional Add On: Whipped cream (2 tbsp - 15c, 1P, 1C, 1F)

SMOOTHIES & SHAKES

FRENCH VANILLA COFFEE

Calories: 350 **Protein: 39** **Carbs: 32** **Fat: 8**

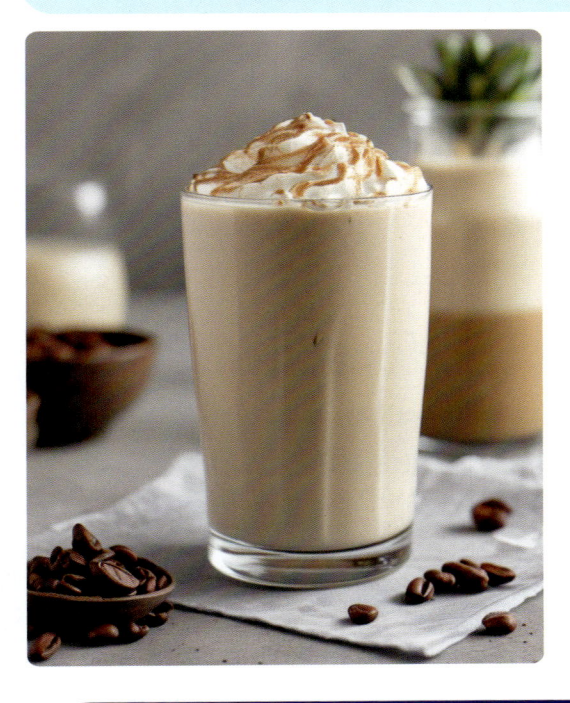

Ingredients — Servings: 1

- 1 scoop Dummy Supps Vanilla Whey
- 1/2 cup unsweetened almond milk
- 1/2 cup iced coffee
- 1/2 cup nonfat plain Greek yogurt
- 1/2 cup frozen sliced banana
- 2 tbsp Lily's white chocolate chips
- 1 tbsp instant espresso

Instructions

1. Add all ingredients to a blender.
2. Blend until smooth.
3. Pour into a glass and enjoy!

VANILLA RASPBERRY

Calories: 510 **Protein: 48** **Carbs: 39** **Fat: 22**

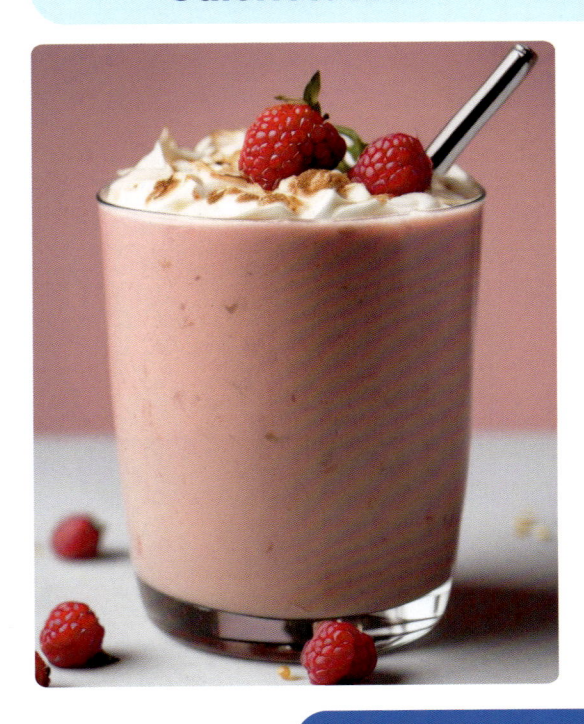

Ingredients — Servings: 1

- 1 scoop Dummy Supps Berry or Vanilla Whey
- 1 cup unsweetened almond milk
- 1/2 cup nonfat plain Greek yogurt
- 1 cup frozen raspberries
- 2 tbsp Lily's white chocolate chips
- 1 tbsp PB&J Dummy Butter

Instructions

1. Add all ingredients to a blender.
2. Blend until smooth.
3. Pour into a glass and enjoy!

Optional Add On: Whipped cream (2 tbsp – 15c, 1P, 1C, 1F)

SMOOTHIES & SHAKES

CHOCOLATE PEANUT BUTTER

Calories: 530 **Protein: 49** **Carbs: 32** **Fat: 22**

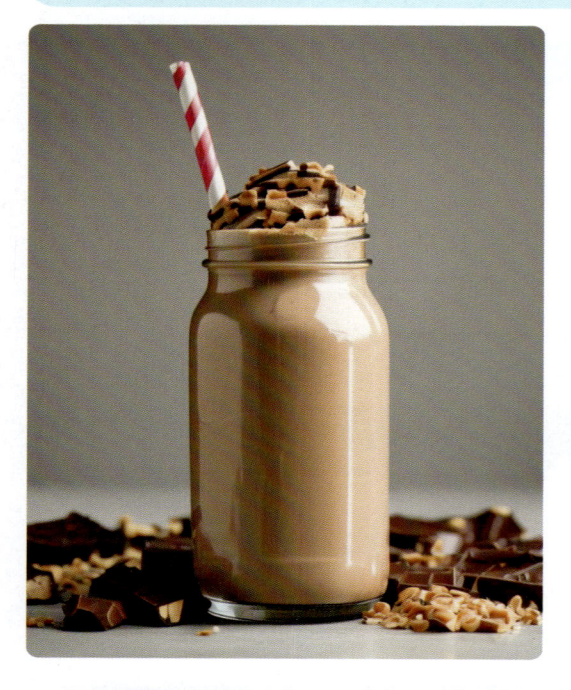

Ingredients — Servings: 1

- 1 scoop Dummy Supps Chocolate Whey
- 1 cup unsweetened almond milk
- 1/2 cup nonfat plain Greek yogurt
- 1/2 cup frozen sliced banana
- 1 tbsp cocoa powder
- 2 tbsp powdered peanut butter

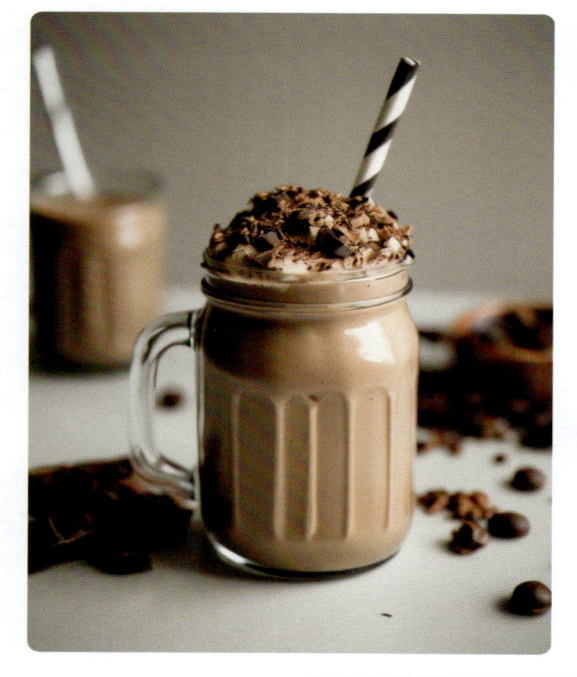

Dummy Supps Whey Protein — SCAN ME

Instructions

1. Add all ingredients to a blender.
2. Blend until smooth.
3. Pour into a glass and enjoy!

CHOCOLATE COFFEE

Calories: 350 **Protein: 39** **Carbs: 32** **Fat: 8**

Ingredients — Servings: 1

- 1 scoop Dummy Supps Chocolate Whey
- 1/2 cup unsweetened almond milk
- 1/2 cup iced coffee
- 1/2 cup nonfat plain Greek yogurt
- 1/2 cup frozen sliced banana
- 2 tbsp Lily's dark chocolate chips
- 1 tsp instant espresso

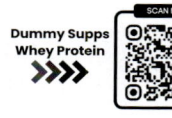

Dummy Supps Whey Protein — SCAN ME

Instructions

1. Add all ingredients to a blender.
2. Blend until smooth.
3. Pour into a glass and enjoy!

Optional Add On: Whipped cream (2 tbsp - 15c, 1P, 1C, 1F)

SMOOTHIES & SHAKES

CHOCOLATE RASPBERRY

Calories: 510   **Protein: 48**   **Carbs: 39**   **Fat: 22**

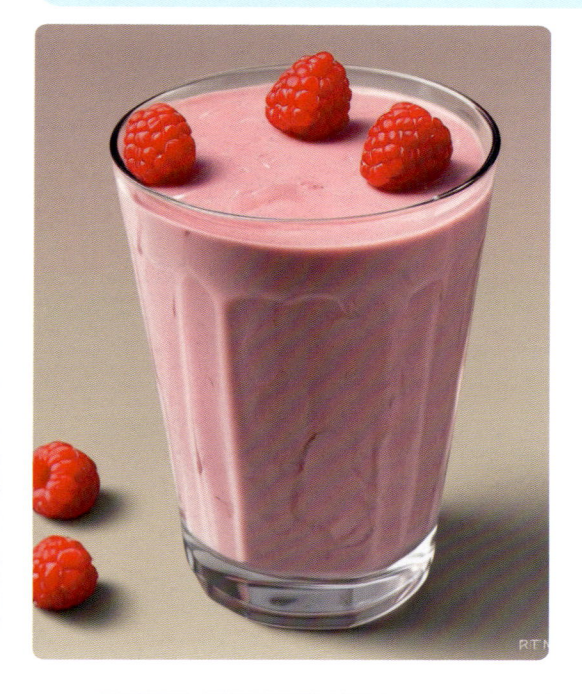

Ingredients   Servings: 1

- 1 scoop Dummy Supps Chocolcte Whey
- 1 cup unsweetened almond milk
- 1/2 cup nonfat plain Greek yogurt
- 1 cup frozen raspberries
- 2 tbsp Lily's dark chocolate chips
- 1 tbsp PB&J Dummy Butter

Dummy Supps Whey Protein

Dummy Butter Peanut Butter

Instructions

1. Add all ingredients to a blender.
2. Blend until smooth.
3. Pour into a glass and enjoy!

BLUEBERRY BASH

Calories: 470   **Protein: 43**   **Carbs: 30**   **Fat: 21**

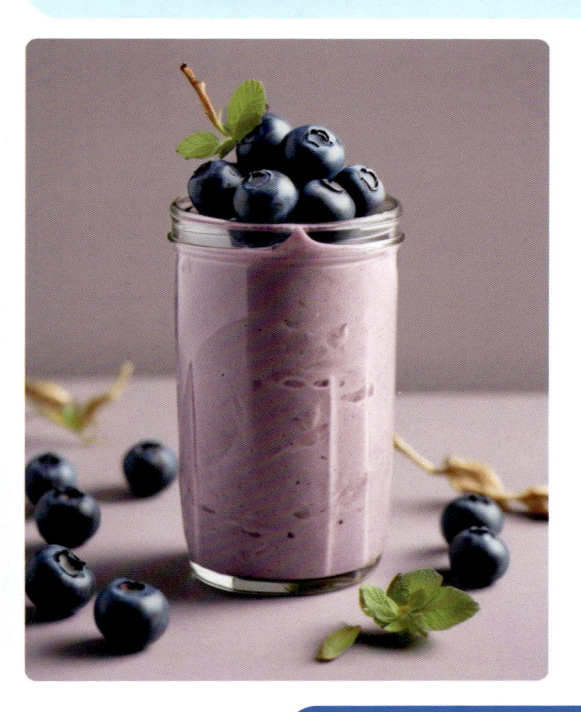

Ingredients   Servings: 1

- 1 scoop Dummy Supps Berry or Vanilla Whey
- 1 cup unsweetened almond milk
- 1/2 cup nonfat plain Greek yogurt
- 1 cup frozen blueberries
- 2 tbsp Lily's white chocolate chips
- 1 tbsp PB&J Dummy Butter

Dummy Supps Whey Protein

Dummy Butter Peanut Butter

Instructions

1. Add all ingredients to a blender.
2. Blend until smooth.
3. Pour into a glass and enjoy!

Optional Add On: Whipped cream (2 tbsp - 15c, 1P, 1C, 1F)

SMOOTHIES & SHAKES

STRAWBERRY BANANA

Calories: 500 **Protein: 47** **Carbs: 37** **Fat: 21**

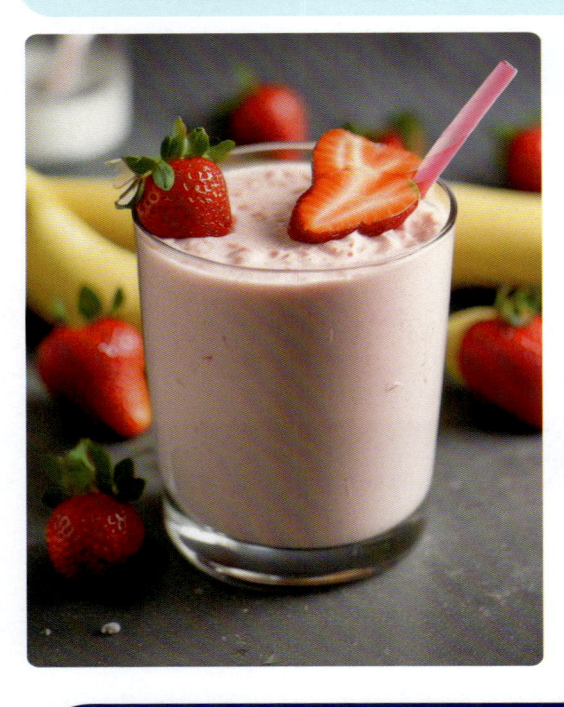

Ingredients — Servings: 1

- 1 scoop Dummy Supps Berry or Vanilla Whey
- 1 cup unsweetened almond milk
- 1/2 cup nonfat plain Greek yogurt
- 1/2 cup frozen strawberries
- 1/2 cup frozen sliced bananas
- 2 tbsp Lily's white chocolate chips
- 1 tbsp PB&J Dummy Butter

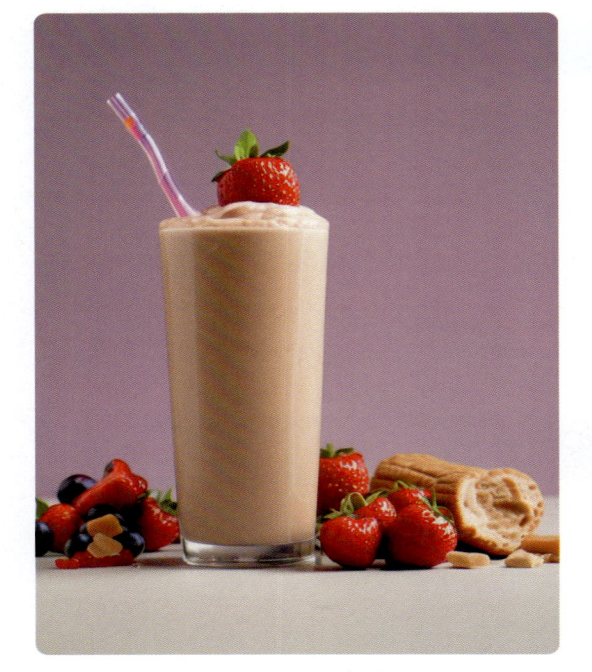

Dummy Supps Whey Protein

Dummy Butter Peanut Butter

Instructions

1. Add all ingredients to a blender.
2. Blend until smooth.
3. Pour into a glass and enjoy!

PEANUT BUTTER & JELLY

Calories: 490 **Protein: 46** **Carbs: 37** **Fat: 21**

Ingredients — Servings: 1

- 1 scoop Dummy Supps Berry or Vanilla Whey
- 1 cup unsweetened almond milk
- 1/2 cup nonfat plain Greek yogurt
- 1 cup frozen strawberries
- 1 tbsp Dummy Butter PB&J
- 1 tbsp sugar-free strawberry jam
- 2 tbsp Lily's dark chocolate chips

Dummy Supps Whey Protein

Dummy Butter Peanut Butter

Instructions

1. Add all ingredients to a blender.
2. Blend until smooth.
3. Pour into a glass and enjoy!

Optional Add On: Whipped cream (2 tbsp - 15c, 1P, 1C, 1F)

SMOOTHIES & SHAKES

PEANUT BUTTER & BANANA

Calories: 530 **Protein: 53** **Carbs: 33** **Fat: 23**

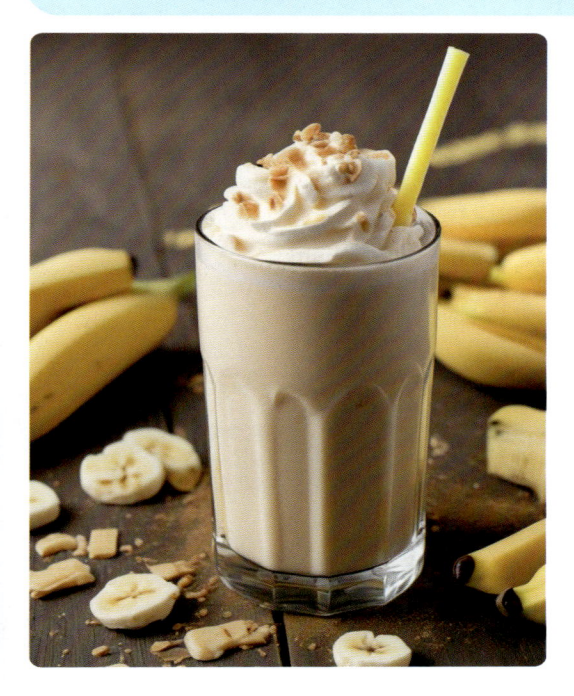

Ingredients   Servings: 1

- 1 scoop Dummy Supps Chocolate Peanut Butter or Chocolate Whey
- 1 cup unsweetened almond milk
- 1/2 cup nonfat plain Greek yogurt
- 1/2 cup frozen sliced bananas
- 2 tbsp Lily's dark chocolate chips
- 2 tbsp powdered peanut butter
- 1 tbsp Mocha Dummy Butter

Dummy Supps Whey Protein

Dummy Butter Peanut Butter

Instructions

1. Add all ingredients to a blender.
2. Blend until smooth.
3. Pour into a glass and enjoy!

S'MORES

Calories: 350 **Protein: 39** **Carbs: 29** **Fat: 11**

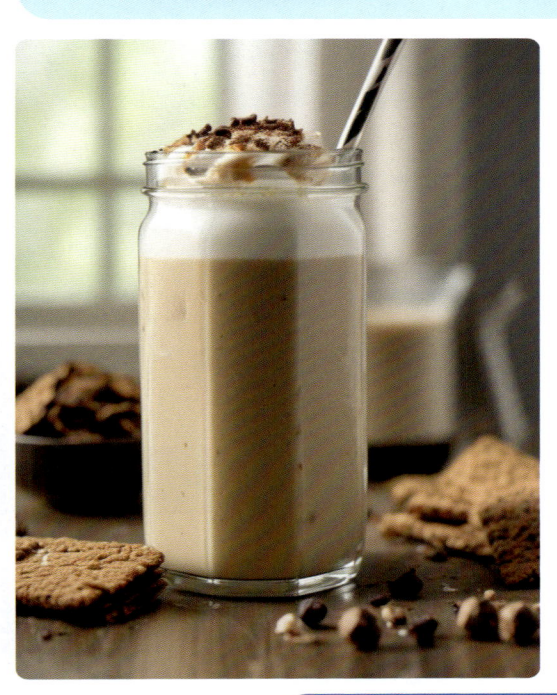

Ingredients   Servings: 1

- 1 scoop Dummy Supps Chocolate Whey
- 1 tsp instant espresso
- 1 cup unsweetened almond milk
- 1/2 cup nonfat plain Greek yogurt
- 1 tbsp cocoa powder
- 2 tbsp Lily's dark chocolate chips
- 1 graham cracker
- 1 cup ice

Dummy Supps Whey Protein

Instructions

1. Add all ingredients to a blender.
2. Blend until smooth.
3. Pour into a glass and enjoy!

Optional Add On: Whipped cream (2 tbsp - 15c, 1P, 1C, 1F)

SMOOTHIES & SHAKES

COOKIES & CREAM

Calories: 430 **Protein: 39** **Carbs: 39** **Fat: 15**

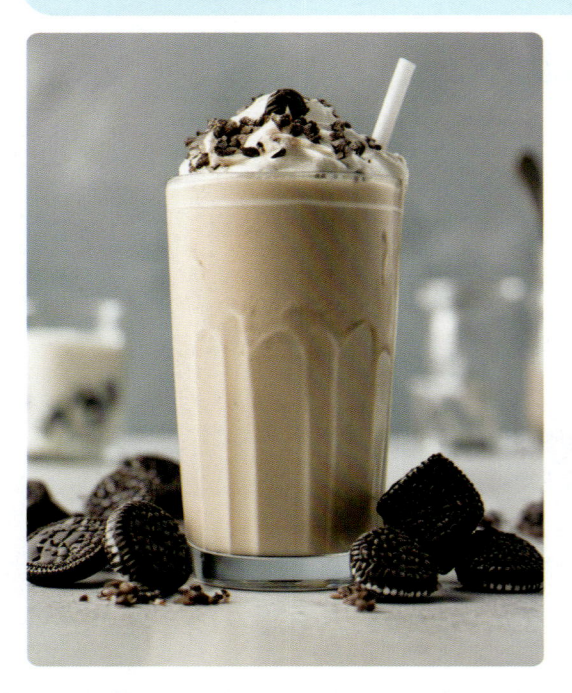

Ingredients — Servings: 1

- 1/2 scoop Dummy Supps Chocolate Whey
- 1/2 scoop Dummy Supps Vanilla Whey
- 1 cup unsweetened almond milk
- 1/2 cup nonfat plain Greek yogurt
- 2 tbsp Lily's dark chocolate chips
- 4 Oreo® Thins
- 1 tbsp cocoa powder
- 1 cup ice

Dummy Supps Whey Protein

Instructions

1. Add all ingredients to a blender.
2. Blend until smooth.
3. Pour into a glass and enjoy!

CHOCOLATE COVERED STRAWBERRY

Calories: 490 **Protein: 48** **Carbs: 37** **Fat: 22**

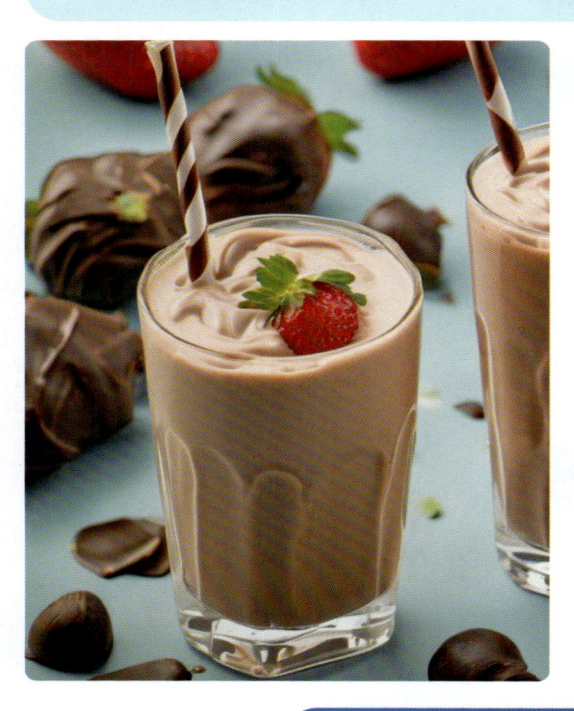

Ingredients — Servings: 1

- 1 scoop Dummy Supps Chocolate Whey
- 1 cup unsweetened almond milk
- 1/2 cup nonfat plain Greek yogurt
- 1 cup frozen strawberries
- 1 tbsp sugar-free strawberry jam
- 1 tbsp cocoa powder
- 2 tbsp Lily's dark chocolate chips
- 1 tbsp PB&J Dummy Butter

Dummy Supps Whey Protein

Dummy Butter Peanut Butter

Instructions

1. Add all ingredients to a blender.
2. Blend until smooth.
3. Pour into a glass and enjoy!

Optional Add On: Whipped cream (2 tbsp - 15c, 1P, 1C, 1F)

SMOOTHIES & SHAKES

VANILLA STRAWBERRY

Calories: 480 **Protein: 47** **Carbs: 35** **Fat: 21**

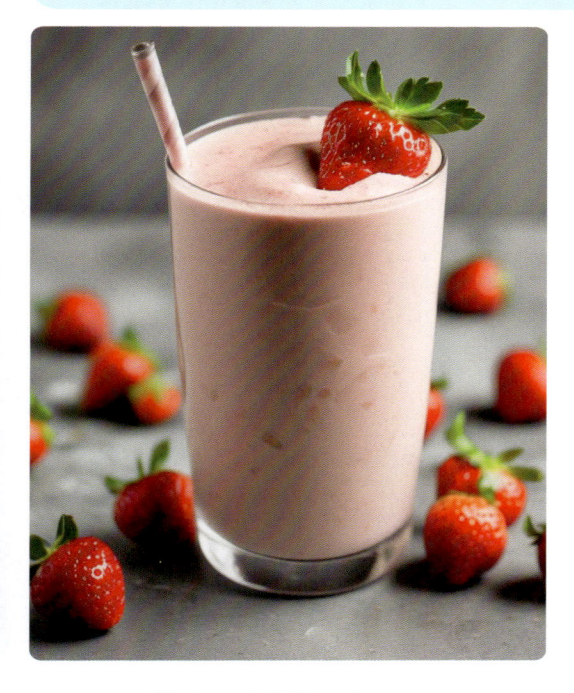

Ingredients — Servings: 1

- 1 scoop Dummy Supps Vanilla Whey
- 1 cup unsweetened almond milk
- 1/2 cup nonfat plain Greek yogurt
- 1 cup frozen strawberries
- 1 tbsp sugar-free strawberry jam
- 2 tbsp Lily's dark chocolate chips
- 1/2 tsp vanilla extract
- 1 tbsp PB&J Dummy Butter

Dummy Supps Whey Protein [QR code]
Dummy Butter Peanut Butter [QR code]

Instructions

1. Add all ingredients to a blender.
2. Blend until smooth.
3. Pour into a glass and enjoy!

PUMPKIN SPICE

Calories: 350 **Protein: 38** **Carbs: 23** **Fat: 12**

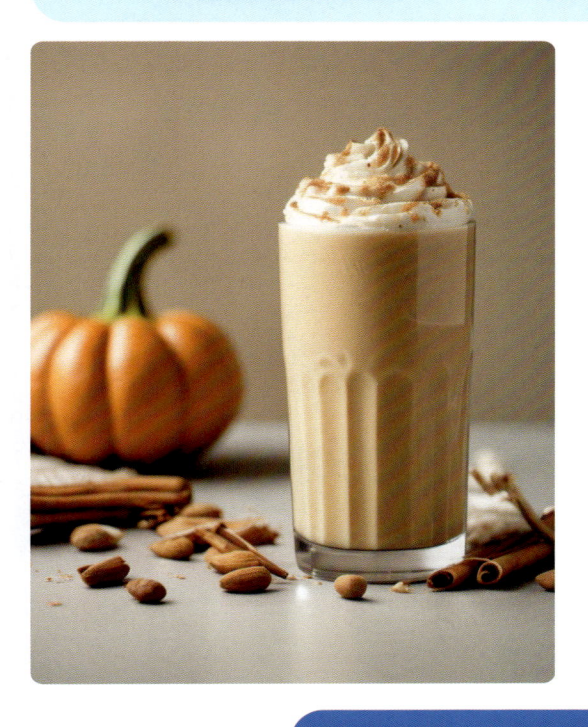

Ingredients — Servings: 1

- 1 scoop Dummy Supps Vanilla Whey
- 1 cup unsweetened almond milk
- 1/2 cup nonfat vanilla or pumpkin Greek yogurt
- 1/2 cup frozen pumpkin puree
- 1/2 tsp vanilla extract
- 2 tbsp Lily's white chocolate chips
- 1 tsp pumpkin pie spice
- 1/4 tsp salt

Dummy Supps Whey Protein [QR code]

Instructions

1. Add all ingredients to a blender.
2. Blend until smooth.
3. Pour into a glass and enjoy!

Optional Add On: Whipped cream (2 tbsp - 15c, 1P, 1C, 1F)

SMOOTHIES & SHAKES

CINNAMON SWIRL

Calories: 340 **Protein: 43** **Carbs: 20** **Fat: 10**

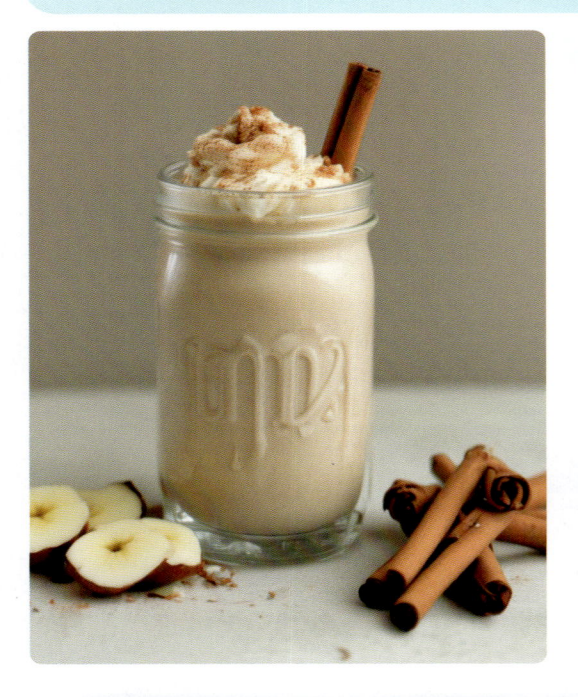

Ingredients   Servings: 1

- 1 scoop Dummy Supps Cinnamon Roll Whey
- 1 cups unsweetened almond milk
- 1/2 cup vanilla Greek yogurt
- 2 tbsp powdered peanut butter
- 2 tbsp Lilly's Dark Chocolate Chips
- 1/2 tsp cinnamon
- 1/2 tsp vanilla extract
- 1/4 tsp salt
- 1 cup ice

Instructions

1. Add all ingredients to a blender.
2. Blend until smooth.
3. Pour into a glass and enjoy!

TIRAMISU

Calories: 400 **Protein: 40** **Carbs: 35** **Fat: 11**

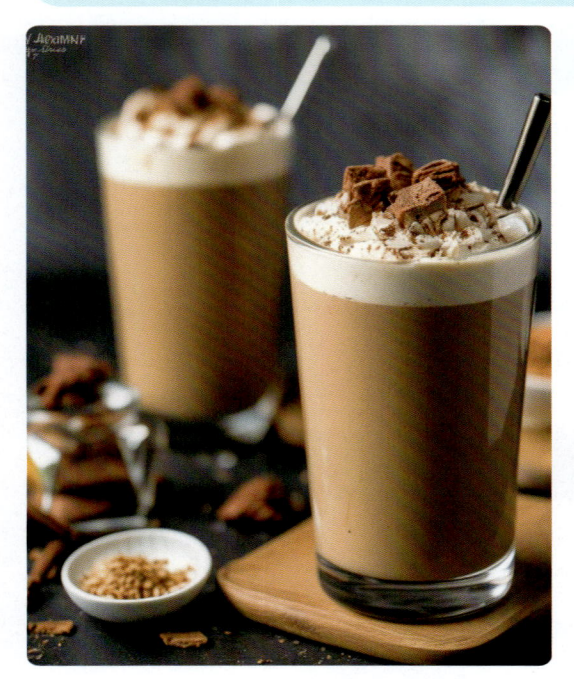

Ingredients   Servings: 1

- 1 scoop Dummy Supps Chocolate Whey
- 1 cup unsweetened almond milk
- 1/2 cup nonfat plain Greek yogurt
- 1/2 cup frozen sliced banana
- 1/2 cup ice
- 1 tbsp cocoa powder
- 1 tsp instant espresso
- 1 graham cracker

Instructions

1. Add all ingredients to a blender.
2. Blend until smooth.
3. Pour into a glass and enjoy!

Optional Add On: Whipped cream (2 tbsp - 15c, 1P, 1C, 1F)

SMOOTHIES & SHAKES

MIXED BERRY

Calories: 470 **Protein: 45** **Carbs: 38** **Fat: 17**

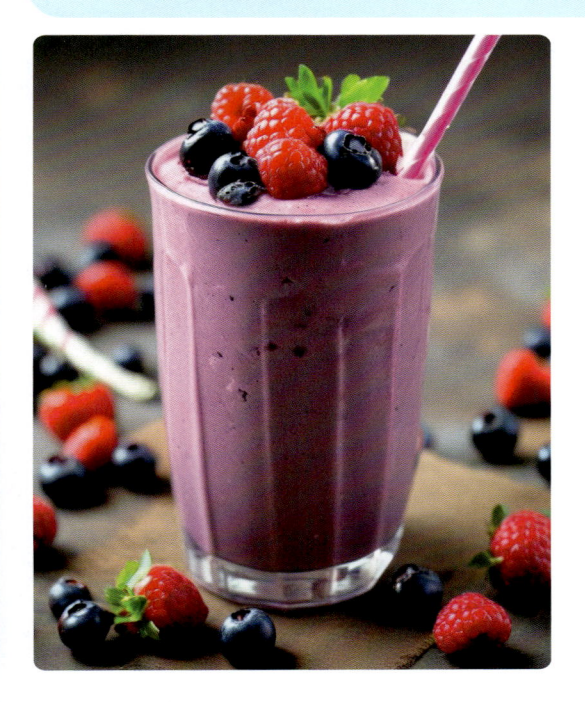

Ingredients — Servings: 1

- 1 scoop Dummy Supps Berry or Vanilla Whey
- 1 cup unsweetened almond milk
- 1/2 cup nonfat vanilla Greek yogurt
- 1 cup frozen mixed berries
- 1 tbsp sugar-free strawberry jam
- 1 tbsp PB&J Dummy Butter

Instructions

1. Add all ingredients to a blender.
2. Blend until smooth.
3. Pour into a glass and enjoy!

BLACKBERRY VANILLA

Calories: 500 **Protein: 47** **Carbs: 42** **Fat: 18**

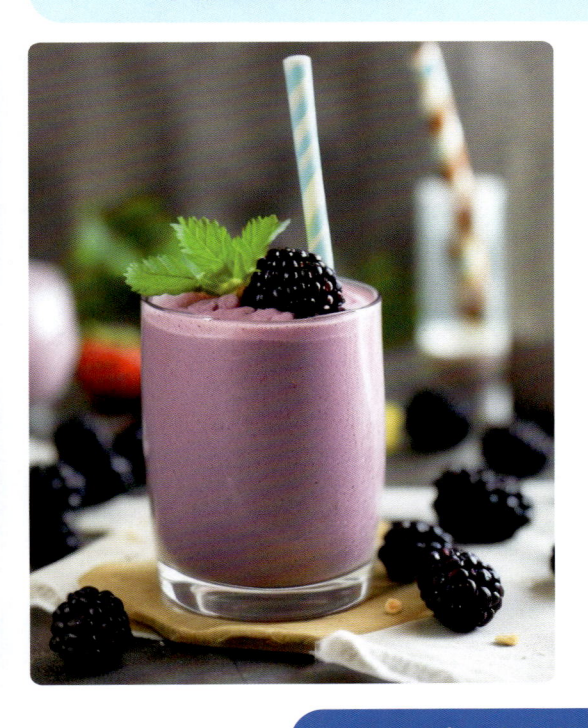

Ingredients — Servings: 1

- 1 scoop Dummy Supps Berry or Vanilla Whey
- 1 cup unsweetened almond milk
- 1/2 cup nonfat vanilla Greek yogurt
- 1 cup frozen blackberries
- 1 tsp vanilla extract
- 1 tbsp sugar-free strawberry jam
- 1 tbsp PB&J Dummy Butter

Instructions

1. Add all ingredients to a blender.
2. Blend until smooth.
3. Pour into a glass and enjoy!

Optional Add On: Whipped cream (2 tbsp - 15c, 1P, 1C, 1F)

SMOOTHIES & SHAKES

CHOCOLATE COCONUT

Calories: 350   **Protein: 40**   **Carbs: 22**   **Fat: 13**

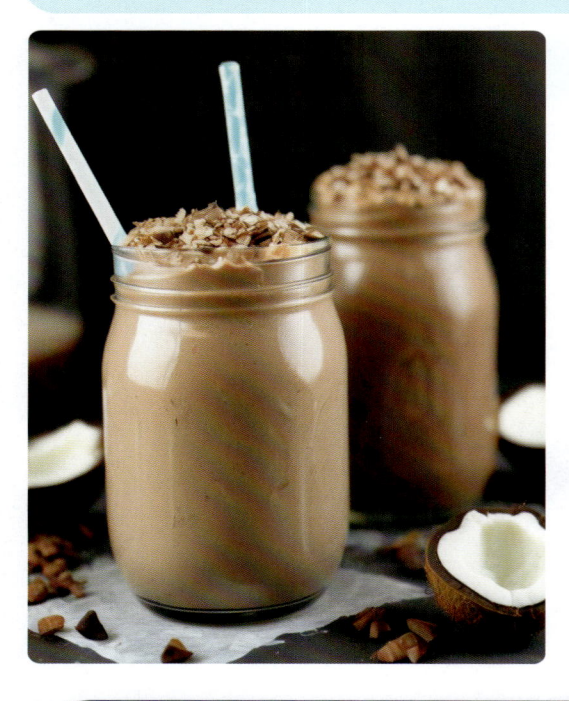

Ingredients   Servings: 1

- 1 scoop Dummy Supps Chocolate Whey
- 1 cup unsweetened almond milk
- 1/2 cup nonfat plain Greek yogurt
- 1 tbsp shredded coconut
- 1 tbsp Mocha Dummy Butter
- 2 tbsp Lily's dark chocolate chips
- 1/2 tsp vanilla extract
- 1/4 tsp salt

Instructions

1. Add all ingredients to a blender.
2. Blend until smooth.
3. Pour into a glass and enjoy!

PINA COLADA

Calories: 420   **Protein: 38**   **Carbs: 42**   **Fat: 13**

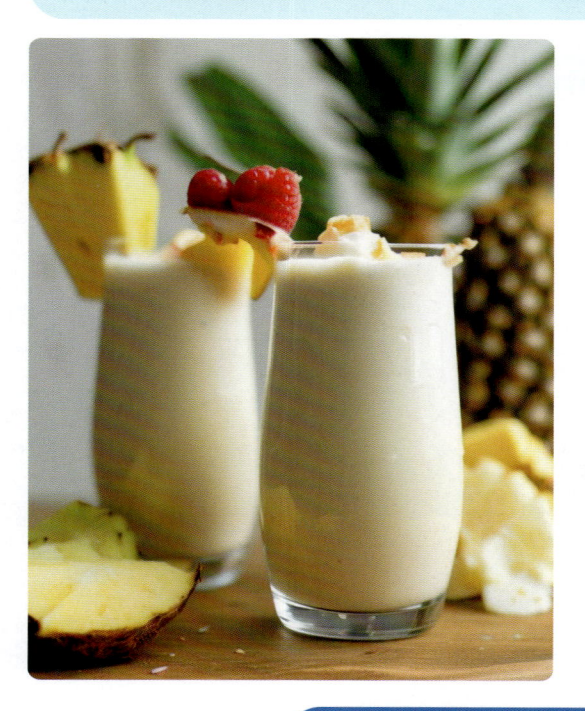

Ingredients   Servings: 1

- 1 scoop Dummy Supps Vanilla Whey
- 1 cup unsweetened almond milk
- 1/2 cup vanilla Greek yogurt
- 1 cup frozen pineapple
- 1 tbsp shredded coconut
- 1/2 tsp vanilla extract
- 1/4 tsp salt

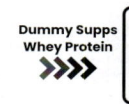

Instructions

1. Add all ingredients to a blender.
2. Blend until smooth.
3. Pour into a glass and enjoy!

Optional Add On: Whipped cream (2 tbsp - 15c, 1P, 1C, 1F)

SMOOTHIES & SHAKES

SALTED CARAMEL MOCHA SHAKE

Calories: 470 **Protein: 47** **Carbs: 25** **Fat: 22**

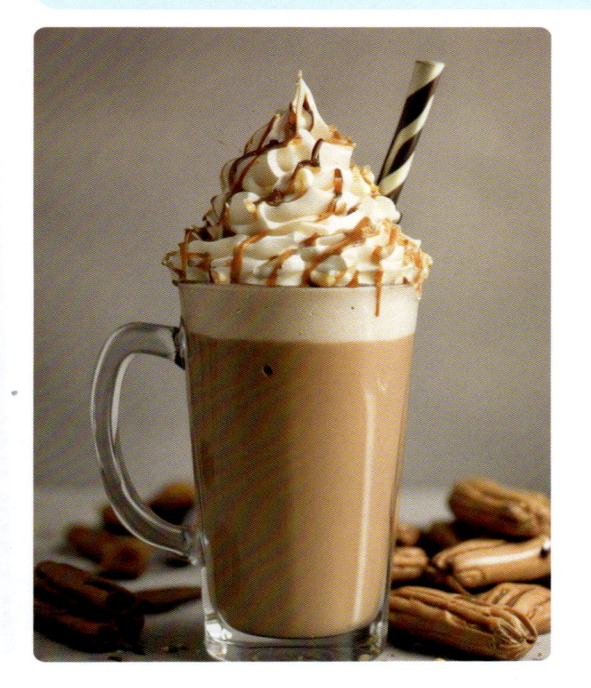

Ingredients — Servings: 1

- 1 scoop Dummy Supps Salted Caramel Whey
- 1 cup unsweetened almond milk
- 1/2 cup nonfat plain Greek yogurt
- 1 tsp instant coffee
- 1 tbsp Mocha Dummy Butter
- 2 tbsp Lilly's Salted Caramel Chips
- 1 tbsp cocoa powder
- 1/4 tsp salt
- 1 cup ice

Dummy Supps Whey Protein

Dummy Butter Peanut Butter

Instructions

1. Add all ingredients to a blender.
2. Blend until smooth.
3. Pour into a glass and enjoy!

CINNAMON ROLL PROTEIN SHAKE

Calories: 490 **Protein: 48** **Carbs: 27** **Fat: 27**

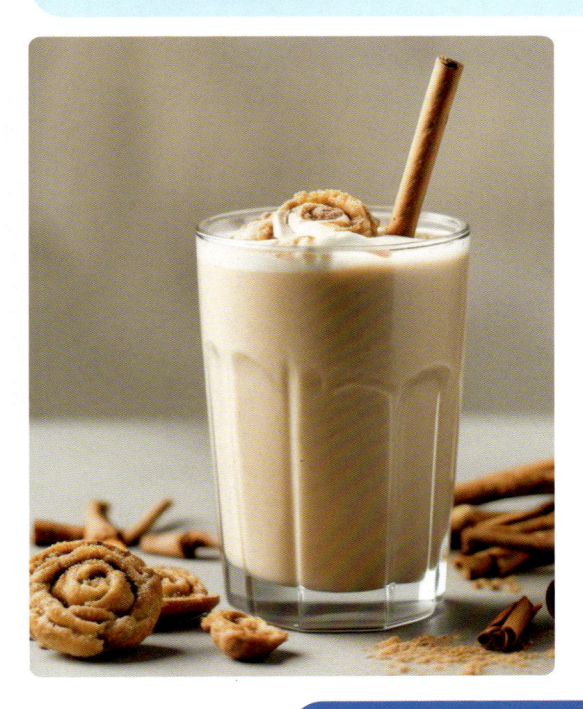

Ingredients — Servings: 1

- 1 scoop Dummy Supps Salted Caramel Whey
- 1 cups unsweetened almond milk
- 1/2 cup nonfat plain Greek yogurt
- 1 tsp instant coffee
- 1 tbsp Mocha Dummy Butter
- 2 tbsp whipped cream cheese
- 1 tbsp cocoa powder
- 1/2 tsp vanilla extract
- 1/4 tsp salt
- 1 cup ice

Dummy Supps Whey Protein

Dummy Butter Peanut Butter

Instructions

1. Add all ingredients to a blender.
2. Blend until smooth.
3. Pour into a glass and enjoy!

Optional Add On: Whipped cream (2 tbsp - 15c, 1P, 1C, 1F)

SMOOTHIES & SHAKES

VANILLA ALMOND CHEESECAKE SHAKE

Calories: 440 **Protein: 46** **Carbs: 24** **Fat: 19**

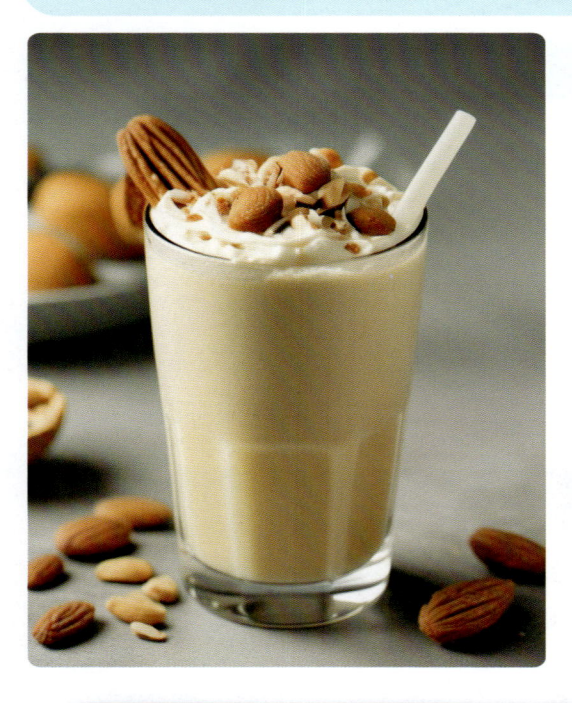

Ingredients Servings: 1

- 1 scoop Dummy Supps Vanilla Whey
- 1 cup unsweetened almond milk
- 1/2 cup nonfat vanilla Greek yogurt
- 2 tbsp powdered peanut butter
- 2 tbsp whipped cream cheese
- 1 tbsp chopped almonds
- 2 tbsp Lilly's White Chocolate Chips
- 1/2 tsp vanilla extract
- 1/4 tsp salt
- 1 cup ice

Dummy Supps Whey Protein

Dummy Butter Peanut Butter

Instructions

1. Add all ingredients to a blender.
2. Blend until smooth.
3. Pour into a glass and enjoy!

STRAWBERRY SHORTCAKE SMOOTHIE

Calories: 530 **Protein: 47** **Carbs: 32** **Fat: 26**

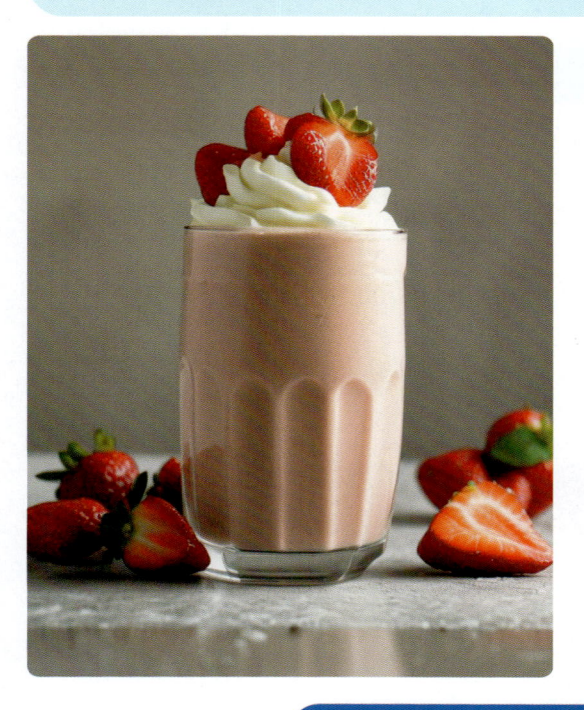

Ingredients Servings: 1

- 1 scoop Dummy Supps Vanilla Whey
- 1 cups unsweetened almond milk
- 1/2 cup vanilla Greek yogurt
- 1 cup frozen strawberries
- 1 tbsp PB&J Dummy Butter
- 2 tbsp Lilly's white chocolate chips
- 1/2 tsp vanilla extract
- 2 tbsp whipped cream cheese

Dummy Supps Whey Protein

Dummy Butter Peanut Butter

Instructions

1. Add all ingredients to a blender.
2. Blend until smooth.
3. Pour into a glass and enjoy!

Optional Add On: Whipped cream (2 tbsp - 15c, 1P, 1C, 1F)

SMOOTHIES & SHAKES

MOCHA CARAMEL SHAKE

Calories: 450   **Protein: 46**   **Carbs: 21**   **Fat: 21**

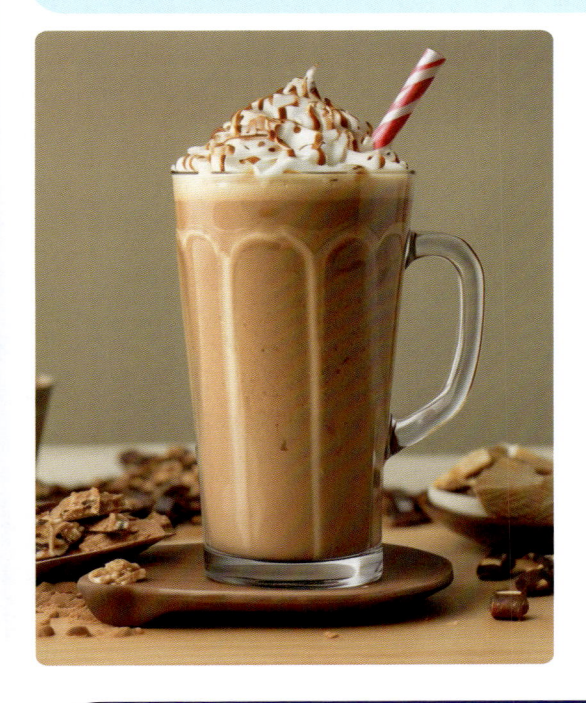

Ingredients   Servings: 1

- 1 scoop Dummy Supps Chocolate Whey
- 1 cup unsweetened almond milk
- 1/2 cup nonfat plain Greek yogurt
- 1 tsp instant coffee
- 1 tbsp Mocha Dummy Butter
- 2 tbsp Lily's Salted Caramel Chips
- 1/4 tsp salt
- 1 cup ice

Dummy Supps Whey Protein

Dummy Butter Peanut Butter

Instructions

1. Add all ingredients to a blender.
2. Blend until smooth.
3. Pour into a glass and enjoy!

BLUEBERRY CHEESECAKE SMOOTHIE

Calories: 540   **Protein: 48**   **Carbs: 34**   **Fat: 26**

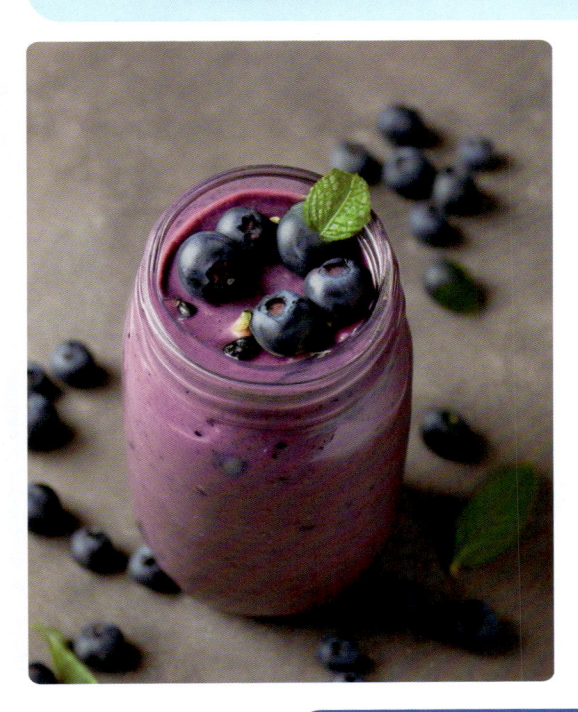

Ingredients   Servings: 1

- 1 scoop Dummy Supps Berry Whey
- 1 cups unsweetened almond milk
- 1/2 cup vanilla Greek yogurt
- 1 cup frozen blueberries
- 1/4 cup whipped cream cheese
- 1 tbsp Dummy Butter PB&J
- 1/2 tsp vanilla extract
- 1/4 tsp salt

Dummy Supps Whey Protein

Dummy Butter Peanut Butter

Instructions

1. Add all ingredients to a blender.
2. Blend until smooth.
3. Pour into a glass and enjoy!

Optional Add On: Whipped cream (2 tbsp - 15c, 1P, 1C, 1F)

SMOOTHIES & SHAKES

STRAWBERRY BOWL

Calories: 480 **Protein: 47** **Carbs: 30** **Fat: 21**

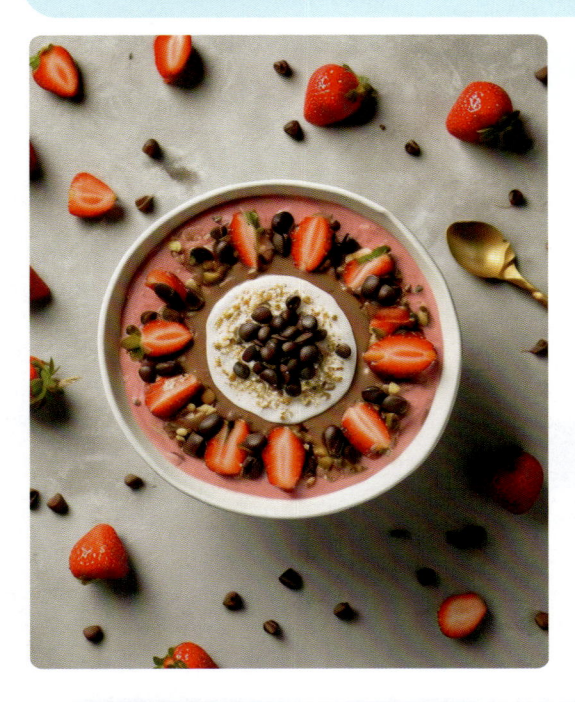

Ingredients — Servings: 1

- 1 cup frozen strawberries
- 3/4 cup unsweetened almond milk
- 1 scoop Dummy Supps Berry/Vanilla Whey
- 1/2 cup nonfat vanilla greek yogurt
- 2 tbsp Lilly's dark chocolate chips
- 1 tbsp PB&J Dummy Butter

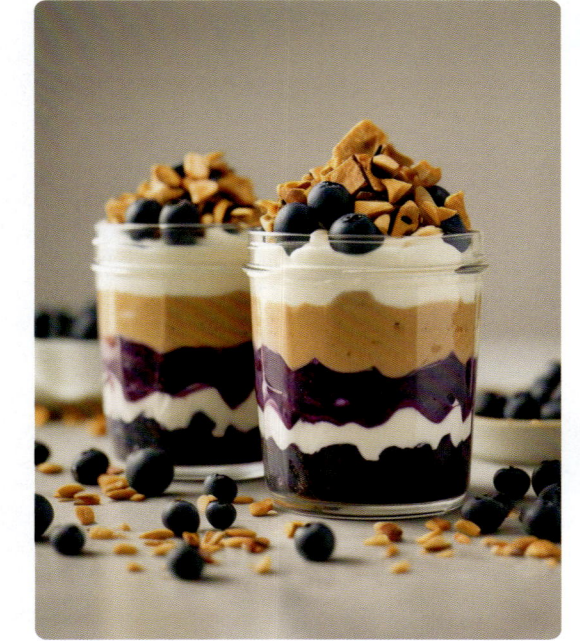

Dummy Supps Whey Protein (QR code)
Dummy Butter Peanut Butter (QR code)

Instructions

1. Add frozen strawberries, almond milk, whey protein, and Greek yogurt to a blender.
2. Blend on high until thick and smooth.
3. Pour into a bowl and top with Lily's dark chocolate chips and PB&J Dummy Butter.

BLUEBERRY PARFAIT

Calories: 460 **Protein: 48** **Carbs: 32** **Fat: 17**

Ingredients — Servings: 1

- 1 cup nonfat vanilla greek yogurt
- 1 scoop Dummy Supps Vanilla/Berry Whey
- 1 cup frozen or fresh blueberries
- 2 tbsp protein granola
- 1 tbsp PB&J Dummy Butter

Dummy Supps Whey Protein (QR code)
Dummy Butter Peanut Butter (QR code)

Instructions

1. In a bowl, mix Greek yogurt with whey protein until smooth.
2. Add blueberries, protein granola, and PB&J Dummy Butter.

Optional Add On: Whipped cream (2 tbsp - 15c, 1P, 1C, 1F)

SMOOTHIES & SHAKES

STRAWBERRY PARFAIT

Calories: 460 **Protein: 48** **Carbs: 30** **Fat: 7**

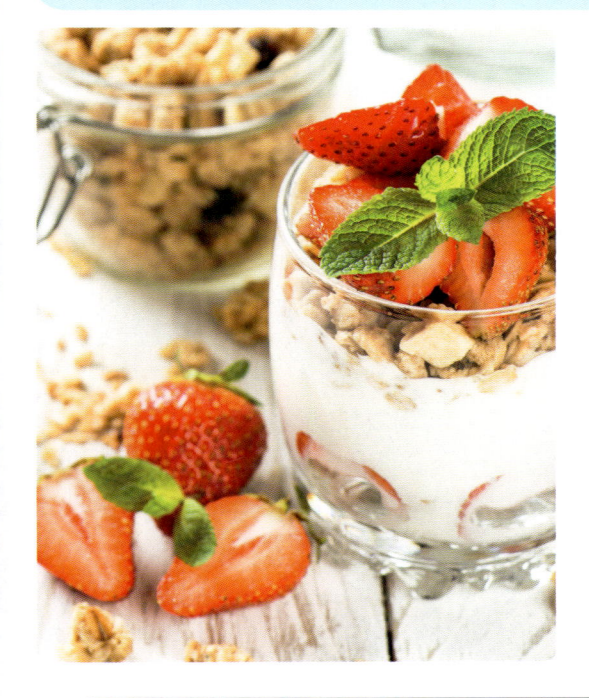

Ingredients — Servings: 1

- 1 cup nonfat vanilla greek yogurt
- 1 scoop Dummy Supps Vanilla/Berry Whey
- 1 cup frozen/fresh sliced strawberries
- 2 tbsp protein granola
- 1 tbsp PB&J Dummy Butter

Instructions

1. In a bowl, mix Greek yogurt with whey protein until smooth.
2. Slice the strawberries.
3. Add sliced strawberries, protein granola, and PB&J Dummy Butter.

BANANA PARFAIT

Calories: 522 **Protein: 48** **Carbs: 48** **Fat: 17**

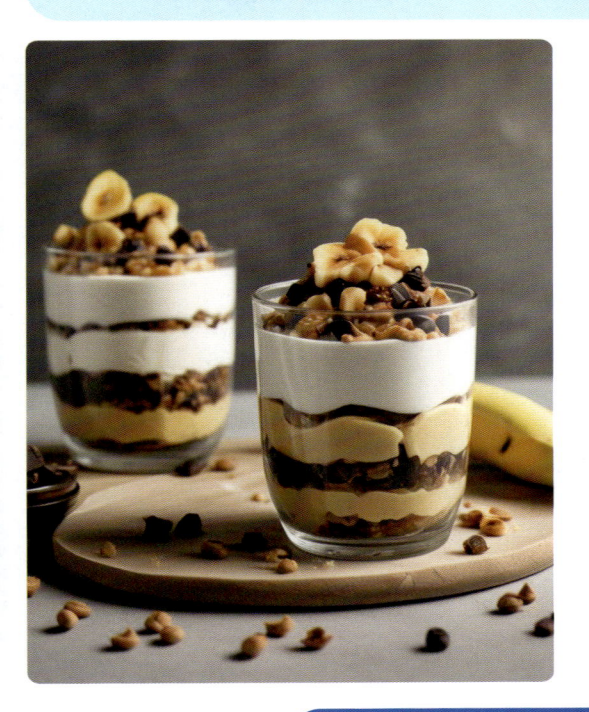

Ingredients — Servings: 1

- 1 cup nonfat vanilla greek yogurt
- 1 scoop Dummy Supps Vanilla/Berry Whey
- 1 banana
- 2 tbsp protein granola
- 1 tbsp PB&J Dummy Butter

Instructions

1. In a bowl, mix Greek yogurt with whey protein until smooth.
2. Slice the banana.
3. Add sliced banana, protein granola, and PB&J Dummy Butter.

Optional Add On: Whipped cream (2 tbsp – 15c, 1P, 1C, 1F)

SMOOTHIES & SHAKES

POWER PARFAIT

Calories: 460 **Protein: 48** **Carbs: 32** **Fat: 17**

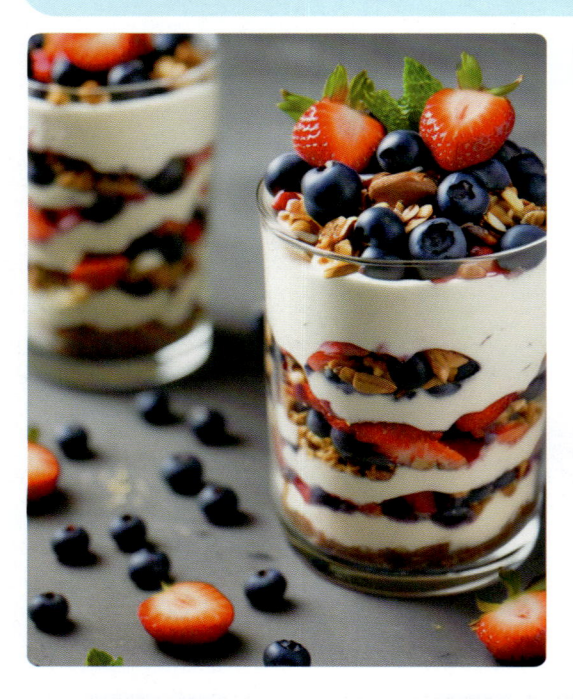

Ingredients — Servings: 1

- 1 cup nonfat vanilla greek yogurt
- 1 scoop Dummy Supps Vanilla/Berry Whey
- 1/2 cup frozen or fresh blueberries
- 1/2 cup frozen or fresh strawberries
- 2 tbsps protein granola
- 1 tbsp PB&J Dummy Butter

Dummy Supps Whey Protein — SCAN ME
Dummy Butter Peanut Butter — SCAN ME

Instructions

1. In a bowl, mix Greek yogurt with whey protein until smooth.
2. Slice strawberries.
3. Add blueberries, sliced strawberries, protein granola, and PB&J Dummy Butter.

SUPER POWER PARFAIT

Calories: 570 **Protein: 49** **Carbs: 59** **Fat: 17**

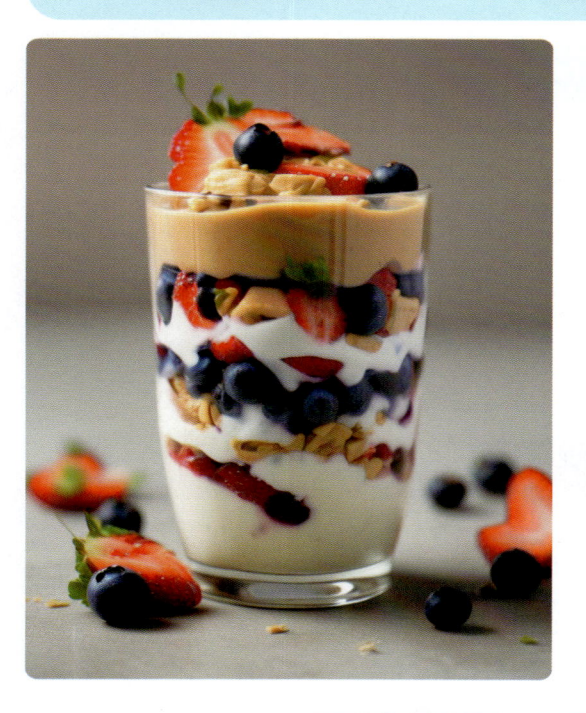

Ingredients — Servings: 1

- 1 cup nonfat vanilla greek yogurt
- 1 scoop Dummy Supps Vanilla/Berry Whey
- 1/2 cup frozen/fresh blueberries
- 1/2 cup frozen or fresh strawberries
- 1 banana
- 2 tbsps protein granola
- 1 tbsp PB&J Dummy Butter

Dummy Supps Whey Protein — SCAN ME
Dummy Butter Peanut Butter — SCAN ME

Instructions

1. In a bowl, mix Greek yogurt with whey protein until smooth.
2. Slice strawberries and banana.
3. Add blueberries, sliced strawberries, sliced banana, protein granola, and PB&J Dummy Butter.

Optional Add On: Whipped cream (2 tbsp - 15c, 1P, 1C, 1F)

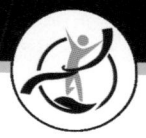

RECIPE INDEX

BREAKFAST

Apple Cobbler French Toast Bake ... 135
Apple Crisp Oatmeal ... 118
Apple Pie Overnight Oats ... 125
Bacon & Cheese Power Scramble ... 74
Bacon Egg & Cheese Bagel ... 89
Bacon Egg & Cheese Burrito ... 96
Bacon Egg & Cheese Muffin ... 106
Bacon Egg & Cheese Muffin Breakfast Sandwich ... 84
Bacon Egg & Cheese Scramble ... 64
Bacon Egg & Cheese Tots ... 81
Bacon Wake Up Wrap ... 102
Bananas Foster Oatmeal ... 117
BBQ Chicken & Cheddar Egg Muffins ... 114
Beef & Eggs ... 72
Beef Breakfast Burrito ... 101
Berry Blast Oatmeal ... 119
Berry Bliss Overnight Oats ... 124
Blueberry French Toast Casserole ... 133
Blueberry Pancakes ... 140
Buffalo Chicken Power Scramble ... 78
Buffalo Chicken Scramble ... 70
Canadian Egg & Cheese Muffin Breakfast Sandwich ... 86
Canadian Bacon Egg and Cheese Bagel ... 91
Chocolate Almond Oatmeal ... 118
Chocolate Brownie ... 119
Chocolate Caramel Dream ... 125
Chocolate Chip Protein Pancakes ... 138
Chocolate Chip Protein Waffles ... 145
Chocolate Coconut Overnight Oats ... 124
Chocolate Espresso Pancakes ... 141
Chocolate Espresso Waffles ... 149
Chocolate PB Banana Pancakes ... 139
Chocolate Peanut Butter Explosion ... 127
Chocolate Peanut Butter Oatmeal ... 116
Chocolate Peanut Butter Waffles ... 146
Chocolate Raspberry Overnight Oats ... 129
Chocolate Strawberry Overnight Oats ... 128
Cinnamon Roll Delight Overnight Oats ... 122
Cinnamon Roll Pancakes ... 143
Cinnamon Roll Waffles ... 147
Classic Cinnamon Oatmeal ... 116
Coconut Chocolate Oatmeal ... 120
Espresso Delight ... 127
Greek Egg Muffin ... 108
Greek Scramble ... 67
Loaded Bagel ... 93
Loaded Beef & Egg Bake ... 80
Loaded Burrito ... 99
Loaded Muffin Breakfast Sandwich ... 88
Loaded Wake Up Wrap ... 104
Maple Pecan Crunch ... 126
Meat Lovers Bagel ... 92
Meat Lovers Burrito ... 98
Meat Lovers Muffin Breakfast Sandwich ... 87
Meat Lovers Egg Muffins ... 111
Meat Lovers Scramble ... 68
Mexican Egg Muffins ... 110
Mocha Chip Overnight Oats ... 123
Parfait & Shake ... 132
PB Chocolate French Toast Bake ... 136
PB&J Overnight Oats ... 126
Peach Cobbler French Toast Bake ... 134
Peanut Butter Banana Overnight Oats ... 123
Pepperoni Pizza Egg Muffins ... 113
Philly Cheesesteak Power Scramble ... 79
Protein Bagels ... 152
Protein Pancakes ... 137
Protein Waffles ... 144
Pumpkin Spice Oatmeal ... 120
Pumpkin Spice Waffles ... 150
Raspberry Vanilla Overnight Oats ... 129
Salted Caramel Crunch Overnight Oats ... 122
Salted Caramel Pancakes ... 142
Salted Caramel Waffles ... 148
Sausage & Cheese Power Scramble ... 62
Sausage Egg & Cheese Bagel ... 90
Sausage Egg & Cheese Burrito ... 97
Sausage Egg & Cheese Muffin ... 107
Sausage Egg & Cheese Scramble ... 65
Sausage Egg & Cheese Tots ... 82
Sausage Muffin Breakfast Sandwich ... 85
Sausage Muffins ... 151
Sausage Wake Up Wrap ... 103
Simple Egg Sandwich ... 94
Southwest Burrito ... 100
Southwest Scramble ... 66
Southwestern Power Scramble ... 77
Steak & Eggs ... 71
Vanilla Blueberry Oatmeal ... 117
Vanilla Strawberry Overnight Oats ... 128
Veggie Egg Muffins ... 112
Western Omelet Egg Muffins ... 109
Western Power Scramble ... 76
Western Scramble ... 69

INDIVIDUAL MEAL PREPS

BBQ Chicken & Rice ... 166
BBQ Chicken & Sweet Potato ... 175
Beef & Rice ... 182
Beef Gyro ... 189
Beef Protein Pasta ... 181
Beef Quesadilla ... 186
Blackened Salmon, Potatoes & Spinach ... 207
Buffalo Chicken Bowl ... 226
Buffalo Chicken Grilled Cheese ... 201
Buffalo Chicken Wrap ... 192
Burger & Fries Bowl ... 184
Cajun Chicken & Rice ... 168
Cheeseburger Bowl ... 185
Chicken Alfredo ... 155
Chicken Bacon Ranch Bowl ... 161
Chicken Bacon Ranch Hash ... 176
Chicken Bacon Ranch Wrap ... 194
Chicken Bruschetta ... 157
Chicken Caesar Wrap ... 193
Chicken Fajita Bowl ... 284
Chicken Gyro ... 195
Chicken Milanese ... 156
Chicken Parmesan ... 154
Chicken Protein Pasta ... 160
Chicken Quesadilla ... 197
Chicken Salad Sandwich ... 200
Chicken Tenders ... 158
Chipotle Chicken Grilled Cheese ... 202
Chipotle Chicken Wrap ... 191
Chipotle-Style Chicken & Rice ... 167
Classic Cheeseburger ... 183
Classic Chicken & Rice ... 164
Garlic Butter Chicken & Rice ... 170
Garlic Herb Chicken & Roasted Potatoes ... 171
Garlic Parmesan Salmon Bites ... 206
Greek Chicken Bowl ... 163
Honey Garlic Chicken & Rice ... 169
Honey Mustard Chicken & Potatoes ... 174
Lemon Pepper Chicken & Rice ... 165
Loaded BLT Sandwich ... 198
Loaded Chicken Sandwich ... 199
Loaded Turkey Sandwich ... 203
Parmesan Crusted Chicken & Roasted Potatoes ... 173
Salmon Rice & Broccoli ... 204
Sausage Peppers Onions ... 208
Southwest Chicken Bowl ... 162
Spicy Korean Beef & Rice ... 188
Spicy Korean Chicken & Rice ... 180
Steak Fajita Bowl ... 190
Sweet & Spicy Salmon ... 205
Sweet and Spicy Bites ... 159
Teriyaki Chicken & Sweet Potatoes ... 172
Teriyaki Chicken Bowl ... 179
Tex-Mex Beef & Potato Skillet ... 187
Turkey Club Wrap ... 196

CROCKPOT MEAL PREPS

BBQ Chicken Sandwiches ... 233
Buffalo Chicken Bowls ... 226
Buffalo Chicken Burritos ... 230
Buffalo Chicken Pasta ... 213
Buffalo Dip Bowls ... 212
Cheesy Chicken and Rice Burritos ... 231
Cheesy Chicken Mac & Cheese ... 218
Chicken Alfredo Pasta ... 214
Chicken Noodle Soup ... 238
Chicken Parm Pasta ... 215
Chicken Tortilla Soup ... 236
Chipotle Chicken Pasta ... 217
Cilantro Lime Burritos ... 228
Cilantro Lime Chicken Bowls ... 225
Classic Beef Stew ... 237
Crack Chicken Soup ... 239
Hot Honey Chicken Bowls ... 219
Momma's Lasagna ... 235
Nacho Soup ... 240
Pulled Buffalo Sandwiches ... 234
Smothered Chipotle Chicken Burritos ... 229
Southwest Chicken Bowls ... 224
Spicy Garlic Pasta ... 216
Spicy Jalapeno Mac & Cheese ... 220
Sweet & Spicy Chicken Bowls ... 227
Sweet & Spicy Sandwiches ... 232
Sweet and Spicy Chicken ... 221
Taco Pasta Salad ... 223
Tinga Taco Bowls ... 222

MULTIPLE MEAL PREPS

Asian Beef Bowls ... 259
Asian Chicken Bowls ... 260
Asian Chicken Slaw Salad ... 306
Avocado Chicken Salad ... 305
Baked Ziti ... 270
BBQ Chicken Pizza ... 313
Beef and Bean Taco Soup ... 293
Beef and Rice ... 258
Beef Burrito Bowls ... 280

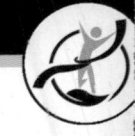

RECIPE INDEX

Beef Nacho Bowls & Protein Queso....257
Beef Taco Salad....307
Beef Tacos & Spicy Chipotle Crema....290
Buffalo Chicken and Fries....247
Buffalo Chicken Patties....298
Buffalo Chicken Pizza....312
Buffalo Chicken Salad....310
Buffalo Mac & Cheese....269
Burger & Fries Bowl....246
Cheeseburger Bowls....245
Cheesy Bacon Ranch Chicken Bowls....262
Cheesy Beef Taquitos....268
Cheesy Lasagna Bakes....282
Chicken Alfredo Bowls....287
Chicken and Rice....261
Chicken Bacon Ranch Pizza....311
Chicken Burrito Bowls....281
Chicken Caesar Salad....309
Chicken Cobb Salad....308
Chicken Fajita Bowls....284
Chicken Nacho Bowls & Protein Queso....263
Chicken Noodle Soup....292
Chicken Parm Bowls....286
Chicken Parm Patties....299
Chicken Patties....297
Chicken Riggies....273
Chicken Stir Fry Bowls....283
Chicken Tacos & Cilantro Lime Crema....285
Chipotle Mac + Cheese....277
Chipotle Steak & Fries....248
Cilantro Lime Chicken....253
Classic Chili....264
Creamy Protein Pasta....272
Greek Pasta Salad....251
Hamburger Helper....244
Italian Stuffed Peppers....304
Lemon Chicken and Rice....256
Loaded Classic Nachos....267
Pasta Bolognese....276
Pasta Salad....250
Penne Alla Vodka....274
Philly Cheesesteak Bowls....255
Popcorn Chicken Mac & Cheese....279
Protein Goulash....271
Rotisserie BBQ Chicken Sandwiches....296
Rotisserie BBQ Chicken Stuffed Sweet Potatoes....300
Rotisserie Buffalo Salad Sandwiches....295
Rotisserie Chicken Enchiladas....288
Rotisserie Chicken Greek Bowls....287
Rotisserie Chicken Salad Sandwiches....295
Southern Dirty Rice....266
Southwest Mac & Cheese....249
Spaghetti and Meatballs....278
Spicy Nacho Cheese Taquitos....265
Spicy Riggatoni....275
Steak Fajita Bowls....289
Steak Stir Fry Bowls....288
Steak Tacos & Guacamole....291
Stuffed Peppers....303
Teriyaki Chicken....254
Thai Peanut Chicken Pasta Salad....252

DESSERTS

Almond Joy Cheesecake....324
Apple Fritter Donut....345
Apple Pie Cheesecake....320
Banana Cream Pie Cheesecake....327
Bananas Foster Cheesecake....330
Berry Banana Bread....368
Berry Blast Cheesecake....323
Blueberry Cheesecake....334
Blueberry Glazed Donut....346
Blueberry Muffins....360
Bulk Protein Brownies....356
Chewy Protein Bars....354
Chocolate Almond Cheesecake....331
Chocolate Banana Bread....366
Chocolate Berry Lava Cake....358
Chocolate Cheesecake....318
Chocolate Chip Banana Bread....370
Chocolate Chip Cheesecake....319
Chocolate Chip Cookies....355
Chocolate Chip Muffins....363
Chocolate Coffee Cheesecake....332
Chocolate Covered Strawberry Cheesecake....333
Chocolate Espresso Ice Cream....339
Chocolate Frosted Donut....344
Chocolate Glazed Donut....347
Chocolate Ice Cream....338
Chocolate Lava Cake....360
Chocolate Mocha Banana Bread....369
Chocolate Mocha Muffins....362
Chocolate PB Brownies....357
Chocolate PB Lava Cake....358
Chocolate Peanut Butter Cheesecake....319
Chocolate Peanut Butter Ice Cream....339
Chocolate Strawberry Lava Cake....359
Cinnamon Bun Donuts....348
Cinnamon Roll Cheesecake....329
Cinnamon Rolls....371
Cinnamon Swirl Cheesecake....329
Cinnamon Swirl Ice Cream....342
Classic Vanilla Ice Cream....338
Coconut Cream Pie Cheesecake....328
Double Chunk Chocolate Muffins....365
Key Lime Pie Cheesecake....323
Lemon Blueberry Cheesecake....336
Lemon Coconut Cheesecake....336
Lemon Vanilla Cheesecake....335
Maple Bacon Donut....351
Maple Pecan Cheesecake....324
Mint Chocolate Cheesecake....321
Mint Chocolate Ice Cream....341
Mixed Berry Cheesecake....325
Mixed Berry Muffins....361
Mocha Cheesecake....322
Mocha Lava Cake....359
Mocha Peanut Butter Cheesecake....325
Oatmeal Cream Pies....372
PB&J Ice Cream....340
Peanut Butter and Jelly Cheesecake....322
Peanut Butter Cup Ice Cream....342
Pineapple Upside Down Cake Cheesecake....330
Pumpkin Banana Bread....367
Pumpkin Glazed Donuts....349
Pumpkin Roll Cheesecake....329
Pumpkin Spice Muffins....364
Pumpkin Spiced Donuts....350
Raspberry Cheesecake....334
S'Mores Cheesecake....328
Salted Caramel Cheesecake....320
Salted Caramel Pretzel Ice Cream....341
Strawberry Cheesecake....333
Strawberry Ice Cream....340
Strawberry Shortcake Cheesecake....327
Tiramisu Cheesecake....321
Vanilla Cheesecake....318
Vanilla Almond Cheesecake....331
Vanilla Banana Cheesecake....335
Vanilla Cheesecake....318
Vanilla Coffee Cheesecake....332
Vanilla Peanut Butter Cheesecake....326

SMOOTHIES & SHAKES

Banana Parfait....389
Blackberry Vanilla Smoothie....283
Blueberry Bash Smoothie....377
Blueberry Cheesecake Smoothie....387
Blueberry Parfait....388
Chocolate Coconut Smoothie....384
Chocolate Coffee Smoothie....376
Chocolate Covered Strawberry Smoothie....380
Chocolate Peanut Butter Smoothie....376
Chocolate Raspberry Smoothie....377
Cinnamon Roll Protein Shake....385
Cinnamon Swirl Smoothie....382
Classic Chocolate Smoothie....374
Classic Vanilla Smoothie....374
Cookies & Cream....380
French Vanilla Coffee Smoothie....375
Mixed Berry Smoothie....383
Mocha Caramel Shake....387
Peanut Butter & Banana Smoothie....379
Peanut Butter & Jelly Smoothie....378
Pina Colada Smoothie....384
Power Parfait....390
Pumpkin Spice Smoothie....381
S'Mores Smoothie....379
Salted Caramel Mocha Shake....385
Strawberry Banana Smoothie....378
Strawberry Bowl....388
Strawberry Parfait....389
Strawberry Shortcake Smoothie....386
Super Power Parfait....390
Tiramisu Smoothie....382
Vanilla Almond Cheesecake Shake....386
Vanilla Raspberry Smoothie....375
Vanilla Strawberry Smoothie....381